Handbook of Autism Spectrum Disorder

Handbook of Autism Spectrum Disorder

Editor: Harold Herrera

AMERICAN
MEDICAL PUBLISHERS
www.americanmedicalpublishers.com

AMERICAN
MEDICAL PUBLISHERS
www.americanmedicalpublishers.com

Cataloging-in-Publication Data

Handbook of autism spectrum disorder / edited by Harold Herrera.
p. cm.
Includes bibliographical references and index.
ISBN 978-1-63927-295-2
1. Autism spectrum disorders. 2. Autism. 3. Developmental disabilities. I. Herrera, Harold.
RC553.A88 H36 2022
616.858 82--dc23

American Medical Publishers,
41 Flatbush Avenue,
1st Floor, New York,
NY 11217, USA

ISBN 978-1-63927-295-2 (Hardback)

Contents

Preface

Autism spectrum disorder (ASD) refers to a set of neurodevelopmental disorders, comprising of autism, Asperger syndrome, childhood disintegrative disorder and pervasive developmental disorder not otherwise specified. Individuals with ASD experience problems with social interaction and communication, and exhibit restricted and repetitive patterns of behavior, activities and interests. Certain factors are associated with a high risk for ASD, such as having a family history of autism, certain genetic conditions, and having an older parent. A diagnosis of ASD can be established by the age of two. In autistic individuals, comorbidity is seen to increase with age. Autism Diagnostic Observation Schedule and Autism Diagnostic Interview-Revised are considered the fundamental standards of diagnosis. There is no cure for autism, but behavior therapy and special education programs early in life can impart the necessary skills. Different approaches, evaluations, methodologies and advanced studies on autism spectrum disorder have been included herein. Some of the diverse topics covered in this book address the varied conditions that fall under this category. This book is a vital tool for all researching and studying autism spectrum disorder.

This book is the end result of constructive efforts and intensive research done by experts in this field. The aim of this book is to enlighten the readers with recent information in this area of research. The information provided in this profound book would serve as a valuable reference to students and researchers in this field.

At the end, I would like to thank all the authors for devoting their precious time and providing their valuable contribution to this book. I would also like to express my gratitude to my fellow colleagues who encouraged me throughout the process.

Editor

Preface

Autism spectrum disorder (ASD) refers to a set of neurodevelopmental disorders, comprising of autism, Asperger syndrome, childhood disintegrative disorder and pervasive developmental disorder not otherwise specified. Individuals with ASD experience problems with social interaction and communication, and exhibit restricted and repetitive patterns of behavior, activities and interests. Certain factors are associated with a high risk for ASD, such as having a family history of autism, certain genetic conditions, and having an older parent. A diagnosis of ASD can be established by the age of two. In autistic individuals, comorbidity is seen to increase with age. Autism Diagnostic Observation Schedule and Autism Diagnostic Interview-Revised are considered the fundamental standards of diagnosis. There is no cure for autism, but behavior therapy and special education programs early in life can impart the necessary skills. Different approaches, evaluations, methodologies and advanced studies on autism spectrum disorder have been included herein. Some of the diverse topics covered in this book address the varied conditions that fall under this category. This book is a vital tool for all researching and studying autism spectrum disorder.

This book is the end result of constructive efforts and intensive research done by experts in this field. The aim of this book is to enlighten the readers with recent information in this area of research. The information provided in this profound book would serve as a valuable reference to students and researchers in this field.

At the end, I would like to thank all the authors for devoting their precious time and providing their valuable contribution to this book. I would also like to express my gratitude to my fellow colleagues who encouraged me throughout the process.

Editor

1

Atypical lateralization of motor circuit functional connectivity in children with autism is associated with motor deficits

Dorothea L. Floris[1,2*], Anita D. Barber[3,4,5], Mary Beth Nebel[3,4,5], Mary Martinelli[3,4,5], Meng-Chuan Lai[1,6,7], Deana Crocetti[3,4,5], Simon Baron-Cohen[1,8,9,10], John Suckling[8,9,10,11], James J. Pekar[12,13] and Stewart H. Mostofsky[3,4,5]

Abstract

Background: Atypical lateralization of language-related functions has been repeatedly found in individuals with autism spectrum conditions (ASC). Few studies have, however, investigated deviations from typically occurring asymmetry of other lateralized cognitive and behavioural domains. Motor deficits are among the earliest and most prominent symptoms in individuals with ASC and precede core social and communicative symptoms.

Methods: Here, we investigate whether motor circuit connectivity is (1) atypically lateralized in children with ASC and (2) whether this relates to core autistic symptoms and motor performance. Participants comprised 44 right-handed high-functioning children with autism (36 males, 8 females) and 80 typically developing control children (58 males, 22 females) matched on age, sex and performance IQ. We examined lateralization of functional motor circuit connectivity based on homotopic seeds derived from peak activations during a finger tapping paradigm. Motor performance was assessed using the Physical and Neurological Examination for Subtle Signs (PANESS).

Results: Children with ASC showed rightward lateralization in mean motor circuit connectivity compared to typically developing children, and this was associated with poorer performance on all three PANESS measures.

Conclusions: Our findings reveal that atypical lateralization in ASC is not restricted to language functions but is also present in circuits subserving motor functions and may underlie motor deficits in children with ASC. Future studies should investigate whether this is an age-invariant finding extending to adolescents and adults and whether these asymmetries relate to atypical lateralization in the language domain.

Keywords: Autism, Lateralization, Hemispheric specialization, Intrinsic functional connectivity, Motor deficits

Background

The macroscopic functional organization of the human brain is characterized by lateralized specialization of the two cerebral hemispheres for cognitive and behavioural abilities. The left hemisphere exhibits dominance for language and motor control, whereas the right hemisphere is specialized for visuospatial attention [1, 2]. This division of function has been explained as an evolutionary advantage to avoid the duplication of cognitive processing and cortical representations [3]. In line with this, we previously showed that leftward lateralization of functional motor circuit connectivity is associated with better motor performance in typically developing children [4] and others have shown that the degree of language and visuospatial lateralization relates to enhanced cognitive functioning [5, 6].

Studies converge to show that this typical pattern of hemispheric specialization is not seen in individuals with autism spectrum conditions (ASC). A consistent finding is that language-related structures such as the planum temporale [7] and inferior frontal gyrus [8] are atypically rightward asymmetric in both children and adults with ASC. These findings are corroborated by functional studies reporting atypical lateralization on linguistic tasks in individuals with ASC [9–15]. Early development of atypical

* Correspondence: dorothea.floris@nyumc.org
[1]Autism Research Centre, Department of Psychiatry, University of Cambridge, Cambridge, UK
[2]Department of Child and Adolescent Psychiatry, the Child Study Center, New York University Langone Medical Center, New York, NY, USA

language lateralization might potentially serve as a biomarker and be clinically relevant if it precedes atypical language development in children with ASC [16]. Language is not the only lateralized functional domain in which individuals with ASC exhibit deficits. Clumsiness and impaired fine motor control are among the most prevalent and earliest identifiable symptoms in individuals with ASC [17–19]. Imaging studies report atypical activation of the premotor cortex [20] and the cerebellum [21–23] during motor execution and decreased connectivity of the motor execution network [22]. However, functional studies of atypical lateralization in ASC have mainly been confined to the language domain. Only a few studies have explored lateralized activation during motor tasks in ASC during imitation [24], sequence [25] or procedural learning [26].

Motor symptoms are of considerable functional and clinical relevance in ASC, given that they are among the earliest detectable behavioural problems, preceding social and language deficits and have been found to be correlated with core social and communicative impairments in ASC [27, 28]. Indeed, the neural contributions to motor skill impairments in ASC may parallel those underlying the broader range of autistic features, leading to impaired development of skills necessary for motor, social and communicative behaviours [29]. Thus, identifying the neurobiological underpinnings of motor signs in ASC is of upmost importance in view of their potential role as biological markers of the condition.

Lateralized functions are subserved by functional coordination among regions in a network rather than by individual brain loci separately. Recent advances in neuroimaging have provided tools to measure the synchronization of cortical regions that share functional properties and thus form complex neural networks. Coherent temporal correlations in slow, spontaneous low-frequency fluctuations in the blood-oxygen-level-dependent (BOLD) signal are the basis for functional resting-state connectivity, which may reflect the intrinsic organization of the human brain [30–32]. Recent resting-state studies have confirmed the presence of lateralized brain functions and have helped to elucidate differential patterns of connectivity. Left hemisphere functions such as language and fine motor control have been suggested to be more focal preventing conduction delays and enabling rapid processing [33, 34], whereas visuospatial functions require more interhemispheric integration to represent the bilateral visual space [35]. Consistent with this, Gotts et al. [5] showed that functional lateralization differs between the two hemispheres, with left-lateralized hubs including language and motor control networks showing a bias towards intrahemispheric interactions, whereas right-lateralized hubs including those subserving attention tending to operate in a more integrative manner between the two hemispheres.

Mounting evidence suggests that the neural substrates of ASC involve atypical neural connectivity and deficient neural synchronization of multiple functional networks [36–38]. Many recent studies in ASC have moved away from task-based fMRI, instead focusing on aberrant functional connectivity of networks subserving cognitive and social functions, such as the default mode network [39–42]. To date, only a few studies have explored atypical motor circuit connectivity in ASC in association with motor performance [22, 43, 44] or atypical lateralization of resting-state (motor) networks in ASC [45, 46]. This is despite the accumulated evidence of autism-associated impairments in motor control and learning [18, 28, 47–49]. Cardinale et al. [45] reported atypical rightward lateralization of multiple functional brain networks in individuals with ASC, including language, motor and visuospatial circuits, concluding that rightward lateralization constitutes a fundamental characteristic of cerebral organization in ASC.

Here, we extend the current literature on atypical cerebral lateralization in ASC to examine the lateralization of functional motor circuit connectivity. We focus on atypical intrahemispheric functional connectivity, based on studies showing greater within-hemisphere interactions for left-lateralized functions [5] and previous studies applying a similar rationale [4, 46, 50]. We hypothesized that children with ASC would show reduced leftward or increased rightward lateralization of motor connectivity, associated with poorer performance on motor tasks.

Methods

Participant characteristics

Participants comprised 44 right-handed children with ASC (36 males, 8 females) and 80 right-handed typically developing children (58 males, 22 females) between 8 and 12 years of age (ASC mean = 10.23, standard deviation (SD) = 1.51, range = 8.01–12.99; controls mean = 10.15, SD = 1.08, range = 8.07–12.76) (see Additional file 1; for participant characteristics of the final sample, see Table 1). Individuals with ASC were recruited through advertisements placed within community-wide service groups, schools and hospitals, as well as from outpatient clinics at the Kennedy Krieger Institute in Baltimore. Participants with ASC received a clinical diagnosis according to the criteria of the Diagnostic and Statistical Manual of Mental Disorders–IV [51], and diagnoses were confirmed using the Autism Diagnostic Interview–Revised (ADI-R; [52]) and Module 3 of the Autism Diagnostic Observation Schedule (ADOS-G; [53]). Participants were excluded if they met any of the following criteria: (1) a history of seizures and/or traumatic brain injury; (2) a full-scale IQ (FIQ) less than 80 (in cases where the FIQ was less than 80, participants were still included if their verbal comprehension index (VCI) or perceptual reasoning index (PRI) was higher than 80), as assessed by the Wechsler

Table 1 Participant characteristics of final sample

Characteristics	ASC ($n = 42$)			Controls ($n = 76$)			Statistics
	Mean	SD	Range	Mean	SD	Range	
Sex	34 males; 8 females	–	–	54 males; 22 females	–	–	$\chi^2(1) = 0.925$, $p = 0.336$
Age[a]	10.18	(1.51)	8.01–12.99	10.16	(1.03)	8.07–12.58	$t = -0.092$, $p = 0.927$
Full-scale IQ[b]	104.67	(15.10)	73–141	112.89	(10.78)	85–140	$t = 3.136$, $p = 0.003$
VCI[b]	107.95	(15.53)	79–134	117.29	(12.37)	85–140	$t = 3.353$, $p = 0.001$
PRI[a]	107.45	(14.31)	79–135	109.30	(11.44)	79–133	$t = 0.768$, $p = 0.444$
Handedness[a]	86.5	(Median)	50–100	88.00	(Median)	41–100	$U = 1590.5$, $p = 0.974$
ADI-R[c]							
Social	20.62	(5.82)	10–30		–		–
Communication	15.95	(4.68)	4–25		–		–
RSB	6.64	(2.15)	3–12		–		–
ADOS-G[c]							
Communication	3.40	(1.06)	1–7		–		–
Social	7.48	(1.98)	4–12		–		–
RSB	3.05	(1.70)	0–6		–		–

Abbreviations: *PRI* perceptual reasoning index, *VCI* verbal comprehension index
[a]There were no significant differences between the ASC and control groups in age, sex, PRI or handedness ($p > 0.05$)
[b]The two groups significantly differed in FIQ and VCI ($p < 0.001$)
[c]Information was available for all 42 individuals with ASC

Intelligence Scale for Children- fourth edition (WISC-III/IV; [54, 55]); (3) a developmental language disorder; (4) reading disability; (5) visual impairment and (6) neurologic disorder such as epilepsy. The Diagnostic Interview for Children and Adolescents, fourth edition (DICA-IV; [56]) was used to determine the presence of additional psychiatric diagnoses. Children with ASC met the following additional DICA-IV diagnoses: ADHD (16), OCD (4), specific phobia (9), generalized anxiety disorder (GAD) (4) and oppositional defiant disorder (ODD) (8). Twenty-four children with ASC were actively taking psychoactive medications, including stimulants (13), selective serotonin reuptake inhibitors (SSRI) (6), clonidine (2), risperidone (2) and lithium (2). Stimulant medications were discontinued the day prior to testing; all other medications were taken as prescribed. There was no diagnosis or family history of ASC in the typically developing control group. We included only individuals in the current sample with less than 3 mm translational and 3° rotational movement over the course of the resting scan.

Cognitive and behavioural measures

Physical and Neurological Examination of Subtle Signs

Motor skills were assessed outside the scanner using the Physical and Neurological Examination of Subtle Signs (PANESS; [57]), a battery of motor control tasks designed for children and standardized for age, sex and handedness. It is sensitive to children's developmental changes in motor skills such as balance, coordination and speed and has adequate test-retest reliability, inter-rater reliability and internal consistency. Motor signs are quantified as *dysrhythmia* (inappropriate timing or sequencing of movements) and *overflow* (unintended and unnecessary movements) examined while performing gait, station and timed limb movements. *Gaits and station* measures are based on gait and balance assessment (gaits on heels, toes and sides of feet and tandem, standing and hopping on one foot, etc.). *Timed limb movements* are assessed during performance of repetitive and sequential movements of the hands and feet such as finger tapping, hand patting and toe tapping. *Speed*, *overflow* and *dysrhythmia* are incorporated into the *total timed score*. In addition to examining the *total gait score* and *total timed score*, the *total PANESS score* was also examined. For all three measures, better performance is associated with lower scores.

Handedness

Handedness was assessed using the Edinburgh Handedness Inventory (EHI; [58]), a self-completed questionnaire for determining hand preference. The sample comprised only right-handed individuals with EHI scores >40.

Structural and functional magnetic resonance imaging acquisition

All participants performed a mock scan the day before the actual scan. All individuals underwent scanning on one of two 3-T Philips scanners (2D-SENSE EPI, 8-channel head coil, SENSE acceleration = 2.0), and axially oriented volumes were acquired using T2*-weighted echo-planar imaging (field of view: 256 × 256 mm, matrix size 64 × 64, repetition time = 2500 ms, echo time = 30 ms, flip angle = 75°). Resting-state scans were acquired for 5 min and 20 s. Children were asked to stay as still as possible and fixate on a centre cross. T1-weighted high-resolution anatomical images were acquired coronally (field of view 256 × 200 mm^2, matrix size 256 × 256, repetition time = 7.99 ms, echo time = 3.76 ms, flip angle = 8°, 1 mm isotropic voxels, slice thickness = 1 mm). These were used to generate age- and gender-matched symmetrical tissue priors.

Image preprocessing

Functional T2*-weighted images were preprocessed using statistical parametric mapping (SPM12; Wellcome Department of Imaging Neuroscience Group, London, UK; http://www.fil.ion.ucl.ac.uk/spm). Images were slice-time corrected using the middle slice as reference slice and realigned relative to their mean. The high-resolution anatomical images were then co-registered to the functional images, segmented and normalized using a symmetrical, age- and gender-matched tissue prior generated with the Template-O-Matic toolbox [59]. The use of a symmetrical template prevents an additional introduction of anatomical asymmetries that might potentially interfere with functional asymmetries [60]. The normalization transformation was then applied to the functional images. Further steps included linear detrending at each voxel in the brain to correct for scanner drift, removal of nuisance variables such as the white matter (WM) and cerebrospinal fluid (CSF) using CompCor [61] (note that we did not use global signal regression (GSR) to avoid introduction of spurious anticorrelations in the data [62]) and six absolute and six differential motion parameters, spatial smoothing (6-mm full width at half maximum (FWHM)), and temporal band-pass filtering constraining the frequency window to 0.01–0.1 Hz. To minimise the confounding influence of micromovement, we computed the average framewise displacement (FD) (based on the median due to a non-normal distribution of movement) according to Power et al. [63] and excluded any participant with a z score of >2.58 [64].

Creation of seed regions

Mostofsky et al. [22] identified the right hemisphere (RH) and left hemisphere (LH) circuits involved in motor execution during a finger-sequencing paradigm in both children with ASC and neurotypical controls between 8 and 12 years. They identified regions of interest by single-group, whole-brain random effects analyses across both groups by executing one-sample t tests on the individual subject's right- and left-rest contrast images. Individual within-group whole-brain activation analyses were then run for the two groups separately identifying peak activations by group. Here, peak coordinates were derived from typical children and served as centres of seeds.

Based on the 'left hemisphere dysfunction' theory of autism, which states that neural impairments are lateralized to the LH in individuals with ASC, we selected peak coordinates from this LH motor circuit (see Table 2). The LH motor circuit (right-sided movement) included the left sensorimotor cortex (SMC), left thalamus (TH), left putamen (PUT), bilateral supplementary motor area (SMA)-rostral (SMA-r), bilateral SMA-dorsal (SMA-d) and right anterior cerebellum (AC) seeds [4].

Six-millimetre-radius 3D seeds were then created using the SPM toolbox PickAtlas (http://fmri.wfubmc.edu/software/PickAtlas) with the peak coordinates as the centre of spheres. All seeds were flipped across the midline ($x = 0$) in order to obtain a set of homotopic RH and LH seeds (see Fig. 1). Time series were then extracted from the seed regions of interest, and pairwise Pearson's correlations were performed for the LH and RH circuits separately. Correlation coefficients were transformed to a normal distribution via Fisher's z transform. Standardized correlations between all seed pairs were then averaged to obtain mean connectivity in the motor circuit in each hemisphere (RH connectivity (R_{con}); LH connectivity (L_{con})) using MATLAB. For the assessment of functional lateralization, we calculated a laterality index (LI) for each pairwise connection and for the overall mean network connectivity by subtracting the connections in the LH from homotopic connections in the right hemisphere: $R_{con} - L_{con}$. Contrary to the usually applied formula for the calculation of structural asymmetry indices ($(R - L)/(R + L)$), here we did not include a denominator as functional connectivity measures comprise both positive and negative values, adversely influencing the index values [50].

Control networks

To test whether atypical lateralization is specific to the motor network and its underlying lateralized functions, we selected two control networks: the default mode network

Table 2 Motor coordinates (mm) based on Mostofsky et al. [22]

	x	y	z
Sensorimotor	−38	−30	51
Putamen	−30	−3	−6
Thalamus	−18	−27	9
B_SMA-d	−9	9	46
	9	9	46
B_SMA-r	−12	−1	66
	12	−1	66
Anterior cerebellum	16	−51	−25

Coordinates in MNI space
Abbreviations: *SMA-d* dorsal SMA, *SMA-r* rostral SMA

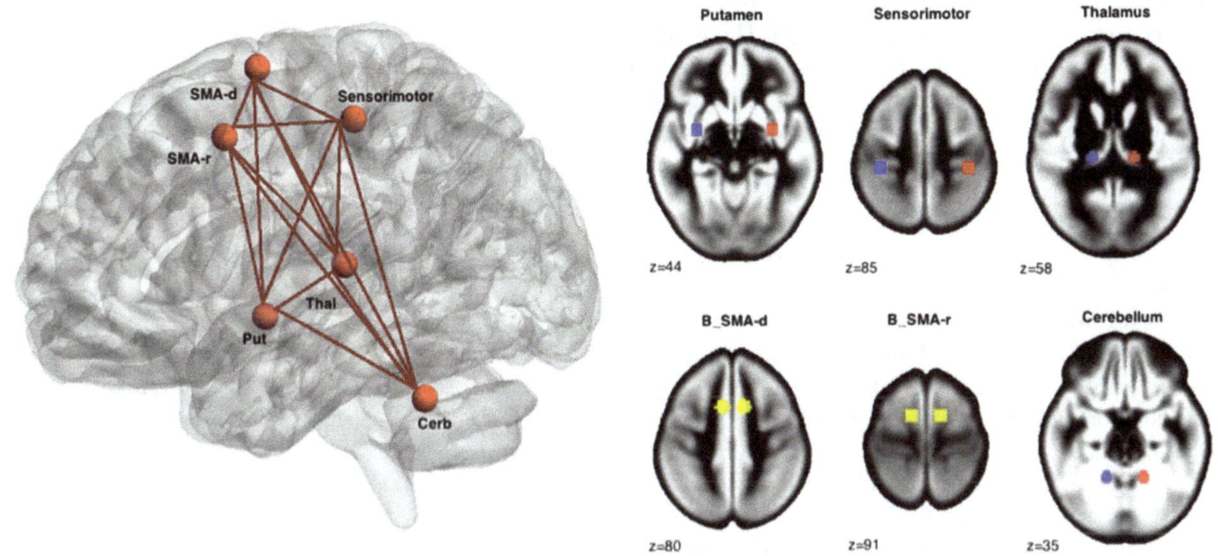

Fig. 1 Homotopic motor seeds derived from Mostofsky et al. [22]. Abbreviations: *SMA-d* dorsal SMA, *SMA-r* rostral SMA, *Put* putamen, *Thal* thalamus, *Cerb* cerebellum. *Red*: left hemisphere seeds; *Blue* right hemisphere seeds

(DMN) and a visual network (VN). DMN seeds were based on peak seed regions of the task-negative network identified by Fox et al. [65] using resting-state connectivity. Seeds were located in the cerebellum, posterior cingulate cortex (PCC), medial prefrontal cortex (MPFC), retrosplenial cortex (RSC), lateral parietal cortex (LP), superior frontal gyrus (SFG), inferior frontal gyrus (IFG) and parahippocampal gyrus (PHG). The VN seeds were based on visual seeds applied by Yeo et al. [66] and were comprised of the central and peripheral primary visual cortex ($V1_c$ and $V1_p$), the central and peripheral regions near the visual area $V3_v$ ($V3_{pv}$ and $V3_{cv}$) and the extrastriate regions of the central and peripheral visual subnetworks (ExP and ExC).

Statistical analyses

Group differences in mean connectivity and individual connection pairs

Participants were excluded as outliers if the average FD or laterality values had a z score of >2.58 [64, 67, 68]. For the analysis of the between-group differences in mean network connectivity, a univariate analysis of covariance (ANCOVA) was conducted. To compare the LIs of all the individual connectivity pairs between the two groups (ASC vs. controls), separate ANCOVAs were conducted with each individual connectivity pair as dependent variables (DV) and the global mean of the LIs of the remaining individual connectivity pairs of the network (Global-Mean$_{\text{network}}$) as nuisance covariates in order to discount their global effect. ANCOVAs were corrected for multiple comparisons by controlling the false discovery rate (FDR) at $q = 0.05$. Age and scanning machine were included as nuisance variables in all models. To control for micromovements, average FD was included as an additional covariate [67]. Furthermore, results were re-evaluated controlling for FIQ to observe if they remained significant. To determine whether significant group differences were driven by rightward over-connectivity or leftward under-connectivity, we also compared the Fisher transformed correlation coefficients of the LH and RH circuits (R_{con} and L_{con}) between the groups with the same model as that exploring the LI differences. To determine the direction of within-group circuit laterality, one-sample t tests were carried out. In an additional step, analyses were repeated in sex-stratified samples. Effect sizes were calculated based on Cohen's d.

Association with cognitive measures within ASC

To test whether atypical lateralization was related to function, we conducted one-tailed (based on our hypothesis that stronger rightward lateralization would be related to more symptoms and poorer performance) Pearson's correlations controlling for scanner, age and average FD within individuals with ASC. For individual connectivity pairs, the Global-Mean$_{\text{network}}$ was additionally included as a covariate. Motor LIs showing group differences were correlated with (a) the repetitive behaviour subscores of the ADI-R (ADI-C) and ADOS (ADOS-D) and (b) the total PANESS score, total gait score (composite measure of speed, overflow and dysrhythmia during gaits and stations) and total timed score (composite measure of speed, overflow and dysrhythmia during all timed movements). Level of significance was set at $p = 0.05$, as all correlation analyses were targeted. All statistical analyses were carried out in SPSS (version 21, SPSS Inc.).

Based on previous reports showing a linkage between motor and social development [69, 70] and the hypothesis that motor deficits might underpin some of the core social-communicative symptoms in ASC [71], an additional, exploratory analysis was conducted posing the question whether lateralization of motor circuit connectivity was related to core social and communicative symptoms, with stronger rightward lateralization being related to more deficits as measured by the ADOS-A, ADOS-B, ADI-A and ADI-B.

Results

Participant characteristics and task performance

Four control individuals and one individual with ASC were excluded due to z values of >2.58 on average FD. One additional individual with ASC was excluded due to z values of >2.58 on more than three laterality measures. The final sample consisted of 42 individuals with ASC (34 males, 8 females) and 76 controls (54 males, 22 females). After exclusion, the two groups were matched on age ($t(62.51) = -0.092$, $p = 0.927$), handedness ($U = 1590.5$, $z = -0.032$, $p = 0.974$), sex ($\chi^2(1) = 0.925$, $p = 0.336$), average FD ($U = 1481$, $z = -0.646$, $p = 0.518$) and PRI ($t(116) = 0.768$, $p = 0.444$). There were, however, significant differences in FIQ ($t(64.87) = 3.136$, $p = 0.003$) and VCI ($t(70.10) = 3.353$, $p = 0.001$). Individuals with ASC had significantly poorer performance on the total score of the PANESS ($F(1,115) = 45.081$, $p < 0.001$), and on the two sub-measures: total gait ($F(1,115) = 36.804$, $p < 0.001$) and total timed ($F(1,115) = 32.339$, $p < 0.001$).

Group differences in lateralization of motor circuit connectivity

There was a significant difference for the LI of mean motor circuit connectivity between the ASC and control group ($F(1,113) = 6.814$, $p = 0.010$; Cohen's $d = 0.506$), with children with ASC being more strongly rightward lateralized (see Fig. 2a). The result remained significant when controlling for FIQ ($F(1,112) = 6.094$, $p = 0.015$; Cohen's $d = 0.479$). This difference was driven by both rightward over- and leftward under-connectivity in mean motor connectivity in children with ASC (group difference R_{con} $F(1,113) = 1.110$, $p = 0.294$; group difference L_{con} $F(1,113) = 0.536$, $p = 0.466$). A one-sample t test revealed that children with ASC were rightward lateralized ($t(41) = 2.390$, $p = 0.022$), whereas control children showed a symmetrical organization ($t(75) = -1.255$, $p = 0.213$). Individual LIs of 'motor' connections were not significantly different or did not survive correction for multiple comparisons (see Table 3). After stratifying analyses by sex, the result was trending in males only ($F(1,83) = 3.920$, $p = 0.051$; Cohen's $d = 0.438$; FIQ $F(1,82) = 2.512$, $p = 0.117$; Cohen's $d = 0.351$) and not significant in females ($F(1,25) = 1.311$, $p = 0.263$; Cohen's $d = 0.489$; FIQ $F(1,24) = 3.701$, $p = 0.066$; Cohen's $d = 0.822$) (for a distribution of values across sex, see Fig. 2b).

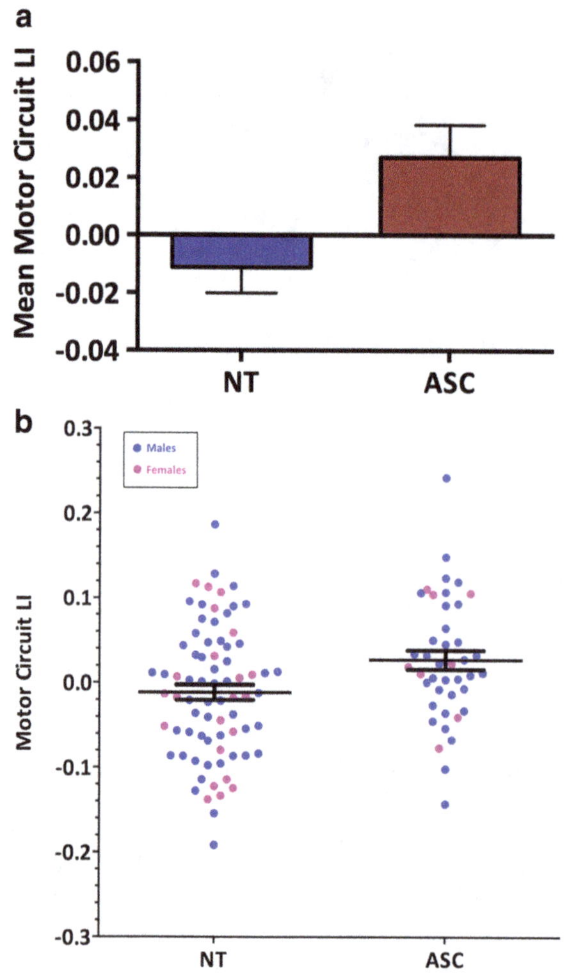

Fig. 2 a Group differences in LIs of mean motor network connectivity. Abbreviations: *NT* neurotypicals (controls). Positive values indicate rightward lateralization, negative values indicate leftward lateralization. Children with ASC show reversed rightward lateralization of mean motor connectivity. **b** LIs of motor network connectivity across sexes

Association with cognitive measures in children with ASC

The LI of total mean motor connectivity was positively associated with the total PANESS scores ($r = 0.455$, $p = 0.002$), total gait subscores ($r = 0.434$, $p = 0.003$) and total timed subscores ($r = 0.357$, $p = 0.013$) (see Table 4). In each case, stronger rightward lateralization was associated with worse performance on the motor task (see Fig. 3a–c). There were no associations with either the ADOS-D ($r = 0.117$, $p = 0.238$) or ADI-C ($r = -0.026$, $p = 0.438$). There were no significant associations between the LI of mean motor connectivity and the ADOS-A ($r = 0.127$, $p = 0.220$), ADOS-B ($r = 0.217$, $p = 0.093$), ADI-A ($r = 0.065$, $p = 0.348$) and ADI-B ($r = -0.075$, $p = 0.325$). Correlations with the PANESS were not significant in typical children (total PANESS score $r = -0.059$, $p = 0.310$; total gait subscores $r = 0.094$, $p = 0.215$; total timed subscores $r = -0.132$, $p = 0.133$).

Table 3 Group differences in LIs of individual motor connections

Connection	ASC Mean (SD)	Controls Mean (SD)	F (1,112)	p	q
SMA-d-AC	0.006 (0.17)	−0.409 (0.14)	1.555	0.215	0.50
SMA-d-M1	0.072 (0.20)	0.001 (0.19)	3.756	0.055	0.35
SMA-d-Put	0.025 (0.18)	0.033 (0.17)	0.902	0.344	0.63
SMA-d-Thal	0.029 (0.19)	−0.044 (0.19)	0.583	0.447	0.63
SMA-r-AC	0.009 (0.15)	−0.026 (0.16)	0.667	0.416	0.63
SMA-r-M1	0.074 (0.22)	−0.004 (0.16)	3.126	0.08	0.35
SMA-r-Put	−0.005 (0.15)	0.049 (0.17)	7.634	0.007	0.098
SMA-r-Thal	0.003 (0.19)	−0.034 (0.18)	0.006	0.939	0.94
AC-M1	0.032 (0.22)	−0.005 (0.21)	0.161	0.689	0.80
AC-Put	0.013 (0.18)	−0.002 (0.17)	0.099	0.754	0.81
AC-Thal	0.042 (0.22)	−0.048 (0.18)	2.388	0.125	0.35
M1-Put	0.037 (0.22)	−0.009 (0.24)	0.221	0.639	0.80
M1-Thal	0.077 (0.18)	−0.019 (0.20)	2.627	0.108	0.35
Put-Thal	−0.008 (0.18)	−0.017 (0.24)	0.577	0.449	0.63

Abbreviations: *SMA-d* dorsal SMA, *SMA-r* rostral SMA, *SMC* sensorimotor cortex, *Put* putamen, *Thal* thalamus, *AC* anterior cerebellum

Control networks

Default mode network

There was no significant difference in LI of mean DMN connectivity ($F(1,113) = 2.12$, $p = 0.143$) between individuals with ASC and controls. Individual LIs of DMN connections were not significantly different or did not survive correction for multiple comparisons (for details, see Additional file 1).

Visual network

There was no significant difference in the LI of mean VN connectivity ($F(1,113) = 0.467$; $p = 0.496$) between individuals with ASC and controls. Individual LIs of VN connections were not significantly different (for details, see Additional file 1).

Discussion

In the current study, we investigated whether the functional motor execution network shows an atypical pattern of hemispheric specialization in ASC. Consistent with our hypothesis, we found stronger rightward lateralization in children with ASC compared to typically developing children.

Table 4 Correlations between the LI of mean motor circuit connectivity and motor-related symptoms

Motor measure	LI mean motor circuit connectivity
PANESS total	*r = 0.455, p = 0.002*, q = 0.008*
PANESS gait	*r = 0.434, p = 0.003*, q = 0.008*
PANESS timed	*r = 0.357, p = 0.013*, q = 0.021*
ADI-C	r = -0.026, p = 0.438, q = 0.438
ADOS-D	r = 0.117, p = 0.238, q = 0.298

* = significant at q<0.05

Disturbance in motor functioning in children with ASC has been linked to dysfunction in multiple motor regions/systems, including the fronto-striatal and cerebellar systems [22, 43, 72–74]. However, few studies have explored the resting-state functional connectivity within the motor execution system in children with ASC [22, 43, 44]. Mostofsky et al. [22] report the overall under-connectivity, which is more pronounced during motor execution than during rest. Nebel et al. [44] focused specifically on M1 connectivity, examining autism-associated differences in regional M1 functional parcellation; they found organizational differentiation in the motor homunculus pointing to an early failure in functional specialization in the motor cortex in children with ASC. Here, we further show that the neurobiological underpinnings of motor impairments in ASC are related to atypical hemispheric lateralization in motor circuits.

Our finding is particularly interesting in the light of rising theories suggesting that autism is a condition of atypical connectivity involving multiple cerebral networks deficient in synchronization and information integration [36, 37]. However, so far, most functional connectivity studies in ASC have focused on under- or over-connectivity of networks critically involved in cognitive and social functions such as the default mode network [39–42] but have not addressed atypical lateralization of these circuits. Our findings are in line with Cardinale et al.'s [45] report of rightward lateralization of the motor networks. They reported on a wider range of networks, raising the question whether atypical rightward asymmetry is a more fundamental feature of network organization in ASC and not restricted to specific functions such as language and motor behaviour. However, we did not find atypical lateralization patterns across all networks; that is, we observed no group differences in the visual and default mode networks. These discrepancies might be due to differences in methodology between the two studies; Cardinale et al. [45] applied a model-free whole-brain approach aggregating information across many regions, whereas we took a hypothesis-driven approach, focusing on specific regions and their interconnections using seed-based analysis. While seed-based and ICA-based analyses yield similar results [75], using a model-free exploratory approach may identify additional unexpected patterns at the network level without making prior assumptions about functional localization.

Rightward asymmetry of motor circuit functional connectivity is associated with motor performance in children with ASC

This study is the first to report a relationship between autistic symptoms and hemispheric lateralization outside the language domain in individuals with ASC; namely, the more rightward asymmetry of the functional correspondence within the motor circuit, the poorer motor performance on three different measures of the PANESS.

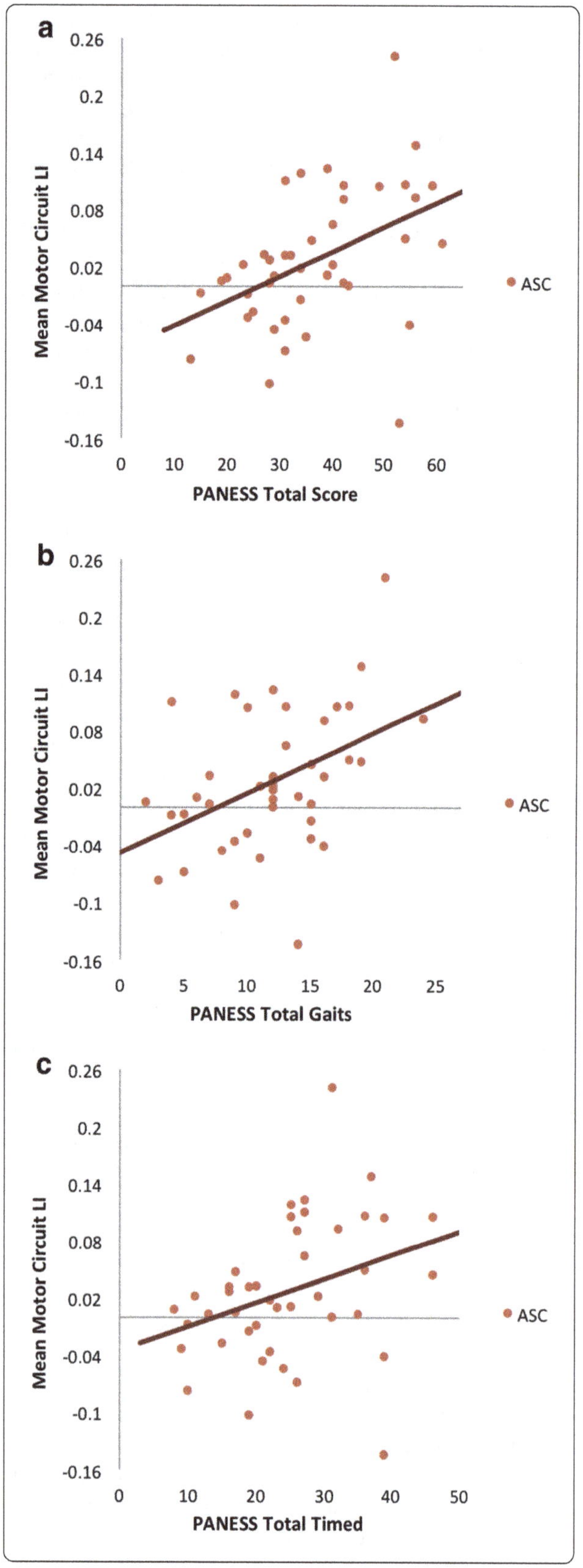

Fig. 3 Association between LI of mean motor network connectivity and motor-related symptoms. **a** Association between LI of mean motor network connectivity and PANESS total scores. **b** Association between LI of mean motor network connectivity and PANESS total gaits scores. **c** Association between LI of mean motor network connectivity and PANESS total timed scores

Both Nielsen et al. [46], who reported atypical lateralization in a language-related network, and Cardinale et al. [45], who reported rightward lateralization of the motor network, did not find such brain-behavioural association. Here, we highlight the importance of their findings by showing functional relevance in children with ASC. Lateralization has been linked to fine motor skills, primarily in relation to handedness. Interestingly, here, we showed that, in addition to fine motor skills, gross motor performances such as gait, balance, timing and sequencing of movements were also associated with atypical hemispheric specialization in children with ASC. Therefore, rightward lateralization may underlie gross motor deficits and atypical gait commonly found in individuals with ASC.

Leftward lateralization of the same circuit has previously been shown to be associated with better motor performance in typically developing children [4]; however, we did not replicate this result here. It remains to be established whether this is due to differing sample characteristics and methods (note that Barber et al. used a different registration approach and laterality index) and whether lateralization of this network constitutes the biological underpinnings for typical motor development or for motor deficits in ASC specifically.

Lateralization in the motor system is present in both structure and function, although it is generally less pronounced compared to the language system lateralization, which would explain why typical children show a subtle shift only towards left here. Structurally, this is characterized by a deeper left central sulcus, increased leftward neuropil in BA4 [76] and expansion of the left hand motor cortex in right-handers [77]. Guye et al. [78] show that whole-brain functional connectivity is more extensive with the left than with the right primary motor cortex. Left premotor and parietal regions are more strongly implicated in higher order actions [79]. Also, the planning of complex, sequential movements [79–81], bimanual coordination [82, 83] and response selection [84] have been attributed to the left hemisphere, which is interesting considering the problems individuals with ASC experience with fine motor skills [85] and planned sequencing of actions [86]. In contrast, sensory processing and spatial aspects of sensorimotor actions have been reported to show right hemisphere dominance [87–89]. It has been suggested that posture and limb position [90], as well as the use of proprioceptive feedback [91, 92], are preferentially lateralized to the right hemisphere in right-handed individuals. Interestingly, we have previously reported that individuals with ASC rely to a much greater extent on proprioceptive feedback during motor learning, which is related to more severe motor impairments and other social symptoms [93]. Atypical rightward lateralization of motor circuits might constitute a neural mechanism contributing to this finding.

Reports of disturbance in establishing typical patterns of hemispheric specialization in ASC date back to the consistently replicated observation of increased rates of left-handedness among individuals with ASC [94–101]. Left-handers activate the right premotor cortex during contra- and ipsilateral finger movements [102] and have increased intrasulcal surface in the right precentral gyrus [76]. Interestingly, our results are not driven by differences in handedness, as participants were matched on a measure of handedness and were right-handed. Still, it will be interesting to explore whether the observed pattern is even more pronounced in left-handed individuals with ASC.

Implications of motor deficits in ASC

Motor deficits are present in at least 80 % of children with ASC [28, 103, 104] comprising some of the earliest signs, such as delays in motor milestones [105, 106]. Later on in development, motor-related deficits persist and become more apparent, with deficits in gross and fine motor coordination [19, 47, 107, 108], atypical gait and posture [109, 110] and particularly difficulty with performance of skilled gestures (i.e. praxis) [18, 27, 28].

In line with this, it has been argued that core social and communicative symptoms in autism might be subserved by the same neural systems underpinning motor-related dysfunction [111, 112]. In fact, there is a close relationship between motor and social-communicative behaviours: motor development is the prerequisite for speech, articulation and engagement in the social world through directing attention, grasping and sharing things, and approaching, imitating and responding to others. In line with this, Iverson and Braddock [113] have shown that children with language deficits have poorer fine and gross motor skills. At the same time, production and understanding of actions, such as performance of sequences of actions and following verbal commands, are dependent on the development of language skills. Thus, atypical lateralization in related cognitive domains such as language might be influenced by the same developmental mechanisms [114, 115]. Notably, here, we did not find a significant association between atypical motor circuit lateralization and social-communicative sub-measures of either the ADOS or ADI. Given that other studies find such relationship [116], future research needs to examine a potential association with more specific measures of atypical social development in ASC and explore the link between motor and social networks directly at the neuronal level.

Limitations and future directions

Here, we report atypical laterality of the motor network in children with ASC. Given that ASC is a neurodevelopmental condition, it remains to be established whether the observed pattern is stable across the lifespan. Many studies show temporal test-retest reliability and reproducibility of functional resting-state networks [117–119]. It has been argued that neural coupling configurations are dynamic and transient over time with fluctuations in connection strengths [120, 121]. As arousal, sleep [122], conscious [123], cognitive [124] and emotional [125] states constitute influencing factors, only replication in independent, longitudinal samples can confirm the stability of the reported findings. Age-related changes have been described in a range of different networks, with decreasing connectivity representing increasing hemispheric specialization and increasing connectivity representing increasing functional cooperation [126]. The same authors also reported not only linear but also quadratic and cubic age effects on changes of functional connectivity, emphasizing the need for longitudinal samples to fully explore the stability and plausible developmental trend of the reported findings.

One limitation concerns the heterogeneity within ASC. Children with ASC frequently have other comorbid conditions, such as ADHD, which is another condition associated with atypical lateralization [127]. Also, Mahajan et al. [128] showed that individuals with ASC with and without ADHD show differences in motor cortex laterality with children with ASC without ADHD exhibiting rightward increases in M1, whereas children with ASC and comorbid ADHD showing left-lateralized increases. Medication exposure is another possible confound which might influence connectivity strength [129–131]. Overall, a large portion of individuals with ASC have psychiatric comorbidities during their lifespan (ADHD 28–44 %; anxiety 42–56 %; depression 12–70 %; oppositional defiant disorder 16–28 %; [132]) and around 70 % of children with ASC use some form of psychoactive medication [133, 134], making any sample that excludes these individuals less representative of the autistic population.

It remains to be established whether these results are restricted to lateralized left hemisphere functions or whether right hemisphere functions such as visuospatial abilities are also affected. Cardinale et al. [45] report rightward asymmetries of more widespread networks including those underlying visuospatial attention, but no other studies have looked at hemispheric specialization of visuospatial information processing in ASC. Future research should explore whether stronger rightward lateralization might underpin superior visual attention and weak central coherence in ASC and whether this potentially differentiates between individuals with ASC with and without enhanced visuospatial processing abilities.

Heterogeneity within the autism spectrum is the biggest challenge in the current research. It will be of interest to explore whether atypical motor network lateralization is characteristic of an as-yet undefined subgroup within ASC, such as language delay, for example, [60]. Other factors constituting heterogeneity include handedness, sex or IQ. We previously showed that handedness can be a marker of rightward lateralization of structural connectivity of regions connecting sensorimotor cortical areas [135]. Whether this also applies to functional lateralization remains to be established. As for sex, our findings here were most pronounced when including both males and females. Sex-stratified analyses show an overlapping functional organization in males and females with ASC regarding lateralization of the motor network. In general, few studies have looked at sex differences in the laterality of resting-state connectivity. Tian et al. [136] reported that males show more locally efficient right hemisphere networks, whereas females have more locally efficient left hemisphere networks. Zuo et al. [126] reported that homotopic resting-state connectivity in the dorsolateral prefrontal cortex and the amygdala show opposite developmental trajectories in males and females. How functional connectivity and its lateralization further differ across genders in ASC awaits investigation. Regarding IQ, our sample was only matched on perceptual reasoning IQ; however, additional analyses showed that results remained largely unaffected by full-scale IQ (i.e. when controlling for FIQ). As motor delay is mostly evident in low-functioning individuals [137, 138], it will be important to explore whether this result is more pronounced in this sub-population with ASC.

The present findings were based on patterns observed in the so-called *resting state*, and it will be interesting to explore whether atypical rightward lateralization remains robust under conditions when the motor execution network is active, as well as whether they are more pronounced in particular parcels underlying the motor homunculus. Lastly, here, we focused on atypical intrahemispheric connectivity. However, many studies have shown that atypical interhemispheric connectivity (such as reduced corpus callosum size) contributes to atypical connectivity in ASC [139–141]. Efficient information processing across the whole brain substantially depends on interhemispheric integration, which may be impaired in ASC [142]. Herbert et al. [143] show that only intrahemispheric connectivity is impaired in ASC, whereas others demonstrate that intra- and interhemispheric connectivities are both affected [141, 144]. Particularly, the right hemisphere regions involved in visuospatial processing have been suggested to rely on more integrative, interhemispheric processing [5]. Thus, future studies need to explore whether atypical lateralization in ASC extends to cross-hemispheric networks, particularly for functions such as visuospatial skills.

Conclusions

Our novel findings show that atypical functional lateralization in ASC extends beyond the language domain to functional circuits underlying motor execution. The deficit in children with ASC in establishing a typical pattern of hemispheric specialization for motor control may contribute to difficulties with motor skill development and might even form the early basis for the development of social and communicative impairments. It remains to be established whether atypical lateralization in functionally related domains (motor and language functions) share common neurodevelopmental origins and trajectories.

Abbreviations

AC, anterior cerebellum; ADI-R, Autism Diagnostic Interview–Revised; ADOS, Autism Diagnostic Observation Schedule; BOLD, blood-oxygen-level-dependent; ASC, autism spectrum conditions; CSF, cerebrospinal fluid; DMN, default mode network; EHI, Edinburgh Handedness Inventory; FD, framewise displacement; FIQ, full-scale IQ; GSR, global signal regression; LH, left hemisphere; LI, laterality index; PANESS, Physical and Neurological Examination of Subtle Signs; PRI, perceptual reasoning index; PUT, putamen; RH, right hemisphere; SMA-d, bilateral supplementary motor area-dorsal segment; SMA-r, bilateral supplementary motor area-rostral segment; SMC, sensorimotor cortex; TH, thalamus; VCI, verbal comprehension index; WM, white matter

Acknowledgements

We would like to thank all the families who participated in the study. This research was supported by grants from the Autism Speaks Foundation (#2506, #2384, #1739); the National Institutes of Health (R01 NS048527-08, R21 MH098228, R01 MH078160-06A1, P41 EB015909); the Clinical and Translational Research (ICTR) (UL1 TR 000424-06, UL1 TR 001079-03); and the Johns Hopkins Institute for Clinical and Translational Research, which is funded in part by grant numbers UL1 TR 000424-06 and UL1 TR 001079-03 from the National Center for Advancing Translational Sciences (NCATS). DLF was funded by Sidney Sussex College, Cambridge; the European Molecular Biology Organization (EMBO); the British Psychological Society; and the Ingelheim Boehringer Foundation. We would like to thank Tibor Auer and Jared Nielsen for the helpful discussion.

Authors' contributions

DLF conducted the analyses and wrote the manuscript. ADB and MBN assisted in carrying out the analyses and revised the manuscript. MM conducted the psychological and behavioural assessments, acquired the data and revised the manuscript. DC acquired and provided the data and revised the manuscript. MCL, JS, SBC and JJP made conceptual suggestions and critically revised the manuscript. SHM designed and obtained funding for the study and edited the manuscript. All authors read and approved the manuscript.

Competing interests

JJP serves as manager of the F.M. Kirby Research Center for Functional Brain Imaging, which receives research support from Philips HealthCare, which manufactured the MRI scanners used in this study. All other authors declare that they have no competing interests.

Author details
[1]Autism Research Centre, Department of Psychiatry, University of Cambridge, Cambridge, UK. [2]Department of Child and Adolescent Psychiatry, the Child Study Center, New York University Langone Medical Center, New York, NY, USA. [3]Center for Neurodevelopmental and Imaging Research, Kennedy Krieger Institute, Baltimore, MD, USA. [4]Department of Neurology, Johns Hopkins School of Medicine, Baltimore, MD, USA. [5]Department of Psychiatry and Behavioral Sciences, Johns Hopkins School of Medicine, Baltimore, MD, USA. [6]Child, Youth and Family Services, Centre for Addiction and Mental Health and Department of Psychiatry, University of Toronto, Toronto, Canada. [7]Department of Psychiatry, College of Medicine, National Taiwan University Hospital, Taipei City, Taiwan. [8]Cambridgeshire and Peterborough NHS Foundation Trust, Cambridge, UK. [9]National Institute of Health Research, Cambridge Biomedical Research Centre, Cambridge, UK. [10]Behavioural and Clinical Neuroscience Institute, University of Cambridge, Cambridge, UK. [11]Brain Mapping Unit, Department of Psychiatry, University of Cambridge, Cambridge, UK. [12]F.M. Kirby Research Center for Functional Brain Imaging, Kennedy Krieger Institute, Baltimore, USA. [13]Department of Radiology, Johns Hopkins School of Medicine, Baltimore, USA.

References

1. Gazzaniga MS. Principles of human brain organization derived from split-brain studies. Neuron. 1995;14(2):217–28.
2. Mesulam MM. Large-scale neurocognitive networks and distributed processing for attention, language, and memory. Ann Neurol. 1990;28(5): 597–613. doi:10.1002/ana.410280502.
3. Hugdahl K. Fifty years of dichotic listening research—still going and going and…. Brain Cogn. 2011;76(2):211–3. doi:10.1016/j.bandc.2011.03.006.
4. Barber AD, Srinivasan P, Joel SE, Caffo BS, Pekar JJ, Mostofsky SH. Motor "dexterity"?: evidence that left hemisphere lateralization of motor circuit connectivity is associated with better motor performance in children. Cereb Cortex. 2012;22(1):51–9. doi:10.1093/cercor/bhr062.
5. Gotts SJ, Jo HJ, Wallace GL, Saad ZS, Cox RW, Martin A. Two distinct forms of functional lateralization in the human brain. Proc Natl Acad Sci U S A. 2013;110(36):E3435–44. doi:10.1073/pnas.1302581110.
6. Mellet E, Zago L, Jobard G, Crivello F, Petit L, Joliot M, et al. Weak language lateralization affects both verbal and spatial skills: an fMRI study in 297 subjects. Neuropsychologia. 2014;65:56–62. doi:10.1016/j.neuropsychologia. 2014.10.010.
7. Rojas DC, Bawn SD, Benkers TL, Reite ML, Rogers SJ. Smaller left hemisphere planum temporale in adults with autistic disorder. Neurosci Lett. 2002; 328(3):237–40.
8. Herbert MR, Ziegler DA, Deutsch CK, O'Brien LM, Kennedy DN, Filipek PA, et al. Brain asymmetries in autism and developmental language disorder: a nested whole-brain analysis. Brain. 2005;128(Pt 1):213–26. doi:10.1093/brain/awh330.
9. Dawson G, Finley C, Phillips S, Lewy A. A comparison of hemispheric asymmetries in speech-related brain potentials of autistic and dysphasic children. Brain Lang. 1989;37(1):26–41.
10. Seery AM, Vogel-Farley V, Tager-Flusberg H, Nelson CA. Atypical lateralization of ERP response to native and non-native speech in infants at risk for autism spectrum disorder. Dev Cogn Neurosci. 2013;5:10–24. doi:10. 1016/j.dcn.2012.11.007.
11. Boddaert N, Belin P, Chabane N, Poline JB, Barthélémy C, Mouren-Simeoni MC, et al. Perception of complex sounds: abnormal pattern of cortical activation in autism. Am J Psychiatry. 2003;160(11):2057–60.
12. Müller RA, Behen ME, Rothermel RD, Chugani DC, Muzik O, Mangner TJ, et al. Brain mapping of language and auditory perception in high-functioning autistic adults: a PET study. J Autism Dev Disord. 1999;29(1):19–31.
13. Knaus TA, Silver AM, Kennedy M, Lindgren KA, Dominick KC, Siegel J, et al. Language laterality in autism spectrum disorder and typical controls: a functional, volumetric, and diffusion tensor MRI study. Brain Lang. 2010; 112(2):113–20. doi:10.1016/j.bandl.2009.11.005.
14. Eyler LT, Pierce K, Courchesne E. A failure of left temporal cortex to specialize for language is an early emerging and fundamental property of autism. Brain. 2012;135(Pt 3):949–60. doi:10.1093/brain/awr364.
15. Kleinhans NM, Müller RA, Cohen DN, Courchesne E. Atypical functional lateralization of language in autism spectrum disorders. Brain Res. 2008; 1221:115–25. doi:10.1016/j.brainres.2008.04.080.
16. Lombardo MV, Pierce K, Eyler LT, Carter Barnes C, Ahrens-Barbeau C, Solso S, et al. Different functional neural substrates for good and poor language outcome in autism. Neuron. 2015;86(2):567–77. doi:10.1016/j.neuron.2015.03.023.
17. Teitelbaum P, Teitelbaum O, Nye J, Fryman J, Maurer RG. Movement analysis in infancy may be useful for early diagnosis of autism. Proc Natl Acad Sci U S A. 1998;95(23):13982–7.
18. Mostofsky SH, Dubey P, Jerath VK, Jansiewicz EM, Goldberg MC, Denckla MB. Developmental dyspraxia is not limited to imitation in children with autism spectrum disorders. J Int Neuropsychol Soc. 2006;12(3):314–26.
19. Green D, Charman T, Pickles A, Chandler S, Loucas T, Simonoff E, et al. Impairment in movement skills of children with autistic spectrum disorders. Dev Med Child Neurol. 2009;51(4):311–6. doi:10.1111/j.1469-8749.2008.03242.x.
20. Müller RA, Kleinhans N, Kemmotsu N, Pierce K, Courchesne E. Abnormal variability and distribution of functional maps in autism: an FMRI study of visuomotor learning. Am J Psychiatry. 2003;160(10):1847–62.
21. Allen G, Courchesne E. Differential effects of developmental cerebellar abnormality on cognitive and motor functions in the cerebellum: an fMRI study of autism. Am J Psychiatry. 2003;160(2):262–73.
22. Mostofsky SH, Powell SK, Simmonds DJ, Goldberg MC, Caffo B, Pekar JJ. Decreased connectivity and cerebellar activity in autism during motor task performance. Brain. 2009;132(Pt 9):2413–25. doi:10.1093/brain/awp088.
23. Allen G, Müller RA, Courchesne E. Cerebellar function in autism: functional magnetic resonance image activation during a simple motor task. Biol Psychiatry. 2004;56(4):269–78. doi:10.1016/j.biopsych.2004.06.005.
24. Dawson G, Warrenburg S, Fuller P. Hemisphere functioning and motor imitation in autistic persons. Brain Cogn. 1983;2(4):346–54.
25. Müller RA, Cauich C, Rubio MA, Mizuno A, Courchesne E. Abnormal activity patterns in premotor cortex during sequence learning in autistic patients. Biol Psychiatry. 2004;56(5):323–32. doi:10.1016/j.biopsych.2004.06.007.
26. D'Cruz AM, Mosconi MW, Steele S, Rubin LH, Luna B, Minshew N, et al. Lateralized response timing deficits in autism. Biol Psychiatry. 2009;66(4): 393–7. doi:10.1016/j.biopsych.2009.01.008.
27. Dowell LR, Mahone EM, Mostofsky SH. Associations of postural knowledge and basic motor skill with dyspraxia in autism: implication for abnormalities in distributed connectivity and motor learning. Neuropsychology. 2009; 23(5):563–70. doi:10.1037/a0015640.
28. Dziuk MA, Gidley Larson JC, Apostu A, Mahone EM, Denckla MB, Mostofsky SH. Dyspraxia in autism: association with motor, social, and communicative deficits. Dev Med Child Neurol. 2007;49(10):734–9. doi:10.1111/j.1469-8749.2007.00734.x.
29. Mostofsky SH, Ewen JB. Altered connectivity and action model formation in autism is autism. Neuroscientist. 2011;17(4):437–48. doi:10.1177/1073858410392381.
30. Biswal B, Yetkin FZ, Haughton VM, Hyde JS. Functional connectivity in the motor cortex of resting human brain using echo-planar MRI. Magn Reson Med. 1995;34(4):537–41.
31. Buckner RL, Andrews-Hanna JR, Schacter DL. The brain's default network: anatomy, function, and relevance to disease. Ann N Y Acad Sci. 2008;1124: 1–38. doi:10.1196/annals.1440.011.
32. Fox MD, Raichle ME. Spontaneous fluctuations in brain activity observed with functional magnetic resonance imaging. Nat Rev Neurosci. 2007;8(9): 700–11. doi:10.1038/nrn2201.
33. Lackner JR, Teuber HL. Alterations in auditory fusion thresholds after cerebral injury in man. Neuropsychologia. 1973;11(4):409–15.
34. Semmes J. Hemispheric specialization: a possible clue to mechanism. Neuropsychologia. 1968;6(1):11–26.
35. Corbetta M, Shulman GL. Spatial neglect and attention networks. Annu Rev Neurosci. 2011;34:569–99. doi:10.1146/annurev-neuro-061010-113731.
36. Belmonte MK, Allen G, Beckel-Mitchener A, Boulanger LM, Carper RA, Webb SJ. Autism and abnormal development of brain connectivity. J Neurosci. 2004;24(42):9228–31. doi:10.1523/jneurosci.3340-04.2004.
37. Courchesne E, Pierce K. Why the frontal cortex in autism might be talking only to itself: local over-connectivity but long-distance disconnection. Curr Opin Neurobiol. 2005;15(2):225–30. doi:10.1016/j.conb.2005.03.001.
38. Just MA, Cherkassky VL, Keller TA, Minshew NJ. Cortical activation and synchronization during sentence comprehension in high-functioning autism: evidence of underconnectivity. Brain. 2004;127(Pt 8):1811–21. doi:10. 1093/brain/awh199.

39. Weng SJ, Wiggins JL, Peltier SJ, Carrasco M, Risi S, Lord C, et al. Alterations of resting state functional connectivity in the default network in adolescents with autism spectrum disorders. Brain Res. 2010;1313:202–14. doi:10.1016/j.brainres.2009.11.057.
40. Lynch CJ, Uddin LQ, Supekar K, Khouzam A, Phillips J, Menon V. Default mode network in childhood autism: posteromedial cortex heterogeneity and relationship with social deficits. Biol Psychiatry. 2013;74(3):212–9. doi:10.1016/j.biopsych.2012.12.013.
41. Assaf M, Jagannathan K, Calhoun VD, Miller L, Stevens MC, Sahl R, et al. Abnormal functional connectivity of default mode sub-networks in autism spectrum disorder patients. Neuroimage. 2010;53(1):247–56. doi:10.1016/j.neuroimage.2010.05.067.
42. Spencer MD, Chura LR, Holt RJ, Suckling J, Calder AJ, Bullmore ET, et al. Failure to deactivate the default mode network indicates a possible endophenotype of autism. Mol Autism. 2012;3(1):15. doi:10.1186/2040-2392-3-15.
43. Nebel MB, Eloyan A, Barber AD, Mostofsky SH. Precentral gyrus functional connectivity signatures of autism. Front Syst Neurosci. 2014;8:80. doi:10.3389/fnsys.2014.00080.
44. Nebel MB, Joel SE, Muschelli J, Barber AD, Caffo BS, Pekar JJ, et al. Disruption of functional organization within the primary motor cortex in children with autism. Hum Brain Mapp. 2014;35(2):567–80. doi:10.1002/hbm.22188.
45. Cardinale RC, Shih P, Fishman I, Ford LM, Müller RA. Pervasive rightward asymmetry shifts of functional networks in autism spectrum disorder. JAMA Psychiatry. 2013;70(9):975–82. doi:10.1001/jamapsychiatry.2013.382.
46. Nielsen JA, Zielinski BA, Fletcher PT, Alexander AL, Lange N, Bigler ED, et al. Abnormal lateralization of functional connectivity between language and default mode regions in autism. Mol Autism. 2014;5(1):8. doi:10.1186/2040-2392-5-8.
47. Jansiewicz EM, Goldberg MC, Newschaffer CJ, Denckla MB, Landa R, Mostofsky SH. Motor signs distinguish children with high functioning autism and Asperger's syndrome from controls. J Autism Dev Disord. 2006;36(5):613–21. doi:10.1007/s10803-006-0109-y.
48. Fournier KA, Hass CJ, Naik SK, Lodha N, Cauraugh JH. Motor coordination in autism spectrum disorders: a synthesis and meta-analysis. J Autism Dev Disord. 2010;40(10):1227–40. doi:10.1007/s10803-010-0981-3.
49. Izawa J, Pekny SE, Marko MK, Haswell CC, Shadmehr R, Mostofsky SH. Motor learning relies on integrated sensory inputs in ADHD, but over-selectively on proprioception in autism spectrum conditions. Autism Res. 2012;5(2):124–36. doi:10.1002/aur.1222.
50. Nielsen JA, Zielinski BA, Ferguson MA, Lainhart JE, Anderson JS. An evaluation of the left-brain vs. right-brain hypothesis with resting state functional connectivity magnetic resonance imaging. PLoS One. 2013;8(8):e71275. doi:10.1371/journal.pone.0071275.
51. American Psychiatric Association. Diagnostic and statistical manual of mental disorders: DSM-IV-TR. 4th ed., Text revision. ed. Washington, DC: American Psychiatric Association; 2000.
52. Lord C, Rutter M, Le Couteur A. Autism Diagnostic Interview-Revised: a revised version of a diagnostic interview for caregivers of individuals with possible pervasive developmental disorders. J Autism Dev Disord. 1994;24(5):659–85.
53. Lord C, Risi S, Lambrecht L, Cook Jr EH, Leventhal BL, DiLavore PC, et al. The autism diagnostic observation schedule-generic: a standard measure of social and communication deficits associated with the spectrum of autism. J Autism Dev Disord. 2000;30(3):205–23.
54. Wechsler D. Wechsler intelligence scale for children—III. 3rd ed. San Antonio: The Psychological Corporation; 1991.
55. Wechsler D. Wechsler intelligence scale for children—IV. 4th ed. San Antonio: The Psychological Corporation; 2003.
56. Reich W. Diagnostic interview for children and adolescents (DICA). J Am Acad Child Adolesc Psychiatry. 2000;39(1):59–66. doi:10.1097/00004583-200001000-00017.
57. Denckla MB. Revised neurological examination for subtle signs (1985). Psychopharmacol Bull. 1985;21(4):773–800.
58. Oldfield RC. The assessment and analysis of handedness: the Edinburgh inventory. Neuropsychologia. 1971;9(1):97–113.
59. Wilke M, Holland SK, Altaye M, Gaser C. Template-O-Matic: a toolbox for creating customized pediatric templates. Neuroimage. 2008;41(3):903–13. doi:10.1016/j.neuroimage.2008.02.056.
60. Floris DL, Lai MC, Auer T, Lombardo MV, Ecker C, Chakrabarti B, et al. Atypically rightward cerebral asymmetry in male adults with autism stratifies individuals with and without language delay. Hum Brain Mapp. 2016;37(1):230–53. doi:10.1002/hbm.23023.
61. Behzadi Y, Restom K, Liau J, Liu TT. A component based noise correction method (CompCor) for BOLD and perfusion based fMRI. Neuroimage. 2007;37(1):90–101. doi:10.1016/j.neuroimage.2007.04.042.
62. Gotts SJ, Saad ZS, Jo HJ, Wallace GL, Cox RW, Martin A. The perils of global signal regression for group comparisons: a case study of autism spectrum disorders. Front Hum Neurosci. 2013;7:356. doi:10.3389/fnhum.2013.00356.
63. Power JD, Barnes KA, Snyder AZ, Schlaggar BL, Petersen SE. Steps toward optimizing motion artifact removal in functional connectivity MRI; a reply to Carp. Neuroimage. 2013;76:439–41. doi:10.1016/j.neuroimage.2012.03.017.
64. Di Martino A, Zuo XN, Kelly C, Grzadzinski R, Mennes M, Schvarcz A, et al. Shared and distinct intrinsic functional network centrality in autism and attention-deficit/hyperactivity disorder. Biol Psychiatry. 2013;74(8):623–32. doi:10.1016/j.biopsych.2013.02.011.
65. Fox MD, Snyder AZ, Vincent JL, Corbetta M, Van Essen DC, Raichle ME. The human brain is intrinsically organized into dynamic, anticorrelated functional networks. Proc Natl Acad Sci U S A. 2005;102(27):9673–8. doi:10.1073/pnas.0504136102.
66. Yeo BT, Krienen FM, Sepulcre J, Sabuncu MR, Lashkari D, Hollinshead M, et al. The organization of the human cerebral cortex estimated by intrinsic functional connectivity. J Neurophysiol. 2011;106(3):1125–65. doi:10.1152/jn.00338.2011.
67. Di Martino A, Yan CG, Li Q, Denio E, Castellanos FX, Alaerts K, et al. The autism brain imaging data exchange: towards a large-scale evaluation of the intrinsic brain architecture in autism. Mol Psychiatry. 2014;19(6):659–67. doi:10.1038/mp.2013.78.
68. Gonzalez-Gadea ML, Baez S, Torralva T, Castellanos FX, Rattazzi A, Bein V, et al. Cognitive variability in adults with ADHD and AS: disentangling the roles of executive functions and social cognition. Res Dev Disabil. 2013;34(2):817–30. doi:10.1016/j.ridd.2012.11.009.
69. Brian J, Bryson SE, Garon N, Roberts W, Smith IM, Szatmari P, et al. Clinical assessment of autism in high-risk 18-month-olds. Autism. 2008;12(5):433–56. doi:10.1177/1362361308094500.
70. Sutera S, Pandey J, Esser EL, Rosenthal MA, Wilson LB, Barton M, et al. Predictors of optimal outcome in toddlers diagnosed with autism spectrum disorders. J Autism Dev Disord. 2007;37(1):98–107. doi:10.1007/s10803-006-0340-6.
71. Bhat AN, Landa RJ, Galloway JC. Current perspectives on motor functioning in infants, children, and adults with autism spectrum disorders. Phys Ther. 2011;91(7):1116–29. doi:10.2522/ptj.20100294.
72. Sears LL, Vest C, Mohamed S, Bailey J, Ranson BJ, Piven J. An MRI study of the basal ganglia in autism. Prog Neuropsychopharmacol Biol Psychiatry. 1999;23(4):613–24.
73. Siegel BV, Asarnow R, Tanguay P, Call JD, Abel L, Ho A, et al. Regional cerebral glucose metabolism and attention in adults with a history of childhood autism. J Neuropsychiatry Clin Neurosci. 1992;4(4):406–14.
74. McAlonan GM, Daly E, Kumari V, Critchley HD, van Amelsvoort T, Suckling J, et al. Brain anatomy and sensorimotor gating in Asperger's syndrome. Brain. 2002;125(Pt 7):1594–606.
75. Joel SE, Caffo BS, van Zijl PC, Pekar JJ. On the relationship between seed-based and ICA-based measures of functional connectivity. Magn Reson Med. 2011;66(3):644–57. doi:10.1002/mrm.22818.
76. Amunts K, Schlaug G, Schleicher A, Steinmetz H, Dabringhaus A, Roland PE, et al. Asymmetry in the human motor cortex and handedness. Neuroimage. 1996;4(3 Pt 1):216–22. doi:10.1006/nimg.1996.0073.
77. Volkmann J, Schnitzler A, Witte OW, Freund H. Handedness and asymmetry of hand representation in human motor cortex. J Neurophysiol. 1998;79(4):2149–54.
78. Guye M, Parker GJ, Symms M, Boulby P, Wheeler-Kingshott CA, Salek-Haddadi A, et al. Combined functional MRI and tractography to demonstrate the connectivity of the human primary motor cortex in vivo. Neuroimage. 2003;19(4):1349–60.
79. Haaland KY, Elsinger CL, Mayer AR, Durgerian S, Rao SM. Motor sequence complexity and performing hand produce differential patterns of hemispheric lateralization. J Cogn Neurosci. 2004;16(4):621–36. doi:10.1162/089892904323057344.
80. Verstynen T, Diedrichsen J, Albert N, Aparicio P, Ivry RB. Ipsilateral motor cortex activity during unimanual hand movements relates to task complexity. J Neurophysiol. 2005;93(3):1209–22. doi:10.1152/jn.00720.2004.
81. Schluter ND, Rushworth MF, Passingham RE, Mills KR. Temporary interference in human lateral premotor cortex suggests dominance for the selection of movements. A study using transcranial magnetic stimulation. Brain. 1998;121(Pt 5):785–99.

82. Jäncke L, Specht K, Shah JN, Hugdahl K. Focused attention in a simple dichotic listening task: an fMRI experiment. Brain Res Cogn Brain Res. 2003;16(2):257–66.
83. Serrien DJ, Cassidy MJ, Brown P. The importance of the dominant hemisphere in the organization of bimanual movements. Hum Brain Mapp. 2003;18(4):296–305. doi:10.1002/hbm.10086.
84. Weissman DH, Banich MT. The cerebral hemispheres cooperate to perform complex but not simple tasks. Neuropsychology. 2000;14(1):41–59.
85. Dawson G, Watling R. Interventions to facilitate auditory, visual, and motor integration in autism: a review of the evidence. J Autism Dev Disord. 2000; 30(5):415–21.
86. Greenspan SI, Wieder S. Developmental patterns and outcomes in infants and children with disorders in relating and communicating: a chart review of 200 cases of children with autistic spectrum diagnoses. J Dev Learn Disord. 1997;1(1):87–141.
87. Ghilardi M, Ghez C, Dhawan V, Moeller J, Mentis M, Nakamura T, et al. Patterns of regional brain activation associated with different forms of motor learning. Brain Res. 2000;871(1):127–45.
88. Wenderoth N, Debaere F, Sunaert S, van Hecke P, Swinnen SP. Parieto-premotor areas mediate directional interference during bimanual movements. Cereb Cortex. 2004;14(10):1153–63. doi:10.1093/cercor/bhh075.
89. Haaland KY, Harrington DL. Hemispheric control of the initial and corrective components of aiming movements. Neuropsychologia. 1989;27(7):961–9.
90. Sainburg RL. Evidence for a dynamic-dominance hypothesis of handedness. Exp Brain Res. 2002;142(2):241–58. doi:10.1007/s00221-001-0913-8.
91. Goble DJ, Brown SH. The biological and behavioral basis of upper limb asymmetries in sensorimotor performance. Neurosci Biobehav Rev. 2008; 32(3):598–610. doi:10.1016/j.neubiorev.2007.10.006.
92. Goble DJ, Noble BC, Brown SH. Proprioceptive target matching asymmetries in left-handed individuals. Exp Brain Res. 2009;197(4):403–8. doi:10.1007/s00221-009-1922-2.
93. Haswell CC, Izawa J, Dowell LR, Mostofsky SH, Shadmehr R. Representation of internal models of action in the autistic brain. Nat Neurosci. 2009;12(8): 970–2. doi:10.1038/nn.2356.
94. Colby KM, Parkison C. Handedness in autistic children. J Autism Child Schizophr. 1977;7(1):3–9.
95. Barry RJ, James AL. Handedness in autistics, retardates, and normals of a wide age range. J Autism Child Schizophr. 1978;8(3):315–23.
96. Gillberg C. Autistic children's hand preferences: results from an epidemiological study of infantile autism. Psychiatry Res. 1983;10(1):21–30.
97. Ricks DM, Wing L. Handedness subtypes in autism. Psychiatric Annals. 1985; 15(7):447–50.
98. Soper HV, Satz P, Orsini DL, Henry RR, Zvi JC, Schulman M. Handedness patterns in autism suggest subtypes. J Autism Dev Disord. 1986;16(2):155–67.
99. McManus IC, Murray B, Doyle K, Baron-Cohen S. Handedness in childhood autism shows a dissociation of skill and preference. Cortex. 1992;28(3):373–81.
100. Cornish KM, McManus IC. Hand preference and hand skill in children with autism. J Autism Dev Disord. 1996;26(6):597–609.
101. Preslar J, Kushner HI, Marino L, Pearce B. Autism, lateralisation, and handedness: a review of the literature and meta-analysis. Laterality. 2014; 19(1):64–95. doi:10.1080/1357650X.2013.772621.
102. Kawashima R, Inoue K, Sato K, Fukuda H. Functional asymmetry of cortical motor control in left-handed subjects. Neuroreport. 1997;8(7):1729–32.
103. Ghaziuddin M, Butler E. Clumsiness in autism and Asperger syndrome: a further report. J Intellect Disabil Res. 1998;42(Pt 1):43–8.
104. David FJ, Baranek GT, Giuliani CA, Mercer VS, Poe MD, Thorpe DE. A pilot study: coordination of precision grip in children and adolescents with high functioning autism. Pediatr Phys Ther. 2009;21(2):205–11. doi:10.1097/PEP.0b013e3181a3afc2.
105. Iverson JM, Wozniak RH. Variation in vocal-motor development in infant siblings of children with autism. J Autism Dev Disord. 2007;37(1):158–70. doi:10.1007/s10803-006-0339-z.
106. Ming X, Brimacombe M, Wagner GC. Prevalence of motor impairment in autism spectrum disorders. Brain Dev. 2007;29(9):565–70. doi:10.1016/j.braindev.2007.03.002.
107. Ament K, Mejia A, Buhlman R, Erklin S, Caffo B, Mostofsky S, et al. Evidence for specificity of motor impairments in catching and balance in children with autism. J Autism Dev Disord. 2015;45(3):742–51. doi:10.1007/s10803-014-2229-0.
108. Noterdaeme M, Mildenberger K, Minow F, Amorosa H. Evaluation of neuromotor deficits in children with autism and children with a specific speech and language disorder. Eur Child Adolesc Psychiatry. 2002;11(5):219–25. doi:10.1007/s00787-002-0285-z.
109. Minshew NJ, Sung K, Jones BL, Furman JM. Underdevelopment of the postural control system in autism. Neurology. 2004;63(11):2056–61.
110. Rinehart NJ, Tonge BJ, Bradshaw JL, Iansek R, Enticott PG, McGinley J. Gait function in high-functioning autism and Asperger's disorder : evidence for basal-ganglia and cerebellar involvement? Eur Child Adolesc Psychiatry. 2006;15(5):256–64. doi:10.1007/s00787-006-0530-y.
111. Nayate A, Bradshaw JL, Rinehart NJ. Autism and Asperger's disorder: are they movement disorders involving the cerebellum and/or basal ganglia? Brain Res Bull. 2005;67(4):327–34. doi:10.1016/j.brainresbull.2005.07.011.
112. Leary MR, Hill DA. Moving on: autism and movement disturbance. Ment Retard. 1996;34(1):39–53.
113. Iverson JM, Braddock BA. Gesture and motor skill in relation to language in children with language impairment. J Speech Lang Hear Res. 2011;54(1):72–86. doi:10.1044/1092-4388(2010/08-0197).
114. Knecht S, Dräger B, Deppe M, Bobe L, Lohmann H, Flöel A, et al. Handedness and hemispheric language dominance in healthy humans. Brain. 2000;123(Pt 12):2512–8.
115. Pujol J, Deus J, Losilla JM, Capdevila A. Cerebral lateralization of language in normal left-handed people studied by functional MRI. Neurology. 1999; 52(5):1038–43.
116. Nebel MB, Eloyan A, Nettles CA, Sweeney KL, Ament K, Ward RE, et al. Intrinsic visual-motor synchrony correlates with social deficits in autism. Biol Psychiatry. 2016;79(8):633–41. doi:10.1016/j.biopsych.2015.08.029.
117. Shehzad Z, Kelly AM, Reiss PT, Gee DG, Gotimer K, Uddin LQ, et al. The resting brain: unconstrained yet reliable. Cereb Cortex. 2009;19(10):2209–29. doi:10.1093/cercor/bhn256.
118. Dosenbach NU, Nardos B, Cohen AL, Fair DA, Power JD, Church JA, et al. Prediction of individual brain maturity using fMRI. Science. 2010;329(5997): 1358–61. doi:10.1126/science.1194144.
119. Chou YH, Panych LP, Dickey CC, Petrella JR, Chen NK. Investigation of long-term reproducibility of intrinsic connectivity network mapping: a resting-state fMRI study. AJNR Am J Neuroradiol. 2012;33(5):833–8. doi:10.3174/ajnr.A2894.
120. Chang C, Glover GH. Time-frequency dynamics of resting-state brain connectivity measured with fMRI. Neuroimage. 2010;50(1):81–98. doi:10.1016/j.neuroimage.2009.12.011.
121. Hutchison RM, Womelsdorf T, Gati JS, Everling S, Menon RS. Resting-state networks show dynamic functional connectivity in awake humans and anesthetized macaques. Hum Brain Mapp. 2013;34(9):2154–77. doi:10.1002/hbm.22058.
122. Fukunaga M, Horovitz SG, van Gelderen P, de Zwart JA, Jansma JM, Ikonomidou VN, et al. Large-amplitude, spatially correlated fluctuations in BOLD fMRI signals during extended rest and early sleep stages. Magn Reson Imaging. 2006;24(8):979–92. doi:10.1016/j.mri.2006.04.018.
123. Greicius MD, Kiviniemi V, Tervonen O, Vainionpää V, Alahuhta S, Reiss AL, et al. Persistent default-mode network connectivity during light sedation. Hum Brain Mapp. 2008;29(7):839–47. doi:10.1002/hbm.20537.
124. Waites AB, Stanislavsky A, Abbott DF, Jackson GD. Effect of prior cognitive state on resting state networks measured with functional connectivity. Hum Brain Mapp. 2005;24(1):59–68. doi:10.1002/hbm.20069.
125. Harrison BJ, Pujol J, Ortiz H, Fornito A, Pantelis C, Yücel M. Modulation of brain resting-state networks by sad mood induction. PLoS One. 2008;3(3): e1794. doi:10.1371/journal.pone.0001794.
126. Zuo XN, Kelly C, Di Martino A, Mennes M, Margulies DS, Bangaru S, et al. Growing together and growing apart: regional and sex differences in the lifespan developmental trajectories of functional homotopy. J Neurosci. 2010;30(45):15034–43. doi:10.1523/JNEUROSCI.2612-10.2010.
127. Reid HM, Norvilitis JM. Evidence for anomalous lateralization across domain in ADHD children as well as adults identified with the Wender Utah rating scale. J Psychiatr Res. 2000;34(4-5):311–6.
128. Mahajan R, Dirlikov B, Crocetti D, Mostofsky SH. Motor circuit anatomy in children with autism spectrum disorder with or without attention deficit hyperactivity disorder. Autism Res. 2015. doi:10.1002/aur.1497.
129. Bolding MS, White DM, Hadley JA, Weiler M, Holcomb HH, Lahti AC. Antipsychotic drugs alter functional connectivity between the medial frontal cortex, hippocampus, and nucleus accumbens as measured by H215O PET. Front Psychiatry. 2012;3:105. doi:10.3389/fpsyt.2012.00105.
130. Sambataro F, Blasi G, Fazio L, Caforio G, Taurisano P, Romano R, et al. Treatment with olanzapine is associated with modulation of the default mode network in patients with Schizophrenia. Neuropsychopharmacology. 2010;35(4):904–12. doi:10.1038/npp.2009.192.

131. Lui S, Li T, Deng W, Jiang L, Wu Q, Tang H, et al. Short-term effects of antipsychotic treatment on cerebral function in drug-naive first-episode schizophrenia revealed by "resting state" functional magnetic resonance imaging. Arch Gen Psychiatry. 2010;67(8):783–92. doi:10.1001/archgenpsychiatry.2010.84.
132. Lai MC, Lombardo MV, Baron-Cohen S. Autism. Lancet. 2014;383(9920):896–910. doi:10.1016/S0140-6736(13)61539-1.
133. Esbensen AJ, Greenberg JS, Seltzer MM, Aman MG. A longitudinal investigation of psychotropic and non-psychotropic medication use among adolescents and adults with autism spectrum disorders. J Autism Dev Disord. 2009;39(9):1339–49. doi:10.1007/s10803-009-0750-3.
134. Oswald DP, Sonenklar NA. Medication use among children with autism spectrum disorders. J Child Adolesc Psychopharmacol. 2007;17(3):348–55. doi:10.1089/cap.2006.17303.
135. Floris DL, Chura LR, Holt RJ, Suckling J, Bullmore ET, Baron-Cohen S, et al. Psychological correlates of handedness and corpus callosum asymmetry in autism: the left hemisphere dysfunction theory revisited. J Autism Dev Disord. 2013;43(8):1758–72. doi:10.1007/s10803-012-1720-8.
136. Tian L, Wang J, Yan C, He Y. Hemisphere- and gender-related differences in small-world brain networks: a resting-state functional MRI study. Neuroimage. 2011;54(1):191–202. doi:10.1016/j.neuroimage.2010.07.066.
137. Jeste SS. The neurology of autism spectrum disorders. Curr Opin Neurol. 2011;24(2):132–9. doi:10.1097/WCO.0b013e3283446450.
138. Hilton CL, Zhang Y, Whilte MR, Klohr CL, Constantino J. Motor impairment in sibling pairs concordant and discordant for autism spectrum disorders. Autism. 2012;16(4):430–41. doi:10.1177/1362361311423018.
139. Hardan AY, Minshew NJ, Keshavan MS. Corpus callosum size in autism. Neurology. 2000;55(7):1033–6.
140. Frazier TW, Hardan AY. A meta-analysis of the corpus callosum in autism. Biol Psychiatry. 2009;66(10):935–41. doi:10.1016/j.biopsych.2009.07.022.
141. Just MA, Cherkassky VL, Keller TA, Kana RK, Minshew NJ. Functional and anatomical cortical underconnectivity in autism: evidence from an FMRI study of an executive function task and corpus callosum morphometry. Cereb Cortex. 2007;17(4):951–61. doi:10.1093/cercor/bhl006.
142. Nydén A, Carlsson M, Carlsson A, Gillberg C. Interhemispheric transfer in high-functioning children and adolescents with autism spectrum disorders: a controlled pilot study. Dev Med Child Neurol. 2004;46(7):448–54.
143. Herbert MR, Ziegler DA, Makris N, Filipek PA, Kemper TL, Normandin JJ, et al. Localization of white matter volume increase in autism and developmental language disorder. Ann Neurol. 2004;55(4):530–40. doi:10.1002/ana.20032.
144. Hahamy A, Behrmann M, Malach R. The idiosyncratic brain: distortion of spontaneous connectivity patterns in autism spectrum disorder. Nat Neurosci. 2015;18(2):302–9. doi:10.1038/nn.3919.

2

Initial evidence that non-clinical autistic traits are associated with lower income

William J. Skylark[1*] and Simon Baron-Cohen[1,2]

Abstract

Among non-clinical samples, autistic traits correlate with a range of educational and social outcomes. However, previous work has not investigated the relationship between autistic traits and income, a key determinant of socio-economic status and well-being. In five studies (total N = 2491), we recruited participants without a diagnosis of autism from the general US population via an online platform and administered the short-form Autism Spectrum Quotient (AQ) as well as asked a range of demographic questions. We found a negative association between AQ and household income, which remained robust after controlling for age, gender, education, employment status, ethnicity, and socially desirable responding. The effect was primarily driven by the participant's own income and was mainly due to the social subscale of the AQ. These results provide initial evidence that income is negatively related to autistic traits among the general population, with potential implications for a range of social, psychological, and health outcomes.

Background

Autism spectrum conditions (henceforth autism) represent the upper end of a distribution of traits found in the general population [1–3]. Building on the observation that the relatives of people with autism often show the broader autism phenotype (BAP) (that is, sub-clinical levels of the atypical social, communicative, and repetitive behaviours that characterize autism [4, 5]), researchers have employed a number of self-report measures to gauge the presence of autistic traits in representative, typical samples. These include the Autism Spectrum Quotient (AQ; [1]), the Broad Autism Phenotype Questionnaire (BAPQ; [6]), the Subthreshold Autism Trait Questionnaire (SATQ; [7]) and the Social Responsiveness Scale (SRS; [8]) (see [9] for a review). These measures show high sensitivity and specificity for detecting formally diagnosed cases of autism and provide a useful tool for identifying people who might benefit from clinical assessment [1, 10]. In addition, typical samples with high levels of autistic traits have a socio-cognitive profile similar to that of people with autism, including greater emphasis on local information during perceptual processing [11–13], more consistent decision-making [14], impaired face-recognition [15], and reduced prosociality [16].

* Correspondence: wjm22@cam.ac.uk
[1]Department of Psychology, University of Cambridge, Cambridge CB2 3EB, UK
Full list of author information is available at the end of the article

Autistic traits also correlate with socio-economic outcomes. For example, university students studying science subjects have higher AQ scores than students taking arts and humanities subjects, and within the sciences, students of mathematics score higher than those taking physical science or engineering, who in turn score higher than biologists and medics [1] (see also [17]). AQ scores are also higher in those who work in science, technology, engineering, and mathematics (STEM) [10]. Other studies have found a negative relationship between autistic traits and school performance [18, 19]. High AQ scores also predict lower relationship satisfaction [20] and greater loneliness [21] (here and throughout, we use "predict" in the statistical sense of regression analysis, where the dependent variable can be predicted from one or more independent variables, or "predictors"; this does not, of course, establish the causal direction of any relationship between variables, as we discuss below).

This paper investigates the link between autistic traits and another key socio-economic variable: income. In industrialized, market-based economies, income is a key determinant of one's ability to acquire goods and services. It therefore plays a fundamental role in determining a person's material circumstances, including their possessions, accommodation, neighbourhood, and access to technology, and predicts a wide variety of social, economic, and health outcomes. Broadly speaking, higher levels of income predict longer life [22], better physical and mental health [23, 24], and greater reported life-satisfaction [25], although the advantages of increasing income may plateau beyond a certain point [25] and there is mounting evidence that how a person's income compares with a relevant reference group is more important than its absolute value [26]. Income can be difficult to measure, but even broad, categorical reports of household income provide a valid predictor of important outcomes [27–29].

The current paper provides an initial investigation of whether, among typical samples, income is related to a person's position on the autism spectrum, after controlling for demographic and situational variables. The research comprises five studies: Studies 1 and 2 were not intended as tests of the link between autistic traits and income; rather, income was recorded as a demographic control variable. Because analysis of these preliminary studies found a consistent and unexpected association between autistic traits and income, studies 3–5 were conducted to probe this relationship further.

Methods

All studies were conducted online using participants recruited via Amazon's Mechanical Turk (MTurk). MTurk does not perfectly represent the US population, but it is more representative than the student and convenience samples used in many studies [30] and has been used in studies of the cognitive and social correlates of autistic traits [10, 14, 31–34].

Study 1 investigated whether autistic traits predict the tendency to make social comparisons [35]; study 2 investigated whether autistic traits modulate contextual effects on financial decisions [36]. Both studies concluded by requesting demographic information: age, gender, and two simple measures of socio-economic status taken from previously published work: education level, measured on a 4-point scale, and annual pre-tax household income, measured using a 7-point scale [37, 38]. As described below, both studies found an unanticipated negative correlation between income and autistic traits, which led to studies 3–5 being conducted as "purpose-built" explorations of this association.

Whereas studies 1 and 2 used relatively coarse measures of income and education, study 3 elicited a more precise measure of the participant's household income by using a 16-point scale and adjusted this by the size of the household to obtain a better measure of affluence [26]. Study 4 fractionated household income by asking participants separate questions about their personal income and the income of the rest of their household. Both studies also employed a fine-grained assessment of educational attainment and employment status, and both also examined participants' subjective socioeconomic status (SSS)—their sense of how they stand relative to the rest of the US population. SSS is positively related to income, but is distinct: an affluent person can believe herself to be relatively poorly off, and vice-versa [39], and these subjective assessments predict many social and psychological outcomes over and above the effects of objective income or wealth [40, 41]. Finally, study 5 examined whether the association between autistic traits and income arises because people with high AQ scores are less likely to exaggerate their wealth. Wealth is often regarded as socially desirable, but people with autism may be less concerned with social reputation [42, 43] and therefore less inclined to overstate their income. Study 5 therefore tested whether the negative relationship between AQ and income persists after controlling for the tendency to make socially desirable responses; it also controlled for the effects of ethnicity.

Ethical approval for all five studies was granted by the University of Cambridge Psychology Research Ethics Committee (PRE.2015.070). Informed consent was obtained from all participants included in the studies. The datasets generated and analysed during the current study are available in the University of Cambridge data repository (https://doi.org/10.17863/CAM.13942).

Measures

Autistic traits were measured with the AQ-Short [44] (hereafter AQ), which consists of 28 items (item order was randomized in all studies). The total score across the 28 items gives an overall assessment of the level of autistic traits. Studies 1, 2, and 5 followed Hoekstra et al. [44] and used a 4-point scale (definitely agree, slightly agree, slightly disagree, definitely disagree). Studies 3 and 4 used a 6-point scale (from "definitely disagree" to "definitely agree"); the labels for the intermediate points on this response scale did not display properly, but the consistency scores were near identical to those reported by Hoekstra et al. [44], indicating that this was not a problem. In studies 3–5, an additional attention check item was included ("Attention check: Please select strongly disagree for this item") to eliminate unengaged participants. Participants in study 1 also completed the SATQ, comprising 24 items answered on a 4-point scale (not at all true, slightly true, mainly true, very true, coded 1–4 with 15 items reverse-scored).

Income

All studies measured household income using an approach found in many previous studies. In studies 1 and 2, participants were asked "What is your annual household income (before taxes)?" with response options: less than \$15,000; \$15,001 to \$25,000; \$25,001 to \$35,000; \$35,001 to \$50,000; \$50,001 to \$75,000; \$75,001 to \$100,000; \$100,001 to \$150,000; and greater than \$150,000 (e.g. [37]).

Study 3 used a more refined 16-point scale ranging from "less than $10,000" to "more than $150,000" in steps of $10,000, with the option to select "This question is not applicable to me". This was followed by questions asking how many adults and how many children are in the household. Studies 4 and 5 gave a definition of "household" and asked for the number of adults and children in the household, followed by a question about the participant's personal pre-tax annual income. If there were other people in the household, the participant was then asked to report the total income of all other members of the household. Both questions used the same 16-point scale as study 3, and both gave the option to indicate that the participant or other householders did not have an income.

Income responses were coded using the mid-point of each category with a median-based Pareto-curve estimator used for the unbounded top category [45, 46]; responses indicating no income for a person or household were coded as $0. For studies 4 and 5, net household income was computed as the sum of own income and other householders' income.

Education

Studies 1 and 2 asked "What is your highest level of educational attainment?" with four response options: did not finish high school, high school graduation, college graduation, and postgraduate degree, coded 1–4. Studies 3–5 asked "What is the highest degree or level of school you have completed? If currently enrolled, mark the previous grade or highest degree received", with responses on a 12-point scale ranging from "No schooling completed" to "Doctorate degree (for example: PhD, EdD)" coded 1–12.

Employment

Participants in studies 3–5 were asked "Which of the following best describes your current situation?" with response options: employed for wages, self-employed, out of work and looking for work, out of work but not currently looking for work, a homemaker, a student, retired, unable to work, other.

Subjective socioeconomic status (SSS)

Participants in studies 3–5 completed a widely used measure of subjective status in which they were shown a cartoon ladder representing "where people stand in the United States", with "the best off – those who have the most money, the most education and the most respected jobs" at the top and "the worst off – who have the least money, least education, and the east respected jobs or no job" at the bottom. Participants selected one of the 10 rungs to indicate where they stand relative to other people in the USA at this time [47].

Social Desirability Scale (SDS)

Participants in study 5 completed Stober's Social Desirability Scale (SDS-17; [48]) by answering True (coded 1) or False (coded 0) to 17 statements such as "I sometimes litter" (6 items are reverse-scored). Higher scores indicate a stronger tendency to make socially desirable responses.

Social comparison tendency

Study 1 included the short-form Iowa-Netherlands Comparison Orientation Measure (INCOM; [35]) with responses on a 6-point scale from strongly disagree to strongly agree (coded 1–6; one item reverse-scored). Full details are in the Additional file 1.

Financial judgment task

Participants in study 2 completed a simple task, adapted from previous studies [49], in which they were told that they had $80 to invest and rated the attractiveness of different savings accounts. Full details are given in Additional file 1.

Demographics

Participants in all studies indicated their gender (male, female; studies 3–5 added the option "prefer not to say"), age (using a slider from 0 to 100), and whether they had ever been diagnosed with autism spectrum disorder or one of its constituents (autism, Asperger's syndrome, or PPD-NOS; response options: yes, no, prefer not to say). In study 5, participants selected indicated their ethnicity by selecting from eight categories; participants who indicated more than one category were coded as "mixed ethnicity".

Design and procedure

In study 1, participants completed the SATQ, INCOM, and AQ, in random order, then indicated their household income, education, and demographics. In study 2, participants completed the financial judgment task followed by the AQ, then household income, education, and demographics. Participants in study 3 completed the AQ followed by the education, employment, and income questions in random order, and finally the SSS followed by the demographic questions. In study 4, participants completed the AQ, education, employment, income, and SSS questions in random order, followed by demographics. Study 5 was intended to be identical to study 4 but with the addition of the Social Desirability Scale and the inclusion of ethnicity in the demographics section. Unfortunately, the survey software malfunctioned: the intention was that participants would complete the AQ, SDS, education, employment, income, and SSS measures in random order. However, one of these items was randomly dropped for each participant. (All participants completed the demographic questions, which appeared at the end of the survey.) Because AQ, income, and SDS were the primary variables of interest, only participants who completed these three items were included in the analyses. Because none of these participants had data for all of the education, employment, and SSS measures, these variables were excluded from the analyses.

Participants

Eligible participants were respondents who completed the task, who indicated their age as over 18, and whose ID/ip address had not occurred earlier in series of studies (see, e.g. [50]). Participants were excluded prior to data analysis for failing the attention check ($N_{Study\_1} = 17$; $N_{Study\_2} = 12$; $N_{Study\_3} = 22$; $N_{Study\_4} = 43$; $N_{Study\_5} = 25$), answering "yes" or "prefer not to say" when asked if they had an ASC ($N_{Study\_1} = 4$; $N_{Study\_2} = 4$; $N_{Study\_3} = 7$; $N_{Study\_4} = 23$; $N_{Study\_5} = 9$), for reporting confusion about the AQ response scale ($N_{Study\_3} = 1$; $N_{Study\_4} = 1$) or for indicating a household, including themselves, of size zero ($N_{Study\_2} = 2$). The final sample sizes and participant information are presented in Table 1. The commonest employment status was "employed for wages" (study 3: 66.75%; study 4, 63.02%, followed by "self-employed" (study 3: 14.25%; study 4: 13.48%). In studies 1 and 2, the modal level of education was "college graduate" (study 1 = 46.99%; study 2 = 56.00%); in studies 3 and 4, it was "bachelor's degree" (study 3 = 39.75%; study 4 = 40.76%). In study 5, 77% of participants reported being white. Full details about employment, education, and ethnicity are reported in Additional file 1.

Data analysis

The data provide several measures of income. *Net household income* is the total reported pre-tax income for the household. To obtain a better measure of spending power, for studies 3–5 net income was divided by (number of adults + 0.5 × number of children) (e.g. [26]) to give *adjusted household income* (the unadjusted net income values are also reported, for comparison with the studies 1 and 2). Studies 4 and 5 provide separate measures of the participant's own income (*personal income*) and of the other people in their household, if any (*others' income*). All four of these income measures were log transformed (as $\ln(x + 1)$) to improve normality (e.g. [26, 46]).

The data were analysed with Pearson's correlations and multiple linear regressions. In the regression analyses, continuous predictors were standardized and categorical predictors were weighted-effect coded, such that each coefficient tests the effects of category membership against the sample mean (e.g. whether being employed for wages raises or lowers income relative to the overall

Table 1 Participant information

	Study 1	Study 2	Study 3	Study 4	Study 5
N	183	350	400	979	579
Male	64.5%	60.9%	60.5%	51.4%	46.5%
Gender not given	–	–	0.5%	0.2%	0.9%
Age range and mean	18–64 32.53 (9.91)	19–75 36.52 (11.12)	20–75 37.34 (12.17)	18–79 37.43 (12.09)	19–84 36.80 (11.91)
Net household income	$36,709 ($2256)	$41,273 ($2139)	$40,257 ($2392)	$60,744 ($2337)	$59,689 ($2335)
Adjusted household income	–	–	$21,666 ($2260)	$29,018 ($2051)	$27,827 (2125)
Personal income	–	–	–	$26,641 ($2919)	$24,798 ($2932)
Others' income	–	–	–	$32,939 ($3785)	$35,950 ($3268)
SSS	–	–	4.69 (1.65)	4.91 (1.76)	–
AQ	65.18 (11.73)	66.23 (11.16)	92.15 (16.04)	93.82 (15.22)	66.92 (9.83)
% live alone	–	–	29.75%	22.98%	21.93%
Adults	–	–	1.97 (0.91)	2.15 (1.01)	2.16 (1.04)
Children	–	–	0.42 (0.91)	0.50 (0.92)	0.63 (1.04)

Values in parentheses are standard deviations. AQ refers to scores on the short-form Autism Spectrum Quotient. For income measures, the values are geometric means calculated by exponentiating the arithmetic mean of $\ln(x + 1)$ where x is the income in thousands per year; similarly, the income standard deviations are the exponentiated standard deviation of $\ln(x + 1)$. Others' income is the net income of all other members of the household, for those participants who do not live alone ($N = 754$ and $N = 452$ for studies 4 and 5, respectively). Studies 3 and 4 used a 6-point response scale for the AQ, which is why the means are much higher than for other studies. % live alone indicates the proportion of participants whose household consists of just one person; adults and children are the mean number of adults (including the participant) and children in the household mean income) [51]. All confidence intervals are 95% confidence intervals.

Results

Studies 1 and 2

In study 1, the two measures of autistic traits (AQ scores and SATQ scores) were strongly correlated, $r = .825$, CI = [0.772, 0.866], $p < .001$. Both AQ and SATQ scores were negatively correlated with INCOM-Opinion, indicating that people with higher levels of autistic traits are less concerned about the beliefs of others: $r_{AQ} = -.193$, CI = [−0.329, −0.049], $p = .009$; $r_{SATQ} = -.189$, CI = [−0.325, −0.045], $p = .011$. In contrast, autistic traits were not meaningfully associated with INCOM-Ability, $r_{AQ} = -.040$, CI = [−0.184, 0.106], $p = .592$; $r_{SATQ} = .050$, CI = [−0.096, −0.193], $p = .505$, indicating little relation between autistic traits and comparison with other people's abilities. In study 2, there was no effect of AQ on the financial judgment task (Additional file 1).

More importantly for the present paper, both studies found an unexpected negative correlation between AQ and net household income (Table 2). This association remained robust after controlling for age, gender, and education (Table 3). In study 1, the same pattern was found for SATQ scores: SATQ negatively correlated with net household income, $r = -.232$, CI = [−0.364, −0.90], $p = .002$, and this effect held when SATQ, age, gender, and education were entered as simultaneous predictors in a regression analysis, $B_{SATQ} = -0.176$, CI = [−0.292, −0.060], $p = .003$.

These studies provided preliminary evidence that autistic traits among the non-clinical population negatively predict income. Because these studies were not intended as test of this relationship, the results must be treated as exploratory. All subsequent results refer to studies 3–5, which used better measures of income and were specifically intended to test the association between income and AQ.

Table 2 Correlations between AQ and other variables

Variable	Study	r	95% CI	p
Net household income	1	−.250	−0.381, −0.109	.001
	2	−.152	−0.253, −0.048	.004
	3	−.120	−0.216, −0.022	.016
	4	−.204	−0.263, −0.143	< .001
	5	−.125	−0.204, −0.044	.003
Adjusted household income	3	−.130	−0.225, −0.032	.009
	4	−.194	−0.254, −0.133	< .001
	5	−.121	−0.200, −0.039	.004
Personal income	4	−.156	−0.217, −0.095	< .001
	5	−.153	−0.232, −0.073	< .001
Others' income	4	−.096	−0.166, −0.025	.008
	5	−.051	−0.143, 0.041	.279
SSS	3	−.171	−0.265, −0.074	.001
	4	−.243	−0.301, −0.183	< .001
Age	1	.009	−0.137, 0.153	.908
	2	−.064	−0.168, 0.041	.229
	3	.039	−0.059, 0.137	.433
	4	−.079	−0.141, −0.016	.014
	5	−.070	−0.151, 0.011	.092
Gender	1	.116	−0.030, 0.257	.118
	2	.040	−0.065, 0.144	.460
	3	−.026	−0.124, 0.073	.607
	4	.081	0.018, 0.143	.012
	5	−.022	−0.104, 0.060	.599
Education	1	−.126	−0.266, 0.020	.090
	2	.030	−0.075, 0.134	.578
	3	.009	−0.090, 0.107	.865
	4	−.094	−0.156, −0.031	.003
	5	.027	−0.071, 0.125	.587

Others' income refers to the net income of all other members of the household, calculated for those participants who live with other people ($N = 754$ and $N = 452$ for studies 4 and 5, respectively)

SSS subjective socioeconomic status

Household income

In studies 3–5, net and adjusted household income were negatively correlated with AQ (Table 2). To see whether AQ predicted household income over and above the effects of other demographic variables, household income was regressed on AQ, age, gender, education, and employment status. (This analysis was only applied to studies 3 and 4 because study 5 did not have complete education and employment data for all participants.) The coefficients for the AQ predictor are shown in Table 3: for both studies, net income and adjusted income were negatively related to AQ, but the effects were only significant in study 4. To test whether this represents a meaningful difference between the studies, the data from studies 3 and 4 were combined in a regression analysis that included the original variables as well as study and its interactions with all other predictors. Study was weighted-effect coded (with study 3 coded −1), and interactions were computed as described in [52]. With adjusted household income as the dependent variable, the study coefficient was positive, $B_{Study} = 0.086$, CI = [0.064, 0.108], $p < .001$, indicating that incomes were higher than average in study 4. However, none of the interactions involving study were significant (all $ps > .250$) suggesting that the effects of the predictors were consistent across studies. In particular, income was negatively related to AQ, $B_{AQ} = -0.086$, CI = [−0.121, −0.051], $p < .001$, and this effect was not modulated by

Table 3 Regression coefficients for AQ predictor

Dependent variable	Study	Control variables	B_{AQ}	95% CI	p	R^2_{adj}	R^2_{change}
Net household income	1	Age, gender, education	− 0.186	[− 0.300, − 0.071]	.002	.099	.050
	2	Age, gender, education	− 0.121	[− 0.197, − 0.044]	.002	.095	.025
	3	Age, gender, education, employment	− 0.068	[− 0.149, 0.014]	.103	.150	.006
	4	Age, gender, education, employment	− 0.139	[− 0.189, − 0.089]	< .001	.148	.026
	5	Age, gender, ethnicity, socially desirable responding	− 0.115	[− 0.185, − 0.044]	.001	.022	.017
Adjusted household income	3	Age, gender, education, employment	− 0.058	[− 0.132, 0.016]	.127	.197	.005
	4	Age, gender, education, employment	− 0.098	[− 0.138, − 0.058]	< .001	.254	.018
	5	Age, gender, ethnicity, socially desirable responding	− 0.092	[− 0.154, − 0.030]	.004	.049	.014
Personal income	4	Age, gender, education, employment	− 0.105	[− 0.159, − 0.052]	< .001	.395	.009
	5	Age, gender, ethnicity, socially desirable responding	− 0.141	[− 0.228, − 0.055]	.001	.084	.016
Others' income	4	Age, gender, education, employment	− 0.120	[− 0.215, − 0.024]	.015	.042	.008
	5	Age, gender, ethnicity, socially desirable responding	− 0.086	[− 0.200, 0.027]	.137	.010	.005
SSS	3	Age, gender, education, employment, adjusted household income	− 0.191	[− 0.334, − 0.048]	.009	.275	.013
	4	Age, gender, education, employment, adjusted household income	− 0.222	[− 0.312, − 0.132]	< .001	.376	.015

All regression entered AQ and the control variables simultaneously. Continuous predictors were standardized
SSS subjective socioeconomic status, R^2_{adj} adjusted *R*-squared for the regression model, R^2_{change} difference in (unadjusted) R^2 between models that do/do not include AQ as a predictor (i.e. the proportion of variance accounted for by AQ, after controlling for other variables)

study, $B_{Study.AQ} = -0.014$, CI = − 0.038, 0.010], $p = .260$. The same pattern was found when net household income was the dependent variable ($B_{Study} = 0.118$, CI = [0.091, 0.145], $p < .001$; $B_{AQ} = -0.118$, CI = [− 0.160, − 0.075], $p < .001$; $B_{Study.AQ} = -0.024$, CI = [− 0.053, 0.005], $p = .108$). Thus, there is a consistent negative association between both income measures and AQ scores, after controlling for other demographic variables.

Socially desirable responding

The tendency to give socially desirable responses, which was measured in study 5, was negatively related to AQ, $r = -.179$, CI = [− 0.257, − 0.099], $p < .001$. However, the negative relationship between AQ and household income remained after controlling for age, gender, ethnicity, and socially desirable responding (Table 3), suggesting that the association is not purely due to greater honesty from people with high AQ scores (that is, the association between AQ and income is not simply due to people with high levels of autistic traits being less likely to over-state their income in order to inflate their social status).

Deconstructing household income

In studies 4 and 5, participants separately reported their personal income and, where applicable, the income of the rest of their household (others' income). In both studies, personal income was negatively related to AQ (Table 2); this effect remained after controlling for age, gender, education, and employment (study 4) and after controlling for age, gender, ethnicity, and socially desirable responding (study 5) (Table 3).

AQ also negatively correlated with others' income, but the relationship was only significant in study 4 (Table 2); the same pattern was found after controlling for other variables (Table 3). (Cross-study comparison is not possible here because the studies had different predictors.) Notably, the overall variation explained by the predictors is markedly less than for the participant's own income, as would be expected given that the predictors—including AQ— are likely to have much more relevance to a person's own economic performance than to the incomes other people in their household.

Subjective socioeconomic status

SSS was also negatively correlated with AQ (Table 2), and the association remained when SSS was regressed onto AQ, age, gender, education, employment, and adjusted household income (Table 3). That is, after controlling for demographic variables and objective determinants of socio-economic status, people with higher levels of autistic traits put themselves lower on the "socioeconomic ladder" than did people with low AQ scores.

Subscales

The AQ is intended to capture five distinct types of trait: social skills, preference for routine, task-switching, imagination, and an interest in numbers and patterns. The first four of these constitute a higher-order "social behaviour" factor. To explore the contributions of these different components of the autistic profile, scores for the social behaviour and numbers-and-patterns dimensions were computed by summing the responses to the relevant items [44] and used as the independent variables in a series of regression analyses, one for each of the key dependent variables: adjusted household income, personal income, and subjective socioeconomic status. The regression results are shown in Table 4. The social behaviour dimension was a consistent negative predictor of household income, personal income, and subjective socioeconomic status across all three studies. In contrast, the numbers-and-patterns dimension showed little relationship with household income and was positively related to personal income and subjective socioeconomic status.

Robustness checks

The regression results were unchanged when education was treated as a factor rather than a continuous variable, and when Box-Cox transformations were used in place of logarithmic transformations of income, except that in the latter case the weak relation between AQ and others' income in study 5 became significant, $B = -0.591$, CI = [1.139, − 0.043], $p = .034$. Similarly, repeating the analyses using binary coding of responses to the AQ items [1] made little difference to the effects of AQ, except that, in study 3, the negative association between AQ and household income became significant (for net household income, $B = -0.082$, CI = [− 0.164, − 0.001], $p = .047$; for adjusted household income, $B = -0.077$, CI = [− 0.151, − 0.003], $p = .041$) and, in study 4, the positive effect of the numbers-and-patterns subscale on adjusted household income became significant, $B = 0.045$, CI = [0.000, 0.089], $p = .048$.

We also examined whether the effects of AQ on income and SSS are explained by a higher propensity for people with high AQ to live in single-member households. In studies 3 and 5, people living alone had similar AQ scores to those living with others: study 3, $M_{alone} = 91.8$ (SD = 15.1), $M_{with\_others} = 92.3$ (SD = 16.4), $t(398) = 0.26, p = .795$; study 5, $M_{alone} = 66.8$ (SD = 10.2), $M_{with\_others} = 67.0$ (SD = 9.8), $t(577) = 0.16$, $p = .876$, although there was evidence for elevated AQ scores among people living alone in study 4, $M_{alone} = 96.1$ (SD = 15.2), $M_{with\_others} = 93.1$ (SD = 15.2), $t(977) = 2.54$, $p = .011$. We re-ran the regression analyses for net and adjusted household income, own income, and SSS, with living alone included as a categorical predictor; including this variable made little difference to the coefficients for AQ shown in Table 3, and the pattern of significance was identical.

Excluding participants with the highest AQ scores

To see whether the effects of autistic traits were driven by the participants with the highest AQ scores (who might represent undiagnosed cases of autism), the regression analyses were re-run after excluding participants with AQ scores more than 1.5 SD above the mean of the sample for the relevant study. (Recall that participants who reported a diagnosis of an ASC, or who preferred not to indicate this, were excluded from the samples prior to analysis, so the calculation of mean and SD were based on the scores of participants who did not have an ASC diagnosis. Participant exclusion occurred after standardizing/weighted-effect coding of predictor variables.) The only changes to the pattern of significance in Tables 3 and 4 were that, in study 3, the negative association between AQ and SSS became non-significant, $B = -0.094$, CI = [− 0.262, 0.074], $p = .272$, as did the negative association between the social behaviour subscale and adjusted household income, $B = -0.078$, CI = [− 0.159, 0.003], $p = .061$, and in study 4, AQ was no longer a significant predictor of others' income, $B = -0.055$, CI = [− 0.168, 0.057], $p = .336$. The pattern of effects for net household income, adjusted household income, and personal income was unchanged. Thus, the negative association between AQ and income is not entirely driven by the participants with the highest AQ scores.

Table 4 Regression coefficients for social behaviour and numbers-and-patterns sub-traits

Dependent variable		Social behaviour			Patterns-and-numbers			R^2_{adj}
	Study	*B*	95% CI	*p*	B	95% CI	*p*	
Adjusted household income	3	− 0.120	− 0.200, − 0.040	.003	0.030	− 0.050, 0.110	.462	.019
	4	− 0.153	− 0.197, − 0.109	< .001	0.023	− 0.021, 0.068	.301	.046
	5	− 0.096	− 0.158, − 0.035	.002	− 0.002	− 0.063, 0.060	.955	.013
Personal income	4	− 0.194	− 0.260, − 0.128	< .001	0.074	0.008, 0.140	.029	.039
	5	− 0.191	− 0.278, − 0.105	< .001	0.052	− 0.035, 0.138	.243	.032
SSS	3	− 0.328	− 0.488, − 0.168	< .001	0.113	− 0.046, 0.273	.164	.042
	4	− 0.481	− 0.588, − 0.374	< .001	0.120	0.013, 0.226	.028	.082

Predictors were standardized and entered simultaneously

SSS subjective socioeconomic status, R^2_{adj} adjusted R-squared for the regression model

Discussion

Income is a complex, multiply-determined variable whose relation to any biological or socio-cognitive predictor cannot be definitively established in a single paper. Nonetheless, the present studies provide an important first step in investigating a potentially crucial functional consequence of non-clinical autistic traits. The studies found a robust negative association between autistic traits and income among people with no reported diagnosis of an autism spectrum condition. We focused on household income because this is a widely used index of a person's financial well-being that predicts many important outcomes. When household income was dissected in studies 4 and 5, the association with autistic traits was primarily due to the participant's own income, with some indication that AQ also predicts the probability of living with other highly paid individuals. The link between AQ and income remained after controlling for employment status, as well as age, gender, and education (studies 3 and 4) and ethnicity and socially desirable responding (study 5).

These effects are not large in absolute terms, which is unsurprising given how many variables affect financial success [53]. For example, one meta-analysis found that the correlation between salary and gender was only .18 and that for ethnicity was .11 (3.2 and 1.2% of variance explained, respectively); even the best predictor, education, only correlated at .29 (8.4% variance explained) [54]. Against this background, and given the importance of income to well-being, the correlations and R^2_{change} values in Tables 2 and 3 suggest that AQ has a modest but meaningful relationship with income.

The generality of these findings is an open question. The online samples used here are more similar to the general population than many of the samples used in studies of autistic traits, but they are not perfectly representative. In addition, there is evidence that autistic traits—and other psychopathological traits—are more pronounced in participants recruited through MTurk than in other samples [55]. The mean AQ-Short scores in the current studies are higher than those in some other studies [44], although they are similar to results from Nishiyama et al. [9] who used a diverse sample of students and employees. Very few studies of autistic traits accurately represent a particular national population, and it will obviously be important to test whether the pattern found here generalizes to other samples. Likewise, it will be instructive to use more fine-grained measures of financial circumstances, such as those that correct for regional costs of living [26]. Nonetheless, the population sampled comprises people from widely varying backgrounds and with diverse personal attributes and circumstances [30, 56–58], and the present results generate several important directions and questions.

The first concerns the causal status of the relationship between income and AQ. One possibility is that AQ and income are both caused by an unmeasured confounding variable, such as the presence of other psychiatric conditions: although we excluded participants with a diagnosis of autism, AQ is elevated in conditions including schizophrenia, social anxiety disorder, and obsessive compulsive disorder [59, 60], all of which might negatively affect income. Another is that the social and cognitive consequence of lower income shape a person's social attitudes and cognitive style in a way that elevates their AQ score. For example, reduced income may lead to reduced opportunity for social interaction, less opportunity to develop imaginative pursuits, poorer nutrition (which could impair task switching), and a more chaotic lifestyle (such that one values routine). All of these would boost a person's self-reported scores on subdomains of the AQ. However, given that AQ is argued to measure stable socio-cognitive dispositions with a heritable basis [1, 61], the most likely causal direction is for autistic traits to influence a person's financial circumstances.

This might arise because even subclinical levels of the social atypicalities that characterize autism limit a person's career progression. Some jobs—such as selling for commission—directly link income to interpersonal interaction and social skills; more generally, "social capital" is an important component of career progression in many fields [62]. In keeping with this, the analysis of subscales suggested that the negative association between AQ and income is driven by atypical social behaviour; in contrast, personal income was positively correlated with the "numbers and patterns" component of the AQ. This accords with evidence that autistic traits are more pronounced among people working in fields such as mathematics and engineering [10], which often offer very high remuneration. Autistic traits may therefore represent something of a double-edged sword.

Autistic traits could also influence income via their effects on economic decision-making. Decision-making is an under-researched aspect of autism [63], but there is emerging evidence that people with autism have a different decision-making style from the general population [64, 65]. For example, Farmer et al. [14] found that people with autism, and non-clinical samples with high levels of autistic traits, show a more conventionally "rational" decision-making style which may not be adaptive in real environments. This atypical profile could limit a person's financial success. Alternatively, people with high levels of autistic traits may simply have priorities and preferences that do not lead to material wealth.

Establishing the causal relationship between autistic traits and income will require longitudinal studies in which a cohort is followed from early in life, to determine whether and how subclinical autistic traits correlate with subsequent financial outcomes after controlling for other variables, and to see whether changes in income (for example, in response to a pay-cut) lead to changes in AQ score. However, whatever the basis for the negative association between AQ and income, it has important implications because low incomes predict poorer mental and physical well-being and lower life satisfaction [22, 24]. The AQ-income association might therefore partially explain why people with high levels of non-clinical autistic traits are more likely to report socio-psychological problems [18, 66], although it could also be that the problems associated with high levels of autistic traits limit people's ability to gain control of financial resources. As a broader point, the current data suggest that whenever a researcher finds a link between income and some socio-psychological variable such as materialism [67], interpersonal hostility [38], or prosociality [68], the effects may be due to the greater prevalence of autistic traits among the low-income participants.

A final observation is that AQ was negatively associated with subjective socioeconomic status, even after controlling for objective socioeconomic indicators (education, employment status, and income). This is concerning because negative health, social, and psychological outcomes are often better predicted by a person's beliefs about their income and social class than by their objective circumstances [26]. However, subjective socioeconomic status per se is less important than the extent to which a person resents his or her relative position [37], so it will be important to explore the link between these reactions and autistic traits.

Conclusions

These studies provide a first exploration of the link between autistic traits and socio-economic status, and it would be premature to draw firm conclusions at this point. Nonetheless, the negative correlation is sufficiently robust and potentially important that exploring the association will be an important direction for researchers interested in the causes and consequences of subclinical autistic traits.

Abbreviations

AQ: Autism Spectrum Quotient; INCOM: Iowa-Netherlands Comparison Orientation Measure; MTurk: Amazon's Mechanical Turk; SATQ: Subthreshold Autism Trait Questionnaire; SDS: Social Desirability Scale; SSS: Subjective socioeconomic status; STEM: Science, technology, engineering, and mathematics

Acknowledgements

Not applicable.

Funding

WJS was supported by Wellcome Trust grant RG76641 and Isaac Newton Trust grant RG70368. SBC was supported by the Autism Research Trust.

Authors' contributions

WJS conceived, designed, and conducted the studies and analysed the data. WJS and SBC wrote the paper. Both authors read and approved the final manuscript.

Competing interests

The authors declare that they have no competing interests.

Author details

[1]Department of Psychology, University of Cambridge, Cambridge CB2 3EB, UK. [2]Autism Research Centre, Department of Psychiatry, University of Cambridge, Cambridge CB2 8AH, UK.

References

1. Baron-Cohen S, Wheelwright S, Skinner R, Martin J, Clubley E. The Autism Spectrum Quotient : evidence from Asperger syndrome/high functioning autism, males and females, scientists and mathematicians. J Autism Dev Disord. 2001;31:5–17.
2. Constantino JN, Todd RD. Autistic traits in the general population. Arch Gen Psychiatry. May 2003;2003(60):524–30.
3. Constantino JN, Todd RD. Intergenerational transmission of subthreshold autistic traits in the general population. Biol Psychiatry. 2005;57:655–60.
4. Wheelwright S, Auyeung B, Allison C, Baron-Cohen S. Defining the broader, medium and narrow autism phenotype among parents using the Autism Spectrum Quotient (AQ). Mol Autism. 2010;1:10. doi:10.1186/2040-2392-1-10.
5. Landa R, Piven J, Wzorek MM, Gayle JO, Chase GA, Folstein SE. Social language use in parents of autistic individuals. Psychol Med. 1992;22:245–54.
6. Hurley RSE, Losh M, Parlier M, Reznick JS, Piven J. The Broad Autism Phenotype Questionnaire. J Autism Dev Disord. 2007;37:1679–90.
7. Kanne SM, Wang J, Christ SE. The Subthreshold Autism Trait Questionnaire (SATQ): development of a brief self-report measure of subthreshold autism traits. J Autism Dev Disord. 2012;42:769–80.
8. Constantino JN. Social Responsiveness Scale—adult version (SRS). Los Angeles, CA: Western Psychological Services; 2002.
9. Nishiyama T, Suzuki M, Adachi K, Sumi S, Okada K, Kishino H, et al. Comprehensive comparison of self-administered questionnaires for measuring quantitative autistic traits in adults. J Autism Dev Disord. 2014;44:993–1007.
10. Ruzich E, Allison C, Chakrabarti B, Smith P, Musto H, Ring H, et al. Sex and STEM occupation predict Autism-Spectrum Quotient (AQ) scores in half a million people. PLoS One. 2015;10:e0141229. doi:10.1371/journal.pone.0141229.
11. Almeida RA, Dickinson JE, Maybery MT, Badcock JC, Badcock DR. A new step towards understanding Embedded Figures Test performance in the autism spectrum: the radial frequency search task. Neuropsychologia. 2010;48:374–81.
12. Stewart ME, Watson J, Allcock A-J, Yaqoob T. Autistic traits predict performance on the block design. Autism. 2009;13:133–42. doi:10.1177/1362361308098515.
13. Grinter EJ, Maybery MT, Van Beek PL, Pellicano E, Badcock JC, Badcock DR. Global visual processing and self-rated autistic-like traits. J Autism Dev Disord 2009;39:1278–1290.
14. Farmer GD, Baron-Cohen S, Skylark WJ. People with autism spectrum conditions make more consistent decisions. Psychol Sci. 2017;28:1067-76. doi:10.1177/0956797617694867.
15. Wyer NA, Martin D, Pickup T, Neil MC. Individual differences in (non-visual) processing style predict the face inversion effect. Cogn Sci. 2012;36:373–84.
16. Jameel L, Vyas K, Bellesi G, Cassell D, Channon S. Great expectations: the role of rules in guiding pro-social behaviour in groups with high versus low autistic traits. J Autism Dev Disord. 2015;45:2311–22. doi:10.1007/s10803-015-2393-x.

17. Billington J, Baron-Cohen S, Wheelwright S. Cognitive style predicts entry into physical sciences and humanities: questionnaire and performance tests of empathy and systemizing. Learn Individ Differ. 2007;17:260–8.
18. Kanne SM, Christ SE, Reiersen AM. Psychiatric symptoms and psychosocial difficulties in young adults with autistic traits. J Autism Dev Disord. 2009;39:827–33.
19. Hsiao M-N, Tseng W-L, Huang H-Y, Gau SSF. Effects of autistic traits on social and school adjustment in children and adolescents: the moderating roles of age and gender. Res Dev Disabil. 2013;34:254–65. doi:10.1016/j.ridd.2012.08.001.
20. Pollmann MMH, Finkenauer C, Begeer S. Mediators of the link between autistic traits and relationship satisfaction in a non-clinical sample. J Autism Dev Disord. 2010;40:470–8.
21. Jobe LE, Williams WS. Loneliness, social relationships, and a broader autism phenotype in college students. Pers Individ Dif. 2007;42:1479–89.
22. Chetty R, Stepner M, Abraham S, Lin S, Scuderi B, Turner N, et al. The association between income and life expectancy in the United States, 2001–2014. Clin Rev Educ. 2016;315:1750–66. doi:10.1001/jama.2016.4226.
23. Muntaner C, Eaton WW, Miech R, O'Campo P. Socioeconomic position and major mental disorders. Epidemiol Rev. 2004;26:53–62.
24. Subramanian SV, Kawachi I. Being well and doing well: on the importance of income for health. Int J Soc Welf. 2006;15:13–22.
25. Kahneman D, Deaton A. High income improves evaluation of life but not emotional well-being. Proc Natl Acad Sci U S A. 2010;107:16489–93. doi:10.1073/pnas.1011492107.
26. Boyce CJ, Brown GDA, Moore SC. Money and happiness. Psychol Sci. 2010; 21:471–5. doi:10.1177/0956797610362671.
27. Avendano M, Kawachi I, Van Lenthe F, Boshuizen HC, Mackenbach JP, Van Den Bos GAM, et al. Socioeconomic status and stroke incidence in the US elderly: the role of risk factors in the EPESE study. Stroke 2006;37:1368–1373.
28. Operario D, Adler NE, Williams DR. Subjective social status: reliability and predictive utility for global health. Psychol Health. 2004;19:237–46.
29. Senn TE, Walsh JL, Carey MP. The mediating roles of perceived stress and health behaviors in the relation between objective, subjective, and neighborhood socioeconomic status and perceived health. Ann Behav Med. 2014;48:215–24.
30. Berinsky AJ, Huber GA, Lenz GS. Evaluating online labor markets for experimental research: Amazon.com's Mechanical Turk. Polit Anal. 2012;20:351–68.
31. Eriksson K. Autism-spectrum traits predict humour styles in the general population. Humour. 2013;26:461–75.
32. Foulkes L, Bird G, Gökçen E, McCrory E, Viding E. Common and distinct impacts of autistic traits and alexithymia on social reward. PLoS One. 2015; 10:e0121018.
33. Yang DYJ, Baillargeon R. Brief report: difficulty in understanding social acting (but not false beliefs) mediates the link between autistic traits and ingroup relationships. J Autism Dev Disord. 2013;43:2199–206.
34. Banerjee K, Bloom P. Why did this happen to me? Religious believers' and non-believers' teleological reasoning about life events. Cognition. 2014;133: 277–303.
35. Schneider SM, Schupp J. Individual differences in social comparison and its consequences for life satisfaction: introducing a short scale of the Iowa-Netherlands Comparison Orientation Measure. Soc Indic Res. 2014; 115:767–89.
36. Brown GDA, Matthews WJ. Decision by sampling and memory distinctiveness: range effects from rank-based models of judgment and choice. Front Psychol. 2011;2:1-4. Article 299.
37. Callan MJ, Kim H, Matthews WJ. Predicting self-rated mental and physical health: the contributions of subjective socioeconomic status and personal relative deprivation. Front Psychol. 2015; 6 September:Article 1415. doi:10.3389/fpsyg.2015.01415.
38. Kraus MW, Horberg EJ, Goetz JL, Keltner D. Social class rank, threat vigilance, and hostile reactivity. Personal Soc Psychol Bull. 2011;37:1376–88. doi:10.1177/0146167211410987.
39. Callan MJ, Kim H, Gheorghiu AI, Matthews WJ. The interrelations between social class, personal relative deprivation, and prosociality. Soc Psychol Personal Sci. 2017;8:660-9.
40. Demakakos P, Nazroo J, Breeze E, Marmot M. Socioeconomic status and health: the role of subjective social status. Soc Sci Med. 2008;67:330–40.
41. Nobles J, Weintraub MR, Adler NE. Subjective socioeconomic status and health: relationships reconsidered. Soc Sci Med. 2013;82:58–66. doi:10.1016/j.socscimed.2013.01.021.
42. Chevallier C, Molesworth C, Happé F. Diminished social motivation negatively impacts reputation management: autism spectrum disorders as a case in point. PLoS One. 2012;7:e31107.
43. Izuma K, Matsumoto K, Camerer CF, Adolphs R. Insensitivity to social reputation in autism. Proc Natl Acad Sci U S A. 2011;108:17302–7. doi:10.1073/pnas.1107038108.
44. Hoekstra RA, Vinkhuyzen AAE, Wheelwright S, Bartels M, Boomsma DI, Baron-Cohen S, et al. The construction and validation of an abridged version of the autism-spectrum quotient (AQ-short). J Autism Dev Disord. 2011;41:589–96.
45. Parker RN, Fenwick R. The pareto curve and its utility for open-ended income distributions in survey research. Soc Forces. 1983;61:872–85.
46. Matthews WJ, Gheorghiu AI, Callan MJ. Why do we overestimate others' willingness to pay? Judgm Decis Mak. 2016;11:21–39.
47. Adler NE, Epel ES, Castellazzo G, Ickovics JR. Relationship of subjective and objective social status with psychological and physiological functioning: preliminary data in healthy white women. Health Psychol. 2000;19:586–92.
48. Stöber J. The Social Desirability Scale-17 (SDS-17): convergent validity, discrimant validity, and relationship with age. Eur J Psychol Assess. 2001;17:222–32.
49. Matthews WJ. How much do incidental values affect the judgment of time? Psychol Sci. 2012;23:1432–4. doi:10.1177/0956797612441609.
50. Matthews WJ, Dylman AS. The language of magnitude comparison. J Exp Psychol Gen. 2014;143:510–20.
51. te Grotenhuis M, Pelzer B, Eisinga R, Nieuwenhuis R, Schmidt-Catran A, Konig R. When size matters: advantages of weighted effect coding in observational studies. Int J Public Health 2017;62:163–167.
52. Nieuwenhuis R, te Grotenhuis M, Pelzer B. Weighted effect coding for observational data with wec. R J 2017;9:477–485.
53. Strenze T. Intelligence and socioeconomic success : a meta-analytic review of longitudinal research. Intelligence. 2007;35:401–26.
54. Ng TWH, Eby LT, Sorensen KL, Feldman DC. Predictors of objective and subjective career success: a meta-analysis. Pers Psychol. 2005;58:367–408.
55. Chandler J, Shapiro DN. Conducting clinical research using crowdsourced convenience samples. Annu Rev Clin Psychol. 2016;12 January:53–81.
56. Huff C, Tingley D. "Who are these people?" Evaluating the demographic characteristics and political preferences of MTurk survey respondents. Res Polit. 2015;2:1–12. doi:10.1177/2053168015604648.
57. Mason W, Suri S. Conducting behavioral research on Amazon's Mechanical Turk. Behav Res Methods. 2012;44:1–23. doi:10.3758/s13428-011-0124-6.
58. Paolacci G, Chandler J. Inside the Turk: understanding Mechanical Turk as a participant pool. Curr Dir Psychol Sci. 2014;23:184–8. doi:10.1177/0963721414531598.
59. Wouters SGM, Spek AA. The use of the Autism-spectrum Quotient in differentiating high-functioning adults with autism, adults with schizophrenia and a neurotypical adult control group. Res Autism Spectr Disord. 2011;5:1169–75. doi:10.1016/j.rasd.2011.01.002.
60. Hoekstra RA, Bartles M, Cath DC, Boomsma DI. Factor structure, reliability and criterion validity of the Autism-Spectrum Quotient (AQ): a study in Dutch population and patient groups; 2008. p. 1555–66.
61. Hoekstra R, Bartels M, CJH V, Boomsma DI. Heritability of autistic traits in the general population. Arch Pediatr Adolesc Med. 2007;161:372–7. doi:10.1001/archpedi.161.4.372.
62. Seibert SE, Kraimer ML, Liden RC. A social capital theory of career success. Acad Manag J. 2001;44:219–37.
63. Davis G, Plaisted-Grant K. Low endogenous neural noise in autism. Autism. 2014;19:351–62. doi:10.1177/1362361314552198.
64. Luke L, Clare ICH, Ring H, Redley M, Watson P. Decision-making difficulties experienced by adults with autism spectrum conditions. Autism. 2012;16: 612–21. doi:10.1177/1362361311415876.

3

No preliminary evidence of differences in astrocyte density within the white matter of the dorsolateral prefrontal cortex in autism

Ting Ting Lee[1,2*], Efstratios Skafidas[1,2,7], Mirella Dottori[2,3,9], Daniela Zantomio[4], Christos Pantelis[1,2,6,7], Ian Everall[1,2,7,8†] and Gursharan Chana[1,2,5,7†]

Abstract

Background: While evidence for white matter and astrocytic abnormalities exist in autism, a detailed investigation of astrocytes has not been conducted. Such an investigation is further warranted by an increasing role for neuroinflammation in autism pathogenesis, with astrocytes being key players in this process. We present the first study of astrocyte density and morphology within the white matter of the dorsolateral prefrontal cortex (DLPFC) in individuals with autism.

Methods: DLPFC formalin-fixed sections containing white matter from individuals with autism ($n = 8$, age = 4–51 years) and age-matched controls ($n = 7$, age = 4–46 years) were immunostained for glial fibrillary acidic protein (GFAP). Density of astrocytes and other glia were estimated via the optical fractionator, astrocyte somal size estimated via the nucleator, and astrocyte process length via the spaceballs probe.

Results: We found no evidence for alteration in astrocyte density within DLPFC white matter of individuals with autism versus controls, together with no differences in astrocyte somal size and process length.

Conclusion: Our results suggest that astrocyte abnormalities within the white matter in the DLPFC in autism may be less pronounced than previously thought. However, astrocytic dysregulation may still exist in autism, even in the absence of gross morphological changes. Our lack of evidence for astrocyte abnormalities could have been confounded to an extent by having a small sample size and wide age range, with pathological features potentially restricted to early stages of autism. Nonetheless, future investigations would benefit from assessing functional markers of astrocytes in light of the underlying pathophysiology of autism.

Keywords: Astrocytes, Glia, Autism, Dorsolateral prefrontal cortex (DLPFC), Cell density, White matter

Background

Autism is a highly complex and heritable neurodevelopmental disorder with prevalence rates soaring from 1 in 5000 children in the 1970s [1] to 1 in 132 global prevalence reported in recent years [2]. The majority of post-mortem brain studies in autism have focused on uncovering neuronal abnormalities; however, recent evidence has demonstrated alterations in both microglial and astrocytic markers within the autistic brain [3]. Microglia and astrocytes are known to have crucial roles in neurodevelopment, including regulation of synapse formation as well as neuroinflammatory and immune pathways. As both synaptogenesis disruption and neuroinflammation are reported in autism, a role for microglial and astrocyte involvement in the pathophysiology of autism has begun to receive an increasing amount of attention [3–5].

Astrocytes represent the most abundant glia cell type in the brain, and in their mature state, form tripartite

* Correspondence: tingtl@unimelb.edu.au
†Equal contributors
[1]Department of Psychiatry, The University of Melbourne, Parkville, Australia
[2]Centre for Neural Engineering, The University of Melbourne, Parkville, Australia

synapses together with presynaptic and postsynaptic neurons in a three-way interaction to regulate neuronal signaling via neurotransmitter/gliotransmitter receptors and ion channels at the level of a single synapse or a neuronal network [3, 6–8]. Astrocytes have also been shown to play a critical role in oligodendrocyte survival and maturation, including influencing the ability of oligodendrocytes to myelinate axons [9, 10]. In addition, glial fibrillary acidic protein (GFAP), a major structural component of astrocytes, has been shown to be necessary for the integrity of CNS white matter as well as long-term maintenance of myelination [11]. This is of interest given post-mortem studies have revealed axonal thinning within the white matter in individuals with autism as well as reduced myelin thickness in the anterior cingulate cortex (ACC) and prefrontal cortex (PFC) [12]. While neuroimaging studies have shown accelerated maturation of white matter within the frontal cortex [13, 14], increased gray and white matter volume in the frontal and temporal regions [15–18], as well as hyper-connectivity in prefrontal, amygdala, and temporal regions [18, 19]. Along with the ACC, the dorsolateral prefrontal cortex (DLPFC) is responsible for higher level executive functioning, including attention, emotional processing, learning and memory, domains that are impaired in individuals with autism [20]. This is evidenced by several studies reporting impairments in individuals with autism compared to controls when performing tasks known to be mediated by the DLPFC, including poor performance in the Wisconsin Card Sorting Test (WCST), as well as decreased functional activity as measured by magnetic resonance spectroscopy (MRS) and functional magnetic resonance imaging (fMRI) [21–23].

Evidence for astrocyte dysfunction have also come from a post-mortem brain investigation in autism demonstrating increased mRNA levels of *GFAP* as well as the excitatory amino acid transporter 1 (*EAAT1*) via microarray profiling within the cerebellum, with upregulation confirmed at the protein level via western blotting [24]. Subsequently, Vargas et al. demonstrated increased GFAP in the cerebellum, middle frontal gyrus, and ACC within individuals with autism compared to controls [25]. This was followed by Laurence and Fatemi's results, also demonstrating increased protein levels of GFAP in the superior frontal, parietal and cerebellar cortex in autism [26]. Further support for prefrontal and cerebellar changes were demonstrated by a quantitative real-time polymerase chain reaction (qPCR) investigation showing increased *GFAP* expression in both regions in autism compared to controls [27]. In addition, Crawford et al. demonstrated increased GFAP at the protein level via western blotting within the white matter of the anterior cingulate gyrus, but not in the gray matter [28]. In contrast to increased GFAP levels within the brain in autism, Morgan et al. demonstrated no difference in density and size of astrocytes between autism and controls following a stereological study of the amygdala [29]. Other astrocytic abnormalities have also been observed in the brains of individuals with autism, including reduced protein levels of aquaporin 4 (AQP4) within the cerebellum together with elevated connexin 43 (CNX43) seen in the superior frontal cortex [30].

Astrocytes are known to be intimately involved in the inflammatory response within the CNS [31], with growing evidence implicating neuroinflammation in the pathophysiology of autism, especially via dysregulation of neurogenesis and neuronal physiology related to activation of microglia and astrocytes [5, 32, 33]. Astrocyte activation in autism has been suggested to occur due to observations of astrogliosis in the cerebellar white matter and subcortical white matter within the frontal lobe [25–27]. Given that astrocytes are known to be involved in neurodevelopment, potential changes in their activation state and/or functioning due to inflammation during development might have consequences for disrupted connectivity and neuropathological changes in autism [34]. Activation of astrocytes and the subsequent pro-inflammatory cytokines release, including interleukin 6 (IL-6), tumor necrosis factor alpha (TNFα), and interleukin 1B (IL-1B), has also been observed in autism within the brain as well as peripherally in the cerebrospinal fluid [25, 35].

Given the growing body of evidence for astrocytic involvement in autism, and their known functioning in maintaining myelin, together with disruptions in myelin integrity seen within the brain of individuals with autism, a more detailed investigation of astrocytic neuropathology within the white matter is warranted. The aim of this investigation was to assess astrocyte density and morphology within the white matter of the DLPFC in autism compared to age- and gender-matched controls using GFAP as a cellular astrocyte marker. This was achieved using the optical fractionator, nucleator, and spaceballs probes to investigate density, somal size, and overall process length respectively.

Methods

Brain tissue

Formalin-fixed DLPFC tissue blocks restricted to BA9 and BA46 from individuals with autism ($n = 11$) and controls ($n = 10$) were provided by the NICHD Brain and Tissue Bank for Developmental Disorders (NBTBD), Baltimore, Maryland upon request (University of Melbourne ethics approval ID: 1339835.1). Tissue was matched as closely as possible for age between autism (range = 4–51 years) and controls (range = 4–46 years). Tissue blocks were serially sectioned using a Leica VT1000s Vibratome (Leica Biosystems, Germany) in phosphate-buffered saline (PBS) at 50 μM and stored in PBS with 0.5% sodium azide at 4 °C. Six samples (3 autism, 3 controls) were excluded from analysis due to poor tissue morphology following immunohistochemistry, thereby reducing the number of cases available to 8 autism and 7 controls (Table 1).

Immunohistochemistry

Four sections from each subject were chosen via systematic random sampling (every 14 sections) spanning the entire tissue blocks and processed for immunohistochemistry using a Vectastain ABC Kit (Vector Laboratories, USA) and a rabbit polyclonal antibody against GFAP (DAKO, Denmark) [1:4000]. For detailed methods, please refer to Additional file 1.

Astrocyte density and morphological measurement

All density quantitation was performed using a ×100 oil immersion objective lens (numerical aperture = 1.4) and a Nikon Eclipse 80i (Nikon Instruments, Japan) together with StereoInvestigator 11 (MBF Biosciences, USA) as described previously [33]. A pilot study was conducted to determine sampling parameters of probes including disector depth, size of sampling contour, and numbers of sampling fields in order to achieve coefficient of error (CE) below 0.05 [36]. Three regions of interest defined by 1 mm × 2 mm (optical fractionator and nucleator) or 1 mm × 1 mm (spaceballs) were drawn using ×4 objective lens within the white matter for each section and systematic random sampling (SRS) grid applied for data collection. Within StereoInvestigator, we utilized the optical fractionator probe to estimate astrocyte and glia density, with simultaneous application of the nucleator probe for astrocyte somal size estimation. The spaceballs probe was used to estimate total astrocyte process length. For detailed methods, please refer to Additional file 1.

Statistical analysis

All measures were tested for normality using a Shapiro-Wilk test, with Pearson or Spearman correlations, carried out between our outcome measures, age, and post-mortem interval (PMI). Any significant correlation at $p < 0.05$ were considered as covariates during analysis for group differences. A general linear model was used to test differences between groups for normally distributed measures while a Mann-Whitney *U* test was utilized for non-parametrically distributed measures.

Results

Identification of adjustment variables

Shapiro-Wilk normality tests demonstrated that nucleator area ($p = 0.023$) was not normally distributed within the autism group; however, all other measures including age, post-mortem interval (PMI), astrocytes density, negative glia density, total glia density, spaceballs length, and IOD were normally distributed. No significant correlations were observed (Table 2).

Table 1 Brain tissue demographics

Sample ID	Age		Cause of death	Sex	PMI (h)	Diagnosis
	Years	Days				
5308	4	182	Skull fractures	M	21	ASD
5144	7	55	Complications from cancer	M	3	ASD
4899	14	126	Drowning	M	9	ASD
5403	16	266	Cardiac arrhythmia	M	35	ASD
4999	20	274	Cardiac arrhythmia	M	14	ASD
5578	35	294	Accident	M	22	ASD
5115	46	135	Complications of pseudomyxoma peritonei	M	29	ASD
5137	51	91	Pneumonia	M	72	ASD
1185	4	258	Drowning	M	17	Control
1500	6	320	Multiple injuries	M	18	Control
917	14	217	Accident/multiple injuries	M	10	Control
1158	16	63	Cardiomegaly	M	15	Control
4916	19	47	Accident/drowning	M	5	Control
4593	33	24	Cardiac arrhythmia	M	8	Control
1936	46	35	Arteriosclerotic cardiovascular disease	M	13	Control

Table 2 Statistical analysis of normality test, correlation test, and group comparison between autism and control

	Diagnosis	Shapiro-Wilk normality test			Correlation age		Correlation PMI		Group differences (ASD vs control)		
		Statistic	df	Sig.	Pearson (*r*)	Spearman (rho)	Pearson (*r*)	Spearman (rho)	Mean	SE	*p* value
Age	ASD	0.907	8	0.335					24.612	5.803	0.604[a]
	Control	0.907	7	0.374					20.092	6.204	
PMI (h)	ASD	0.864	8	0.133					25.625	5.673	0.132[a]
	Control	0.954	7	0.766					12.286	6.065	
Population (all glia)	ASD	0.950	8	0.715	0.205 ($p = 0.463$)		−0.390 ($p = 0.150$)		2,401,704.83	121,494.58	0.415[a]
	Control	0.873	7	0.196					2,351,803.21	129,883.17	
Population (astrocyte)	ASD	0.969	8	0.894	−0.267 ($p = 0.337$)		0.168 ($p = 0.549$)		100,669.51	8557.62	0.202[a]
	Control	0.978	7	0.949					117,513.34	9148.48	
Population (other glia)	ASD	0.951	8	0.718	0.219 ($p = 0.433$)		−0.392 ($p = 0.149$)		2,401,035.25	124,249.39	0.376[a]
	Control	0.868	7	0.178					2,234,289.88	132,828.19	
Nucleator (area)	ASD	0.791	8	0.023		−0.093 ($p = 0.742$)		−0.118 ($p = 0.676$)	92.475	4.556	0.397[b]
	Control	0.866	7	0.170					87.423	4.870	
Spaceballs length (all) (um)	ASD	0.901	8	0.298	−0.289 ($p = 0.296$)		−0.206 ($p = 0.461$)		51,228,155.8	6,563,846.09	0.923[a]
	Control	0.982	7	0.970					52,176,610.3	7,017,046.63	
IOD (mean)	ASD	0.938	8	0.591	−0.681 ($p = 0.007$)		−0.517 ($p = 0.059$)		143.083	4.159	0.066[c]
	Control	0.922	7	0.487					156.127	4.809	

[a]General linear model
[b]Non-parametric independent sample *t* test
[c]General linear model with covariate "age"

Astrocyte and total glial densities

No significant differences in the density of astrocytes were seen between autism and controls (autism = $10.07 \times 10^4 \pm 85.58 \times 10^2$, control = $11.75 \times 10^4 \pm 91.48 \times 10^2$ (mean ± SEM); $p = 0.202$, Fig. 1a). In addition, no group differences were seen for GFAP negative glia (autism = $24.01 \times 10^5 \pm 12.42 \times 10^4$, control = $23.34 \times 10^5 \pm 13.28 \times 10^4$ (mean ± SEM); $p = 0.376$, Fig. 1b), or total glia (autism = $24.02 \times 10^4 \pm 12.15 \times 10^4$, control = $23.52 \times 10^4 \pm 12.99 \times 10^4$ (mean ± SEM); $p = 0.415$, Fig. 1c).

Astrocyte somal size and process length

As somal sizes were not normally distributed within the autism group, we employed a Mann-Whitney *U* nonparametric test to compare differences between autism and control groups. No significant difference between autism and controls were seen for somal area of white matter astrocytes (autism = 92.475 ± 4.56 μm^2, control = 87.423 ± 4.87 μm^2 (mean ± SEM); $p = 0.397$, Fig. 2a). Furthermore, spaceballs analysis showed no significant difference between autism and control group for total length of astrocytes processes in the white matter (autism = $51.23 \times 10^6 \pm 65.64 \times 10^5$ μm, control = $52.18 \times 10^6 \pm 70.17 \times 10^5$ μm (mean ± SEM); $p = 0.923$, Fig. 2c).

Discussion

This study provides the first investigation of astrocyte density, morphology, and activation status within the white matter of the DLPFC in autism. Based on previous evidence demonstrating increased GFAP within the brain in autism, we hypothesized that we would observe an increased density of astrocytes in the white matter of the DLPFC of individuals with autism. In contrast, our results demonstrate no difference in the density and cellular morphology of GFAP-positive astrocytes in the white matter of the DLPFC of autism when compared to age-matched controls. Our findings are in keeping with recent studies demonstrating no alteration in astrocyte number and astrocyte somal size in the amygdala in autism, as well as no increase in GFAP mRNA and protein in the anterior PFC and ACC [28, 29].

During severe reactive astrogliosis, a marked increase in astrocytic size, arborization, GFAP expression, and proliferation are observed [37, 38]. Therefore, the current study investigated the population of GFAP-positive astrocytes along with other glial cells using StereoInvestigator to obtain an estimation of astrocyte and glial density, as well as astrocytic somal size and process length. Our results provide support for no alteration in astrocyte or glial density in the autism brain, consistent with Morgan et al. reporting no alteration of astrocyte numbers in autism within the amygdala [29]. In addition, our results demonstrated no evidence for increased astrocytic reactivity within the DLPFC white matter of individuals with autism compared to controls, as indicated by no changes in morphology, including cell somal size and process length. Similar to our findings for astrocyte somal size, Morgan et al. also found no evidence for differences in astrocyte somal size between autism and controls within the amygdala [29].

Our lack of findings for alterations in astrocyte density and activation status within the DLPFC white matter in autism represent an absence in gross astrocyte morphological changes in this brain region. However, another possibility is that any astrocyte activation may be present at a less pronounced level and that our employed strategies for investigating activation may have not been sensitive enough to detect such changes. This is in keeping with a lack of stark neuropathological changes observed in the autism brain. Yet another possible explanation is that astrocytes measured for our investigation may have resolved their reactivity and activation status, with morphological changes potentially taking place much earlier in disease progression [38]. Given the early developmental nature of autism and likely heterogeneity in autism pathophysiology, the latter two possibilities are equally likely to potentially explain the lack of astrocyte reactivity within our samples. Our results therefore highlight the need for more sensitive measures of assessing astrocyte activation as well as potentially assessing temporal and regional changes in astrocyte activation.

Despite a lack of evidence in our study to suggest activation of astrocytes, their contribution to the pathophysiology of autism might still be very significant.

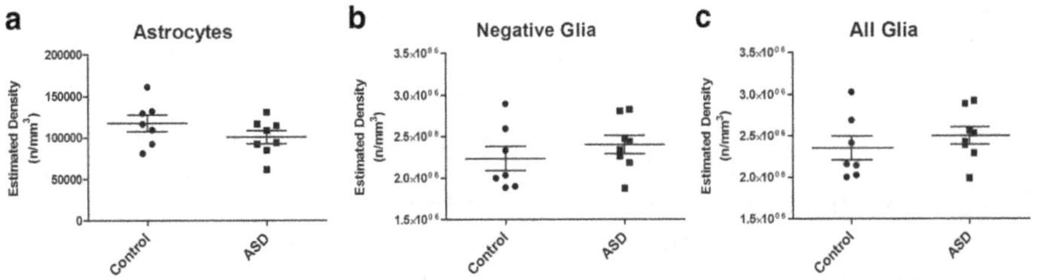

Fig. 1 Optical fractionator results of ASD and controls. Estimated density of **a** astrocytes (GFAP positive), **b** negative glia (GFAP-negative glia), and **c** total glia, in the DLPFC of ASD and control subjects

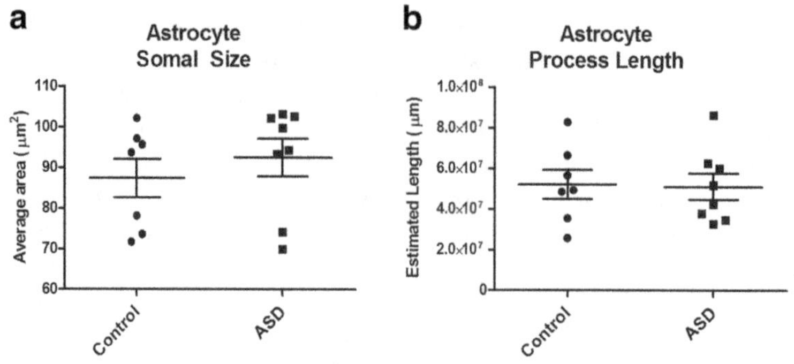

Fig. 2 Astrocyte morphology estimates. Astrocytes reactivity measures of **a** cell somal area via nucleator probe, and **b** cell processes length using spaceballs probe

Given astrocytes play a central role in regulating the functions of other cell types in the brain, any loss or gain of function of astrocytes could have a direct or indirect effect on brain physiology. Astrocytes contribute to synaptic functioning, especially clearing of glutamate via transporter EAAT2. A disturbance of this function could potentially be detrimental to neuronal health and functioning due to excitotoxicity caused by excess glutamate within the extracellular space [39]. Developmentally, astrocytes contribute to synaptic pruning by actively removing synapses via MEFG10 and MERTK pathways [40], or by tagging synapses for elimination by microglia via upregulation of C1q protein, loss of this function could lead to over- or under-pruning of synapses as observed in autism [41]. Within the white matter, disturbance of astrocytic physiology could also lead to perturbation of myelination, which has also been observed in autism [42, 43]. Therefore, potential functional alterations in astrocytes due to neuroinflammation and change in their activation may warrant a more detailed investigation in an attempt to tease out the mechanistic roles of astrocytes in the neuropathology of autism.

Due to the limitation of post-mortem brain samples available, autism studies including the current one are often limited by sample size. This also contributed to a relatively large age range within the cohort investigated. Consequently, our lack of astrocyte abnormalities in the current study could to a certain extent have been masked by an age-related effect, whereby abnormalities present in early developmental stages may be normalized later in life. This is particularly interesting given age-related cortical thinning has been reported within the temporal and parietal cortices of autism brain during adolescence and early adulthood, despite evidence of cortical overgrowth earlier in life [44]. In addition, findings from several longitudinal neuroimaging studies also suggest that brain abnormalities such as overgrowth is pronounced within the first few years of life and subsequently found to normalize towards controls during aging [45–47]. Furthermore, it is not uncommon for individuals with autism to have comorbid neurological disorders such as epilepsy, which may additionally represent a confounding factor, with potential brain changes due to an underlying neurodegenerative disease. With regard to epilepsy, this would be particularly pertinent for our investigation as individuals with epilepsy are known to have increased astrocyte numbers and activation [48].

For this study, we employed a strict protocol of sampling whereby we ensured the CE for all cases was below 0.05, in attempt to increase our precision in estimating density, size, and process length measurements. As the spaceballs probe was used to estimate all astrocyte processes present within the ROI regardless of the presence of the cell body, our results reflect more global increases in astrocyte length as opposed to arborization characteristics of individual astrocytes. Nevertheless, our data provides a reliable 3D estimate of overall length of astrocyte processes as a measure of potential astrocyte activation. Future studies may benefit from investigating an extended suite of astrocyte markers, including aldehyde dehydrogenase 1 family member L1 (ALDH1L1), glutamate synthetase (GS), and S100 calcium-binding protein B (S100B), to obtain a more complete perspective on structural and functional astrocyte abnormalities in the autism brain.

Conclusions

In conclusion, our results suggest that gross morphological changes in astrocyte density and activation status are not present in the DLPFC white matter. This could suggest a lack of astrogliosis, but does not rule out astrocytic abnormalities, that may be present in the absence of gross morphological changes. In addition, regional differences in the reactivity of astrocytes in the brain in autism may also be present and should be considered. Further post-mortem investigations within the autism brain should be aimed at assessing astrocyte abnormalities utilizing more functional markers of astrocytes to further understand the role that astrocytes play in the pathophysiology of autism and their impact on other cell types in the brain including neurons, microglia, and oligodendrocytes, with these cells also likely contributing to the underlying etiology of the disorder.

Abbreviations

ABC: Avidin-biotin complex; ACC: Anterior cingulate cortex; ALDH1L1: Aldehyde dehydrogenase 1 family member L1; AOI: Area of interest; AQP4: Aquaporin 4; CE: Coefficient of error; CNS: Central nervous system; CNX43: Connexin 43; DAB: Diaminobenzadine; DLPFC: Dorsolateral prefrontal cortex; EAAT1: Excitatory amino acid transporter 1; GFAP: Glial fibrillary acidic protein; GS: Glutamate synthetase; IL-1B: Interleukin 1B; IL-6: Interleukin 6; IOD: Integrated optical density; MRI: Magnetic resonance imaging; NGS: Normal goat serum; PBS: Phosphate-buffered saline; PFC: Prefrontal cortex; qPCR: Quantitative real-time polymerase chain reaction; S100B: S100 calcium binding protein B; SEM: Standard error of mean; SRS: Systematic random sampling; TNFα: Tumor necrosis factor alpha

Acknowledgements

The authors would like to acknowledge the brain donors and their families; this work would not be possible without the brain tissues.

Funding

This work was supported by funds obtained through the Melbourne Grant Support Scheme run by the University of Melbourne. Prof Christos Pantelis was supported by a NHMRC Senior Principal Research Fellowship (ID: 628386 and 1105825) and the Brain and Behavior Research Foundation (NARSAD) Distinguished Investigator Award. Prof Efstratios Skafidas (The Clifford Chair in Neural Engineering) and the Centre for Neural Engineering received funding from Mr. Leigh Clifford and family.

Authors' contributions

TL conducted the experiment and contributed to study design, data analysis, and manuscript writing. ES contributed to study design, data analysis, and manuscript editing. MD, DZ, and CP contributed to study design and manuscript editing. IE and GC contributed to study design, acquisition of samples, data analysis, and manuscript writing. All authors read and approved the final manuscript.

Competing interests

The authors declare that they have no competing interests.

Author details

[1]Department of Psychiatry, The University of Melbourne, Parkville, Australia. [2]Centre for Neural Engineering, The University of Melbourne, Parkville, Australia. [3]Department of Biomedical Engineering, The University of Melbourne, Parkville, Australia. [4]Department of Clinical Haematology, Austin Hospital, Heidelberg, Australia. [5]Department of Medicine, The University of Melbourne, Parkville, Australia. [6]Melbourne Neuropsychiatry Centre, The University of Melbourne & Melbourne Health, Parkville, Australia. [7]Florey Institute of Neuroscience and Mental Health, The University of Melbourne, Parkville, Australia. [8]The Institute of Psychiatry, Psychology and Neuroscience, King's College London, London, UK. [9]Illawarra Health and Medical Research Institute, University of Wollongong, Wollongong, Australia.

References

1. Weintraub K. The prevalence puzzle: autism counts. Nature. 2011; 479(7371):22–4.
2. Baxter AJ, et al. The epidemiology and global burden of autism spectrum disorders. Psychol Med. 2015;45(3):601–13.
3. Petrelli F, Pucci L, Bezzi P. Astrocytes and microglia and their potential link with autism spectrum disorders. Front Cell Neurosci. 2016;10:21.
4. Voineagu I, et al. Transcriptomic analysis of autistic brain reveals convergent molecular pathology. Nature. 2011;474(7351):380–4.
5. Fan LW, Pang Y. Dysregulation of neurogenesis by neuroinflammation: key differences in neurodevelopmental and neurological disorders. Neural Regen Res. 2017;12(3):366–71.
6. Panatier A, Robitaille R. Astrocytic mGluR5 and the tripartite synapse. Neuroscience. 2016;323:29–34.
7. Fiacco TA, McCarthy KD. Astrocyte calcium elevations: properties, propagation, and effects on brain signaling. Glia. 2006;54(7):676–90.
8. Popoli M, et al. The stressed synapse: the impact of stress and glucocorticoids on glutamate transmission. Nat Rev Neurosci. 2011;13(1):22–37.
9. Moore CS, et al. How factors secreted from astrocytes impact myelin repair. J Neurosci Res. 2011;89(1):13–21.
10. Kiray H, et al. The multifaceted role of astrocytes in regulating myelination. Exp Neurol. 2016;283(Pt B):541–9.
11. Liedtke W, et al. GFAP is necessary for the integrity of CNS white matter architecture and long-term maintenance of myelination. Neuron. 1996;17(4): 607–15.
12. Zikopoulos B, Barbas H. Changes in prefrontal axons may disrupt the network in autism. J Neurosci. 2010;30(44):14595.
13. Ben Bashat D, et al. Accelerated maturation of white matter in young children with autism: a high b value DWI study. NeuroImage. 2007;37(1):40–7.
14. Ouyang M, et al. Atypical age-dependent effects of autism on white matter microstructure in children of 2–7 years. Hum Brain Mapp. 2016;37(2):819–32.
15. Herbert MR, et al. Dissociations of cerebral cortex, subcortical and cerebral white matter volumes in autistic boys. Brain. 2003;126(Pt 5):1182–92.
16. Schumann CM, et al. Longitudinal MRI study of cortical development through early childhood in autism. J Neurosci. 2010;30(12):4419–27.
17. Bigler ED, et al. Volumetric and voxel-based morphometry findings in autism subjects with and without macrocephaly. Dev Neuropsychol. 2010; 35(3):278–95.
18. Ameis SH, Catani M. Altered white matter connectivity as a neural substrate for social impairment in autism spectrum disorder. Cortex. 2015;62:158–81.
19. Di Martino A, et al. Functional brain correlates of social and nonsocial processes in autism spectrum disorders: an activation likelihood estimation meta-analysis. Biol Psychiatry. 2009;65(1):63–74.
20. Logue SF, Gould TJ. The neural and genetic basis of executive function: attention, cognitive flexibility, and response inhibition. Pharmacol Biochem Behav. 2014;0:45–54.
21. Sawa T, et al. Dysfunction of orbitofrontal and dorsolateral prefrontal cortices in children and adolescents with high-functioning pervasive developmental disorders. Ann General Psychiatry. 2013;12:31.
22. Fujii E, et al. Function of the frontal lobe in autistic individuals
: a proton magnetic resonance spectroscopic study. J Med Investig. 2010; 57(1,2):35–44.
23. Christakou A, et al. Disorder-specific functional abnormalities during sustained attention in youth with attention deficit hyperactivity disorder (ADHD) and with autism. Mol Psychiatry. 2013;18(2):236–44.
24. Purcell AE, et al. Postmortem brain abnormalities of the glutamate neurotransmitter system in autism. Neurology. 2001;57(9):1618–28.
25. Vargas DL, et al. Neuroglial activation and neuroinflammation in the brain of patients with autism. Ann Neurol. 2005;57(1):67–81.
26. Laurence JA, Fatemi SH. Glial fibrillary acidic protein is elevated in superior frontal, parietal and cerebellar cortices of autistic subjects. Cerebellum. 2005; 4(3):206–10.
27. Edmonson C, Ziats MN, Rennert OM. Altered glial marker expression in autistic post-mortem prefrontal cortex and cerebellum. Mol Autism. 2014;5(1):3.

28. Crawford JD, et al. Elevated GFAP protein in anterior cingulate cortical white matter in males with autism spectrum disorder. Autism Res. 2015; 8(6):649–57.
29. Morgan JT, et al. Stereological study of amygdala glial populations in adolescents and adults with autism spectrum disorder. PLoS One. 2014; 9(10):e110356.
30. Fatemi SH, et al. Expression of astrocytic markers aquaporin 4 and connexin 43 is altered in brains of subjects with autism. Synapse. 2008;62(7):501–7.
31. Kimelberg HK. Functions of mature mammalian astrocytes: a current view. Neuroscientist. 2010;16(1):79–106.
32. Zantomio D, et al. Convergent evidence for mGluR5 in synaptic and neuroinflammatory pathways implicated in ASD. Neurosci Biobehav Rev. 2015;52:172–7.
33. Chana G, et al. Decreased expression of mGluR5 within the dorsolateral prefrontal cortex in autism and increased microglial number in mGluR5 knockout mice: pathophysiological and neurobehavioral implications. Brain Behav Immun. 2015;49:197–205.
34. Chung WS, Allen NJ, Eroglu C. Astrocytes control synapse formation, function, and elimination. Cold Spring Harb Perspect Biol. 2015;7(9):a020370.
35. Gupta S, et al. Transcriptome analysis reveals dysregulation of innate immune response genes and neuronal activity-dependent genes in autism. Nat Commun. 2014;5(2041–1723 (Electronic)):5748.
36. Gundersen HJ, et al. The efficiency of systematic sampling in stereology—reconsidered. J Microsc. 1999;193(Pt 3):199–211.
37. Koob AO. Astrogenesis versus astrogliosis. Neural Regen Res. 2017;12(2):203–4.
38. Sofroniew MV, Vinters HV. Astrocytes: biology and pathology. Acta Neuropathol. 2010;119(1):7–35.
39. Lin C.L., et al., Glutamate transporter EAAT2: a new target for the treatment of neurodegenerative diseases. 2012; (1756–8927 (Electronic)).
40. Chung W-S, et al. Astrocytes mediate synapse elimination through MEGF10 and MERTK pathways. Nature. 2013;504(7480):394–400.
41. Stevens, B., et al., The classical complement cascade mediates CNS synapse elimination. (0092–8674 (Print)).
42. Ameis, S.H. and M. Catani, Altered white matter connectivity as a neural substrate for social impairment in autism spectrum disorder. 2015; (1973–8102 (Electronic)).
43. Li T, Giaume Fau-Xiao C, and L. Xiao, Connexins-mediated glia networking impacts myelination and remyelination in the central nervous system. 2014(1559–1182 (Electronic)).
44. Wallace GL, et al. Age-related temporal and parietal cortical thinning in autism spectrum disorders. Brain. 2010;133(Pt 12):3745–54.
45. Lange N, et al. Longitudinal volumetric brain changes in autism Spectrum disorder ages 6–35 years. Autism Res. 2015;8(1):82–93.
46. Hazlett HC, et al. Early brain overgrowth in autism associated with an increase in cortical surface area before age 2. Arch Gen Psychiatry. 2011; 68(5):467–76.
47. Hazlett HC, et al. Early brain development in infants at high risk for autism spectrum disorder. Nature. 2017;542(7641):348–51.
48. Steinhäuser C, Grunnet M, Carmignoto G. Crucial role of astrocytes in temporal lobe epilepsy. Neuroscience. 2016;323:157–69.

4

Advanced glycation endproducts, dityrosine and arginine transporter dysfunction in autism

Attia Anwar[1†], Provvidenza Maria Abruzzo[2,4†], Sabah Pasha[1], Kashif Rajpoot[3], Alessandra Bolotta[2,4], Alessandro Ghezzo[2], Marina Marini[2,4], Annio Posar[5,6], Paola Visconti[5], Paul J. Thornalley[1,7] and Naila Rabbani[1,7,8*]

Abstract

Background: Clinical chemistry tests for autism spectrum disorder (ASD) are currently unavailable. The aim of this study was to explore the diagnostic utility of proteotoxic biomarkers in plasma and urine, plasma protein glycation, oxidation, and nitration adducts, and related glycated, oxidized, and nitrated amino acids (free adducts), for the clinical diagnosis of ASD.

Methods: Thirty-eight children with ASD (29 male, 9 female; age 7.6 ± 2.0 years) and 31 age-matched healthy controls (23 males, 8 females; 8.6 ± 2.0 years) were recruited for this study. Plasma protein glycation, oxidation, and nitration adducts and amino acid metabolome in plasma and urine were determined by stable isotopic dilution analysis liquid chromatography-tandem mass spectrometry. Machine learning methods were then employed to explore and optimize combinations of analyte data for ASD diagnosis.

Results: We found that children with ASD had increased advanced glycation endproducts (AGEs), N_ε-carboxymethyl-lysine (CML) and N_ω-carboxymethylarginine (CMA), and increased oxidation damage marker, dityrosine (DT), in plasma protein, with respect to healthy controls. We also found that children with ASD had increased CMA free adduct in plasma ultrafiltrate and increased urinary excretion of oxidation free adducts, alpha-aminoadipic semialdehyde and glutamic semialdehyde. From study of renal handling of amino acids, we found that children with ASD had decreased renal clearance of arginine and CMA with respect to healthy controls. Algorithms to discriminate between ASD and healthy controls gave strong diagnostic performance with features: plasma protein AGEs—CML, CMA—and 3-deoxyglucosone-derived hydroimidazolone, and oxidative damage marker, DT. The sensitivity, specificity, and receiver operating characteristic area-under-the-curve were 92%, 84%, and 0.94, respectively.

(Continued on next page)

* Correspondence: n.rabbani@warwick.ac.uk
†Equal contributors
[1]Warwick Medical School, University of Warwick, Clinical Sciences Research Laboratories, University Hospital, Coventry, UK
[7]Zeeman Institute for Systems Biology & Infectious Disease Epidemiology Research, Senate House, University of Warwick, Coventry CV4 7AL, UK
Full list of author information is available at the end of the article

(Continued from previous page)

Conclusions: Changes in plasma AGEs were likely indicative of dysfunctional metabolism of dicarbonyl metabolite precursors of AGEs, glyoxal and 3-deoxyglucosone. DT is formed enzymatically by dual oxidase (DUOX); selective increase of DT as an oxidative damage marker implicates increased DUOX activity in ASD possibly linked to impaired gut mucosal immunity. Decreased renal clearance of arginine and CMA in ASD is indicative of increased arginine transporter activity which may be a surrogate marker of disturbance of neuronal availability of amino acids. Data driven combination of these biomarkers perturbed by proteotoxic stress, plasma protein AGEs and DT, gave diagnostic algorithms of high sensitivity and specificity for ASD.

Keywords: Autism spectrum disorder (ASD), Advanced glycation endproducts (AGEs), Oxidative stress, Amino acid metabolome, Machine learning

Background

Autism spectrum disorders (ASD) are defined as developmental disorders mainly affecting social interactions and range of interests and causing a wide spectrum of other disabilities, such as speech disturbances, repetitive and/or compulsive behaviors, hyperactivity, anxiety, and difficulty to adapt to new environments, with or without cognitive impairment [1]. The high heterogeneity of the clinical presentation makes diagnosis of ASD difficult and uncertain, particularly at the early stages of development. Discovery and development of robust biomarkers for diagnosis and progression of severity of ASD is expected to facilitate earlier diagnosis and intervention. It will also likely reveal new causative factors [2, 3]. In particular, alteration in the metabolome and specific damaging biochemical modifications may reveal the presence of a shared metabolic impairment in children with an otherwise highly heterogeneous background, thus shedding some light on the etiopathogenesis of ASD. Genetic causes of ASD are evident in about 30–35% of cases. For the remaining 65–70% of patients, it is generally agreed that ASD results from the combination of environmental factors with multiple de novo mutations, copy number variation, and rare genetic variants, each possibly lending to additive effects. Environmental factors may also be involved and reflected in epigenetic modifications [4]. Transcriptomic, proteomic, and metabolomic profiling have been proposed for diagnosis of ASD, with diagnostic performance judged by area under-the-curve of receiver operating characteristic (AUROC) plot of 0.73–0.91 [5–7]. It is expected that improved diagnostic performance may be achieved with a relatively small number of biomarker analytes linked to the pathogenic mechanism of ASD.

Impairment of protein homeostasis leading to proteotoxic stress and activation of the unfolded protein response (UPR) has been implicated in ASD [8]. Drivers of impaired protein quality are increased spontaneous modifications by glycation, oxidation, and nitration [9]. Glycation of proteins occurs by spontaneous reaction of proteins with glucose, reactive dicarbonyl metabolites, glyoxal, methylglyoxal (MG), and 3-deoxyglucosone (3-DG), and other saccharides and saccharide derivatives. Protein glycation adducts are classified as early stage glycation adducts—such as N_ε-fructosyl-lysine (FL) residues formed by glycation of proteins by glucose—and late-stage adducts, advanced glycation endproducts (AGEs)—such as N_ε-carboxymethyl-lysine (CML) and glucosepane (GSP) residues—formed by the degradation of FL residues, hydroimidazolones G-H1, MG-H1, and 3DG-H formed by the modification of arginine residues by glyoxal, MG and 3-DG, respectively, N_ω-carboxymethylarginine (CMA)—also formed by the reaction of glyoxal with arginine residues, and methylglyoxal-derived lysine crosslink (MOLD). Protein oxidation occurs by the reaction of proteins with reactive oxygen species (ROS) and is increased in oxidative stress. Examples of protein oxidation adducts are dityrosine (DT), *N*-formylkynurenine (NFK), α-aminoadipic semialdehyde (AASA), and glutamic semialdehyde (GSA) residues. Oxidative stress has been implicated as a contributory factor in the development of ASD [10–12]. Increased oxidative damage associated with oxidative stress and neuroinflammation may be common features of ASD in children. Protein nitration occurs by the reaction of proteins with reactive nitrogen species such as peroxynitrite. The main adduct formed by protein nitration is 3-nitrotyrosine (3-NT) residues (Fig. 1). Increased protein damage by these mechanisms may lead to activation of the UPR to counter the proteotoxic threat and related inflammatory response [13, 14].

Glycated, oxidized, and nitrated proteins undergo proteolysis to form related glycated, oxidized, and nitrated amino acids—also called glycation, oxidation, and nitration free adducts. Glycated, oxidized, and nitrated amino acids are released into plasma and are excreted in urine. Urinary excretion of glycation, oxidation, and nitration free adducts are approximate measures of whole body fluxes of protein glycation, oxidation, and nitration, respectively. There are also minor contributions to the pool of these metabolites by direct glycation, oxidation, and nitration of amino acids and absorption from food after digestion of damaged proteins therein [9]. Insight into renal handling of amino acids by the kidney is gained by deducing the renal clearance (CL) of amino acids from plasma to urine. For low

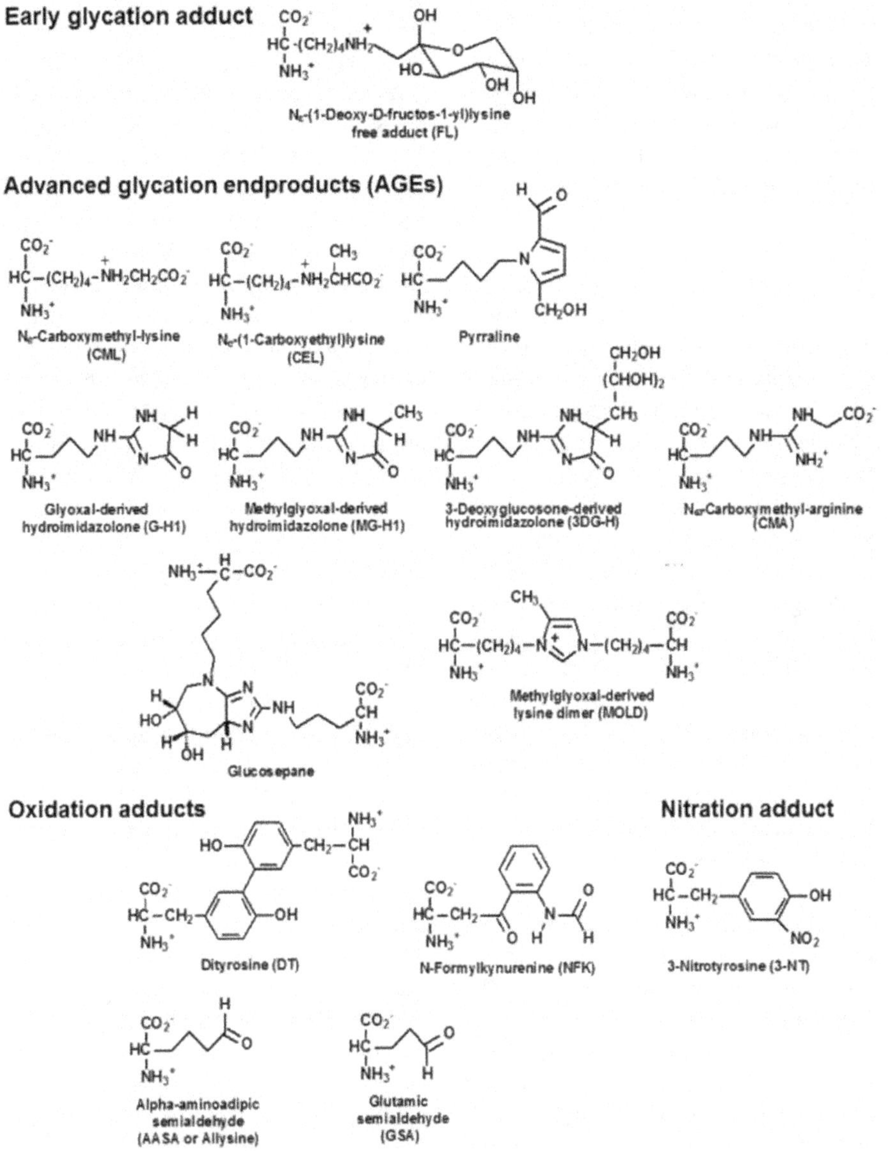

Fig. 1 Protein glycation, oxidation, and nitration free adducts. Ionization status at physiological pH is shown. For related adduct residues of proteins, alpha-amino-NH_3^+ and terminal carboxylate $-CO_2^-$ groups are moieties of as peptide bonds –NH–CO– with amino acid residues immediately before and after in the peptide backbone

molecular weight metabolites such as amino acids, CL is mainly influenced by renal tubule reuptake of amino acids mediated by amino acid membrane transporters. ASD has been previously associated with homozygous mutations in gene solute carrier family 7, member 5 (SLC7A5) which encodes the large neutral amino acid transporter subunit-1 (hLAT-1); and in males, with rare holomorphic variants of cationic amino acid transporter-3 (CAT-3) mediating uptake of arginine, ornithine, and lysine. These transporters mediate amino acid uptake into the cells, including neurons [15].

In this study, we explore the association of proteotoxic damage with ASD by quantifying levels of protein glycation, oxidation, and nitration adducts in plasma protein and related free adducts in plasma and urine of children with ASD and healthy controls. We also quantify the conventional plasma amino acid metabolome [16] and CL of glycation, oxidation, and nitration free adducts and unmodified amino acids. We then explore the diagnostic potential of these biomarkers by development of diagnostic algorithms with optimum combinations of analyte features. We found evidence of increase of selected plasma protein AGEs and DT in children with ASD and also decreased CL of arginine and CMA. These findings implicate a disturbance of metabolism of dicarbonyl precursors of AGEs and activation of dual oxidase (DUOX) in ASD. The initial evidence given herein suggests combination of plasma protein AGE and DT levels may provide a blood-based test for diagnosis of ASD. Decreased CL of arginine and CMA is proposed to be linked to amino acid transporter dysfunction in ASD, building on increasing evidence of neuronal amino acid availability as a driver in ASD development.

Methods

Subject recruitment

A total of 69 children were recruited. Of these, 38 had a diagnosis of ASD (29 males and 9 females) and 31 were classified as typically developing (TD) children (23 males and 8 females)—Fig. 2. The age of the two subject groups was not significantly different. Subject age was as follows: ASD group, 7.6 years ±2.0 years, range 5–12 years and TD group, 8.6 ± 2.0 years, range 5–12 years. All ASD subjects received a diagnosis of ASD by two child development experts at the Child Neurology and Psychiatry Unit of the Bellaria Hospital of Bologna (IRCCS Institute of Neurological Sciences), according to the Diagnostic and Statistical Manual of Mental Disorders V (DSM 5 [1] criteria, Autism Diagnostic Observation Schedule (ADOS) [10], Childhood Autism Rating Scale (CARS) [17] and characteristics of onset pattern of ASD defined according to Ozonoff et al. [18]. Developmental and cognitive levels were assessed by Psychoeducational Profile-3 (PEP-3) [19] and Leiter International Performance Scale–Revised (Leiter-R) [20]. For both ASD and TD subjects, exclusion criteria were presence of inflammatory or infective disease and taking antioxidant supplements at the time of study. No subject underwent any surgery intervention in the 4 months prior to blood and urine collection. None of the ASD subjects had active epilepsy at the time of blood and urine sampling. Subjects with ascertained medical and neurological comorbidity were excluded, through a medical work up including electroencephalography (recorded during awake and sleep), cerebral magnetic resonance imaging, standard clinical and neurological examination, neurometabolic, and genetic investigations (including comparative genomic hybridization array, molecular assay for Fragile X and MECP2). Subjects recruited for this study were not taking any medication. TD children were recruited in the local community, with no sign of cognitive, learning, and psychiatric involvement. They were attending mainstream school and had not been subjected to stressful events. Dietary habits were assessed by a Food Questionnaire, built according to the guidelines issued by the Emilia-Romagna Health Authority. No ASD child was on a diet free of gluten or casein. Both patients and controls were on a typical Mediterranean diet, as defined by the prevalence of both simple and complex carbohydrates, use of olive oil, and plenty of fruit [21]. The consumption of vegetables was less than desirable in both patients and controls, although vegetable intake was more limited in ASD patients. Demographic and clinical features of ASD are summarized in Table 1. All subjects were recruited at the Child Neurology and Psychiatry Unit of the Bellaria Hospital of Bologna, Bologna, Italy.

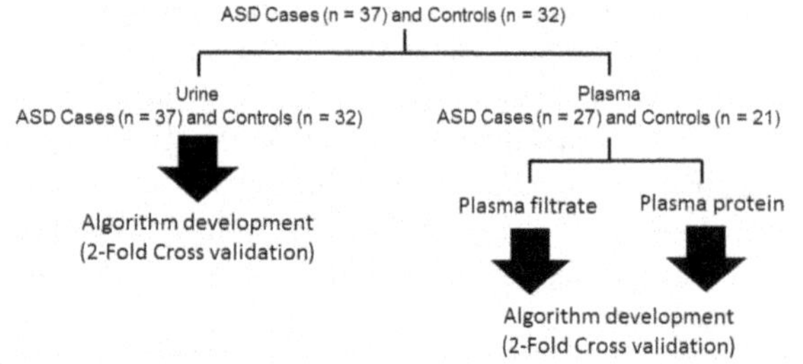

Fig. 2 Training and validation subject groups of diagnostic algorithms for detection of autistic spectrum disorder

Blood and urine sampling

Blood was withdrawn in the morning from fasting children. Spot urine samples were the first ones in the morning. Blood samples were collected using ethylenediaminetetra-acetic acid (EDTA) as anticoagulant. Plasma and blood cells were separated immediately by centrifugation (2000*g*, 10 min) and plasma samples stored at − 80 °C until analysis and transferred between collaborating laboratories on dry ice.

Assay of markers of protein glycation, oxidation, and nitration

The content of glycated, oxidized, and nitrated adduct residues in plasma protein was quantified in exhaustive enzymatic digests by stable isotopic dilution analysis liquid chromatography-tandem mass spectrometry (LC-MS/MS), with correction for autohydrolysis of hydrolytic enzymes [22]. The concentrations of related glycated, oxidized, and nitrated amino acids related free adducts (glycated, oxidized, and nitrated amino acids) in plasma and urine were determined similarly in plasma and urine ultrafiltrate, respectively. Ultrafiltrate of plasma (50 μL) was collected by microspin ultrafiltration (10 kDa cut-off) at 4 °C. Retained protein was diluted with water to 500 μL and washed by 4 cycles of concentration to 50 μL and dilution to 500 μL with water over the microspin ultrafilter at 4 °C. The final washed protein (100 μL) was delipidated and hydrolysed enzymatically as described [22, 23]. Ultrafiltrate of urine (50 μL) was collected by microspin ultrafiltration (3 kDa cut-off) at 4 °C.

Protein hydrolysate (25 μL, 32 μg equivalent) or ultrafiltrate (5 μL) was mixed with stable isotopic standard analytes (amounts as given previously [24]) and analyzed by LC-MS/MS using an Acquity™ UPLC system with a Xevo-TQS tandem mass spectrometer (Waters, Manchester, UK). Samples are maintained at 4 °C in the

Table 1 Demographic and clinical features of the autistic children group

No	Age (years)	Gender	ADOS score	CARS total score	CARS activity level item score (hyperactivity)	CARS body use item score (stereotypes)	CARS total number of items with score ≥ 3	Autism severity level	Cognitive/ developmental impairment	Onset pattern (1, early; 2, regressive; 3, mixed)†	Probability of autism‡ from algorithm no.			
											1	2	3	4
1	6.0	m	22	41.0	2.0	3.0	9	Severe	Severe	1	0.93	0.79	0.82	0.80
2	5.6	m	14	34.0	2.0	2.0	2	Mild	Mild	1	1.00	0.71	0.99	0.77
3	5.5	m	18	40.5	2.5	3.5	9	Severe	Moderate	1	1.00	0.86	1.00	0.29
4	5.4	f	17	31.5	2.0	2.0	1	Mild	Mild	3	0.88	0.69	0.55	0.27
5	8.5	m	22	36.5	2.0	2.5	6	Mild	Mild	3	0.98	0.64	1.00	0.88
6	8.7	m	19	44.5	3.0	3.0	11	Severe	Moderate	2	1.00	0.69	1.00	0.74
7	6.8	m	19	36.5	2.5	2.0	7	Mild	Normal IQ	1	1.00	0.63	1.00	0.91
8	5.5	f	15	41.5	2.5	2.0	9	Severe	Borderline IQ	1	0.73	0.77	0.72	0.92
9	11.9	m	22	44.5	2.5	3.0	11	Severe	Severe	2	0.20	0.91	0.34	0.45
10	9.2	f	15	47.5	3.5	3.0	13	Severe	Moderate	1	0.84	0.88	0.94	0.36
11	12.0	m	20	39.0	3.0	3.5	8	Severe	Severe	3	0.94	0.68	0.82	0.63
12	6.2	m	22	42.5	3.0	2.5	10	Severe	Severe	1	1.00	0.69	1.00	0.98
13	6.7	m	21	40.5	2.5	3.0	9	Severe	Severe	2	0.83	0.51	0.85	0.56
14	6.6	m	19	37.0	2.5	3.0	7	Severe	Moderate	1	0.83	0.63	0.74	0.97
15	5.5	m	22	40.5	3.0	3.0	9	Severe	Moderate	3	0.68	0.57	0.82	0.98
16	5.7	m	20	41.5	2.5	3.0	11	severe	severe	1	0.98	0.81	0.98	0.81
17	7.8	m	21	46.0	3.5	4.0	11	Severe	Severe	1	0.83	0.35	0.52	0.79
18	5.7	f	20	43.5	2.5	3.0	10	Severe	Normal IQ	3	0.85	0.39	0.58	0.68
19	7.8	m	20	48.5	3.0	4.0	12	Severe	Severe	2	0.95	0.58	0.93	0.57
20	6.8	m	19	42.0	3.0	3.0	9	Severe	Moderate	2	0.67	0.61	0.54	0.77
21	9.6	m	19	39.5	3.0	3.0	7	Severe	Severe	1	0.55	0.44	0.62	0.51
22	6.2	m	19	41.0	2.5	3.0	9	Severe	Severe	3	0.81	0.32	0.78	0.73
23	8.3	m	16	35.0	2.5	2.0	3	Moderate	Moderate	1	0.70	0.35	0.63	0.56
24	7.1	m	22	41.0	2.5	2.0	7	Severe	Moderate	1	0.83	1.00	0.99	1.00
25	6.2	f	17	38.0	2.0	2.5	7	Severe	Severe	1	0.28	0.82	0.15	0.79
26	10.3	f	21	33.5	2.0	2.0	4	Moderate	Normal IQ	3	0.89	0.55	0.82	0.86
27	10.7	m	19	39.0	2.0	2.5	7	Moderate	Normal IQ	1	0.89	0.60	0.97	0.52
28	6.5	m	17	39.0	3.0	2.5	6	Moderate	Normal IQ	3	ND	ND	ND	0.76
29	8.0	m	22	44.0	2.5	3.0	11	Severe	Moderate	1	ND	ND	ND	0.54
30	7.0	m	18	39.5	2.5	3.0	8	Moderate	Normal IQ	1	ND	ND	ND	0.96
31	9.5	m	21	47.0	3.0	3.5	13	Severe	Severe	1	ND	ND	ND	0.29
32	8.6	m	16	41.5	4.0	2.0	10	Severe	Moderate	3	ND	ND	ND	0.33
33	10.9	m	18	35.0	2.0	3.0	3	Mild	Normal IQ	1	ND	ND	ND	0.28
34	5.8	f	18	43.0	2.5	3.0	11	Severe	Moderate	2	ND	ND	ND	0.30
35	5.3	f	17	39.5	2.5	2.5	6	Moderate	Normal IQ	1	ND	ND	ND	0.62
36	5.3	f	17	41.0	2.5	2.5	7	Severe	Normal IQ	1	ND	ND	ND	0.77
37	8.2	m	20	41.0	2.0	3.5	9	Severe	Moderate	1	ND	ND	ND	0.58
38	11.1	m	13	34.0	2.0	1.5	2	Mild	Normal IQ	3	ND	ND	ND	0.87

†Onset pattern was defined according to Ozonoff et al. [18]

‡Probability the subject has autism estimated from diagnostic algorithms derived from experimental biomarker data—see Table 7

autosampler during batch analysis. The columns were 2.1 × 50 mm and 2.1 mm × 250 mm, 5 μm particle size Hypercarb™ (Thermo Scientific), in series with programmed switching, at 30 °C. Chromatographic retention was necessary to resolve oxidized analytes from their amino acid precursors to avoid interference from partial oxidation of the latter in the electrospray ionization source of the mass spectrometric detector. Analytes were detected by electrospray positive ionization and mass spectrometry multiple reaction monitoring (MRM) mode where analyte detection response was specific for mass/charge ratio of the analyte molecular ion and major fragment ion generated by collision-induced dissociation in the mass spectrometer collision cell. The ionization source and desolvation gas temperatures were 120 and 350 °C, respectively; cone gas and desolvation gas flow rates were 99 and 900 L/h; and the capillary voltage was 0.60 kV. Argon gas (5.0×10^{-3} mbar) was in the collision cell. For MRM detection, molecular ion and fragment ion masses and collision energies optimized to ± 0.1 Da and ± 1 eV, respectively, were programmed [22]—Additional file 1: Table S1. Analytes determined were glycation adducts—FL, and AGEs, CML, N_ε-(1-carboxyethyl)lysine (CEL), pyrraline, CMA, G-H1, MG-H1, 3DG-H, MOLD and GSP; oxidation adducts—DT, NFK, AASA, GSA; nitration adduct, 3-NT; and all major amino acids. Oxidation, nitration, and glycation adduct residues are normalized to their amino acid residue precursors and given as millimoles/mole amino acid modified, and related free adducts are given in nanomolar. Chemical structures and biochemical and clinical significance of these analytes have been described elsewhere [9, 25]. Renal clearance (CL) of glycation, oxidation, and nitration free adducts and unmodified amino acids was deduced from plasma and spot urine collections: CL (μL/mg creatinine or mL/mg creatinine) = $[\text{analyte}]_{\text{Urine}}$ (nmol/mg creatinine)/$[\text{analyte}]_{\text{Plasma}}$ (pmol/mL or nmol/mL).

Machine learning analysis

The objective was to distinguish between children with ASD and healthy controls. In all cases, the diagnostic algorithms were trained on 50% of the cases and controls (training subset) before being used to predict the disease class for each sample in the remaining subjects (test set), twofold cross-validation. The outcome was to assign, for each test set sample, a set of probabilities corresponding to each of the ASD/control groups—the group assignment being that for which the probability is highest. Test data were held separate from algorithm training; algorithm settings were not adjusted once we began to analyze the test set data—thereby guarding against overfitting and hence providing a rigorous estimate of predictive performance. Four algorithm types were tested for performance: random forests, logistic regression, ensemble classifier, and support vector machines (SVMs) [26–28]. During the algorithm training, we used the complete panel of protein glycation, oxidation, and nitration adducts as features and developed algorithms for each analyte type: plasma protein adduct residues, plasma free adducts, and urinary free adducts. For the latter two, unmodified amino acids were also included as features. The aim during the training was to select the set of features that accomplishes the highest performance. The machine learning experiments initially explored using all metabolite features. Subsequent selection of a subset of discriminant biomarker features improved the algorithm performance. For the biomarker selection, we used a sequential feature selection approach. The biomarker feature selection and classifier selection were made on the basis of algorithm performance defined by classification accuracy, sensitivity, specificity, area under-the-curve of the receiver operating characteristic curve (AUROC), positive likelihood ratio, negative likelihood ratio, positive predictive value, negative predictive value, and *F*-measure. For each performance metric, the mean and 95% CI was determined and reported. The algorithm training and testing was repeated 10 times, without altering the algorithm parameters, with 50% data split, to test for algorithm's robustness against any bias towards data split. We developed our computer programs using Statistics and Machine Learning Toolbox of MATLAB® (MathWorks, Inc., Natick, USA), with a linear kernel SVM and sequential minimal optimization (SMO).

Statistical analysis

Data are presented as mean ± SD for parametric distributions and median (lower–upper quartile) for nonparametric distributions. The test for normality of data distribution applied was the Kolmogorov–Smirnov test. Significance was evaluated by Student's *t* test or by Mann–Whitney *U* test for parametrically or nonparametrically distributed data, respectively. Bonferroni correction was made for analysis of multiple analytes without preconceived hypothesis. Correlation analysis was performed by Spearman's rho method with continuous variables. For clinical categorical variables with ≥ 6 categories, Spearman correlation was performed—assuming approximation to a continuous variable [29]; for other categorical variables, significance of difference of biomarker data distributions between categories was assessed by oneway ANOVA for parametric data and Kruskal—Wallis *H* test. Data were analyzed using SPSS, version 24.0.

For power analysis in the study design, we chose the level of the irreversible oxidative damage marker DT in plasma protein. In healthy human subjects, plasma protein DT was 0.0287 ± 0.0027 mmol/mol tyr ($n = 29$) in previous studies [30]. We designed our study to detect a 50% increase in plasma protein DT at the 0.01% significance level, for which ≥ 18 case and control samples were required. Post hoc analysis revealed an 88% increase with $P = 0.00017$, after Bonferroni correction of 14, 15 or 20 as appropriate with 27 cases and 21 controls, suggesting the study was adequately powered for this key target analyte.

Results

Children with autistic spectrum disorder recruited for this study

Thirty-eight children with ASD were recruited for this study. The distribution of severity of ASD in this subject group recruited was (number of cases) mild (6), moderate (6), and severe (26). The distribution of cognitive/developmental impairment was (number of cases) normal/borderline IQ (11), mild (3), moderate (12), and severe (12). The distribution of onset pattern of ASD was (number of cases) early (22), regressive (6), and mixed (10). The ADOS score ranged from 13 to 22 and the CARS total score from 31.5 to 48.5.

Plasma protein glycation, oxidation, and nitration

In plasma protein, protein content of AGEs—CML, MG-H1 and CMA—were increased in children with ASD, with respect to healthy controls, whereas plasma protein content of AGE, 3DG-H, was decreased in children with ASD, with respect to healthy controls. Plasma protein content of the oxidative damage adduct, DT, was increased in children with ASD, with respect to healthy controls. Only changes in CML, CMA, and DT remained significant after Bonferroni correction for measurement of multiple analytes (Table 2). In correlation analysis, highly significant positive correlations ($P < 0.01$, Spearman) were of CML with DT, G-H1 with MG-H1 and DT, MG-H1 with CMA, CMA with DT, and AASA with GSA—Additional file 1: Table S2. No correlation or association of glycation, oxidation, and nitration adduct residues was found with demographic and clinical features. There was no significant difference of these variables between subject groups of different genders with and without ASD.

Plasma glycated, oxidized, and nitrated amino acids and amino acid metabolome

For glycated, oxidized, and nitrated amino acid concentration in plasma, FL, G-H1, and NFK were decreased whereas CMA, AASA, and GSA were increased in children with ASD, with respect to healthy controls. Only increase in CMA remained significant after Bonferroni correction (Table 3). In correlation analysis, highly significant positive correlations were of pyrraline with MG-H1 and 3DG-H, FL with CML, G-H1 and MG-H1, CEL with MG-H1 and CMA, MG-H1 with 3DG-H, and CMA with AASA. There were highly significant negative correlations of pyrraline with NFK, CMA with MOLD, and MOLD with AASA—Additional file 1: Table S3.

For the conventional amino acid metabolome, there were increases in arg, gln, glu, and thr and decrease in trp in children with ASD, with respect to healthy controls. None of these changes remained significant after Bonferroni correction (Table 4). There were many highly significant positive correlations between plasma amino acid concentrations—Additional file 1: Table S4. No correlation or association of glycation, oxidation, and nitration free adducts and amino acids

Table 2 Glycation, oxidation, and nitration adduct residue content of plasma protein

Glycation markers	Healthy controls	ASD	*P* value
FL (mmol/mol lys)	1.27 ± 0.39	1.41 ± 0.53	NS
CML (mmol/mol lys)	0.158 ± 0.026	0.190 ± 0.038	0.0018*
CEL (mmol/mol lys)	0.117 ± 0.044	0.092 ± 0.054	NS
G-H1 (mmol/mol arg)	0.012 ± 0.005	0.016 ± 0.011	NS
MG-H1 (mmol/mol arg)	0.473 ± 0.074	0.535 ± 0.100	0.021
3DG-H (mmol/mol arg)	0.165 ± 0.037	0.138 ± 0.027	0.0052
CMA (mmol/mol arg)	0.054 (0.043–0.067)	0.077 (0.066–0.101)	0.000082**
MOLD (mmol/mol lys)	0.027 ± 0.011	0.025 ± 0.016	NS
GSP (mmol/mol lys)	0.514 ± 0.111	0.571 ± 0.206	NS
DT (mmol/mol tyr)	0.025 (0.019–0.031)	0.047 (0.035–0.094)	0.000012***
NFK (mmol/mol trp)	15.6 ± 1.7	15.0 ± 1.5	NS
AASA (mmol/mol lys)	0.154 ± 0.048	0.152 ± 0.081	NS
GSA (mmol/mol arg)	0.639 ± 0.327	0.713 ± 0.350	NS
3-NT (mmol/mol tyr)	0.0056 (0.0045–0.0069)	0.0053 (0.0045–0.0064)	NS

Data are median (lower–upper quartile); healthy controls, $n = 21$, and ASD, $n = 27$. Significance (Mann-Whitney *U*)
$^*P < 0.05$, $^{**}P < 0.01$, and $^{***}P < 0.001$ after Bonferroni correction of 14 applied

Table 3 Plasma and urinary glycation, oxidation, and nitration free adduct in plasma filtrate

Amino acid	Plasma (nM)			Urine (nmol/mg creatinine)		
	Healthy controls	ASD	*P* value	Healthy controls	ASD	*P* value
FL	1489 (987–1863)	751 (361–1.570)	0.047	56.7 (33.8–128.7)	90.8 (42.4–167.9)	
CML	807 (587–1051)	853 (219–1222)		26.2 (19.7–34.7)	33.1 (26.6–42.6)	0.016
CEL	402 (298–477)	420 (310–599)		0.435 (0.202–0.848)	0.472 (0.180–0.940)	
G-H1	0.819 (0.553–1.26)	0.527 (0.366–0.959)	0.037	1.88 (1.11–3.04)	2.57 (1.53–3.75)	0.024
MG-H1	271 (176–475)	335 (213–500)		18.6 (8.00–27.4)	24.5 (9.14–37.6)	
3DG-H	413 (303–637)	360 (280–434)		2.06 (0.587–4.38)	2.92 (1.09–6.26)	
CMA	9.18 (6.67–12.5)	17.7 (13.2–24.8)	0.00052**	1.46 (0.636–1.97)	1.78 (1.14–2.91)	0.037
GSP	12.8 (7.4–17.1)	12.9 (9.3–22.0)		1.58 (1.15–1.98)	1.53 (1.20–1.98)	
MOLD	1.79 (0.800–3.42)	1.10 (0.503–0.2.21)		0.025 (0.013–0.050)	0.040 (0.017–0.068)	0.027
Pyrraline	22.0 (12.2–30.4)	24.2 (19.4–40.6)		20.6 (14.9–44.2)	34.2 (22.7–72.5)	0.047
DT	0.501 (0.286–0.771)	0.676 (0.500–0.847)		0.070 (0.058–0.085)	0.086 (0.075–0.109)	0.0022*
NFK	15.2 (12.5–18.1)	11.3 (6.23–14.3)	0.030	0.117 (0.084–0.231)	0.179 (0.107–0.238)	0.037
AASA	19.7 (16.9–29.1)	30.6 (21.1–46.4)	0.0063	1.08 (0.805–2.76)	1.80 (1.13–2.89)	0.040
GSA	73.9 (53.2–129)	109 (80.1–203)	0.039	17.3 (13.2–22.7)	34.5 (12.7–48.0)	0.0018*
3-NT	1.10 (0.90–1.26)	1.17 (0.79–1.58)		0.0044 (0.001–0.010)	0.0077 (0.003–0.014)	

Data are median (lower – upper quartile); healthy controls, $n = 21–31$, and ASD, $n = 27–38$. Significance (Mann-Whitney *U*)
*$P < 0.05$ after Bonferroni correction of 15 applied

Table 4 Plasma and urinary amino acid metabolome

Amino acid	Plasma (μM)			Urine (nmol/mg creatinine)		
	Healthy controls	ASD	*P* value	Healthy controls	ASD	*P* value
Ala	294 ± 71.5	330 ± 98.3		301 (224–432)	392 (305–533)	0.030
Arg	39.4 ± 10.3	48.4 ± 16.6	0.016	52.1 ± 17.1	64.0 ± 18.0	0.014
Asn	33.2 ± 4.57	34.3 ± 10.6		92.4 (72.1–132)	169 (123–236)	0.0012*
Asp	35.5 ± 7.37	37.0 ± 10.0		142 (112–179)	160 (117–241)	
Cys (total)	41.7 ± 10.4	46.1 ± 15.0		25.3 (20.4–35.9)	28.3 (21.1–43.3)	
Gln	463 ± 38.6	496 ± 61.2	0.024	529 (452–704)	741 (609–876)	0.0048
Glu	1672 ± 324	1999 ± 619	0.034	373 (254–495)	475 (367–690)	0.010
Gly	272 (187–1061)	241 (121–515)		1.12 (1.19–2.78)	2.58 (1.84–3.45)	0.019
His	68.0 ± 8.51	72.8 ± 9.96		2.19 ± 0.88	2.90 ± 1.21	0.027
Ile	50.7 ± 15.3	51.6 ± 12.4		13.0 ± 4.37	18.1 ± 6.50	0.0059
Leu	126 ± 34.4	132 ± 25.6		43.1 ± 13.6	52.0 ± 13.5	0.028
Lys	132 ± 20.3	146 ± 36.7		136 (83.3–264)	171 (117–352)	
Met	23.1 ± 6.41	26.2 ± 5.84		17.9 ± 7.98	23.1 ± 7.20	0.0037
Phe	68.9 ± 11.3	68.8 ± 16.8		101 ± 38.9	110 ± 32.9	
Pro	195 ± 65.4	223 ± 94.7		14.5 ± 6.21	20.7 ± 5.37	0.00073**
Ser	128 ± 23.5	132 ± 18.7		461 (413–621)	677 (519–910)	0.0021*
Thr	116 ± 36.0	141 ± 46.8	0.041	216 (170–265)	283 (221–405)	0.0039
Trp	5.22 ± 1.26	3.92 ± 2.40	0.0055	114 ± 73.6	164 ± 48.6	0.0043
Tyr	84.4 ± 21.3	87.9 ± 26.8		204 (133–255)	240 (173–317)	
Val	125 ± 31.3	120 ± 26.0		25.6 ± 9.52	34.8 ± 10.9	0.00073**

Data are Mean ± SD or median (lower–upper quartile); healthy controls, $n = 21$, and ASD, $n = 27$. Significance: *t* test for parametric data and Mann-Whitney *U* for non-parametric data
*$P < 0.05$ and **$P < 0.01$ after Bonferroni correction of 20 applied

was found with demographic and clinical features. There was no significant difference of these variables between genders.

Urinary glycated, oxidized, and nitrated amino acids and amino acid metabolome and renal clearance

For the urinary flux of glycated, oxidized, and nitrated amino acids, children with ASD showed increased urinary excretion of CML, G-H1, CMA, MOLD, pyrraline, DT, NFK, AASA, and GSA. Only urinary excretions of DT and GSA remained significant after Bonferroni correction (Table 3). For the urinary flux of unmodified amino acids, children with ASD showed increased urinary excretion of all amino acids except asp, cys, lys, phe, and tyr. Only increases in urinary excretion of asn, pro, ser, and val remained significant after Bonferroni correction (Table 4). There were several highly significant positive correlations between urinary excretions of glycation, oxidation, and nitration adducts and amino acids—see Additional file 1: Table S5 and Table S6.

Renal clearance of CMA, GSP, DT, arg, glu, leu, phe, and thr were decreased and renal clearance of NFK and trp were increased in children with ASD, with respect to healthy controls. Only decreases in renal clearance of arg and CMA remained significant after Bonferroni correction: CL_{arg} decreased 32% and CL_{CMA} decreased 50% in children with ASD, compared to healthy control; $P < 0.001$ (Tables 5 and 6). No correlation or association of these glycation, oxidation, and nitration free adduct and amino acid variables was found with demographic and clinical features. There was no significant difference of these variables between genders.

Changes of glycation, oxidation, and nitration adducts and amino acid metabolome in plasma and urine are summarized in heat maps (Fig. 3a, b). Data distributions of biomarker with significantly different change in the ASD study group after Bonferroni correction are given in Fig. 4.

Table 5 Renal clearance of glycation, oxidation, and nitration free adducts

Amino acid	Renal clearance (μL/mg creatinine)		
	Healthy controls	ASD	*P* value
FL#	0.696 (0.375–1.16)	0.866 (0.384–2.31)	
CML	0.297 (0.249–0.387)	0.259 (0.171–0.782)	
CEL	0.0068 (0.003–0.019)	0.0042 (0.002–0.011)	
G-H1	21.2 (13.1–34.7)	23.9 (15.0–57.7)	
MG-H1#	0.718 (0.496–1.04)	0.628 (0.363–0.912)	
3DG-H	0.067 (0.033–0.163)	0.087 (0.042–0.131)	
CMA	1.57 (0.997–2.08)	0.791 (0.465–1.36)	0.0011*
GSP	0.121 (0.083–0.274)	0.112 (0.067–0.195)	
MOLD	0.214 (0.075–0.487)	0.269 (0.153–0.656)	
Pyrraline	0.81 (0.58–1.17)	1.07 (0.64–1.96)	
DT	0.119 (0.657–2.02)	0.747 (0.545–0.107)	0.0025
NFK	0.062 (0.038–0.109)	0.096 (0.049–0.139)	0.030
GSA	29.9 (11.1–45.8)	17.8 (1.96–26.1)	
3-NT	0.068 (0.034–0.100)	0.042 (0.036–0.129)	

Data are mean ± SD or median (lower–upper quartile); healthy controls, $n = 21$, and ASD, n = 27. Significance: t-test for parametric data and Mann-Whitney *U* for non-parametric data
*$P < 0.05$, after Bonferroni correction of 14 applied
#mL/mg creatinine

Development of diagnostic algorithms for ASD

To explore diagnostic utility of protein glycation, oxidation, and nitration measurements for ASD, we analyzed plasma and urinary amino acid analyte data by a machine learning approach. SVMs was the best-performing method out of the four algorithms that were investigated. Algorithm optimized from twofold cross-validation were as below.

(i) Algorithm-1, developed from plasma protein glycation, oxidation, and nitration adduct residue analytes.

It has the following features: CML, 3DG-H, CMA, and DT. Classification accuracy was 88%, sensitivity 92%, specificity 84%, and AUROC 0.94. A random outcome is 0.50.

(ii) Algorithm-2, developed from plasma glycated, oxidized, and nitrated amino acids and conventional amino acid metabolome.

It has the following features: CML and CMA. Classification accuracy was 75%, sensitivity 81%, and specificity 67% and AUROC 0.80.

(iii) Algorithm-3, developed from plasma protein glycation, oxidation, and nitration adduct residues and plasma glycated, oxidized, and nitrated amino acids and conventional amino acid metabolome combined.

It has the following features: plasma protein CML, 3DG-H, CMA and DT residues, and plasma G-H1 and GSA free adducts. Classification accuracy was 89%, sensitivity 90%, specificity 87%, and AUROC 0.95.

(iv) Algorithm-4, developed from urinary glycated, oxidized, and nitrated amino acids.

It has the following features: GSA and pyrraline free adducts. Classification accuracy was 77%, sensitivity 77%, specificity 76%, and AUROC 0.79 (Fig. 5, Table 7, and Additional file 1: Table S7).

The diagnostic algorithms were used to deduce the probability of having ASD for each patient diagnosed with ASD by clinical symptoms (Table 1). The association and

Table 6 Renal clearance of amino acids

Amino acid	Renal clearance (mL/mg creatinine)		
	Healthy controls	ASD	*P* value
Ala	1.03 (0.746–1.712)	1.27 (0.890–1.65)	
Arg	0.011 (0.009–0.015)	0.008 (0.006–0.010)	0.0019*
Asn	2.80 (2.22–4.76)	4.30 (3.05–7.14)	0.0055
Asp	3.81 (3.04–4.96)	4.73 (2.92–7.82)	
Cys (total)	0.646 (0.518–0.812)	0.629 (0.452–1.133)	
Gln	1.18 (0.913–1.53)	1.54 (1.14–1.96)	0.025
Glu	0.210 (0.158–0.304)	0.243 (0.179–0.357	0.049
Gly	0.0050 (0.002–0.009)	0.0067 (0.004–0.029)	0.018
His	0.029 (0.024–0.040)	0.040 (0.027–0.053)	
Ile	0.262 (0.192–0.347)	0.354 (0.256–0.441)	0.0116
Leu	0.358 ± 0.135	0.402 ± 0.105	
Lys	0.011 (0.005–0.018)	0.0071 (0.005–0.011)	
Met	0.0066 ± 0.0015	0.0056 ± 0.0023	
Phe	1.32 (0.959–2.02)	1.65 (1.33–1.95)	
Pro	0.077 ± 0.031	0.104 ± 0.039	0.0138
Ser	3.66 (2.95–4.79)	5.22 (3.99–6.78)	0.0081
Thr	2.023 ± 0.765	2.44 ± 1.05	
Trp	0.209 (0.155–0.242)	0.287 (0.166–0.497)	0.010
Tyr	0.0209 (0.016–0.025)	0.015 (0.012–0.025)	
Val	0.0017 (0.0014–0.0022)	0.0016 (0.0013–0.0026)	

Data are mean ± SD or median (lower-upper quartile); healthy controls, $n = 21$, and ASD, $n = 27$. Significance: *t* test for parametric data and Mann-Whitney *U* for non-parametric data

*$P < 0.05$, after Bonferroni correction of 20 applied

correlation of these probabilities with clinical features was explored. No significant association or correlation of these probabilities with clinical features (age, ADOS, total CARS, CARS hyperactivity and CARS body use scores, autism severity, cognitive/developmental impairment, and ASD onset pattern) was found.

Discussion

In this study, we identified changes in plasma protein AGE and oxidation adducts, increased CML, CMA, and DT and decreased 3DG-H in ASD. Combined in an algorithm, these features provided diagnostic performance improved over that previously achieved in transcriptomic, proteomic, and metabolomic studies [5–7]—with AUROC 0.94 and classification efficiency 88%. This was slightly improved by combination with plasma G-H1 and GSA free adducts, with AUROC 0.95 and classification efficiency 89%. This novel biomarker approach focused to protein damage or proteotoxic stress may lead to biochemical-based diagnosis of ASD and suggests that protein AGE and oxidation may be linked to ASD pathogenesis.

Change in AGE and oxidation adduct content of plasma proteins relates to the rate of protein modification in the plasma compartment and, to a lesser extent, to modifications of plasma proteins in interstitial fluid. The major plasma protein albumin makes repeated cycles from plasma to interstitial fluid and lymph before degradation [31]. CML residues in plasma protein are mainly produced by the oxidative degradation of FL with a usually minor contribution from glycation by glyoxal. CML is also considered to be a marker of oxidative damage [32]. CMA is

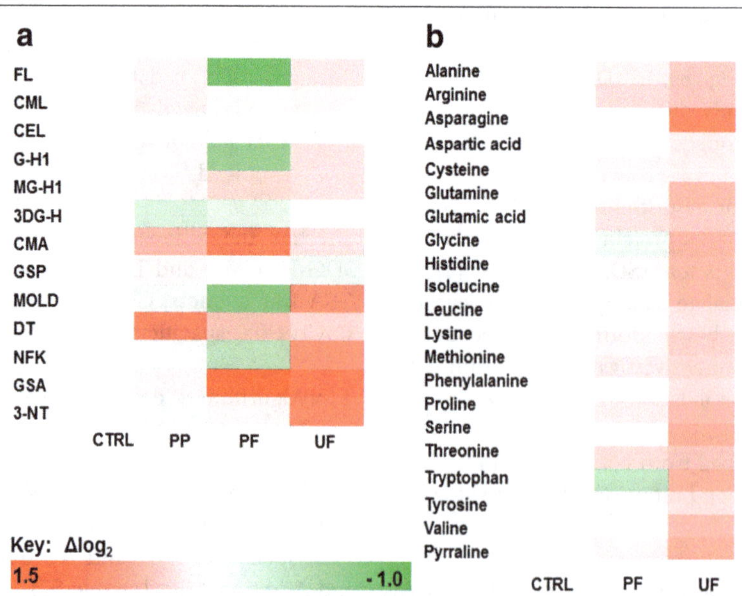

Fig. 3 Heat map of changes in glycated, oxidized, and nitrated proteins and amino acids in plasma and urine of subjects with autistic spectrum disorder. **a** Trace level protein glycation, oxidation, and nitration adducts. **b** Amino acid metabolome. Key: CTRL control, PP plasma protein (adduct residues), PF plasma filtrate (free adducts), and UF urine filtrate (free adducts). Data are given in Tables 2, 3, 4, and 5

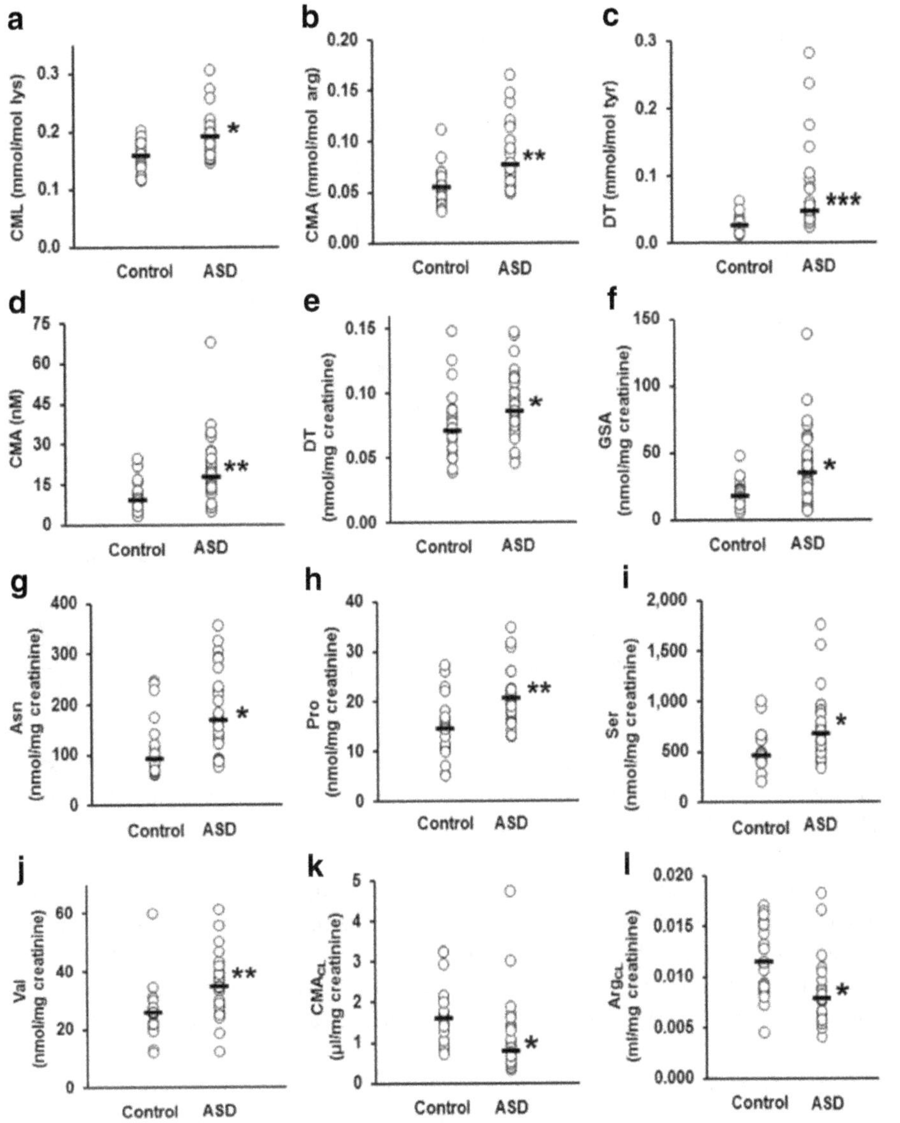

Fig. 4 Scatter plots for protein damage biomarker variables changed in children with ASD. Protein adduct residues: **a** CML, **b** CMA, and **c** DT. Plasma free adduct: **d** CMA. Urine free adduct and amino acids: **e** DT, **f** GSA, **g** Asn, **h** Pro, **i** Ser, and **j** Val. Renal clearance: **k** CMA and **l** Arg (an outlier point, 0.0565, was excluded from the ASD data). Significance: One asterisk, two asterisks, and three asterisks indicate $P < 0.05$, $P < 0.01$, and $P < 0.001$, respectively

produced exclusively by the glycation of proteins by glyoxal [9]. Increased formation of glyoxal, mainly sourced from lipid peroxidation, in ASD may explain increases in plasma protein CML and CMA (Fig. 6a). Markers of lipid peroxidation, plasma and red blood cell malondialdehyde, urinary 8-isoprostane-F2a, and hexanoyl-lysine adduct were elevated in ASD [33–35].

DT residue content of plasma proteins was increased in subjects with ASD whereas other oxidative damage markers, NFK, AASA, and GSA, were not. DT residue formation occurs by reaction of tyrosine residues in proteins with ROS and DUOX [36]. The selective increase in DT may suggest a role of increased DUOX activity in subjects with ASD. DUOX expression is increased through activating transcription factor 2 in inflammatory signaling [37]. DUOX has an important role in gut mucosal immunity, host–microbe homeostasis, and signaling for neutrophil recruitment into allergic airways [38, 39]. Gut microbiota may be influential in the development of the behavioral phenotype in ASD children [40] (Fig. 6a).

Decrease of 3DG-H content of plasma protein in subjects with ASD likely reflects decreased concentration of plasma 3-DG. 3-DG is formed by degradation of fructosamine-3-phosphate in the repair of early glycated proteins and degradation of fructose-3-phosphate formed by fructosamine-3-phosphokinase [41, 42] and the slow, non-enzymatic

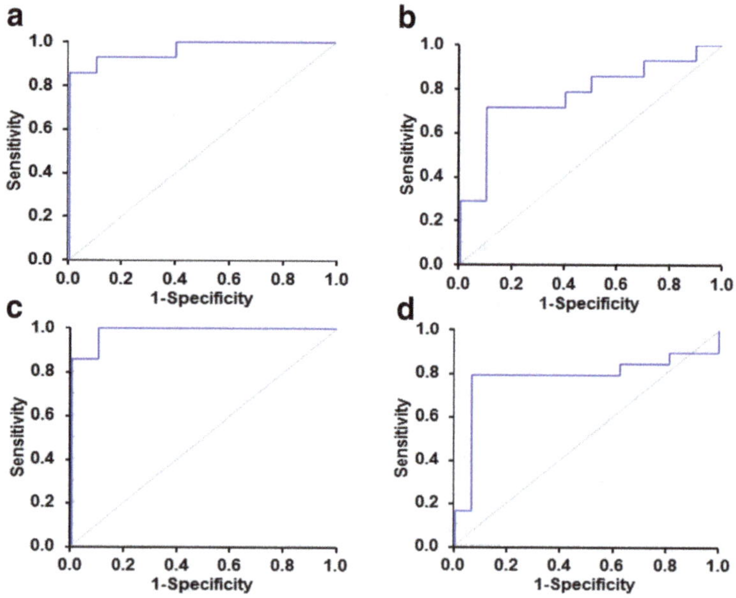

Fig. 5 Receiver operating characteristic plots of diagnostic algorithms for detection of autistic spectrum disorder by protein glycation and oxidation adducts. **a** Algorithm-1, plasma protein adduct residues. AUROC = 0.96. **b** Algorithm-2, plasma free adducts. AUROC = 0.78. **c** Algorithm-3, plasma protein adduct residues and free adducts. AUROC = 0.99. **d** Algorithm-4, urine free adducts. AUROC = 0.78. ROC plots are representative results from one run of the classification experiment. A random outcome is AUROC = 0.50

oxidative degradation of glucose and proteins glycated by glucose [43]. It is metabolized to 3-deoxyfructose by aldo-keto reductases 1A4, 1B1, and 1B3 which together constitute 3-DG reductase activity [44]. Since FL residue content of subjects with ASD was unchanged, with respect to healthy controls, there is unlikely to be decreased activity of fructosamine-3-phosphokinase in ASD. Rather, increased 3-DG reductase activity may explain decrease in plasma protein 3DG-H residue content in ASD (Fig. 6a).

Combination of markers of oxidative metabolism, DNA oxidation, and methylation in multivariate statistical models was recently found to distinguish between children with ASD and healthy controls [12]. Herein, oxidative damage markers, plasma protein CML and DT and plasma GSA free adduct, emerged as features of diagnostic algorithms for ASD. Measurement of multiple chemically defined markers of protein oxidative damage in plasma and urine compartments in subjects with and

Table 7 Diagnostic algorithms developed for autistic spectrum disorder from plasma and urinary analytes

Algorithm no	1	2	3	4
Compartment and analyte	Plasma protein adduct residues	Plasma amino acids	Plasma protein adduct residues and amino acids	Urinary amino acids
Features	CML, 3DG-H, CMA, and DT	CML and CMA	CML, 3DG-H, CMA, and DT residues with G-H1 and GSA free adducts	GSA and pyrraline free adducts
Accuracy (%)	88.3 (85.5–91.2)	74.8 (71.7–77.9)	89.0 (87.0–91.0)	76.8 (74.6–79.0)
Sensitivity (%)	91.9 (89.1–94.6)	80.5 (75.1–86.0)	90.4 (87.7–93.1)	77.1 (73.4–80.8)
Specificity (%)	83.9 (79.3–88.4)	67.1 (58.9–75.4)	87.3 (84.1–90.5)	76.4 (72.0–80.8)
AUROC	0.94 (0.91–0.96)	0.80 (0.77–0.83)	0.95 (0.94–0.96)	0.79 (0.76–0.81)
Positive likelihood ratio	5.69 (4.49–6.89)	2.85 (2.16–3.55)	7.23 (6.09–8.38)	4.16 (2.88–5.44)
Negative likelihood ratio	0.10 (0.07–0.13)	0.28 (0.21–0.35)	0.11 (0.08–0.14)	0.30 (0.25–0.34)
Positive predictive value (%)	88.2 (85.0–91.4)	77.1 (72.9–81.4)	90.2 (87.9–92.5)	80.6 (77.6–83.5)
Negative predictive value (%)	89.1 (85.5–92.6)	75.0 (70.6–79.4)	88.0 (85.1–91.0)	73.7 (71.0–76.5)
F score	0.90 (0.87–0.92)	0.78 (0.75–0.81)	0.90 (0.88–0.92)	0.78 (0.76–0.81)

Algorithm outcomes for twofold cross-validation (10 randomized repeat trials for robustness) using SVMs (95% CI given in brackets)

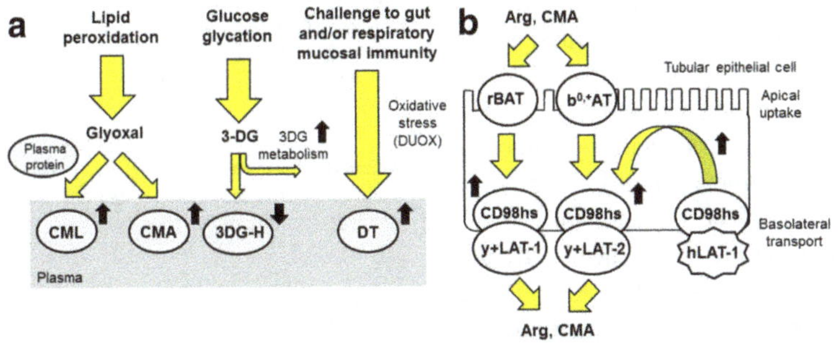

Fig. 6 Schematic explanation for changes found in protein damage and amino acids in ASD. **a** Proposed mechanism for observed changes found in plasma protein glycation and oxidation adducts. **b** Transport of arg and CMA across the renal tubular epithelium and proposed mechanism for increased renal CL (increased arg and CMA reuptake). Key: yellow-filled arrows show processes; black-filled arrows show changes observed (**a**) and changes expected (**b**) in ASD

without ASD has provided evidence of changes specific to oxidative damage marker type and sample compartment that likely contributed to algorithm development for ASD with improved diagnostic performance.

For unmodified amino acids, we found no changes after correction for multiple measurements in plasma but there were significant increases in urinary excretion of asn, pro, ser, and val. This may relate to impaired tissue uptake and retention of these amino acids in ASD. For modified amino acids, only increased CMA remained significantly increased in plasma for children with ASD. This may relate to proteolysis of plasma proteins and potentially other proteins of increased CMA residue content in ASD. For modified amino acids in urine, urinary excretions of oxidative damage markers, DT and GSA free adducts, were increased in children with ASD after correction for multiple analytes. This may relate to proteolysis of plasma proteins and other proteins with increased oxidative damage and DUOX-catalyzed modification in ASD. The amino acid metabolome in plasma and urine has been explored previously for biomarkers of ASD [7, 45–47]. We confirmed the reported minor increase in plasma arg in ASD, compared to healthy controls, but significance was lost after correction for multiple measurements [48].

Pyrraline is an AGE sourced only from food [49]. Increased urinary pyrraline is indicative of increased food consumption and/or permeability of the gastrointestinal tract to pyrraline. The positive correlation of pyrraline with CML, MG-H1, CMA, DT, and GSA free adducts in urine suggests that increase of these free adducts may be partly due to food consumption.

Exploring changes in renal CL of amino acids provides insight in functional activity of amino acid transporters in the renal tubular epithelium. The deduction of CL herein was an indirect measure based on estimates of urinary analyte/creatinine ratio rather than urinary analyte excretion rate determined in urine collection made over a fixed time interval, usually 24 h. This was done because of difficulties in timed collection of urine in children [50]. Decreased CL relates to increased tubular reuptake and increased amino acid transporter activity. Decreased CL of arg and CMA likely reflects increased reuptake of arg and CMA. Arg uptake by the tubular epithelium is mediated by neutral and basic amino acid transport protein rBAT and solute carrier 7, member 9 ($b^{0,+}$AT) [apical uptake] and CD98 heavy subunit (CD98hs)/y+LAT-2 (solute carrier family 7 member 6) and CD98hs/y+LAT-1 (solute carrier family 7 member 7) complexes [basolateral transport] [51] and this likely mediates renal tubule uptake of arginine derivative CMA too (Fig. 6b). Homozygous mutations of SLC7A5 gene were associated with ASD. SLC7A5 encodes protein hLAT-1 which, together with CD98hs, form the large neutral amino acid transporter involved in maintaining normal levels of brain branched chain amino acids in the brain [52]. Dysfunction of hLAT-1, also found in the renal tubular epithelium in complex with CD98hs [51], may leave the latter more available for complexation with y+LAT-1 and y+LAT-2 and drive increased reuptake and decreased CL of arginine and CMA. In addition, rare holomorphic variants in males of amino acid transporter CAT-3 were associated with ASD [15]. Disturbance in arginine transporter function may be a common feature of ASD and measure of CL of arginine is an accessible biomarker of this.

Combination of AGE and DT residue content of plasma protein in Algorithm-1 and this combined with G-H1 and GSA free adducts in Algorithm-3 gave the best diagnostic performance for detection of ASD from the analytes determined herein. The absence of conventional, unmodified amino acids from optimum features of the diagnostic algorithms suggests that assay of trace level, AGE and oxidised amino acid residues of plasma protein and free adducts in plasma provides a diagnostic advantage which has not been hitherto explored. It also suggests that AGE and oxidation proteotoxic stress may underly the development of ASD, at least in part. Protein glycation and oxidation adducts from dietary protein contribute to levels of plasma and urinary glycation and oxidation free adducts; whereas glycation and oxidation adduct residues of protein reflect rates of endogenous glycation and oxidation of protein in mainly the vascular compartment. The dominance of plasma protein AGE and oxidation adducts in Algorithm-1 and the modest improvement by addition of plasma G-H1 and GSA free adducts (Algorithm-3) may indicate that there is limited influence of dietary glycated and oxidized proteins to the development of ASD. Rather, challenge to proteostasis by changes in endogenous protein modification by AGEs and DT may contribute to the development of ASD.

Conclusions

We identified changes in plasma protein glycation and oxidation markers; increased CML, CMA, and DT and decreased 3DG-H that combined in an algorithm gave improved diagnostic performance over other approaches. Increased levels of DT may indicate induction of increased DUOX activity linked to gut mucosa dysfunction. Disturbance of renal handling of arginine and CMA may indicate dysfunctional arginine transporter function common in ASD. Further clinical validation of plasma protein CML, CMA, DT, and 3DG-H may provide improved diagnosis of ASD. For future studies, we suggest firstly validation of the current findings in an independent clinical study group. Thereafter, priorities are investigation of the biomarkers in children younger than 5 years old to assess their ability to improve diagnosis at earlier stages of ASD development, assessment of the biomarkers in prospective studies for prediction of risk of progression to severe symptoms, study of the association of genetic polymorphisms of DUOX and arginine transporters with clinical ASD, preclinical functional genomics of DUOX and arginine transporters with an ASD-like phenotype, and assessment of the specificity of the algorithms for ASD versus other psychiatric conditions.

Abbreviations

3-DG: 3-Deoxyglucosone; 3DG-H: Hydroimidazolone AGEs derived from 3-deoxyglucosone; 3-NT: 3-Nitrotyrosine; AASA: α-Aminoadipic semialdehyde; ADOS: Autism diagnostic observation schedule; AGE: Advanced glycation endproduct; ASD: Autism spectrum disorder; AUROC: Area under-the-curve of receiver operating characteristic plot; $b^{0,+}$AT: Solute carrier 7, member 9; CARS: Childhood autism rating scale; CAT-3: Cationic amino acid transporter-3; CD98hs: Cluster of differentiation heavy subunit; CEL: N_ε-(1-carboxyethyl)lysine; CL: Renal clearance; CMA: N_ω-carboxymethylarginine; CML: N_ε-carboxymethyl-lysine; DT: Dityrosine; DUOX: Dual oxidase; EDTA: Ethylenediaminetetra-acetic acid; FL: N_ε-fructosyl-lysine; G-H1: Hydroimidazolone AGE derived from glyoxal; GSA: Glutamic semialdehyde; GSP: Glucosepane; hLAT-1: Large neutral amino acid transporter subunit-1; LC-MS/MS: Liquid chromatography-tandem mass spectrometry; Leiter-R: Leiter international performance scale–revised; MG: Methylglyoxal; MG-H1: Hydroimidazolone AGE derived from methylglyoxal MOLD, methylglyoxal-derived lysine crosslink; MRM: Multiple reaction monitoring; NFK: *N*-Formylkynurenine; PEP-3: Psychoeducational profile-3; rBAT: Neutral and basic amino acid transport protein; ROS: Reactive oxygen species; SLC7A5: Solute carrier family 7, member 5; SVM: Support vector machines; TD: Typically developing; UPR: Unfolded protein response; y+LAT-1: Solute carrier family 7 member 7; y+LAT-2: Solute carrier family 7 member 6

Acknowledgements

We thank all the subjects recruited and their parents for agreeing to participate in this study.

Funding

This work received funding from Warwick Impact Fund award to NR and funding from Fondazione del Monte di Bologna e Ravenna, Italy, and from Fondazione Nando Peretti, Rome, Italy, to M.M.

Authors' contributions

MM, PMA, AG, PJT, and NR designed the research; PV and AP chose the autistic and the control subjects, carried out the clinical evaluation, and supervised the blood withdrawal and urine collection; AB organized the handling of biological samples, performed some preliminary experimental procedures, and kept the records; AA and SP analyzed the clinical samples and extracted analytical data, AG, KR, PJT, and NR analyzed the data and checked the data extraction; PJT, NR, MM, and PMA wrote the manuscript. All authors read, edited, and approved the final manuscript.

Competing interests

The authors declare that they have no competing interests.

Author details

[1]Warwick Medical School, University of Warwick, Clinical Sciences Research Laboratories, University Hospital, Coventry, UK. [2]Department of Experimental, Diagnostic and Specialty Medicine, School of Medicine, University of Bologna, Via Belmeloro 8, 40126 Bologna, Italy. [3]Department of Computer Science, University of Birmingham, Birmingham, UK. [4]Don Carlo Gnocchi Foundation ONLUS, IRCCS "S. Maria Nascente", Via Alfonso Capecelatro 66, 20148 Milan, Italy. [5]Child Neurology and Psychiatry Unit, IRCCS Institute of Neurological Sciences, Via Altura, 3, 40139 Bologna, Italy. [6]Department of Biomedical and Neuromotor Sciences, University of Bologna, Via Altura 3, 40139 Bologna, Italy. [7]Zeeman Institute for Systems Biology & Infectious Disease Epidemiology Research, Senate House, University of Warwick, Coventry CV4 7AL, UK. [8]Research Technology Platform–Proteomics, University of Warwick, Coventry, UK.

References

1. American-Psychiatric-Association. Diagnostic and statistical manual of mental disorders. Washington, DC: American Psychiatric Publishing; 2013.
2. Walsh P, Elsabbagh M, Bolton P, Singh I. In search of biomarkers for autism: scientific, social and ethical challenges. Nat Rev Neurosci. 2011;12(10):603–12.
3. Abruzzo PM, Ghezzo A, Bolotta A, Ferreri C, Minguzzi R, Vignini A, Visconti P, Marini M. Perspective biological markers for autism spectrum disorders: advantages of the use of receiver operating characteristic curves in evaluating marker sensitivity and specificity. Dis Markers. 2015;2015:329607.
4. Loke YJ, Hannan AJ, Craig JM. The role of epigenetic change in autism spectrum disorders. Front Neurol. 2015;6:18.
5. Scherer SW, Dawson G. Risk factors for autism: translating genomic discoveries into diagnostics. Hum Genet. 2011;130(1):123–48.
6. Momeni N, Bergquist J, Brudin L, Behnia F, Sivberg B, Joghataei MT, Persson BL. A novel blood-based biomarker for detection of autism spectrum disorders. Transl Psychiatry. 2012;2(3):e91.
7. Diémé B, Mavel S, Blasco H, Tripi G, Bonnet-Brilhault F, Malvy J, Bocca C, Andres CR, Nadal-Desbarats L, Emond P. Metabolomics study of urine in autism spectrum disorders using a multiplatform analytical methodology. J Proteome Res. 2015;14(12):5273–82.

8. Louros SR, Osterweil EK. Perturbed proteostasis in autism spectrum disorders. J Neurochem. 2016;139(6):1081–92.
9. Thornalley PJ, Rabbani N. Detection of oxidized and glycated proteins in clinical samples using mass spectrometry—a user's perspective. Biochim Biophys Acta. 2014;1840(2):818–29.
10. Melnyk S, Fuchs GJ, Schulz E, Lopez M, Kahler SG, Fussell JJ, Bellando J, Pavliv O, Rose S, Seidel L, et al. Metabolic imbalance associated with methylation dysregulation and oxidative damage in children with autism. J Autism Dev Disord. 2012;42(3):367–77.
11. Frye RE, DeLaTorre R, Taylor H, Slattery J, Melnyk S, Chowdhury N, James SJ. Redox metabolism abnormalities in autistic children associated with mitochondrial disease. Transl Psychiatry. 2013;3:e273.
12. Howsmon DP, Kruger U, Melnyk S, James SJ, Hahn J. Classification and adaptive behavior prediction of children with autism spectrum disorder based upon multivariate data analysis of markers of oxidative stress and DNA methylation. PLoS Comput Biol. 2017;13(3):e1005385.
13. Hetz C, Chevet E, Oakes SA. Proteostasis control by the unfolded protein response. Nat Cell Biol. 2015;17(7):829–38.
14. Janssens S, Pulendran B, Lambrecht BN. Emerging functions of the unfolded protein response in immunity. Nat Immunol. 2014;15(10):910–9.
15. Nava C, Rupp J, Boissel J-P, Mignot C, Rastetter A, Amiet C, Jacquette A, Dupuits C, Bouteiller D, Keren B, et al. Hypomorphic variants of cationic amino acid transporter 3 in males with autism spectrum disorders. Amino Acids. 2015;47(12):2647–58.
16. Bala KA, Dogan M, Mutluer T, Kaba S, Aslan O, Balahoroglu R, Cokluk E, Ustyol L, Kocaman S. Plasma amino acid profile in autism spectrum disorder (ASD). European Review for Medical and Pharmacological Sciences. 2016; 20(5):923–9.
17. Schopler E, Reichler RJ, Renner BR. The childhood autism rating scale. Los Angeles: Western Psychological Services; 1994.
18. Ozonoff S, Heung K, Byrd R, Hansen R, Hertz-Picciotto I. The onset of autism: patterns of symptom emergence in the first years of life. Autism research : official journal of the International Society for Autism Research. 2008;1(6): 320–8.
19. Schopler E, Lansing MD, Reichler RJ, Marcus LM. Psychoeducational profile. 3rd ed. Torrance: Western Psychological Services; 2005.
20. Roid G, Miller LJ. Leiter international performance scale-revised: examiners manual. Wood Dale: Stoelting Co.; 1997.
21. Keys A. Epidemiological studies related to coronary heart disease: characteristics of men aged 40–59 in seven countries. Acta Medica Scandinavica. 1966;180:4–5.
22. Rabbani N, Shaheen F, Anwar A, Masania J, Thornalley PJ. Assay of methylglyoxal-derived protein and nucleotide AGEs. Biochem Soc Trans. 2014;42(2):511–7.
23. Ahmed U, Anwar A, Savage RS, Costa ML, Mackay N, Filer A, Raza K, Watts RA, Winyard PG, Tarr J, et al. Biomarkers of early stage osteoarthritis, rheumatoid arthritis and musculoskeletal health. Sci Rep. 2015;5:9259.
24. Ahmed U, Anwar A, Savage RS, Thornalley PJ, Rabbani N. Protein oxidation, nitration and glycation biomarkers for early-stage diagnosis of osteoarthritis of the knee and typing and progression of arthritic disease. Arthritis Res Ther. 2016;18(1):250.
25. Ahmed U, Anwar A, Savage RS, Costa ML, Mackay N, Filer A, Raza K, Watts RA, Winyard PG, Tarr J, et al. Biomarkers of early stage osteoarthritis, rheumatoid arthritis and musculoskeletal health. Sci Rep. 2015;5(9259):9251–7.
26. Breiman L. Random forests. Mach Learn. 2001;45(1):5–32.
27. Friedman J, Hastie T, Tibshirani R. Regularization paths for generalized linear models via coordinate descent. J Statistical Software. 2010;33(1):1–22.
28. Sajda P. Machine learning for detection and diagnosis of disease. Annu Rev Biomed Eng. 2006;8(1):537–65.
29. Rhemtulla M, Brosseau-Liard PE, Savalei V. When can categorical variables be treated as continuous? A comparison of robust continuous and categorical SEM estimation methods under suboptimal conditions. Psychol Methods. 2012;17(3):354–73.
30. Xue M, Weickert MO, Qureshi S, Ngianga-Bakwin K, Anwar A, Waldron M, Shafie A, Messenger D, Fowler M, Jenkins G, et al. Improved glycemic control and vascular function in overweight and obese subjects by glyoxalase 1 inducer formulation. Diabetes. 2016;65(8):2282–94.
31. Margarson MP, Soni N. Serum albumin: touchstone or totem? Anaesthesia. 1998;53(8):789–803.
32. Knecht KJ, Dunn JA, McFarland KF, McCance DR, Lyons TJ, Thorpe SR, Baynes JW. Effect of diabetes and aging on carboxymethyllysine levels in human urine. Diabetes. 1991;40(2):190–6.
33. Chauhan A, Chauhan V, Brown WT, Cohen I. Oxidative stress in autism: increased lipid peroxidation and reduced serum levels of ceruloplasmin and transferrin-the antioxidant proteins. Life Sci. 2004;75(21):2539–49.
34. Ming X, Stein TP, Brimacombe M, Johnson WG, Lambert GH, Wagner GC. Increased excretion of a lipid peroxidation biomarker in autism. Prostaglandins Leukot Essent Fat Acids. 2005;73(5):379–84.
35. Ghezzo A, Visconti P, Abruzzo PM, Bolotta A, Ferreri C, Gobbi G, Malisardi G, Manfredini S, Marini M, Nanetti L, et al. Oxidative stress and erythrocyte membrane alterations in children with autism: correlation with clinical features. PLoS One. 2013;8(6):14.
36. Lévigne D, Modarressi A, Krause K-H, Pittet-Cuénod B. NADPH oxidase 4 deficiency leads to impaired wound repair and reduced dityrosine-crosslinking, but does not affect myofibroblast formation. Free Radic Biol Med. 2016;96:374–84.
37. Ha E-M, Lee K-A, Seo YY, Kim S-H, Lim J-H, Oh B-H, Kim J, Lee W-J. Coordination of multiple dual oxidase-regulatory pathways in responses to commensal and infectious microbes in drosophila gut. Nat Immunol. 2009; 10(9):949–57.
38. Bae YS, Choi MK, Lee W-J. Dual oxidase in mucosal immunity and host-microbe homeostasis. Trends Immunol. 2010;31(7):278–87.
39. Chang S, Linderholm A, Franzi L, Kenyon N, Grasberger H, Harper R. Dual oxidase regulates neutrophil recruitment in allergic airways. Free Radic Biol Med. 2013;65:38–46.
40. Mussap M, Noto A, Fanos V. Metabolomics of autism spectrum disorders: early insights regarding mammalian-microbial cometabolites. Expert Rev Mol Diagn. 2016;16(8):869–81.
41. Delpierre G, Rider MH, Collard F, Stroobant V, Vanstapel F, Santos H, Van Schaftingen E. Identification, cloning, and heterologous expression of a mammalian fructosamine-3-kinase. Diabetes. 2000;49(10):1627–34.
42. Lal S, Randall WC, Taylor AH, Kappler F, Walker M, Brown TR, Szwergold BS. Fructose-3-phosphate production and polyol pathway metabolism in diabetic rat hearts. Metabolism. 1997;46(11):1333–8.
43. Thornalley PJ, Langborg A, Minhas HS. Formation of glyoxal, methylglyoxal and 3-deoxyglucosone in the glycation of proteins by glucose. BiochemJ. 1999;344(1):109–16.
44. Baba SP, Barski OA, Ahmed Y, O'Toole TE, Conklin DJ, Bhatnagar A, Srivastava S. Reductive metabolism of AGE precursors: a metabolic route for preventing AGE accumulation in cardiovascular tissue. Diabetes. 2009;58(11): 2486–97.
45. Ming X, Stein TP, Barnes V, Rhodes N, Guo L. Metabolic perturbance in autism spectrum disorders: a metabolomics study. J Proteome Res. 2012; 11(12):5856–62.
46. West PR, Amaral DG, Bais P, Smith AM, Egnash LA, Ross ME, Palmer JA, Fontaine BR, Conard KR, Corbett BA, et al. Metabolomics as a tool for discovery of biomarkers of autism spectrum disorder in the blood plasma of children. PLoS One. 2014;9(11):e112445.
47. Gevi F, Zolla L, Gabriele S, Persico AM. Urinary metabolomics of young Italian autistic children supports abnormal tryptophan and purine metabolism. Molecular Autism. 2016;7(1):47.
48. Kuwabara H, Yamasue H, Koike S, Inoue H, Kawakubo Y, Kuroda M, Takano Y, Iwashiro N, Natsubori T, Aoki Y, et al. Altered metabolites in the plasma of autism spectrum disorder: a capillary electrophoresis time-of-flight mass spectroscopy study. PLoS One. 2013;8(9):e73814.
49. Foerster A, Henle T. Glycation in food and metabolic transit of dietary AGEs (advanced glycation end-products): studies on the urinary excretion of pyrraline. BiochemSocTrans 2003; 31:1383-1385.

5

Reversed gender ratio of autism spectrum disorder in Smith-Magenis syndrome

Heidi Elisabeth Nag[1,2*], Ann Nordgren[3], Britt-Marie Anderlid[3] and Terje Nærland[4,5]

Abstract

Background: A substantial amount of research shows a higher rate of autistic type of problems in males compared to females. The 4:1 male to female ratio is one of the most consistent findings in autism spectrum disorder (ASD). Lately, the interest in studying ASD in genetic disorders has increased, and research has shown a higher prevalence of ASD in some genetic disorders than in the general population.

Smith-Magenis syndrome (SMS) is a rare and complex genetic syndrome caused by an interstitial deletion of chromosome 17p11.2 or a mutation on the retinoic acid induced 1 gene. The disorder is characterised by intellectual disability, multiple congenital anomalies, obesity, neurobehavioural abnormalities and a disrupted circadian sleep-wake pattern.

Methods: Parents of 28 persons with SMS between 5 and 50 years old participated in this study. A total of 12 of the persons with SMS were above the age of 18 at the time of the study. A total of 11 came from Sweden and 17 were from Norway.

We collected information regarding the number of autism spectrum symptoms using the Social Communication Questionnaire (SCQ) and the Social Responsiveness Scale (SRS). Adaptive behaviour was also measured using the Vineland Adaptive Behavior Scale II. The level of intellectual disability was derived from a review of the medical chart.

Results: We found significant gender differences in ASD symptomatology using the SCQ and SRS questionnaires. We found approximately three females per male above the SCQ cutoff. The same differences were not found in the intellectual level and adaptive behaviour or for behavioural and emotional problems.

Gender had an independent contribution in a regression model predicting the total SCQ score, and neither the Vineland Adaptive Behavior Scale II nor the Developmental Behaviour Checklist had an independent contribution to the SCQ scores.

Conclusion: We found a clear reversed gender difference in ASD symptomatology in persons with SMS. This may be relevant in the search for female protective factors assumed to explain the male bias in ASD.

Keywords: Gender, Autism symptomatology, Smith-Magenis syndrome

Background

A substantial amount of research shows a higher rate of autistic type problems in males compared to females. The 4:1 male to female ratio is one of the most consistent findings in autism spectrum disorder (ASD) research [1–3], and a gender difference has been a part of the description of ASD since the first characterisation of the disorders.

ASD occurs in conditions with X-linked recessive inheritance, but because of the rarity of these disorders, this inheritance cannot explain the male bias in prevalence of ASD [4]. The fact that most ASD risk loci are found in autosomal regions makes the male bias in ASD largely unexplained [5]. Most current data suggest that the male bias is more likely to be due to female protective factors rather than male-specific risk factors, but comprehensive molecular explanations are lacking for both [6].

Gender ratios in ASD differ substantially from study to study. Among individuals with ASD and normal cognitive functioning, gender differences as high as 9:1 have been reported [7]. A newer systematic review and meta-

* Correspondence: hel@frambu.no
[1]Frambu Resource Centre for Rare Disorders, Siggerud, Norway
[2]University of Stavanger, Stavanger, Norway

analysis from Loomes et al. [8] found a male to female ratio closer to 3:1 than 4:1. According to Loomes et al. [8], the main reasons for this change were both how ASD was diagnosed and what population were used to investigate the male to female ratio in ASD in different studies. Loomes [8] found that studies screening the general populations for ASD had a lower male to female ratio than studies investigating population with pre-existing diagnosis. In cohorts with ASD in combination with intellectual disability, the ratio varies between 2:1–7:1 [2, 4]. Loomes et al. [8] also found a lower male to female ratio in their meta-analysis in the subgroup of the studies including participants with lower IQ. Epidemiological studies describe the degree of intellectual disability and the ascertainment approach as major explanations behind the varying ratios that were reported [9].

The particular biological aetiologies of autistic problems are probably also relevant, even when the degree of intellectual disability (ID) is controlled for, but such a line of investigation has not yet been explored. How different biological pathways to ASD differ in the ASD-gender ratio may shed light on basic ASD biology.

ASD is in the Diagnostic and Statistical Manual V (DSM V) referred to as a dyad of impairments; difficulties in social interactions and social communications; and restricted and repetitive behaviour, interests, and activities [10]. Gender differences in profiles of autistic symptoms have a limited research base [11]. Several studies [11–13] have found that males have more restricted and repetitive behaviours than females. Some studies have found that females have more impairment in social reciprocity and communication than males, but these findings are not consistent [13]; others have found that females with ASD have better sociability skills than males with ASD [14].

Lately, the interest in studying ASD in genetic disorders has increased, and research shows a higher prevalence of ASD in some genetic disorders than in the general population [15]. The focus so far has been on the prevalence and phenomenology in different syndromes, and further studies are required to tell us more about the differences in ASD phenomenology between ASD in genetic syndromes and idiopathic autism. Using the Autism Screening Questionnaire (ASQ), Oliver et al. [16] found a high level of autism (> 45%) in individuals with Cornelia de Lange syndrome (CdLS) and fragile X syndrome (FXS) (only males with FXS participated in the study) but lower levels in individuals with cri du chat syndrome (CDCS), Angelman syndrome and Prader Willis syndrome (PWS) (< 20%). Individuals with Lowe syndrome and Smith-Magenis syndrome (SMS) were more in the middle with approximately 35% scoring above the cutoff for autism. No significant gender differences in any of the syndromes were found. Another study concerning tuberous sclerosis (TSC) found no significant differences between females and males regarding ASD [17]. Recently, Nærland et al. [18] published an article regarding gender differences in Down syndrome. The gender ratios in their sample were approximately 2M:1F, which is slightly less than expected in idiopathic ASD with the same degree of ID.

SMS is one of the rare disorders where ASD has been described as a prominent part of the disorder [19] but also a disorder where gender differences in ASD symptoms, favouring females, have been found. Laje et al. [19] found that females had higher *T* scores on the Social Responsiveness Scale (SRS) total and on the 'Social cognition' and 'Autistic mannerisms' subscales. In this study, they did not control for the gender differences already accounted for in the gender-specific norms. They did not find any significant gender differences in Social Communication Questionnaire (SCQ) scores [20].

SMS is a rare and complex genetic syndrome caused by an interstitial deletion of chromosome 17p11.2 [21] or a mutation on the retinoic acid induced 1 (RAI1) gene [22]. Most SMS patients have a deletion containing 76 genes [23], but the patients with mutations in the RAI1 gene also display most of the core features of SMS, which indicates that the RAI1 gene is a dosage-sensitive gene responsible for most of the symptoms in SMS patients [24]. The disorder is characterised by intellectual disability, multiple congenital anomalies, obesity, neurobehavioural abnormalities and a disrupted circadian sleep-wake pattern [25]. The incidence of SMS is estimated to range from 1:15,000–1:25,000 births [26]. Delayed diagnosis is common, although the use of array-CGH and SNP-array analyses in routine clinical practice, together with greater recognition of the syndrome in the last decade, has led to earlier diagnosis [27].

Children and adults with SMS appear to have unique neurobehavioural problems that are challenging for both parents and professionals. These problems include sleep disturbances, self-injurious and maladaptive behaviours, stereotypies, and sensory integration disorders [28]. A thorough investigation of aggressive behaviours of a cohort with SMS showed that self-injurious behaviour, physical aggression and destructive behaviour were all significantly more prevalent in persons with SMS compared with a cohort of persons with IDs of mixed aetiologies [29]. In this study, 96.9% of participants displayed self-injurious behaviour, 87.5% exhibited physical aggression, 81.3% showed destructive behaviour and 43.8% were verbally aggressive [29]. SRS scores consistent with ASD have also been identified in almost 90% of the investigated populations with SMS [19]. A progression of autistic-like behaviour has also been described in young children with SMS [20]. A study comparing several genetic disorders (PWS, FXS, CdLS, CDCS, etc.) found that persons with SMS scored higher (were more impaired) than PWS and CDCS in the social domain, but in the two other domains (communication and repetitive behaviour), they did not differ from the other groups [16].

In addition to the study by Laje [19] mentioned earlier, two other studies have looked at gender differences in SMS [19, 30]. In an animal model study, Huang et al. [24] found a sexually dimorphic phenotype regarding obesity in mice (females were significantly more obese than males) with loss of RAI1 functions, but due to high mortality, they did not investigate this any further and the cause of the sexually dimorphic phenotype is not clear. Edelman et al. [30] found some somatic differences between males and females such as myopia, cold hands and feet, eating/appetite problems and possible hypersensitivity (problems finding shoes to fit) in females; Edelman et al. also found that females had more frustration with communication than males.

Measuring ASD in genetic syndromes is fraught with some difficulties. Individuals with known genetic syndromes are usually excluded from the standardisation of ASD assessment tools, and it is known that degree of intellectual disability influences these tools [31]. Additionally, it is recently documented that the commonly used ASD assessment tools are highly influenced by parent-reported behavioural and emotional problems [32]. In the SMS population with its varying cognitive abilities and high rates of behavioural problems, it is therefore important to control for these factors when making claims about ASD symptomatology.

The main aim of this study was to investigate gender differences in rates and profile of ASD symptoms in SMS when controlling for rates of emotional and behaviour problems and adaptive behaviour as a proxy for developmental level. Based on previous research and our own clinical experiences, we hypothesised that the usual increased rate of ASD symptoms in males (the male bias) would be absent in a sample of individuals with SMS.

Methods

Recruitment and participants

This study was part of a larger assessment study of SMS in Norway and Sweden. The participants were recruited through Frambu Resource Centre for Rare Disorders (Frambu) and the Smith-Magenis Foundations in Norway and Sweden (both family support groups). Both organisations spread information regarding the study via their Facebook sites and email lists. Frambu, which is one of nine publicly funded centres of expertise administered by the Norwegian National Advisory Unit on Rare Disorders, has its own register, which is based on informed consent. Frambu could therefore send invitations to registered families with a child or an adult with a diagnosis of SMS. The Swedish families were recruited through the Swedish Smith-Magenis Foundation both through information via their Facebook site and through information at their annual gathering. The only inclusion criterion was a genetically confirmed diagnosis of SMS. The diagnosis was confirmed by review of the genetic testing reports. The parents and the patients above the age of 16 provided written consent to participate in the study.

Parents of 28 persons with SMS aged between 5 and 50 years participated in this study; 12 of the persons with SMS were above the age of 18 at the time of the study. A total of 11 came from Sweden and 17 were from Norway (all the Norwegian patients were recruited through Frambu). In Norway, we know of 36 patients diagnosed with SMS and in Sweden 20; we have thus included approximately 47% of the Norwegian and approximately 55% of the Swedish SMS population. In Norway, 58% ($n = 21$) are females and in Sweden, 50% ($n = 10$) are females.

The level of ID was derived from a review of the medical charts. Consents were given to collect medical charts from the paediatric/habilitation and pedagogical centres. The levels of ID were collected from these charts. There was a wide variety as to who administered the test, with what instrument and at what age the level of ID was established.

Demographics

The demographics are displayed in Table 1. The mean age was 18.5 with a range from 5.1–50.5. The intellectual disability (ID) level was available from medical charts; seven of the patients did not have ID. It seems that more females had lower levels of ID, but this gender difference was not significant (asympt. $p = 0.07$).

Table 1 Demographics

	Total	Females	Males
N	28	15	13
Mean age	18.5	16.2	22.2
Range	5.1–50.5	5.1–33.9	5.1–50.5
Genetics			
Deletion	25	12	13
Mutation	3	3	0
ID grade			
No ID	7	3	4
Mild	5	1	4
Moderate	15	10	5
Severe/profound	1	1	0

Instruments

The Social Communication Questionnaire (SCQ) is a standardised screening tool for ASD [33]. The SCQ was used to assess the number of autism symptoms [33]. The questionnaire is used from the age of four. It contains 40 items, which are answered with 'Yes' (= 1) or 'No' (= 0) and comes in two versions. SCQ-Current covers the individual's behaviour during the most recent 3 months, whereas SCQ-Lifetime is based on the individual's entire developmental history. Both versions give a single total score, where a score of 15 or above is regarded as an indicator of possible ASD. The SCQ are also scored in three different domains: the reciprocal social interaction domain, communication domain and repetitive domain. In this study, the SCQ-Lifetime questionnaire was used [34]. In the initial standardisation of the assessment tool, a good reliability was reported with a Cronbach's alpha of 0.84–0.93 across the age groups and a Cronbach's alpha of 0.81–0.92 across the diagnostic groups [33]. Rutter et al. [33] also measured the validity and found a correlation of 0.71 between SCQ and the Autism Diagnostic Interview-Revised (ADI-R). In two groups of children with Down syndrome (DS) with ASD and DS without ASD, Magyar et al. [35] investigated the validity of SCQ and found that it did discriminate between the two groups. Children with DS and ASD obtained a significantly higher total score on the SCQ than children with DS only. SCQ is used in research on different genetic disorders [35, 36] including SMS [19].

The Social Responsiveness Scale (SRS) is a 65-item, quantitative parent-reported or adult self-reported measure that assesses social impairment associated with ASD [37]. The SRS enquires about specific and observable elements of reciprocal social behaviour (39 items), social use of language (6 items) and behaviour characteristics of children with autism and other PDDs (20 items), and it generates a standardised score. In addition to a total score, SRS consists of five subscores: Social Awareness, Social Cognition, Social Communication, Social Motivation and Autistic Mannerisms. In the initial standardisation of the questionnaire, the reliability was tested across gender and parents' and teachers' reports and in clinical settings. A good reliability was reported across these groups with a Cronbach's alpha of 0.93–0.97 [37]. The validity of the SRS has also been evaluated and a strong association between the SRS and the ADI-R was found [37]. Recently, in a large sample of idiopathic ASD, the SRS scores were shown to be influenced by rates of behavioural problems [32]. We therefore use both the SCQ and the SRS in this study and we assess the effect of behavioural problems. Since the SRS *T* score norms are different for males and females, we chose to use raw scores in addition to *T* scores when comparing the genders.

The Developmental Behaviour Checklist (DBC) [38, 39] is a questionnaire completed by parents or other primary caretakers or teachers that report problems over a 6-month period. Each behavioural description is scored on a 0, 1 and 2 rating where 0 = 'not true as far as you know', 1 = 'somewhat or sometimes true', and 2 = 'very true or often true'. Five versions of the Checklist are available: the Parent/Carer version (DBC-P), the Teacher version (DBC-T), the Adult version (DBC-A), the Short-form (DBC-P24) and the Monitoring chart (DBC-M). In this study, the DBC-P was used.

The Vineland Adaptive Behavior Scale II (VABS II) [40, 41] is a semi-structured interview or rating form of the parents or caregivers that assesses the everyday behavioural functioning of children and adults from birth throughout life. In this study, both the interview form (Norwegian cohort) and the parent/caregiver rating form (Swedish cohort) were used. The scales yield standard scores (mean = 100: one standard deviation (SD) = 15) in the domains of communication, daily living skills, socialisation and motor function, as well as a total sum score on adaptive behaviour composite. Each domain contains several subdomains. Motor function can only be assessed in children less than 6 years of age. In this study, the Norwegian and Swedish versions of the scales based on Scandinavian normative data were used. VABS II is a standardised and validated tool. Many studies have confirmed its reliability and validity making this measure one of the most widely used assessment tools of adaptive behaviour [42]. This tool has also been used with SMS several times [43, 44].

Table 2 Social Communication Questionnaire scores

	Total ($N = 27^a$)	Females ($N = 15$)	Males ($N = 12$)	p value (Cohen's d)
SCQ total (SD)	16.04 (6.10)	19.07 (4.77)	12.25 (5.55)	0.003 (1.32)
Reciprocal Social Interaction (SD)	5.19 (3.05)	6.87 (2.83)	3.08 (1.78)	0.000290 (1.60)
Communication (SD)	5.07 (2.73)	5.93 (1.98)	4.00 (3.22)	0.086 (0.72)
Repetitive behaviour (SD)	4.81 (2.19)	5.27 (1.91)	4.25 (2.45)	0.252 (0.46)
	N(%)[ratio]	*N*(%)	*N*(%)	
Number above cutoff (≥ 15)	14(52)[2.93]	11(73)	3(25)	0.021

[a]One parent did not return the SCQ questionnaire

The SRS, SCQ and DBC were all mailed to the parents after they consented to participate in the study. The parents filled in the information at home and mailed the questionnaire back to the researchers in a prepaid envelope. The VABS II were conducted in two different ways; the Norwegian cohort was interviewed on the telephone, and the Swedish cohort was mailed the parent/caregiver rating form together with the other questionnaires. The difference in procedure was due to language issues of performing the telephone interview with the Swedish cohort.

These instruments were chosen, instead of the gold-standard instruments ADI-R and Autism Diagnostic Observation Schedule (ADOS), because of their ease of use, because they have been used earlier with SMS, and to assess persons scattered around Norway and Sweden with the least possible burden for the patients.

Statistical analysis

Data were compiled for statistical analysis using the Statistical Package for the Social Sciences (SPSS) version 23 (IBM). Analysis of group differences in the degree of ID was conducted with the Mann-Whitney independent sample test. Descriptive statistics were derived, and the total scores and subscores obtained from the SRS and the SCQ were analysed as continuous dependent variables using t tests. The ratio was calculated as number of females above the cutoff on the SCQ total score divided by the number of males above the cutoff. Effect sizes (Cohen's d) were calculated using Social Science Statistics' online resources. The two-sided Fisher's exact test was used to test the proportion of males and females above the SCQ cutoff and in the different SRS classifications. Multiple regression analyses were conducted to assess the impact of 'gender', 'DBC' and 'VABS II standard scores' on the 'total SCQ score'. The normality of the residuals was checked using the visual inspection of P-P plots. Due to the combination of dichotomous and continuous predictor variables, we report the standardised coefficients (β), in addition to unstandardized B.

Results

Social Communication Questionnaire

The SCQ scores from 27 patients were analysed. A total of 52% scored above the cutoff (≥ 15). The females had higher scores on both the SCQ total score and all domains, but only the total SCQ score and the reciprocal social interaction domain showed a significant gender difference. A total of 25% of the males and 73% of the females scored above the ≥ 15 cutoff ($p = 0.021$). This provides a gender ratio of 3:1 and favours the females. All the SCQ scores are summarised in Table 2. The means for the males and females on each SCQ subdomain score are plotted in Fig. 1. How the ID grades are distributed between the males and females with SCQ scores above versus below the ASD cutoff are displayed in Table 3 (females) and Table 4 (males).

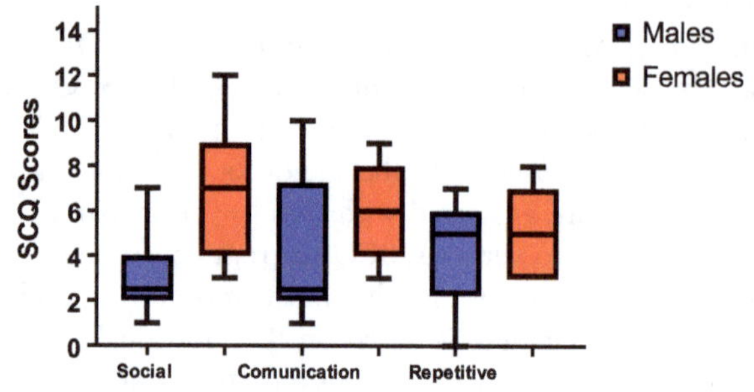

Fig. 1 SCQ subdomain scores divided by males and females

Social Responsiveness Scale

The SRS scores from 28 patients were analysed. A total of 71% of the scores were in the severe range, and 25% were in the mild to moderate range. Only 4% were in the normal range. Total scores and all subscales were higher in females on both standardised and raw scores. The gender difference was significant only in the subscales of Social Awareness and Social Cognition. The total T score and the raw score of Social Awareness and Social Cognition also had between large and very large effect sizes on the differences between males and females. A total of 87% of the females' and 54% of the males' scores were within the severe range, 13% of the females' and 38% of the males' scores fell in the mild to moderate range and 8% of the males' scores was in the normal range. All the SRS scores are summarised in Table 5.

Vineland Adaptive Behavior Scale II

The VABS II scores from 24 patients were analysed. All the VABS II scores are summarised in Table 6. There was a difference in the adaptive behaviour composite score, between males and females, but the differences were not significant.

Table 3 ID grade and SCQ-cutoff crosstabulation males

			SCQ-cutoff		Total
			≤ 15	≥ 15	
ID grade	No ID	Count	3	0	3
		% within ID grade	100.0	0.0	100.0
	Mild	Count	2	2	4
		% within ID grade	50.0	50.0	100.0
	Moderate	Count	4	1	5
		% within ID grade	80.0	20.0	100.0
Total		Count	9	3	12
		% within ID grade	75.0	25.0	100.0

Table 4 ID grade and SCQ-cutoff crosstabulation females

			SCQ-cutoff		Total
			≤ 15	≥ 15	
ID grade	No ID	Count	1	2	3
		% within ID grade	33.3	66.7	100.0
	Mild	Count	0	1	1
		% within ID grade	0.0	100.0	100.0
	Moderate	Count	3	7	10
		% within ID grade	30.0	70.0	100.0
	Severe	Count	0	1	1
		% within ID grade	0.0	100.0	100.0
Total		Count	4	11	15
		% within ID grade	26.7	73.3	100.0

Developmental Behaviour Checklist

The DBC scores from 27 patients were analysed and all scores were above the clinical cutoff (≥ 46). All the DBC scores are summarised in Table 7. The DBC did not have the same gender differences that we observed in the SRS and SCQ, except from the subscale Social Relating, where we found a strong tendency for more problems among the females (Cohen's *d* 0.85).

Effect of gender when controlling for developmental level and behavioural problems

To determine the impact of gender on the SCQ score when controlling for developmental level (VABS II standard score) and amount of emotional and behavioural problems (DBC total score), a linear regression was conducted with the total SCQ score as the dependent variable. Measuring IQ in individuals with SMS is known to be problematic due to their behavioural characteristics. Therefore, we use data from the VABS II as a proxy for developmental level.

When gender, VABS II and DBC were entered as covariates, we obtained a highly significant model of the SCQ score ($R^2 = 0.60$, $F = 8.8$, $p = 0.0008$). Only gender had an independent contribution on the model ($\beta = 0.70$, $p = 0.0003$); VABS II ($\beta = -0.13$, $p = 0.44$) and DBC ($\beta = -0.16$, $p = 0.31$) had no independent contribution.

A similar linear regression was conducted with the SRS total raw score. When gender, VABS II and DBC were entered as covariates, we still obtained a significant model of the SRS total raw score ($R^2 = 0.46$, $F = 5.1$, $p = 0.010$). Both gender ($\beta = 0.46$, $p = 0.022$) and DBC ($\beta = 0.48$, $p = 0.013$) contributed to the model. VABS II ($\beta = 0.04$, $p = 0.836$) had no independent contribution. More details from the models are displayed in Table 8.

Discussion

This study explored a number of ASD symptoms across gender in a Scandinavian SMS sample. The approximately three females per male above the SCQ cutoff is exactly the opposite of what we would expect to find in a sample of idiopathic ASD. It is particularly in the social domain of ASD that females with SMS differ substantially from females with other aetiological pathways to ASD.

The reversed gender ratio of ASD symptoms identified in this study cannot be explained by differences in neither developmental level nor in the amount of emotional and behavioural problems. The clinical diagnoses of intellectual disability differ between the genders, and we found a tendency for poorer development in females (VABS II total 53) than males (VABS II total 62), but this difference was not significant. In the regression model, the VABS II score did not have an independent contribution to the SCQ score. Emotional and behavioural problems, as measured with the DBC, did not differ between the sexes. In the regression model of the SRS, we

Table 5 Social Responsiveness Scale scores

	Total ($n = 28$)	Females ($N = 15$)	Males ($N = 13$)	Significant p value (Cohen's d)
Total T score (SD)	82.29 (12.63)	89.73 (9.88)	73.69 (9.77)	0.000 (1.63)
Social Awareness raw score (SD)	12.43 (2.73)	13.60 (2.53)	11.08 (2.36)	0.011 (1.03)
Social Cognition raw score (SD)	11.68 (5.36)	19.47 (5.00)	13.46 (3.82)	0.001 (1.35)
Social Communication raw score (SD)	27.93 (7.70)	29.60 (6.72)	26.00 (8.56)	0.233 (0.47)
Social Motivation raw score (SD)	13.07 (5.26)	14.47 (4.91)	11.46 (5.36)	0.137 (0.58)
Autistic Mannerisms raw score (SD)	21.14 (5.97)	21.73 (5.99)	20.46 (6.12)	0.585 (0.21)
Total raw score	91.32 (20.60)	98.87(17.65)	82.62(20.93)	0.038 (0.84)
SRS classification	N(%)[ratio]	N(%)	N(%)	
Normal (>60)	1(4)[0]	0	1(8)	a
Mild–moderate (60–75)	7(25)[0.35]	2(13)	5(38)	a
Severe (< 75)	20(71)[1.61]	13(87)	7(54)	0.096

[a]Not applicable due to small sample

Table 6 Vineland Adaptive Behavior Scale II scores

	Total ($N = 24^a$)	Females ($N = 13$)	Males ($N = 11$)	Significant p value (Cohen's d)
VABS II standard score (SD)	56.88 (12.86)	52.85 (12.69)	61.64 (11.89)	0.094 (0.71)
Communication (SD)	57.92 (14.12)	54.38 (13.25)	52.09 (14.59)	0.193 (0.55)
Daily activities (SD)	61.79 (12.79)	62.69 (12.44)	60.73 (13.71)	0.719 (0.15)
Socialisation (SD)	62.54 (10.36)	59.46 (9.03)	66.18 (11.05)	0.123 (0.67)

[a]Four parents were not available for telephone interview

found that DBC contributed in addition to gender. This probably indicates that the SRS is more sensitive to behavioural problems than the SCQ is [32, 45]. The SRS places a heavier emphasis on the reciprocal social interaction trait in ASD, whereas the SCQ places a similar emphasis on all three ASD domains [45].

Neither Oliver [16] nor Vignoli [17] found any significant gender differences in ASD symptomatology in other rare genetic syndromes such as cri du chat syndrome, Cornelia de Lange syndrome, Prader Willis syndrome or tuberous sclerosis complex.

We wanted to investigate whether a difference in ASD symptomatology could be the result of females having more severe phenotypes than males and if it could be linked to levels of ID or whether the emotional and behaviour problems in SMS affected gender differences. We found a strong tendency for lower degrees of ID in females than in males, but the difference was not significant. But as the difference is approaching significance (0.07), it would be interesting to investigate further if there could be a real gender difference in ID levels in SMS. As mentioned before, the accuracy of our ID levels is questionable and therefore not used to draw any conclusions. In general, administering formal psychometric assessments is often reported to be very difficult with people with SMS, due to the maladaptive behaviours, sleep disturbance and difficulties in expressive language skills [46].

The observed gender differences in ASD do not seem to be related to the main genetic mechanisms for SMS. The RAI1 mutations, associated with less severe SMS phenotype, were more frequent in females (3/20%) with more ASD symptoms than in males (0/0%) who had less ASD symptoms. The group of individuals with RAI1 mutations was too small to be tested as a separate subgroup in any of the analyses.

Current research suggest that female protective factors are more important than particular male-linked risk in explaining the male bias in ASD, but the mechanisms behind such female protection are not established [4, 6]. Whatever the female protective factor turns out to be, the current data suggest that it is not present in females with SMS.

We found three other papers presenting gender differences in SMS [19, 24, 30]. In the study from Edelman et al. [30], the authors found some gender differences, with the females showing more problems. Most of them were somatic (myopia, cold hands and feet, eating/appetite problems and possible hypersensitivity (problems finding shoes to fit)), but they also found that females had a significantly higher frustration with communication level. Neither of the questionnaires used in our study found a significant gender difference regarding communication, but a more thorough investigation of communication profiles in this syndrome would be beneficial both to investigate the gender difference more and to propose possible interventions. The study by Laje et al. [19] indicated an absence of the usual gender difference regarding ASD measured with SRS but not SCQ. In our study, we find gender differences both in the SRS and in the SCQ measure, both showing more problems among the females. It is particularly the social domain of ASD that has an unusual male/female ratio. Females with SMS have significantly more social problems than males. We did not find any difference in repetitive behaviour. Laje et al. [19] found a gender difference, favouring the females, in two subscales on the SRS but not in the total raw score or on the SCQ. In our study, we found a

Table 7 Developmental Behaviour Checklist scores

	Total ($N = 27^a$)	Females ($N = 15$)	Males ($N = 12$)	Significant p value (Cohen's d)
DBC total percentiles (SD)	84.44 (13.19)	83.73 (13.87)	85.33 (12.83)	0.759 (0.12)
Disruptive/antisocial percentiles (SD)	85.63 (16.24)	83.47 (18.45)	88.33 (13.26)	0.433 (0.30)
Self-absorbed percentiles (SD)	80.67 (12.47)	80.53 (11.89)	80.83 (13.68)	0.953 (0.02)
Communication disturbance percentiles (SD)	75.93 (20.75)	73.73 (20.76)	78.67 (21.33)	0.551 (0.23)
Anxiety percentiles (SD)	61.11 (28.28)	62.53 (29.15)	59.33 (28.31)	0.776 (0.11)
Social Relating percentiles (SD)	42.96 (24.82)	51.60 (25.28)	32.17 (20.33)	0.036 (0.85)

[a]One parent did not correctly fill out the questionnaire

Table 8 Regression model summary

	SCQ total			SRS raw score		
Factors	*B*	*p*	95%	*B*	*p*	95%
Constant	12.44	0.204	− 7.38/32.25	− 21.43	0.615	− 109.37/66.50
Gender	8.30	0.0003	4.34/12.24	20.95	0.022	3.42/38.48
VABS II	− 0.08	0.44	− 0.21/0.10	0.96	0.836	− 0.74/0.61
DBC	− 0.06	0.31	− 0.25/0.08	− 0.07	0.013	0.23/1.68
Model's R^2		0.60			0.46	
Model's *p* value		0.0008			0.010	

B unstandardized B, *Sig* significant level, *95%* confidence interval for B for each factor

gender difference in ASD symptomatology, but neither in our study nor in the study by Laje et al. [19] could this difference be explained by differences in other traits in the syndrome. IQ level, adaptive behaviour and general emotional and behaviour problems have been investigated. A more thorough investigation of gender differences in adaptive behaviour profiles and the emotional and behaviour problems would be beneficial, alongside further molecular research regarding possible sexually dimorphic processes in SMS.

Limitations

Assigning a formal diagnosis of ASD to individuals with a known genetic syndrome is a matter of some debate [15]. In the current study, we only used the SCQ and the SRS as a measure of the number of ASD symptoms; we did not observe or use diagnostic instruments such as ADI-R or ADOS. Hence, we do not have data on how many actually fulfil the criteria for an ASD diagnosis.

Measuring IQ in individuals with SMS, as mentioned earlier, is known to be problematic due to their behavioural characteristics. Therefore, data from the VABS II were used as a proxy for developmental level. Even though VABS II cannot substitute a formal psychometric assessment such as IQ tests, consistency has been demonstrated between formal IQ tests and the VABS II [41]. In this study, we used developmental level instead of intellectual level/disability in most of our analysis, due to the fact that we ourselves did not collect the ID levels and could not guarantee for their validity.

Conclusion

We found a clear reversed gender difference in the number of ASD symptoms in persons with SMS. This female bias in ASD symptoms is not explained by differences in the developmental level or the amount of emotional and behavioural problems. The deletion that is known to cause SMS is located on chromosome 17 (17p11.2), and there is no known reason to expect gender differences in any traits in this autosomal condition. The finding of a clear gender difference is therefore notable, and the mechanisms behind this require further study. A previous study found a sexually dimorphic phenotype in eating behaviour in mice with loss of RAI1 functions [24]. Whether this is related to our finding should be explored. Knowledge about the biological underpinnings of the reversed ASD gender ratio may be of relevance to understand gender differences in other biological pathways to ASD. The female protective factors assumed to explain the male bias in ASD seems to be lacking in SMS.

Abbreviations

ADI-R: Autistics Diagnostic Interview-Revised; ADOS: Autism Diagnostic Observation Schedule; ASD: Autism spectrum disorder; DBC: Developmental Behaviour Checklist; ID: Intellectual disability; RAI1: Retinoic acid induced 1; SCQ: Social Communication Questionnaire (SCQ); SMS: Smith-Magenis syndrome; SRS: Social Responsiveness Scale; VABSII: Vineland Adaptive Behavior Scale II

Acknowledgements

We are thankful to the participants in the study and the Norwegian and Swedish SMS Foundations. This study is part of the BUPgen study group and the NeuroDevelop research network.

Funding

The study has been funded by Frambu Resource Centre for Rare Disorders and NevSom, Department of Rare Disorders and Disabilities, Oslo University Hospital.

Authors' contributions

HEN, AN and TN planned and designed the study. HEN, BMA and AN collected the clinical information. HEN and TN analysed the data and interpreted the results. HEN wrote the first draft of the manuscript. All the authors contributed to the manuscript and read and approved the final manuscript.

Competing interests

The authors declare that they have no competing interests.

Author details

[1]Frambu Resource Centre for Rare Disorders, Siggerud, Norway. [2]University of Stavanger, Stavanger, Norway. [3]Karolinska Centre for Rare Diseases, Karolinska

University Hospital, Solna, Sweden. [4]NevSom, Department of Rare Disorders and Disabilities, Oslo University Hospital, Oslo, Norway. [5]KG Jebsen Centre for Psychosis Research, NORMENT, University of Oslo, Oslo, Norway.

References

1. Kirkovski M, Enticott PG, Fitzgerald PB. A review of the role of female gender in autism spectrum disorders. J Autism Dev Disord. 2013;43(11):2584–603.
2. Lai MC, Lombardo M, Baron Cohen S. Autism. Lancet. 2014;383:896–910.
3. Halladay AK, Bishop S, Constantino JN, Daniels AM, Koenig K, Palmer K, Messinger D, Pelphrey K, Sanders SJ, Singer AT, et al. Sex and gender differences in autism spectrum disorder: summarizing evidence gaps and identifying emerging areas of priority. Mol Autism. 2015;6(1):36.
4. Jacquemont S, Coe Bradley P, Hersch M, Duyzend Michael H, Krumm N, Bergmann S, Beckmann Jacques S, Rosenfeld Jill A, Eichler Evan E. A higher mutational burden in females supports a "female protective model" in neurodevelopmental disorders. Am J Hum Genet. 2014;94(3):415–25.
5. Sanders SJ, He X, Willsey AJ, Ercan-Sencicek AG, Samocha KE, Cicek AE, Murtha MT, Bal VH, Bishop SL, Dong S, et al. Insights into autism spectrum disorder genomic architecture and biology from 71 risk loci. Neuron. 2015; 87(6):1215–33.
6. Werling DM, Parikshak NN, Geschwind DH. Gene expression in human brain implicates sexually dimorphic pathways in autism spectrum disorders. Nat Commun. 2016;7:107–17.
7. Brugha TS, McManus S, Bankart J, Scott F, Purdon S, Smith J, Bebbington P, Jenkins R, Meltzer H. Epidemiology of autism spectrum disorders in adults in the community in England. Arch Gen Psychiatry. 2011;68(5):459–65.
8. Loomes R, Hull L, Mandy WPL. What is the male-to-female ratio in autism spectrum disorder? A systematic review and meta-analysis. J Am Acad Child Adolesc Psychiatry. 2017;56(6):466–74.
9. Fombonne E. Epidemiology of pervasive developmental disorders. Pediatr Res. 2009;65(6):591–8.
10. Association. AP: Diagnostic and statistical manual of mental disorders (5th ed). Arlington, VA: American Psychiatric Association; 2013.
11. Hartley SL, Sikora DM. Sex differences in autism spectrum disorder: an examination of developmental functioning, autistic symptoms, and coexisting behavior problems in toddlers. J Autism Dev Disord. 2009;39(12):1715–22.
12. Carter AS, Black DO, Tewani S, Connolly CE, Kadlec MB, Tager-Flusberg H. Sex differences in toddlers with autism spectrum disorders. J Autism Dev Disord. 2007;37(1):86–97.
13. Lai MC, Lombardo MV, Pasco G, Ruigrok AN, Wheelwright SJ, Sadek SA, Chakrabarti B, Baron-Cohen S. A behavioral comparison of male and female adults with high functioning autism spectrum conditions. PLoS One. 2011; 6(6):e20835.
14. Head AM, McGillivray JA, Stokes MA. Gender differences in emotionality and sociability in children with autism spectrum disorders. Mol Autism. 2014;5(1):19.
15. Richards C, Jones C, Groves L, Moss J, Oliver C. Prevalence of autism spectrum disorder phenomenology in genetic disorders: a systematic review and meta-analysis. Lancet Psychiatry. 2015;2(10):909–16.
16. Oliver C, Berg K, Moss J, Arron K, Burbidge C. Delineation of behavioral phenotypes in genetic syndromes: characteristics of autism spectrum disorder, affect and hyperactivity. J Autism Dev Disord. 2011;41(8):1019–32.
17. Vignoli A, La Briola F, Peron A, Turner K, Vannicola C, Saccani M, Magnaghi E, Scornavacca GF, Canevini MP. Autism spectrum disorder in tuberous sclerosis complex: searching for risk markers. Orphanet J Rare Dis. 2015;10:154–62.
18. Nærland T, Bakke KA, Storvik S, Warner G, Howlin P: Age and gender-related differences in emotional and behavioural problems and autistic features in children and adolescents with Down syndrome: a survey-based study of 674 individuals. J Intellect Disabil Res 2016:n/a-n/a. doi: https://doi.org/10.1111/jir.12342.
19. Laje G, Morse R, Richter W, Ball J, Pao M, Smith ACM. Autism spectrum features in Smith-Magenis syndrome. Am J Med Genet C Semin Med Genet. 2010;154C(4):456–62.
20. Wolters PL, Gropman AL, Martin SC, Smith MR, Hildenbrand HL, Brewer CC, Smith AC. Neurodevelopment of children under 3 years of age with Smith-Magenis syndrome. Pediatr Neurol. 2009;41:250–8.
21. Smith AC, McGavran L, Robinson J, Waldstein G, Macfarlane J, Zonona J. Interstitial deletion of (17) (p11.2p11.2) in nine patients. Am J Med Genet. 1986;24:393–414.
22. Slager RE, Newton TL, Vlangos CN, Finucane B, Elsea SH. Mutations in RAI1 associated with Smith-Magenis syndrome. Nat Genet. 2003;33(4):466–8.
23. Elsea SH, Girirajan S. Smith-Magenis syndrome. Eur J Hum Genet. 2008;16(4):412–21.
24. Huang WH, Guenthner CJ, Xu J, Nguyen T, Schwarz LA, Wilkinson AW, Gozani O, Chang HY, Shamloo M, Luo L. Molecular and neural functions of Rai1, the causal gene for Smith-Magenis syndrome. Neuron. 2016;92(2):392–406.
25. Williams SR, Zies D, Mullegama SV, Grotewiel MS, Elsea SH. Smith-Magenis syndrome results in disruption of CLOCK gene transcription and reveals an integral role for RAI1 in the maintenance of circadian rhythmicity. Am J Hum Genet. 2012;90(6):941–9.
26. Greenberg F, Guzzetta V, Montes de Oca-Luna R, Magenis RE, Smith AC, Richter SF, Kondo I, Dobyns WB, Patel PI, Lupski JR. Molecular analysis of the Smith-Magenis syndrome: a possible contiguous-gene syndrome associated with del(17)(p11.2). Am J Hum Genet. 1991;49(6):1207–18.
27. Gropman AL, Duncan WC, Smith ACM: Neurologic and developmental features of the Smith-Magenis syndrome (del 17p11.2). Pediatr Neurol 2006, 34(5):337-350.
28. Smith AC, Dykens E, Greenberg F: Behavioral phenotype of Smith-Magenis syndrome (del 17p11.2). Am J Med Genet 1998, 81(2):179-185.
29. Sloneem J, Oliver C, Udwin O, Woodcock KA. Prevalence, phenomenology, aetiology and predictors of challenging behaviour in Smith-Magenis syndrome. J Intellect Disabil Res. 2011;55(2):138–51.
30. Edelman EA, Girirajan S, Finucane B, Patel PI, Lupski JR, Smith AC, Elsea SH. Gender, genotype, and phenotype differences in Smith-Magenis syndrome: a meta-analysis of 105 cases. Clin Genet. 2007;71(6):540–50.
31. Moss J, Howlin P. Autism spectrum disorders in genetic syndromes: implications for diagnosis, intervention and understanding the wider autism spectrum disorder population. J Intellect Disabil Res. 2009;53:852–73.
32. Havdahl KA, Bal VH, Huerta M, Pickles A, Øyen AS, Stoltenberg C, Lord C, Bishop SL. Multidimensional influences on autism symptom measures: implications for use in etiological research. J Am Acad Child Adolesc Psychiatry. 2016;55(12):1054–1063.e1053.
33. Rutter M, Bailey A, Lord C. Social Communication Questionnaire. Los Angeles, CA: Western Psychological Services; 2003.
34. Schjølberg S, Tambs K: Social Communication Questionnaire (Norwegian). Hogrefe Psykologisk Forlag 2005.
35. Magyar CI, Pandolfi V, Dill CA. An initial evaluation of the Social Communication Questionnaire for the assessment of autism spectrum disorders in children with Down syndrome. J Dev Behav Pediatr. 2012;33(2):134–45.
36. Hall SS, Lightbody AA, Hirt M. Autism in fragile X syndrome: a category mistake? J Am Acad Child Adolesc Psychiatry. 2010;49(9):921–33.
37. Constantino JN, CP G: Social Responsiveness Scale (SRS). Los Angeles: Western Psychol Serv; 2005.
38. Einfeld SL, Tonge BJ. Manual for the Developmental Behaviour Checklist. Clayton, Melbourne and Sydney: University of New South Wales: Monash University for Developmental Psychiatry and School of Psychiatry; 1992.
39. Einfeld SL, Tonge BJ: Manual for the Developmental Behaviour Checklist: Primary Carer Version (DBC-P) & Teacher Version (DBC-T) (2nd. ed.). Clayton, Melbourne: Monash University Centre for Developmental Psychiatry and Psychology; 2002.
40. Sparrow SS, Balla DA, Cicchetti DV. Vineland Adaptive Scales. American Guidance Service: Circle Pines, MN; 1984.
41. Sparrow SS, Balla DA, Cicchetti DV. Vineland Adaptive Behavior Scale II. Circle Pines, MN: American Guidance Service; 2005.
42. Sparrow SS, Cicchetti DV: Diagnostic uses of the Vineland Adaptive Behavior Scale. *Pediatric* Psychology 1985, 10:215-225.
43. Martin SC, Wolters PL, Smith ACM. Adaptive and maladaptive behavior in children with Smith-Magenis syndrome. J Autism Dev Disord. 2006;36(4):541–52.
44. Madduri N, Peters SU, Voigt RG, Llorente AM, Lupski JR, Potocki L. Cognitive and adaptive behavior profiles in Smith-Magenis syndrome. J Dev Behav Pediatr. 2006;27(3):188–92.
45. Towbin KE, Pradella A, Gorrindo T, Pine DS, Leibenluft E. Autism spectrum traits in children with mood and anxiety disorders. J Child Adolesc Psychopharmacol. 2005;15(3):452–64.
46. Smith MR, Hildenbrand H, Smith ACM. Sensory motor and functional skills of dizygotic twins: one with Smith-Magenis syndrome and a twin control. Phys Occup Ther Pediatr. 2009;29(3):239–57.

6

Altered reward system reactivity for personalized circumscribed interests in autism

Gregor Kohls[1], Ligia Antezana[2], Maya G. Mosner[3], Robert T. Schultz[4,5,6] and Benjamin E. Yerys[4,6*]

Abstract

Background: Neurobiological research in autism spectrum disorders (ASD) has paid little attention on brain mechanisms that cause and maintain restricted and repetitive behaviors and interests (RRBIs). Evidence indicates an imbalance in the brain's reward system responsiveness to social and non-social stimuli may contribute to both social deficits and RRBIs. Thus, this study's central aim was to compare brain responsiveness to individual RRBI (i.e., circumscribed interests), with social rewards (i.e., social approval), in youth with ASD relative to typically developing controls (TDCs).

Methods: We conducted a 3T functional magnetic resonance imaging (fMRI) study to investigate the blood-oxygenation-level-dependent effect of personalized circumscribed interest rewards versus social rewards in 39 youth with ASD relative to 22 TDC. To probe the reward system, we employed short video clips as reinforcement in an instrumental incentive delay task. This optimization increased the task's ecological validity compared to still pictures that are often used in this line of research.

Results: Compared to TDCs, youth with ASD had stronger reward system responses for CIs mostly within the non-social realm (e.g., video games) than social rewards (e.g., approval). Additionally, this imbalance within the caudate nucleus' responsiveness was related to greater social impairment.

Conclusions: The current data support the idea of reward system dysfunction that may contribute to enhanced motivation for RRBIs in ASD, accompanied by diminished motivation for social engagement. If a dysregulated reward system indeed supports the emergence and maintenance of social and non-social symptoms of ASD, then strategically targeting the reward system in future treatment endeavors may allow for more efficacious treatment practices that help improve outcomes for individuals with ASD and their families.

Keywords: Autism spectrum disorders, Reward, Motivation, Circumscribed interests, Restricted and repetitive behaviors and interests, Functional magnetic resonance imaging, Striatum, Caudate nucleus, Reward system

Background

Neurobiological research in autism spectrum disorders (ASD) has largely focused on social communication impairments, with much less attention on brain mechanisms that cause and maintain restricted and repetitive behaviors and interests (RRBIs) [1]. There is accumulating evidence indicating that both symptom clusters might be mediated, in part, by the same mesocorticolimbic system subserving reward-driven, motivational behaviors [2]. But the reward system's role in both symptom clusters has not been systematically studied in a single sample of youth with ASD to date.

The social motivation hypothesis postulates ASD as a motivation disorder with affected persons preferring to explore and learn from the non-social environment at the expense of the social world [3]. The imbalance between motivation for social versus non-social stimuli is reflected in the responsiveness of the brain's reward system [4]. Specifically, this hypothesis posits that some RRBIs may originate, in part, from the reward system being hyper-reactive for circumscribed interests (CIs)

* Correspondence: yerysb@email.chop.edu
[4]Center for Autism Research, The Children's Hospital of Philadelphia, 3535 Market Street, Ste 860, Philadelphia, PA 19104, USA
[6]Psychiatry Department, Perelman School of Medicine, University of Pennsylvania, Philadelphia, PA, USA

mostly within the non-social realm (e.g., mechanical and physical aspects of the environment), whereas social impairments may result, in part, from the reward system being hypo-reactive for socially rewarding stimuli and encounters such as social interactions with positive or non-negative affect [3]. Consequently, the developing child with ASD becomes deprived of crucial social learning opportunities, leading to aberrant social skill development and failed specialization of brain regions subserving social information processing [5].

Most recently, functional magnetic resonance imaging (fMRI) studies have started to address the neural system of reward responsiveness as a proxy for motivation functioning in ASD (see for a review, [6]). Although there is accumulating evidence of neural reward processing dysfunction in this population, findings are decidedly mixed, i.e., the direction and specificity of the deviations are inconsistent [2]. Thus, any firm conclusions are premature at this point. Several studies, however, report aberrant blood-oxygen-level-dependent (BOLD) responses of crucial reward regions in individuals with ASD, including ventral and dorsal striatum, ventromedial prefrontal cortex (vmPFC), anterior cingulate cortex (ACC), and orbitofrontal cortex (OFC), in response to both social rewards (e.g., smiling face, approval) and monetary rewards (e.g., gain of 0.50$) [7–11]. Findings of altered reward system responsiveness in ASD have generally been interpreted as potential neural signatures of decreased motivation to seek and appreciate these types of "conventional" desires.

In contrast, the pursuit of RRBIs, particularly CIs, are reported to be a source of pleasure by affected people [12], and the use of RRBIs as reward contingencies in behavioral modification programs has been found to be therapeutically effective [13]. Given the sporadic behavioral studies addressing the rewarding value of RRBIs, it is not surprising that there has only been limited neurobiological research on the reward system's potential role in RRBIs [1].

Although the reward system may contribute, at least partially, to all forms of RRBIs [4], CIs may make the ideal candidate for investigating neural reward mechanisms of RRBIs—versus social impairments—in ASD: (1) The non-social quality of CIs stand in stark contrast to the diminished social interests of affected people (i.e., CIs usually are non-socially interesting, not shared, and negatively impact interpersonal relations [12]); (2) CIs can be compared to interests of typically developing controls (TDC); TDCs likely exhibit low rates of other RRBIs during the school age years (e.g., stereotypic body movements); and (3) In practical terms, CIs are relatively easier to recreate and measure in the MRI environment than other RRBI symptoms.

To date, two studies have investigated reward system responsiveness for CIs in ASD [14, 15]. Dichter et al. [6] applied a standardized set of stimuli hypothesized to be "autism-specific objects of high interest" (e.g., pictures of trains, computers) as reward outcomes; their presentation was contingent on accurate task performance in a reaction time task. The study revealed diminished ventral striatal activation for monetary reward in adults with ASD, which was accompanied by enhanced activation in vmPFC for autism-specific object rewards. Because Dichter et al. [6] used standardized object images rather than individualized items, it remains unknown whether the participants' actual interests were covered by the stimulus set used. More importantly, the study did not contrast the interest rewards with social rewards. Thus, the social motivation hypothesis of ASD was tested only indirectly.

Cascio and colleagues [14] used a passive viewing paradigm with personalized CI pictures of each participant with ASD, focusing on youth rather than adults. The authors report heightened BOLD responses in anterior insula as well as mid-dorsal ACC—critical nodes of the "salience network"—when youth with ASD viewed their own versus others' interests. The use of a passive task that did not require an active response to maximize reward outcome might explain the lack of group differences for CIs in reward circuitries. Reliable between-group activation differences within core reward regions (e.g., striatum) appear to be critically dependent on the requirement for an instrumental response [16].

For the current investigation, we leveraged the strengths of both prior imaging studies. Like Dichter, Felder and colleagues [6], we applied an incentive delay task to assess neural reward responsiveness with fMRI. Here, we chose a blocked design that has previously shown robust reward system activation in youth with vs. without ASD [7]. Existing imaging experiments targeting motivation in ASD relied on static pictures to serve as appetitive stimuli, which are, at best, only weakly rewarding and can fail to elicit motivational processes. Therefore, we employed dynamic stimuli that are perceived as more natural and engaging and, thus, may serve as more vital incentives [17]. To this end, for the current study, we developed a novel set of video clips of social and interest rewards [18]. More specifically, for the CI reward condition, we created individualized video stimuli for each participant based on self- and parent-reported CIs similar to Cascio and colleagues [14].

Thus, the present fMRI study aimed to compare the brain's reward system responsiveness to individual CI rewards versus social rewards in youth with ASD relative to TDC. We expected enhanced neural signals in participants with ASD in response to their individual CI reward (in particular, in ventral and dorsal striatum as well as in vmPFC, ACC, and OFC), while neural activation would be reduced for social rewards. Additionally, to specifically test predictions derived from the social motivation hypothesis, we explored correlations between differential reward system responsiveness for CI reward versus social reward and ASD symptom severity.

Methods

Participants

Sixty-seven youth, ages 8–17 years, were enrolled in this study, including 45 with ASD (without intellectual disability) and 22 TDC. Five participants with ASD did not attempt the scan, and one child with ASD was excluded for extreme hydrocephalus. All participants stayed within our head motion thresholds during the scan (i.e., root mean square < 1.75 mm of maximum displacement and .0175 rad of translation). The final imaging sample comprised 39 youth with ASD and 22 TDCs. All participants had a General Conceptual Ability (GCA) ≥ 75, equivalent to full-scale IQ, as measured by the Differential Ability Scales—Second Edition [19].

Youth with ASD received an expert clinical diagnosis based on Diagnostic and Statistical Manual of Mental Disorders–Fourth Edition–Text Revision criteria (DSM-IV-TR) [20]; the Autism Diagnostic Interview-Revised [21], and the Autism Diagnostic Observation Schedule [22] were used by experienced clinicians to inform diagnostic decisions. Youth with ASD were excluded if parents reported any known genetic, current mood or psychotic disorder, neurological disorder, premature birth (gestational age ≤ 37 weeks), or other significant medical conditions that affects brain functioning. Youth on atypical antipsychotics were excluded. Youth on psychostimulants were asked to withhold on the day of the study ($n = 5$), and youth taking other psychoactive medication were included (selective serotonin reuptake inhibitors: $n = 10$, selective norepinephrine reuptake inhibitors: $n = 3$, alpha2a-agonist: $n = 3$).

TDCs were excluded if parents reported any known genetic, language, learning, neurological, or psychiatric disorder, premature birth, or first- or second-degree relative with ASD. Youth were also excluded if parents reported elevated symptoms on any scale from the Child and Adolescent Symptom Inventory (CASI-4R; [23]. Groups did not differ in age and sex ratio, but the ASD group had a marginally lower GCA than TDCs (Table 1).

Table 1 Summary of participant characteristics by diagnostic group

Measure	TDC ($n = 22$)	ASD ($n = 39$)	*p* value*
Age (years) *M*(SD)	12.85 (2.13)	12.58 (2.37)	0.66
Age range	9.08–17.00	8.17–17.58	
VIQ (SS) *M*(SD)	113.5 (15.4)	105.6 (14.4)	0.06
PIQ (SS) *M*(SD)	109.2 (16.2)	101.9 (16.5)	0.10
FSIQ (SS) *M*(SD)	111.9 (18.0)	103.6 (15.7)	0.08
Sex ratio (male:female)	17:5	29:10	0.80
ADOS-2 social affect + RRB	–	11.62 (3.89)	–
ADOS-2 severity	–	6.87 (0.32)	–
ADI-R social Interaction	–	18.39 (5.20)	–
ADI-R communication	–	14.61 (4.87)	–
ADI-R repetitive behaviors	–	6.03 (2.09)	–
RBS-R (total score)	–	17.87 (11.88)	–
SRS-2 (total *T*-score)	39.5 (4.87)	73.41 (10.71)	< 0.001
IS (total score)	9.53 (2.41)	14.2 (3.76)	< 0.001

VIQ verbal IQ, *PIQ* performance/nonverbal IQ, *FSIQ* full-scale IQ, *SS* standard score ($M = 100$; SD = 15), *SRS-2* Social Responsiveness Scale—2nd Edition, *ADOS-2* Autism Diagnostic Observation Schedule Module 3 or 4, *ADI-R* Autism Diagnostic Interview—Revised, *RBS-R* Repetitive Behavior Scale-Revised, *IS* Interests Scale

*p values are based on two-sample t tests and χ^2 test (for sex ratio)

Phenotypic measures

For this study, we developed the Interest Preference Assessment (IPA), a short interview adapted from the Interests Scale [24, 25], to directly evaluate each child's most favorite interest/hobby to be used in the fMRI task (see Additional file 1). The IPA is comprised of two sections: The first section consists of a list of 25 categories of interest (e.g., machines or figuring out how things work, animals, people), and children are asked to rate each interest on a scale from 1 to 5, with 5 indicating "I could do this activity or talk about this topic all the time." The second part of the IPA asks children to identify their primary interest and answer questions assessing the interference and intensity of that interest (e.g., "How much time do you spend doing or thinking about this interest or hobby? Does this get in the way of other responsibilities? Do you get annoyed or upset when you are asked to stop talking or doing this interest or hobby?"). Most children identified a singular primary interest, but a few children identified more than one interest as their "favorite." In these cases, we asked them to pinpoint the interest they would most enjoy having in the upcoming MRI session. Examples of interests include videogames, professional sport teams, musicians/actors, toys, elevators, and movies (Additional file 1: Table S1).

Additionally, all parents were asked to complete the Social Responsiveness Scale-2nd Edition (SRS-2; [26]), the Repetitive Behavior Scale-Revised (RBS-R; [27, 28]), and the Interests Scale (IS; [24, 25]) to dimensionally assess behaviors characteristic of ASD.

Participants were compensated for their participation in this study. Written informed consent was obtained from all participants and their parents. This study was approved by the local Institutional Review Board.

FMRI task

We used an incentive delay task (IDT) in a blocked fMRI design that is an adaptation of the "classic" IDT [29] and aims to examine participants' motivation to receive either a social or a personalized type of reward based on individual interests (vs. neutral outcome). To maximize ecological validity, we utilized short movie clips of actors expressing facial expressions along with other nonverbal gestures in the social reward condition as well as short video clips depicting personalized interests in the interest reward condition (Fig. 1 and Additional file 1 for details).

The IDT is a simple speeded button press task to examine neural responses to rewards that can be gained dependent upon a person's ability to quickly and accurately respond to a target symbol in each trial. An online tracking algorithm was implemented to continuously monitor and adjust the target duration according to individual performance to achieve an accuracy rate of ≥ 50% (see Table 2). In social reward (SR) trials, target hits resulted in a short video clip of a person showing happy facial expressions, including nodding with a smile and a praising nonverbal gesture—the "thumbs up" sign. The outcome for misses was a video clip of a person showing neutral expressions, with slight natural motion (e.g., eye blinks). In personalized interest reward (IR) trials, target hits resulted in a short video clip of a person's favorite interest (e.g., Minecraft©), whereas the outcome for misses was a video clip of a tree with slight natural movement (i.e., breeze gently moves leaves). The outcome in the neutral (NR) condition was always a video clip of "TV static." The SR video clips portrayed six different adult actors (half female, half male, of various races and ethnicities representative of the local region) and six unique clips of personalized interests were presented in the IR condition; each of which was randomly repeated eight times throughout the experiment. Actor's videos were chosen from a larger pool based on ratings of the actor's likability as well as based on her authenticity of depicting approval; only actors who had the highest ratings on both scales were included (see [18]). Interest clips were chosen from various youtube© videos to depict the participants' individual interests. All video clips fulfilled the following criteria: HD quality, multicolored content, disabled audio, .avi format, resolution 720 × 400 pixels, 25 frames/s, and 1500 ms duration; and the actor or interest/hobby is depicted in the center of the screen.

There were two 6 min 44 s runs that presented the three experimental conditions (i.e., SR, NR, and IR) block-wise, with a fixation period interspersed after each block. Altogether, 6 blocks per condition and 18 fixation periods were presented across the two runs. Within each

Table 2 Main performance variables of the incentive delay task by group and incentive condition

	TDC *M*(SD)	ASD *M*(SD)	*p* value*
RT for hits (in ms)			
Neutral	255.3 (29.8)	250.9 (27.7)	0.56
Social reward	206.7 (22.4)	200.7 (20.0)	0.29
Interest reward	242.4 (23.9)	238.4 (28.3)	0.58
Accuracy (in %):			
Neutral	49.5 (11.7)	47.7 (9.9)	0.53
Social reward	56.9 (9.9)	54.8 (6.7)	0.32
Interest reward	45.1 (11.6)	45.7 (7.6)	0.83

**p* values are based on two-sample *t* tests

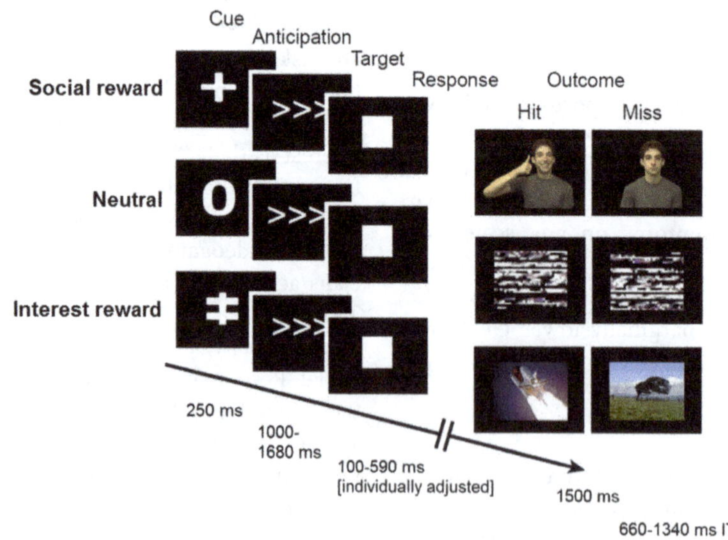

Fig. 1 Illustration of the incentive delay task in a blocked fMRI design, including three different reward conditions: social reward (SR), interest reward (IR), and neutral (NR). To increase the ecological validity of the paradigm, static photos were replaced with short video clips (see text for more details)

run, trial types were designated using intuitive cues signaling the reward type that could be obtained in the ongoing trial for correct performance: a plus sign for SR trials, the numeral zero for NR trials, and a double-plus sign for IR trials. Each block consisted of a total of 7 trials across a total of 3 presentations per run (21 trials per run and 42 trials per condition across both runs). Each trial started with a condition cue for 250 ms, followed by a variable anticipation phase (three arrows were displayed in the middle of the screen; 1000–1669 ms) and the target appearance (white solid square; individually tailored duration of 100–590 ms based on the online tracking algorithm). Feedback was presented immediately after target disappearance for a duration of 1500 ms, followed by a jittered inter-trial interval (660–1340 ms). Jittering was optimized so that each trial lasted exactly two TRs (4.68 s). Block duration was 32.76 s. The fixation period between each block flashed a crosshair in each corner of the screen and then the center of the screen for the duration of a single TR (2.34 s × 5 crosshairs = 11.7 s).

To ensure that all participants fully understood the different cue-outcome relations, i.e., to avoid a learning component during the experiment, each participant received training right before the scan. This was followed by a performance-based test of their understanding as well as a practice session of the task. Only participants who fully understood the task instructions (i.e., remembered each cue-outcome relation in all three reward conditions for hit and miss trials) moved on to the practice session of the task, followed by the real fMRI scan. All participants passed the test with 100% accuracy.

Image acquisition

All imaging data were collected using a Siemens Verio 3T scanner (Erlangen, Germany) and a 32 multichannel headcoil. Functional data consisted of two 6-min 44 s runs of whole-brain T2*-weighted BOLD echo planar images with 173 volumes acquired per run, including two "dummy" scans at run onset allowing for T1 magnetic saturation (40 oblique axial slices, isotropic voxel size = 3.5 mm, TR/TE = 2340 ms/25 ms, flip angle = 60°). Two high-resolution structural MR images were acquired for the registration of fMRI data to MNI space: A T1-weighted MPRAGE sequence of the entire brain (176 sagittal slices, isotropic voxel size = 1 mm, TR/TE = 1900 ms/2.54 ms, flip angle = 9°) and a FLASH sequence collected in the same plane as the fMRI data (number of slices = 40, slice thickness = 3.5 mm, TR/TE = 300 ms/2.46 ms, flip angle = 60°).

Image analysis

Functional image processing and statistical analyses were then carried out using FEAT (FMRIB's Expert Analysis Tool), part of FMRIB's Software Library (FSL) package [30, 31]. Prior to image analysis, the first two images of the functional data set were discarded because of the non-equilibrium state of magnetization. Each time series was despiked using AFNI's 3ddespike program, motion-corrected, temporally filtered (nonlinear high-pass filter with a 1/90 HZ cutoff calculated with FSL's cutoffcalc), and a 3D Gaussian filter (FWHM = 5 mm) was applied to account for individual differences in morphology and local variations in noise. Voxel-wise regression analyses were performed on each of the participant's runs using FILM (FMRIB's Improved Linear Model). Motion parameters (i.e., six parameters corresponding to three directions of translation and three axes of rotation) were entered as nuisance regressors (absolute mean displacement: ASD = 0.13 ± 0.05 mm, TDC = 0.14 ± 0.04 mm, $p = 0.38$; relative mean displacement: ASD = 0.09 ± 0.04 mm, TDC = 0.10 ± 0.04 mm, $p = 0.79$). Each task condition (SR, IR, and NR) was coded as an explanatory variable (EV) and convolved with a double gamma function, along with its temporal derivative. Each EV yielded a per-voxel parameter estimate (β map) that represented the activation magnitude associated with that regressor. In order to create comparisons of interest, β maps were contrasted. Functional data were registered to MNI stereotactic space using affine transformations. Next, within-subject analyses across runs employed a fixed-effects model, whereas group-level inferential statistical analyses were carried out on each contrast of interest (e.g., IR vs. SR, IR vs. NR, and SR vs. NR) using FMIRB's linear analysis of mixed effects (FLAME1+2), followed by two-sample t tests (TDC vs. ASD). Whole-brain Z-statistic (Gaussianized T) maps were thresholded using clusters determined by a voxel level of $Z \geq 3.1$ (i.e., $p \leq 0.001$) and an FWE-corrected cluster-significance threshold of $p \leq 0.05$ to strictly control type I errors [32]. In addition, to test our a priori hypothesis of greater reward system activation for individual CI reward than social reward in ASD vs. TDC, we examined group differences in six regions of interest (ROI), including ventral striatum/nucleus accumbens (Nacc), dorsal striatum/caudate, ACC, vmPFC, OFC, and insula, which were anatomically defined areas from the Harvard-Oxford structural probabilistic atlases [33]. We applied a FWE-corrected threshold of $p \leq 0.05$ across each region using the Randomise v2.1 program as part of FSL [34].

Results

Behavioral task performance

Reaction times (RTs) for hits (in ms) and task accuracy (correct response rate in %) on the IDT were analyzed using a three (reward: NR vs. SR vs. IR) by two (group: ASD vs. TDC) repeated-measures MANOVA model, followed by planned contrasts. This analysis revealed a main effect of reward [$F(4,56) = 143.65$, $p < 0.001$, Cohen's $d > 1.4$], but no main effect of group [$F(2,58) = 0.53$, ns] or group-by-reward interaction effect [$F(4,56) = 1.13$, ns]. This suggests that the different reward conditions similarly affected behavioral performance across groups. The following univariate ANOVAs showed that the significant reward effect was related to both speed ($p < 0.001$, Cohen's $d > 1.4$) and accuracy ($p < 0.001$, Cohen's $d > 1.4$). Regarding RT, post hoc contrasts revealed fastest RTs for SR, slowest RTs for NR and with the IR condition intermediate (all $ps < 0.001$, all Cohen's $ds > 1.06$). This indicates that incentive manipulations within the experimental task were successful. Post hoc contrasts for accuracy revealed the highest the correct response rate for SR, the lowest the correct response rate for IR and the NR condition intermediate (all $ps < 0.004$, all Cohen's $ds > 0.77$) (see Table 2). Although we intended to maintain an equal average accuracy across conditions and participants by adjusting the target duration according to individual trial-by-trial performance, our finding of different accuracy rates for the three incentive conditions is in line with prior studies [11].

Reward system responsiveness across both study groups

Considering reward system responsiveness across both groups for the two high-level contrasts, i.e., SR > NR and IR > NR, the whole-brain analysis revealed robust brain activation (i.e., $k \geq 10$) in ventral striatum (including Nacc), dorsal striatum (including caudate nucleus, and putamen), thalamus, amygdala, ACC, vmPFC, insula, and OFC (Fig. 2). Considering differential reward system activation for the two reward types, the IR > SR comparison showed greater BOLD responses in a cluster, comprising Nacc, caudate, thalamus, ACC, vmPFC, insula and OFC ($MNI_{peak} = -2, 42, 0$; $Z_{max} = 9.16$; $k = 8047$) as well as a cluster within posterior cingulate cortex ($MNI_{peak} = 0, -30, 28$; $Z_{max} = 9.00$; $k = 166$). The reversed comparison (i.e., SR > IR) yielded significant activation differences within right and left insula ($MNI_{right\text{-}peak} = 36, -18, 20$; $Z_{max} = 5.18$; $k = 802$, and $MNI_{left\text{-}peak} = -42, -18, 6$; $Z_{max} = 4.87$; $k = 500$).

Reward system imbalance for interest reward versus social reward in ASD

Following up our hypothesis of reward "imbalance" in ASD (i.e., enhanced reward system activation for CI reward, but diminished responsiveness for social reward), we specifically investigated group activation differences in response to IR versus SR. Using whole-brain cluster thresholding that strictly controls type I errors [32], neither the IR > SR contrast nor the SR > IR contrast revealed significant group activation differences. The additional ROI analyses, however, demonstrated that the right caudate ($MNI_{peak} = 12, 14, 14$; $t_{max} = 3.14$; Cohen's $d = 0.84$; $k = 26$) as well as the left caudate ($MNI_{peak} = -12, 6, 12$; $t_{max} = 3.14$; Cohen's $d = 0.89$; $k = 96$) were more active for IR than SR in youth with ASD relative to TDC; or put differently, the caudate was less active to SR than IR in ASD versus TDC (Fig. 3). None of the other a priori ROIs (i.e., Nacc, vmPFC, ACC, OFC, and insula) revealed significant group differences for IR > SR and SR > IR.

To further examine the differential caudate response, we extracted individual β values from this bilateral cluster, separately for group and reward type (see lower right of Fig. 3). The repeated-measures ANOVA performed on the β values as the dependent variable confirmed the significant group-by-reward interaction effect [$F(1,59) = 10.46$, $p = 0.001$, Cohen's $d = 0.84$]; main effects of reward and group were non-significant ($ps > 0.51$). Follow-up within-group t tests yielded a significantly greater caudate response for interest reward than social

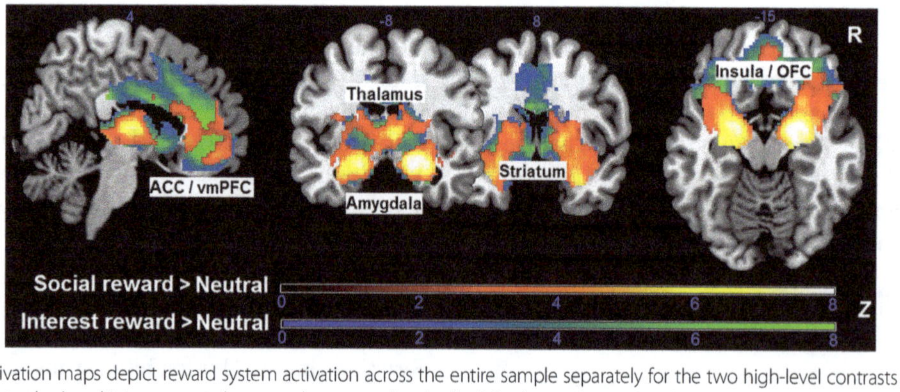

Fig. 2 *Z*-statistic activation maps depict reward system activation across the entire sample separately for the two high-level contrasts social reward > neutral outcome (hot colors) and interest reward > neutral outcome (cool colors). Both social reward and interest reward (versus neutral outcome) strongly activated a widespread reward system, comprising ventral and dorsal striatum, thalamus, amygdala, medial prefrontal areas (ACC, vmPFC) as well as clusters with orbitofrontal cortex (OFC) and anterior insula. Maps were thresholded using clusters determined by a voxel-level of $p \leq 0.001$ and an FWE-corrected cluster-significance threshold of $p \leq 0.05$. Color bars indicate *Z*-scores

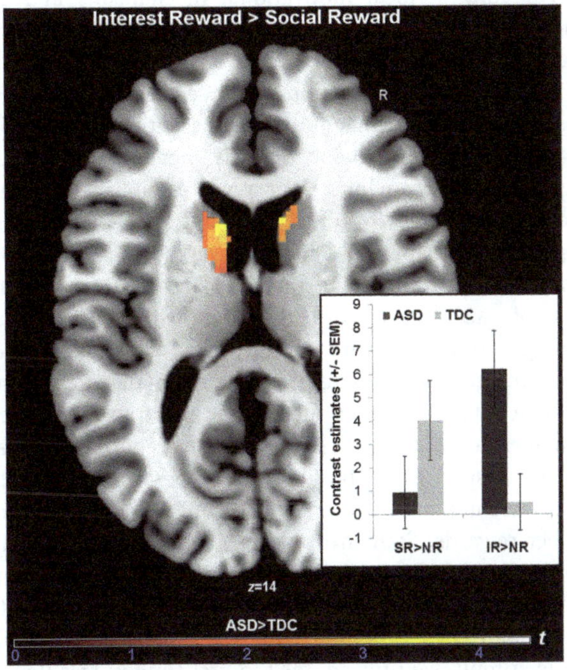

Fig. 3 ROI analyses revealed a significant group-by-reward type interaction effect in the caudate nucleus with greater dorsal striatum activation for interest reward (IR) than social reward (SR) in youth with ASD, while TDCs did not show significant differences—although a reverse direction—in their response pattern to both reward types. Bar graphs depict mean β values from the bilateral caudate cluster identified by the significant interaction effect. The ROI was anatomically defined based on the Harvard-Oxford structural probabilistic atlas. Results are FEW corrected at $p \leq 0.05$ across this particular region. Color bar indicates t-statistics

reward in the ASD group [$t(38) = -3.05$, $p = 0.004$, Cohen's $d = 0.53$], while TDC showed marginally stronger caudate activation for social reward compared to interest reward [$t(21) = 1.83$, $p = 0.081$, Cohen's $d = 0.51$]. Between-group t tests yielded significantly stronger caudate activation for IR in the ASD group compared to TDC [$t(59) = 2.79$, $p = 0.007$, Cohen's $d = 0.74$], but no significant activation differences between groups in response to SR within this cluster [$t(59) = -1.28$, *ns*, Cohen's $d = 0.34$]. The group-by-reward interaction effect remained significant when age and GCA (i.e., FSIQ) were controlled for ($p < 0.001$, Cohen's $d = 0.93$).

Given the nonselective nature of this analysis [35], we additionally investigated unbiased individual β values averaged across an anatomically defined bilateral caudate mask (based on the Harvard-Oxford probabilistic atlas). We found that the group-by-reward interaction effect was still significant, but with a lower, though still medium strong, effect size [$F(1,59) = 4.34$, $p = 0.04$, Cohen's $d = 0.55$]. Please also note that there were no significant between-group differences in brain activation for the neutral condition using whole-brain or ROI analyses (NR > fixation for structurally defined bilateral caudate: $t(59) = -1.04$, *ns*).

Because our study sample comprised of substantially more youth with ASD than TDC, we repeated our structural ROI analyses for right and left caudate in an age- and IQ-matched sub-sample of 22 individuals with ASD (14 males, 8 females; age 12.3 ± 2.4 years; IQ 110.2 ± 17.2) and the initial group of 22 TDC (17 males, 5 females; age 12.9 ± 2.1 years; IQ 111.9 ± 18.0). The results remained virtually the same, with significantly greater bilateral caudate activation for IR than SR in the 22 youth with ASD relative to the 22 TDC (right $MNI_{peak} = 10, 14, 14$; $t_{max} = 3.55$, left $MNI_{peak} = -12, 6, 12$; $t_{max} = 3.24$). Taken together, these results suggest that the caudate nucleus responded differently in ASD versus TDC dependent on the reward type. This effect was driven by particularly greater dorsal striatum responsiveness for personalized interest reward than social reward in ASD, while TDCs did not show significant differences—although a reverse direction—in their response pattern to both reward types.

Correlations between caudate response, clinical symptom severity, and RTs

To specifically test predictions derived from the social motivation hypothesis, we correlated the individual β values from the cluster that distinguished the two groups (i.e., magnitude of caudate response for IR > SR) with the degree of social dysfunction in ASD as assessed by the autism diagnostic observation scale (ADOS) severity score [36] and the SRS-2 social communication and interaction (SCI) subscale's *T*-score [26]. This analysis yielded a significant positive correlation between (right) caudate responses and SRS-2 SCI scores ($r(39) = 0.31$, $p = 0.05$; ADOS: Spearman's $\rho(39) = -0.02$, *ns*), such that stronger caudate activation for interest reward than social reward was related to greater social impairment in the ASD group (Fig. 4). Because of our a priori hypothesis, we did not apply corrections for multiple comparisons.

We further explored associations between bilateral caudate responses for IR > SR and RRBI symptoms in ASD as assessed with the RBS-R (total score), IS (total score), ADI-R (RRB total score), ADOS-2 (RRB total score), and SRS-2 (restricted interests and repetitive behavior subscale *T*-score). This analysis revealed a significant positive correlation with ADOS-2 RRB symptom expression (Spearman's $\rho(39) = 0.41$, $p = 0.011$; Additional file 1: Table S2), such that stronger caudate responsiveness for CI reward than social reward was associated with greater (clinically observed) RRBIs in our ASD sample. This correlation, however, would not survive correction for multiple comparisons.

We additionally found a significant negative correlation between (left) caudate activation differences to IR

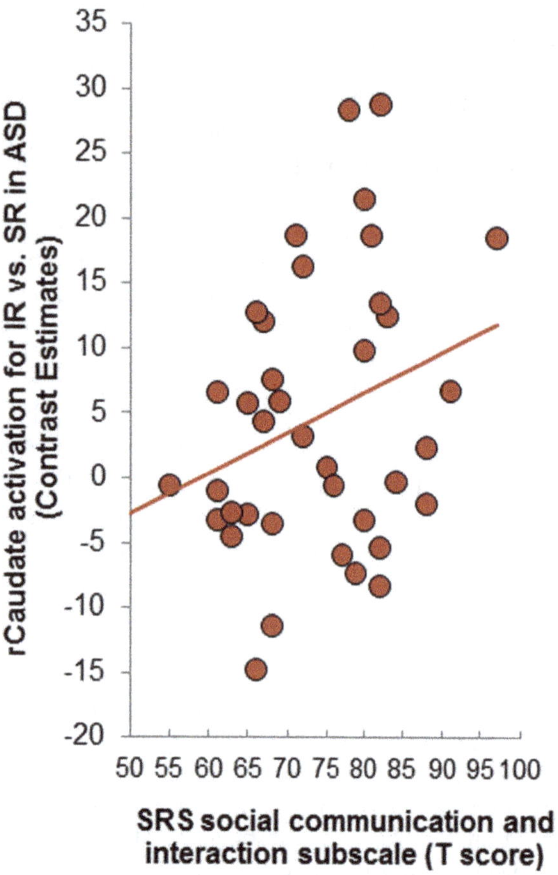

Fig. 4 The magnitude of caudate activation that distinguished the two groups correlated positively with ASD symptom severity as assessed by the SRS-2 social communication and interaction sub-score (for the ASD group only). The stronger the caudate activation for personalized interest reward vs. social reward the greater the social impairment in the ASD group

> NR and ΔRT for IR vs.NR in the ASD group ($r(39) = -0.32$, $p = 0.05$). This suggests that stronger caudate responsiveness to CIs versus neutral outcome was associated with faster behavioral responses by the participants with ASD to attain this individual reward. Please note, though, that this correlation would not survive correction for multiple comparisons.

Discussion

The results of this fMRI study are in line with predictions by the social motivation hypothesis [3, 37]: Compared to TDCs, youth with ASD had stronger reward system responses for CIs mostly within the non-social realm (e.g., video games) than social rewards (e.g., approval). Additionally, aberrant reward system responses—most pronounced within the caudate nucleus-were related to greater social impairment. Behavioral task performance did not differ between the two study groups, emphasizing the power of neurobiological data in revealing atypical motivational mechanisms in ASD and at the same time avoiding a potential confounding factor [38].

The current investigation advanced the strengths of the two preceding imaging studies targeting CIs in ASD [14, 15] by (a) employing a newly created set of video clips as reinforcement in (b) a well-established instrumental reward task to (c) reliably contrast reward system responsiveness for individual CIs versus social approval rewards. Thus, we tested the social motivation hypothesis of ASD more directly, and we applied more ecologically valid reward stimuli. Using a standard set of static images hypothesized to be "autism-specific objects of high interest" versus monetary reward as incentives, Dichter and colleagues [6] previously reported blunted striatal responses to both reward types in adults with ASD, accompanied by enhanced vmPFC activation for object rewards. Standardized objects as a proxy for CIs, however, provide a potentially weaker estimate of the neural reward effects that could be identified with individualized CI items. Moreover, instead of simple static stimuli, we utilized, for the first time in this line of research, dynamic incentives that are commonly experienced as more naturalistic and appealing and, thus, may elicit both stronger and more reliable motivational responses [39].

The aberrant pattern of caudate activation in ASD not only supports prior research but also highlights a potentially fundamental difference in how individuals with ASD prioritize CI stimuli over social stimuli. Our finding of greater BOLD responses for CI rewards than social rewards in youth with ASD compared to a more balanced response pattern in TDCs substantiates the earlier report by Dichter and colleagues [6]. In contrast to our hypothesis, our follow-up analyses did not reveal specifically diminished caudate responses to social reward when directly comparing the two groups, at least with the social incentives used in this study sample. Other recent functional imaging studies, however, did reveal aberrant caudate responses to both social and monetary reward in ASD [7, 11]. Converging evidence from human and nonhuman research links the caudate nucleus directly to decision-making processes, specifically to the selection and initiation of purposeful actions in order to maximize reward outcome [40]. In this regard, we found that greater BOLD responses in the left caudate to CI rewards were associated with faster reaction times by the participants with ASD to obtain this positive outcome (but only at an uncorrected significance level). This suggests that in youth with ASD the caudate nucleus may optimize goal-directed actions for CIs to a greater extent than for social rewards or other types of "conventional" desires (e.g., money). Whether the caudate nucleus is also involved in aberrant instrumental responsiveness to primary rewards, such as food [41], should be investigated in future studies.

Notably, we detected that stronger caudate responsiveness for CIs (versus social reward) was related to greater overall symptom severity among our participants with ASD. Cascio and colleagues [14] recently reported that activation of the insula—as part of the "salience network"—in response to viewing pictures of one's own vs. others' interests was positively correlated with CI severity, but not overall clinical symptomatology, in youth with ASD. As noted in the Introduction, an instrumental task with active response-outcome contingencies is critical for stimulating reward pathways [16]. A passive viewing task may be less optimal for observing reward system responsiveness in relation to ASD symptoms. Thus, our findings emphasize the connection between the caudate nucleus as a core reward region involved in goal-directed behavior and the clinical phenotype of ASD (see also [42]).

Although several plausible models have been advanced to explain RRBIs in ASD (e.g., inhibitory control deficit), the relatively overactive caudate nucleus for CIs, as found in the present study, supports the idea that ASD may be in part a motivational disorder of "behavioral dependency" to RRBIs because of the rewarding effects they induce [4]. Different authors have argued that the rewarding effect of RRBIs, including CIs, may originate from the need of people with ASD for predictability, i.e., lawful and deterministic events in their environment, where they can exert more control [43]; rapid and uncertain moment-by-moment changes of a person's behavior inherent in social encounters are the opposite. The unpredictable nature of social encounters may make them unrewarding or even anxiety-provoking and aversive for individuals with ASD [44]. RRBIs, such as CIs, in turn, may offer a pleasurable compensation for the unpredictable social world.

The exact mechanisms as to how the dominating reward effects of CIs emerge and interfere with the reward value of social engagement in ASD are, however, yet unclear. When CIs are indeed rewarding, their pursuit may be strengthened through self-reinforcement that turns them into rigid habits [45]. The self-reinforcing character of RRBIs, like CIs, may hijack the normal developmental trajectories of entire repertoires of behaviors, including social ones. We suggest that the caudate nucleus—in concert with other frontolimbic structures [46]—may dominate the formation and maintenance of RRBIs. On a daily basis, RRBIs hinder social development and functioning because they absorb resources typically dedicated to social learning opportunities [4]. This view converges with recent evidence demonstrating the role of the caudate nucleus, as part of a cortico-striatal-thalamo-cortical loop [47], in CIs as well as compulsive and ritualistic behaviors in individuals with ASD across different age groups [42, 48–51].

While we could demonstrate robust neural activation differences between ASD and TDC for CI rewards versus social rewards in dorsal striatum, other brain regions that have previously been related to CIs did not emerge in our study (i.e., ventral striatum/Nacc and vmPFC [15] as well as ACC and insula [14]). Despite our specific finding of an imbalance of caudate nucleus responsiveness in ASD, we acknowledge that CIs are not limited to a single anatomical correlate, but are mediated by various distinct yet interacting subcortical and cortical systems [1, 47]. Follow-up studies are warranted to better define how different subcomponents of reward processing—and their neural correlates—contribute to the emergence of and adherence to CIs. Incentive delay tasks, such as the one applied here, can principally be used to test reward learning, reward anticipation and reward valuation as three crucial reward components to consider with regard to CIs and the responsiveness to other "conventional" rewards in ASD [2]. While each reward component has been associated with some distinct (and some interrelated) neural correlates [52], recent human research highlights, however, the difficulty to effectively decompose the neural signals of the various components within a single experimental paradigm (see for a discussion on this issue, [53]). Thus, we foresee that refined inventories of specifically tailored reward measures—preferably grounded in preclinical studies and adequately validated in humans—will benefit this line of research.

Importantly, future fMRI investigations need to control more strictly for multiple comparisons at the whole-brain level. This will help avoiding high degrees of false positive findings and, thus, will ensure that neuroimaging results—particularly between-group findings—are more reliably reproduced. In the present study, we implemented most recent recommendations from the literature using whole-brain cluster thresholding that rigorously controls type I errors [32]; this could also explain why we were not able to replicate some of the previous findings (see Additional file 1: Table S3 for prior analytic approaches in this line of research).

This study had the following limitations: While we presented individually tailored interest clips, we did not utilize personalized social rewards, such as approval clips by caregivers, or preferred peers. Several recent investigations, however, indicate that personally meaningful social incentives hold similar reward value for youth with ASD as unfamiliar social rewards (e.g., [54, 55]); thus, it is unlikely that this potential confound fully accounts for the present findings. An imminent drawback to the use of unique interest items was their diversity among participants, which possibly added noise into the data. We endeavored to strictly equate stimulus properties across participants and conditions. Stimulus diversity (including differential complexity and luminance of video materials), however, may have precluded us from having enough statistical power to reveal additional regions involved in core reward mechanisms of CIs due to BOLD signal heterogeneity (e.g., Nacc, or vmPFC). Moreover, using a blocked design did not allow parsing brain responses for reward learning, anticipation, and consumption. Finally, because we explicitly targeted CIs, our findings are limited to this specific type of RRBI. A logical next step would be to extend this line of research to elucidate reward functions with regard to stereotypies, insistence on sameness, and sensory responses (e.g., [56]) using fMRI as well as other imaging methods, such as event-related brain potentials [57].

Conclusion

In conclusion, the results of this fMRI study add to the emerging clinical and imaging evidence of striatal involvement in the ASD pathophysiology [58]. More precisely, we demonstrated aberrant caudate nucleus responsiveness in ASD, with greater brain responses for CIs relative to social reward that was also associated with social impairment. We did not find, however, specifically diminished reward system responses to social reward when directly comparing youth with ASD to TDC, at least with the social rewards (i.e., approval from unfamiliar adults) used in the present study. We speculate that reward system dysfunction—most pronounced within the caudate nucleus—may contribute to enhanced motivation for RRBIs in ASD, accompanied by diminished motivation for social engagement. If a dysregulated reward system indeed supports the emergence and maintenance of social and non-social symptoms of ASD, then strategically targeting the role of reward mechanisms will allow for the development of more efficacious treatment practices to better support individuals with ASD and their families.

Abbreviations

ACC: Anterior cingulate cortex; ADI-R: Autism Diagnostic Interview-Revised; ADOS: Autism Diagnostic Observation Schedule; ASD: Autism spectrum disorder; avi: Audio video interleave; BOLD: Blood-oxygen-level-dependent; CASI: Child and Adolescent Symptom Inventory; CI: Circumscribed interest; DSM-IV-TR: Diagnostic and Statistical Manual of Mental Disorders-Fourth Edition-Text Revision; EV: Explanatory variable; fMRI: Functional magnetic resonance imaging; FSIQ: Full-scale intelligence quotient; FWE: Family-wise error rate; GCA: General conceptual ability; HD: High definition; IDT: Incentive delay task; IPA: Interest Preference Assessment; IQ: Intelligence quotient; IR: Interest reward; IS: Interests Scale; Nacc: Nucleus accumbens; NR: Neutral; OFC: Orbitofrontal cortex; PIQ: Performance/nonverbal IQ; R: Social reward; RBS-R: Repetitive Behavior Scale-Revised; ROI: Region of interest; RRBI: Restricted and repetitive behaviors and interests; RT: Reaction time; SRS-2: Social Responsiveness Scale—2nd Edition; SS: Standard score; TDC: Typically developing controls; VIQ: Verbal IQ; vmPFC: Ventromedial prefrontal cortex

Acknowledgements

We thank the many youths and families for their participation in the study.

Funding

The study was sponsored by grants from the National Institute of Mental Health (K23MH086111; PI: B.E. Yerys, R21MH092615; PI: B.E. Yerys, RC1MH088791; R.T. Schultz), and a New Program Development Award to B.E. Yerys through the Intellectual and Developmental Disabilities Research Center funded by the National Institute of Child and Human Development (P30HD026979; PI: M. Yudkoff), a grant from the Philadelphia Foundation (co-funded Dr. Yerys' New Program Development Award), a grant from the Pennsylvania Department of Health (SAP #4100042728) to R.T. Schultz, a grant from the Pennsylvania Department of Health (SAP #4100047863) to R.T. Schultz, a grant from Pfizer to R.T. Schultz, and a grant from the Robert Wood Johnson Foundation, #6672 to R.T. Schultz. G. Kohls was supported by funding from the European Community's Seventh Framework Programme (FP7/2007–2013) under Grant Agreement no. 602407 (FemNAT-CD) during manuscript preparation.

Authors' contributions

GK and BEY conceived of the study. LA and MGM recruited participants and carried out assessments and data collection, including MRI acquisition. BEY contributed to consensus clinical diagnosis. GK and BEY performed the statistical analyses and drafted the manuscript. LA contributed to data analyses. RTS contributed to the theoretical approach presented in the manuscript. All authors contributed to writing the manuscript, and they read and approved the final manuscript.

Competing interests

The authors declare that they have no competing interests.

Author details

[1]Department of Child and Adolescent Psychiatry, Psychosomatics and Psychotherapy, RWTH Aachen University, Aachen, Germany. [2]Department of Psychology, Virginia Polytechnic Institute and State University, Blacksburg, VA, USA. [3]Department of Psychology, University of North Carolina at Chapel Hill, Chapel Hill, NC, USA. [4]Center for Autism Research, The Children's Hospital of Philadelphia, 3535 Market Street, Ste 860, Philadelphia, PA 19104, USA. [5]Pediatrics Department, Perelman School of Medicine, University of Pennsylvania, Philadelphia, PA, USA. [6]Psychiatry Department, Perelman School of Medicine, University of Pennsylvania, Philadelphia, PA, USA.

References

1. Yerys BE. An update on the neurobiology of repetitive behaviors in autism. In: International review of research in developmental disabilities. 2015. 91–150.
2. Kohls G, Chevallier C, Troiani V, Schultz RT. Social "wanting" dysfunction in autism: neurobiological underpinnings and treatment implications. J Neurodev Disord. 2012;4:10.
3. Chevallier C, Kohls G, Troiani V, Brodkin ES, Schultz RT. The social motivation theory of autism. Trends Cogn Sci. 2012;16:231–9.
4. Kohls G, Yerys BE, Schultz RT. Striatal development in autism: repetitive behaviors and the reward circuitry. Biol Psychiatry. 2014;76:358–9.
5. Schultz RT. Developmental deficits in social perception in autism: the role of the amygdala and fusiform face area. Int J Dev Neurosci. 2005;23:125–41.
6. Dichter GS, Damiano CA, Allen JA. Reward circuitry dysfunction in psychiatric and neurodevelopmental disorders and genetic syndromes: animal models and clinical findings. J Neurodev Disord. 2012;4:19.
7. Kohls G, Schulte-Rüther M, Nehrkorn B, Müller K, Fink GR, Kamp-Becker I, et al. Reward system dysfunction in autism spectrum disorders. Soc Cogn Affect Neurosci. 2013;8:565–72.
8. Kohls G, Thönessen H, Bartley GK, Grossheinrich N, Fink GR, Herpertz-Dahlmann B, et al. Differentiating neural reward responsiveness in autism versus ADHD. Dev Cogn Neurosci. 2014;10:104–16.

9. Scott-Van Zeeland AA, Dapretto M, Ghahremani DG, Poldrack RA, Bookheimer SY. Reward processing in autism. Autism Res. 2010;3:53–67.
10. Dichter GS, Richey JA, Rittenberg AM, Sabatino A, Bodfish JW. Reward circuitry function in autism during face anticipation and outcomes. J Autism Dev Disord. 2012;42:147–60.
11. Delmonte S, Balsters JH, McGrath J, Fitzgerald J, Brennan S, Fagan AJ, et al. Social and monetary reward processing in autism spectrum disorders. Mol Autism. 2012;3:7.
12. Mercier C, Mottron L, Belleville S. A psychosocial study on restricted interests in high functioning persons with pervasive developmental disorders. Autism. 2000;4:406–25.
13. Charlop-Christy MH, Haymes LK. Using objects of obsession as token reinforcers for children with autism. J Autism Dev Disord. 1998;28:189–98.
14. Cascio CJ, Foss-Feig JH, Heacock J, Schauder KB, Loring WA, Rogers BP, et al. Affective neural response to restricted interests in autism spectrum disorders. J Child Psychol Psychiatry. 2014;55:162–71.
15. Dichter GS, Felder JN, Green SR, Rittenberg AM, Sasson NJ, Bodfish JW. Reward circuitry function in autism spectrum disorders. Soc Cogn Affect Neurosci. 2012;7:160–72.
16. Bjork JM, Hommer DW. Anticipating instrumentally obtained and passively-received rewards: a factorial fMRI investigation. Behav Brain Res. 2007;177:165–70.
17. Risko EF, Laidlaw KEW, Freeth M, Foulsham T, Kingstone A. Social attention with real versus reel stimuli: toward an empirical approach to concerns about ecological validity. Front Hum Neurosci. 2012;6:143.
18. Kohls G, Perino MT, Taylor JM, Madva EN, Cayless SJ, Troiani V, et al. The nucleus accumbens is involved in both the pursuit of social reward and the avoidance of social punishment. Neuropsychologia. 2013;51:2062–9.
19. Elliott CD. Differential Ability Scales-II (DAS-II). San Antonio: Pearson Assessments; 2007.
20. American Psychiatric Association. Diagnostic and statistical manual of mental disorders, fifth edition (DSM-5). Washington: American Psychiatric Association; 2013.
21. Lord C, Rutter M, Le Couteur A. Autism diagnostic interview-revised: a revised version of a diagnostic interview for caregivers of individuals with possible pervasive developmental disorders. J Autism Dev Disord. 1994;24:659–85.
22. Lord C, Risi S, Lambrecht L, Cook EH, Leventhal BL, DiLavore PC, et al. The autism diagnostic observation schedule-generic: a standard measure of social and communication deficits associated with the spectrum of autism. J Autism Dev Disord. 2000;30:205–23.
23. Gadow KD, Sprafkin J. Child symptom inventories manual. Stony Brook: Checkmate Plus; 1994.
24. Anthony LG, Kenworthy L, Yerys BE, Jankowski KF, James JD, Harms MB, et al. Interests in high-functioning autism are more intense, interfering, and idiosyncratic than those in neurotypical development. Dev Psychopathol. 2013;25:643–52.
25. Turner-Brown LM, Lam KSL, Holtzclaw TN, Dichter GS, Bodfish JW. Phenomenology and measurement of circumscribed interests in autism spectrum disorders. Autism. 2011;15:437–56.
26. Constantino J, Gruber C. The Social Responsiveness Scale—second edition (SRS-2) manual. Torrance: Western Psychological Services; 2012.
27. Bodfish JW, Symons FJ, Parker DE, Lewis MH. Varieties of repetitive behavior in autism: comparisons to mental retardation. J Autism Dev Disord. 2000;30:237–43.
28. Lam KSL, Aman MG. The repetitive behavior scale-revised: independent validation in individuals with autism spectrum disorders. J Autism Dev Disord. 2007;37:855–66.
29. Knutson B, Taylor J, Kaufman M, Peterson R, Glover G. Distributed neural representation of expected value. J Neurosci. 2005;25:4806–12.
30. Jenkinson M, Beckmann CF, Behrens TEJ, Woolrich MW, Smith SM. FSL. NeuroImage. 2012;62:782–90.
31. Smith SM, Jenkinson M, Woolrich MW, Beckmann CF, Behrens TEJ, Johansen-Berg H, et al. Advances in functional and structural MR image analysis and implementation as FSL. NeuroImage. 2004;23 S(1):208–19.
32. Eklund A, Nichols TE, Knutsson H. Cluster failure: why fMRI inferences for spatial extent have inflated false-positive rates. Proc Natl Acad Sci U S A. 2016;113:7900–5.
33. Mazziotta J, Toga A, Evans A, Fox P, Lancaster J, Zilles K, et al. A probabilistic atlas and reference system for the human brain: international consortium for brain mapping (ICBM). Philos Trans R Soc Lond B Biol Sci. 2001;356: 1293–322.
34. Winkler AM, Ridgway GR, Webster MA, Smith SM, Nichols TE. Permutation inference for the general linear model. NeuroImage. 2014;92:381–97.
35. Kriegeskorte N, Simmons WK, Bellgowan PSF, Baker CI. Circular analysis in systems neuroscience: the dangers of double dipping. Nat Neurosci. 2009; 12:535–40.
36. Gotham K, Pickles A, Lord C. Standardizing ADOS scores for a measure of severity in autism spectrum disorders. J Autism Dev Disord. 2009;39:693–705.
37. Dawson G, Webb SJ, McPartland J. Understanding the nature of face processing impairment in autism: insights from behavioral and electrophysiological studies. Dev Neuropsychol. 2005;27:403–24.
38. Murphy K, Garavan H. Artifactual fMRI group and condition differences driven by performance confounds. NeuroImage. 2004;21:219–28.
39. Chevallier C, Parish-Morris J, McVey A, Rump KM, Sasson NJ, Herrington JD, et al. Measuring social attention and motivation in autism spectrum disorder using eye-tracking: stimulus type matters. Autism Res. 2015;8:620–8.
40. Balleine BW, Delgado MR, Hikosaka O. The role of the dorsal striatum in reward and decision-making. J Neurosci. 2007;27:8161–5.
41. Cascio CJ, Foss-Feig JH, Heacock JL, Newsom CR, Cowan RL, Benningfield MM, et al. Response of neural reward regions to food cues in autism spectrum disorders. J Neurodev Disord. 2012;4:9.
42. Langen M, Bos D, Noordermeer SDS, Nederveen H, van Engeland H, Durston S. Changes in the development of striatum are involved in repetitive behavior in autism. Biol Psychiatry. 2014;76:405–11.
43. Baron-Cohen S. Autism: the empathizing-systemizing (E-S) theory. Ann N Y Acad Sci. 2009;1156:68–80.
44. Factor RS, Condy EE, Farley JP, Scarpa A. Brief report: insistence on sameness, anxiety, and social motivation in children with autism spectrum disorder. J Autism Dev Disord. 2016;46:2548–54.
45. Bandura A. Self-reinforcement: theoretical and methodological considerations. Behaviorism. 1976;4:135–55.
46. Graybiel AM. Habits, rituals, and the evaluative brain. Annu Rev Neurosci. 2008;31:359–87.
47. Langen M, Durston S, Kas MJH, van Engeland H, Staal WG. The neurobiology of repetitive behavior: …and men. Neurosci Biobehav Rev. 2011;35:356–65.
48. Eisenberg IW, Wallace GL, Kenworthy L, Gotts SJ, Martin A. Insistence on sameness relates to increased covariance of gray matter structure in autism spectrum disorder. Mol Autism. 2015;6:54.
49. Langen M, Schnack HG, Nederveen H, Bos D, Lahuis BE, de Jonge MV, et al. Changes in the developmental trajectories of striatum in autism. Biol Psychiatry. 2009;66:327–33.
50. Qiu T, Chang C, Li Y, Qian L, Xiao CY, Xiao T, et al. Two years changes in the development of caudate nucleus are involved in restricted repetitive behaviors in 2-5-year-old children with autism spectrum disorder. Dev Cogn Neurosci. 2016;19:137–43.
51. Schuetze M, Park MTM, Cho IY, MacMaster FP, Chakravarty MM, Bray SL. Morphological alterations in the thalamus, striatum, and pallidum in autism spectrum disorder. Neuropsychopharmacology. 2016;41:2627–37.
52. Berridge KC, Robinson TE, Aldridge JW. Dissecting components of reward: 'liking', 'wanting', and learning. Curr Opin Pharmacol. 2009;9:65–73.
53. Rizvi SJ, Pizzagalli DA, Sproule BA, Kennedy SH. Assessing anhedonia in depression: potentials and pitfalls. Neurosci Biobehav Rev. 2016;65:21–35.
54. Stavropoulos KKM, Carver LJ. Effect of familiarity on reward anticipation in children with and without autism spectrum disorders. PLoS One. 2014;9:e106667.
55. Pankert A, Pankert K, Herpertz-Dahlmann B, Konrad K, Kohls G. Responsivity to familiar versus unfamiliar social reward in children with autism. J Neural Transm. 2014;

7

Insulin receptor sensitization restores neocortical excitation/inhibition balance in a mouse model of autism

Fu-Sun Lo and Reha S. Erzurumlu*

Abstract

Background: Met receptor tyrosine kinase regulates neurogenesis, differentiation, migration, connectivity, and synaptic plasticity. The human *Met* gene has been identified as a prominent risk factor for autism spectrum disorder (ASD). Met gene-altered mice serve as useful models for mechanistic studies of ASD. Inactivation of *Met* in excitatory cortical neurons in mice (*Emx1*^{cre}/*Met* ^{flox} mice) yields a phenotype in which significantly decreased $GABA_A$ receptor-mediated inhibition shifts the excitation/inhibition (E/I) balance toward excitation in the somatosensory cortex. Further, unlike that seen in wild-type mice, insulin does not increase inhibition in the mutant cortex, suggesting that one of the consequences of kinase inactive *Met* gene could be desensitization of insulin receptors. To test this hypothesis, we investigated the effects of insulin receptor sensitizer, pioglitazone, on inhibition in the somatosensory thalamocortical circuitry.

Methods: We used whole-cell patch clamp electrophysiology and analyzed excitatory and inhibitory responses of cortical layer IV excitatory cells following stimulation of their thalamic input in thalamocortical pathway intact brain slices. We applied insulin alone and insulin + a thiazolidinedione, pioglitazone (PIO), to test the effects of sensitizing insulin receptors on inhibitory responses mediated by $GABA_A$ receptors in the somatosensory cortex of *Emx1*^{cre}/*Met* ^{flox} mice.

Results: In WT brain slices, application of insulin together with PIO did not enhance the effect of insulin alone. In contrast, PIO application induced a much larger inhibition than that of insulin alone in *Met*-defective cortex. Thus, insulin resistance of $GABA_A$ receptor-mediated response in *Met* mutant mice may result from desensitized insulin receptors.

Conclusions: Sporadic clinical studies reported improved behavioral symptoms in children with autism following PIO treatment. We show that PIO can aid in normalization of the E/I balance in the primary somatosensory cortex, a potential physiological mechanism underlying the positive effects of PIO treatment.

Keywords: Met receptor tyrosine kinase, Barrel cortex, Homeostatic plasticity, $GABA_A$ receptors, Pioglitazone, Thalamocortical circuitry

Background

Numerous studies have associated *Met* gene as a of a functional risk allele in autism spectrum disorders (ASD) [1–3]. The Met receptor tyrosine kinase is a multifunctional receptor with diverse biological roles activating various intracellular signaling pathways. *Met* mutations in mice provide models to investigate cellular and molecular deficits in the nervous system. One such line, *Emx1*^{cre}/*Met* ^{flox} mice (from here on referred to as *Met-Emx1* mouse), has kinase-inactive *Met* gene in excitatory neurons of the neocortex, hippocampus, and olfactory bulbs [4, 5]. For cortical studies, these mice may be considered as cortex-specific null mutation of *Met*. Previously, we reported that in thalamocortical brain slices from *Met-Emx1* mice the E/I ratio is biased toward excitation in the primary somatosensory cortex due to decreased $GABA_A$ receptor-mediated inhibition [6]. Excitation-inhibition (E/I) balance in neural circuits is a type of homeostatic synaptic plasticity that is notably affected in various neurological and psychiatric conditions [7, 8].

Insulin receptors are abundant in the brain [9, 10], and insulin regulates GABAergic inhibition by increasing the

* Correspondence: rerzurumlu@som.umaryland.edu
Department of Anatomy and Neurobiology, University of Maryland School of Medicine, 22 Penn Street HSFII-S259, Baltimore, MD 21201, USA

density of $GABA_A$ receptors, consequently augmenting inhibitory postsynaptic currents [11, 12]. In our study, we found that in wild-type (WT, C57BL/6) brain slices insulin enhances $GABA_A$ receptor-mediated response. In contrast, insulin treatment had no effect on slices from *Emx1*^{cre}/*Met*^{flox} mice [6]. To determine whether sensitizing insulin receptors can enhance $GABA_A$ receptor-mediated response, we tested pioglitazone (PIO) treatment. PIO is a widely used thiazolidinedione that acts as an insulin-sensitizer through activation of the peroxisome proliferator-activated receptor-γ [13]. There are two members of the class thiazolidinediones that have been used as insulin sensitizers in treatment of type 2 diabetes: pioglitazone (Actos) and rosiglitazone (Avandia). We have chosen to use PIO because it is the most widely used and rosiglitazone has yielded less-desirable effects. Furthermore, few clinical studies have reported improved symptoms in neurodevelopmental and neurogeriatric conditions following PIO treatment [14–20]. In the future, testing different members of this drug family under in vivo conditions could yield important insights. In WT thalamocortical slices, application of insulin plus PIO did not enhance the effect of insulin alone. However, this treatment induced a much larger inhibition than that of insulin alone in *Met-Emx1* mice. This finding indicates that the insulin resistance of $GABA_A$ receptor-mediated response in *Met-Emx1* mice mainly results from desensitized insulin receptors.

Methods

Animals

The brain slices were derived from *Met-Emx1* mice of both sexes ($n = 5$). We obtained these mice through crossings of the floxed *Met* mouse (*Met-fx*) with the cerebral cortical and hippocampal specific *Emx1-cre* mouse. Our original sources and further details of the mouse lines are detailed in a previous paper [6], currently both lines are commercially available (*Met-fx* stock #016974, *Emx1-Cre*, stock #005628, Jackson Laboratory, Bar Harbor, ME). Control brain slices were from mice with *Met-fx* or *Emx1-cre* alleles alone or C57BL/6 (the background of the mutant line) mice ($n = 5$). There were no differences between the three types of control slices. For mouse use, we followed the National Institute of Health Guide for the Care and Use of Laboratory Animals (ISBN:13:978-0-309-15400-0, revised in 2011) and the UMB SOM Animal Use and Care Committee approved our protocol.

Brain slice preparation

Two- to 4-week-old mice were euthanized and their brains removed into cold sucrose supplemented with artificial cerebrospinal fluid (ACSF, in mM: $NaHCO_3$ 25, glucose 11, sucrose 234, KCl 2.5, $NaHPO_4$ 1.25, $MgSO_4$ 10). Next, we cut 350-μm-thick thalamocortical pathway intact brain slices using a vibratome (Campden 7000msz), at an angle of 50–55° from the mid-sagittal plane and 10° from the coronal plane [21, 22]. In such slices, the connections from the ventrobasal nucleus of the thalamus (VB) to the primary somatosensory, specifically the whisker representation zone, the barrel cortex, remain intact. We kept the slices in normal ACSF (in mM: NaCl 126, KCl 3.0, NaH_2PO_4 1.25, $MgSO_4$ 1.0, $NaHCO_3$ 26, glucose 10, $CaCl_2$ 2, L-ascorbic acid 1.3, pH = 7.4) for at least 1 h, at room temperature. We placed the slice containing the thalamocortical pathway in a submerged-type recording chamber (27 L, Warner Ins.), and continuously perfused (> 2 mL/min) with normal ACSF at room temperature. Under these conditions, intra-cortical circuits are inactivated, and the excitatory thalamocortical synapses on layer IV neurons can be isolated [23].

Thalamocortical slice electrophysiology

We prepared borosilicate glass (WPI, K150F-4) whole-cell-patch micropipettes by pulling them in three stages with a P-87 horizontal puller (Sutter Instrument Co.). We back-filled the electrodes with a Cs-based intracellular solution (in mM: $CsMeSO_3$, 115; NaCl, 10; KCl, 1, $MgCl_2$, 4; $CaCl_2$, 1; EGTA, 11; HEPES, 20; Na_2-ATP, 3; Na_2-GTP, 0.5, pH = 7.25, > 290 mOsm). The electrodes had a tip resistance of 5–9 MΩ. Spiny stellate and star pyramid cells are the excitatory neurons of layer IV barrel cortex. We patched these neurons to form whole-cell configuration. We passed depolarizing current pulses through the patch pipette in current clamp mode to identify the cells by their firing patterns [24–26]. For stimulation of the thalamocortical afferents, we used a concentric electrode (FHC, CBFP J50) either inserted in the VB, which can be visualized in slices or in the internal capsule (IC). We passed 0.33 Hz electrical pulses for 0.3 ms duration, 0.33 Hz to evoke postsynaptic responses in both current- and voltage-clamp modes. We acquired the by Axopatch 200B amplifier and an Instru-TECH ITC-16 interface unit and stored on a Dell DM061 computer with PULSE (HEKA) software program.

Isolation of $GABA_A$ receptor- and AMPA receptor-mediated postsynaptic currents

At − 60 mV holding potential, stimulation of the VB elicits an early inward current (excitatory postsynaptic current, EPSC) followed by an outward current (inhibitory postsynaptic current, IPSC). As we move the holding potential toward more negative values, the outward current becomes smaller, and when this current disappears around − 70 mV holding potential, we define this as the $GABA_A$ receptor reversal potential. In the absence of any NMDA receptor blockade, the remaining inward current is pure AMPA receptor-mediated EPSC. This inward current can be blocked by 10 μM NBQX, but not by 50 μM picrotoxin (PTX). Changing the holding potential toward more positive values decreased the amplitude of the inward current and it disappeared around 0 mV holding potential, which we defined as the reversal potential for glutamate receptors. The resulting outward current could be completely blocked by 50 μM PTX but not by 100 μM DL-APV; thus, it is the isolated $GABA_A$ receptor-mediated IPSC. We calculated the ratio of AMPA/GABA (E/I) for each neuron by averaging 10 traces of EPSCs and IPSCs induced by maximal stimulation.

$GABA_A$ receptor-mediated spontaneous IPSCs (sIPSCs)

We recorded spontaneous IPSCs at 0 mV. We measured the averaged amplitude of sIPSCs using MiniAnalysis Software.

Chemicals

Insulin (500 nM), pioglitazone (PIO, 10 μM), an insulin receptor sensitizer, NBQX (10 μM), an AMPA receptor antagonist, DL-APV (100 μM), a NMDA receptor antagonist, and PTX (50 μM), a $GABA_A$ receptor antagonist were applied as needed. All chemicals are purchased from Sigma-Aldrich Co. (St. Louis, MO).

Data analysis

We used Student's *t* test to determine significance. All data are expressed by mean ± s.e.m. (standard error of the mean). Box and whisker plots were generated in R studio version 1.1.419.

Results

Functional insulin receptors in the barrel cortex of WT mice

Previously, we investigated the thalamocortical synaptic transmission in the barrel cortex of various lines of transgenic and WT mice [6, 27, 28]. In complete agreement with those studies, layer IV excitatory neurons show adapting discharges (regular spikes, RS) upon membrane depolarization (Fig. 1a–c). Stimulation of VB induces an excitatory postsynaptic potential-inhibitory postsynaptic potential (EPSP-IPSP) sequence. At membrane potential of − 60 mV, the IPSP just curtails the

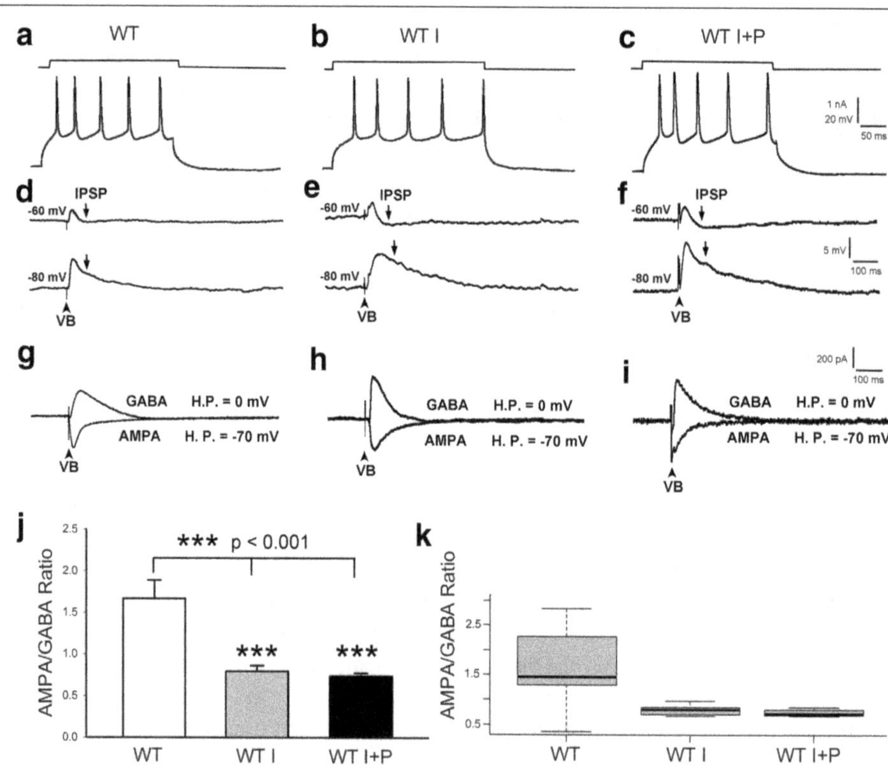

Fig. 1 Insulin and pioglitazone treatment effects on the E/I ratio in WT brain slices. **a–c** Membrane depolarization characteristically leads to regular spiking of layer IV excitatory neurons. This characteristic is evident in control (WT) slices, and after application of insulin (WT I), or insulin + pioglitazone (WT I + P). **d** EPSP-IPSP sequence following VB stimulation. At − 60 mV, the IPSP does not hyperpolarize below − 60 mV (upper trace). The IPSP polarity reverses at − 80 mV, around $GABA_A$ receptor reversal potential (lower trace). **e** 500 nM insulin application results in an increase of IPSP that hyperpolarized below base line at − 60 mV (upper trace). The IPSP is mediated by $GABA_A$ receptor, because it reverses at − 80 mV (lower trace). **f** Addition of pioglitazone to insulin application does not lead to any notable change. **g–i** Representative records of $GABA_A$ receptor- and AMPA receptor-mediated currents under control, insulin, and insulin + pioglitazone application conditions. *HP* holding potential. **j** The averaged AMPA/GABA (E/I) ratios under the three conditions. Note that insulin application significantly reduces the E/I ratio; addition of pioglitazone does not change insulin effects alone. **k** Box and whisker plots showing the population distribution

EPSP but does not hyperpolarize below − 60 mV (Fig. 1d, upper trace). The IPSP is reversed in polarity at − 80 mV, suggesting that it is mediated by $GABA_A$ receptor with a reversal potential around − 70 mV (Fig. 1d, lower trace).

In WT thalamocortical slices, application of 500 nM insulin resulted in an increase of IPSP that hyperpolarized below base line at − 60 mV (Fig. 1e, WT I, upper trace). The IPSP was also mediated by $GABA_A$ receptor, because it reversed at − 80 mV (Fig. 1e, lower trace). In order to quantify the changes in E/I ratio, we voltage-clamped each cell to the reversal potential of $GABA_A$ receptors (around − 70 mV) and AMPA receptors (around 0 mV) so that we could record $GABA_A$ receptor- and AMPA receptor-mediated currents (1; 25). Figure 1g, h are representative records. The averaged AMPA/GABA (E/I) ratio for control WT mice was 1.67 ± 0.22 ($n = 11$, Fig. 1j, k), while insulin significantly ($p < 0.001$) reduced the ratio to 0.79 ± 0.07 ($n = 7$, Fig. 1j, k). To test whether the effect of insulin can be further enhanced by insulin receptor sensitizer PIO, we applied both 500 nM insulin and 10 μM PIO (I+P) to the in vitro preparation. The results were largely similar to those obtained with insulin application alone (Fig. 1c, f, i, j, k). The averaged AMPA/GABA ratio was 0.74 ± 0.03 ($n = 6$, Fig. 1j, k), which is about the same as insulin alone ($p > 0.53$). Thus, PIO did not increase the effect of insulin on $GABA_A$ receptor-mediated response in WT slices, suggesting that insulin receptors are saturated by 500 nM insulin.

To investigate the mechanism underlying insulin-induced increased inhibition, we recorded $GABA_A$ receptor-mediated spontaneous IPSCs (sIPSCs) as shown in Fig. 2a–c. The cumulative fraction curves of the amplitude of sIPSCs (Fig. 2d) show that the amplitude distribution for WT I (medium thickness line) and WT I + P (thick line) is shifted to the right (larger amplitude) than that of no insulin controls (WT, thin line). This indicated that insulin (I) and insulin + PIO (I + P) increased the amplitude of sIPSCs. The difference between WT I

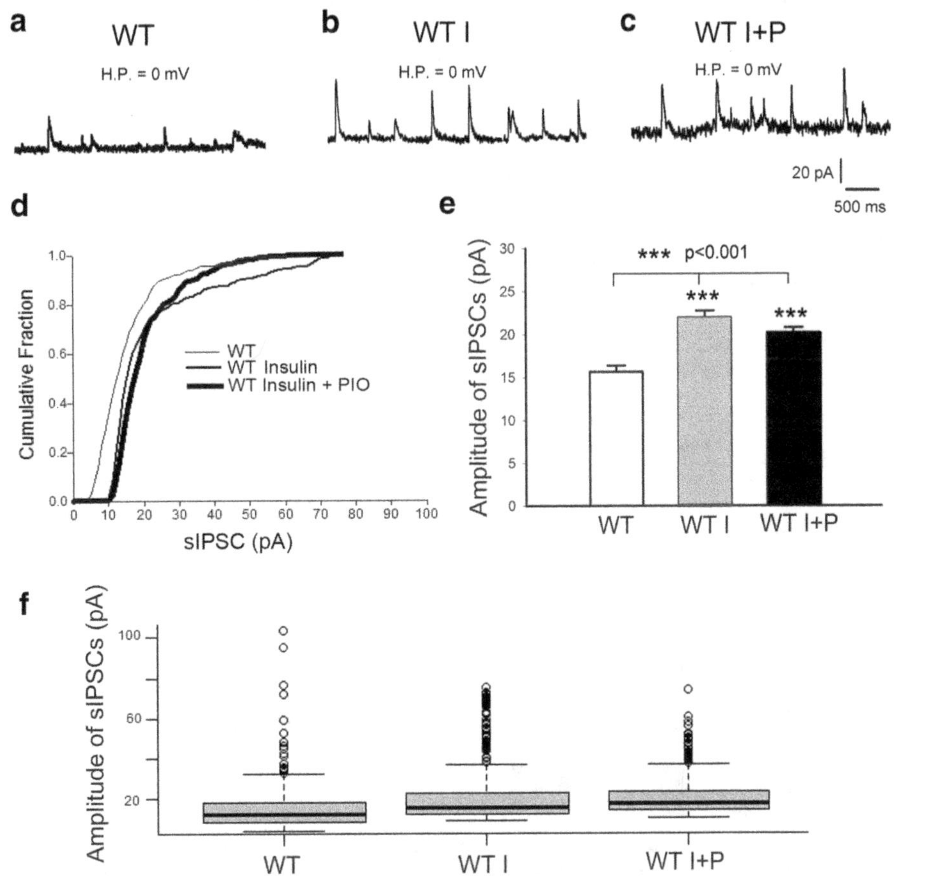

Fig. 2 Insulin-induced increased inhibition. **a**–**c** Example records of $GABA_A$ receptor-mediated sIPSCs. *HP* holding potential. **d** Cumulative fraction curves of the sIPSC amplitudes show that the amplitude distribution for insulin (WT I) and insulin + pioglitazone (WT I + P) are shifted to the right (larger amplitude), indicating that both conditions increase the amplitude of sIPSCs compared to no drug controls. **e** The average amplitude of sIPSCs is higher with either drug application condition compared to the controls, but not different between the two drug application conditions. **f** Box and whisker plots showing the population distribution

and WT I + P curves resulted from the difference in amplitude distribution. WT I + P group had less (12%) larger (> 30 pA) sIPSCs and WT I group had (19%) larger sIPSCs. However, the averaged amplitude of sIPSCs for WT I and WT I + P (Fig. 2e, f) showed no significant difference ($p > 0.08$), because the averaged amplitude of sIPSCs of WT I was 22.00 ± 0.76 ($n = 434$) pA, while that for WT I + P was 20.22 ± 0.56 ($n = 319$). Both of them were significantly ($p > 0.001$) larger than the WT group (15.64 ± 0.68 pA, $n = 320$).

Insulin receptors are desensitized in the barrel cortex of *Met-Emx1* mice

Layer IV of barrel cortex excitatory neurons of *Met-EMx1* mice also show regular spiking upon membrane depolarization (Fig. 3a–c). Stimulation of VB induced mainly an EPSP without a clear cut IPSP in *Me-Emx1* mice (Fig. 3d). Isolated AMPA receptor- and $GABA_A$ receptor-mediated currents revealed a relatively smaller IPSC (Fig. 3g). The averaged AMPA/GABA ratio for *Met-Emx1* mice was 3.53 ± 0.43 ($n = 8$, Fig. 3j, k), which is significantly ($p < 0.001$) larger than that of the WT mice (1.67 ± 0.22). In contrast to the WT slices, application of insulin (*Met-Emx1* I) did not change the magnitude of $GABA_A$ receptor-mediated response (Fig. 3e, h, j, k). The averaged AMPA/GABA ratio was 3.53 ± 0.42 ($n = 5$) that was just the same as without insulin ($p > 0.99$). The failure of insulin effect on inhibition may result from desensitized insulin receptors; thus, we applied PIO together with insulin (*Met* I + P). Representative records (Fig. 3f, i) demonstrated that addition of PIO increased $GABA_A$ receptor-mediated inhibition so that the averaged AMPA/GABA ratio was 0.69 ± 0.08 ($n = 5$), which is significantly ($p < 0.001$) smaller than previous groups (Fig. 3j, k).

We also recorded $GABA_A$ receptor-mediated sIPSCs in *Met-Emx1* mice. Representative records (Fig. 4a–c) showed that the amplitudes of sIPSCs increased only during application of insulin plus PIO (Fig. 4c). The cumulative fraction curves for *Met-Emx1* and *Met-Emx1* I were about the same (Fig. 4d, thin and medium lines). However, the curve for *Met-Emx1* I + P was shifted to the right, the larger amplitude area (Fig. 4d, thick line). The averaged amplitude of sIPSCs for *Met-Emx1* mice

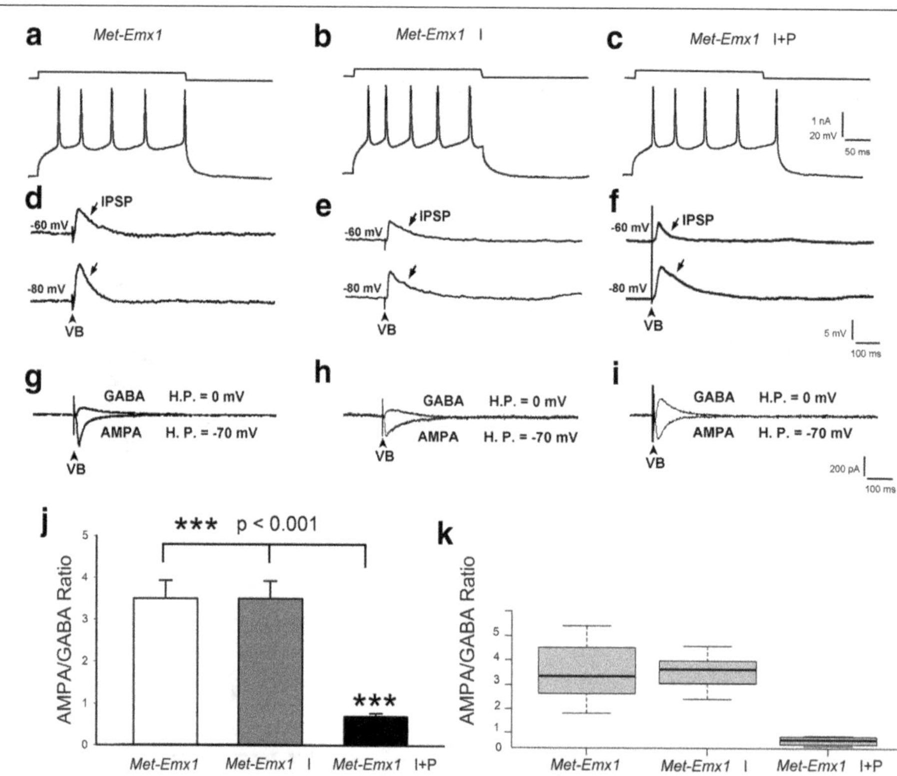

Fig. 3 Insulin and pioglitazone treatment effects on the E/I ratio in *Met-EMx1* brain slices. **a–c** Regular spiking of layer IV excitatory neurons in control (*Met-EMx1*) slices, and after application of insulin (*Met-EMx1* I), or insulin + pioglitazone (*Met-EMx1* I + P). **d, g** In mutant brain slices, stimulation of VB induced mainly an EPSP without a clear cut IPSP. Isolated AMPA receptor- and $GABA_A$ receptor-mediated currents reveal small IPSC. **e, h** Application of insulin (*Met-EMx1* I) did not change the magnitude of $GABA_A$ receptor-mediated response. **f, i** Addition of pioglitazone to insulin application dramatically increased $GABA_A$ receptor-mediated inhibition. **j** The averaged AMPA/GABA (E/I) ratio is similar between no drug treatment and insulin alone treatment conditions, but application of pioglitazone along with insulin dramatically changed this ratio. **k** Box and whisker plots showing the population distribution

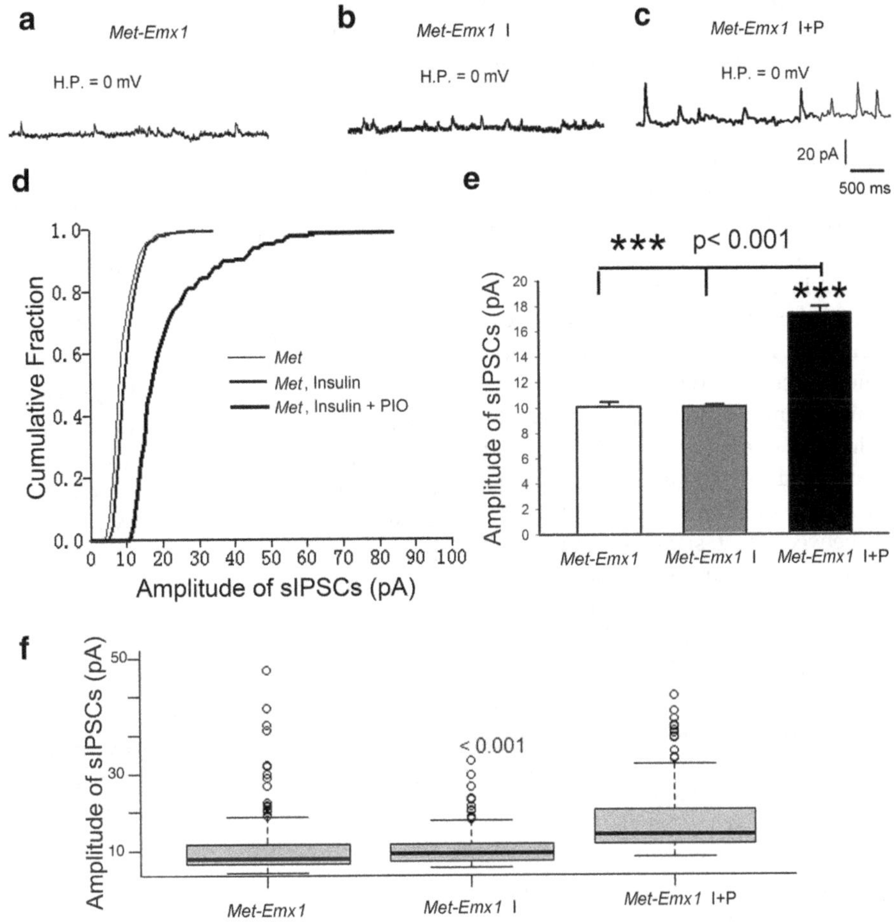

Fig. 4 Insulin sensitization-increased inhibition in *Met-EMx1* brain slices. **a**–**c** Example records of $GABA_A$ receptor-mediated sIPSCs in *Met-EMx1* cortical neurons without drug application, and with insulin alone (I) or insulin + pioglitazone (I + P) applications. **d** Cumulative fraction curves of the sIPSC amplitudes show a significant shift of the amplitude distribution for insulin + pioglitazone condition compared to no drug treatment (*Met-EMx1*) or insulin treatment (*Met-EMx1* I) alone. **e** The average amplitude of sIPSCs is much higher following insulin receptor sensitization with pioglitazone. **f** Box and whisker plots showing the population distribution

was 10.10 ± 0.37 pA (n = 295, Fig. 4e, f) that was significantly ($p < 0.001$) smaller than that of WT mice (15.64 ± 0.68 pA). However, application of insulin (*Met* I) did not change ($p > 0.97$) the averaged amplitude of sIPSCs (10.11 ± 0.17 pA, n = 470, Fig. 4e, f), suggesting insulin resistance of $GABA_A$ receptor-mediated response. Additional PIO together with insulin remarkably ($p < 0.001$) increased the amplitude of sIPSCs to 17.44 ± 0.55 pA (n = 235, Fig. 4e, f) that was still smaller ($p < 0.001$) than WT I + P (20.22 ± 0.56 pA). These suggest that insulin receptors are desensitized in *Met-Emx1* mice. The density of insulin receptors in *Met-Emx1* mice may be lower than that in WT mice.

Discussion

E/I balance in neural circuits is an essential component of homeostatic synaptic plasticity, which is thought to restrain cortical network activity to operate at optimal levels by weakening synaptic efficacy after heightened activity and increasing it after low levels of activation [29]. A disturbed E/I balance, particularly in neocortical circuits, has been proposed and observed in ASD individuals and in animal models [7, 30, 31].

In neurodevelopmental disorders, failure in neuronal differentiation [32], defects in neurotransmitter release, and their postsynaptic receptors [33–35] have been linked to altered E/I balance. In neocortical circuits, interactions between Gamma-aminobutyric acidergic (GABAergic) interneurons and glutamatergic pyramidal neurons that form the corticocortical, callosal, and subcortical connections have been targeted by numerous studies seeking to unveil the circuit defects in disorders with cognitive symptoms. GABAergic neurons are a small population of neocortical residents, but they control inhibition of the most populous excitatory cortical neurons. Defects in differentiation of GABAergic interneurons, GABAergic synaptic transmission, and postsynaptic receptors have been the usual suspects in altered excitability and homeostatic plasticity of neural circuits.

Met receptor tyrosine kinase is a cell surface receptor activated by hepatocyte growth factor (HGF). For obvious reasons, Met and HGF signaling have been extensively studied in the liver. Met is structurally related to the insulin receptor tyrosine kinase and Met signaling is essential in regulation of insulin response by hepatocytes [36]. In fact, a potential therapeutic role for HGF treatment for insulin resistance in type 2 diabetes has been suggested [36]. A more recent study on cell cocultures and in knockout mice brings conclusive evidence for Met regulation of insulin sensitivity [37]. While both Met and HGF are expressed in a spatiotemporal specificity in the brain (reviewed in [1]), there are no studies examining any link between Met signaling and insulin sensitivity in neocortical excitatory neurons and how lack of it might affect GABAergic synaptic transmission.

In the primary somatosensory cortex of mice, with inactive autism-associated Met receptor tyrosine kinase, we found that increased excitation is due to decreased postsynaptic inhibition mediated via the $GABA_A$ receptors [6]. Altered $GABA_A$ receptor function can directly affect the E/I balance. In transgenic mice lacking the β3 subunit of the $GABA_A$ receptor (Gabrb3), seizure susceptibility, hypersensitivity, hyperactivity, learning, and memory deficits have been reported [38, 39]. In fragile X mouse models too, decreased $GABA_A$ receptor expression has been observed [40–42]. A potential strategy to ameliorate decreased $GABA_A$ receptor function is to increase receptor sensitivity. In cultured hippocampal neuron, application of insulin increased $GABA_A$ receptor-mediated response [43, 44]. We confirmed this response in thalamocortical slices taken from WT mice [6]. However, in thalamocortical slices from *Met-Emx1* mice, insulin application did not change $GABA_A$ receptor-mediated response, suggesting that there might be insulin resistance in neocortical neurons that lack Met function [6]. In the present study, we show that insulin resistance of $GABA_A$ receptor-mediated response in *Met-Emx1* mice can be altered by insulin sensitization. We find that application of PIO, a common insulin sensitizer used in diabetes therapy, can significantly alter the $GABA_A$ receptor response and restore E/I balance to levels of normalcy. At the present time, we do not know how Met deficiency in excitatory cortical neurons alters receptor desensitization or the intracellular signaling pathways involving insulin receptors. Further studies are needed to investigate these mechanisms in a cell type-specific manner to determine whether Met signaling through insulin receptors occurs in similar ways between the neocortical excitatory neurons and hepatocytes.

Conclusions

Excitation/inhibition balance is altered in favor of excitation in the primary somatosensory cortex of mice with inactive autism-associated Met receptor tyrosine kinase. Altered E/I balance, in favor of excitation, in the somatosensory cortex of mice with inactive autism-associated Met receptor tyrosine kinase may relate to somatic sensory hypersensitivity of children with ASD to shoes and clothing. We applied insulin alone and insulin + pioglitazone (PIO) to test the effects of sensitizing insulin receptors on inhibitory responses mediated by $GABA_A$ receptors in the thalamocortical circuitry of $Emx1^{cre}/Met^{flox}$ mice. We show that PIO can aid in normalization of the E/I balance in the primary somatosensory cortex, a potential physiological mechanism underlying the positive effects of PIO treatment in ASD patients. Our results shed light to the underlying mechanisms and suggest that decreased $GABA_A$ receptor activity is the major culprit in scaling E/I balance to more excitation and that insulin sensitization can help in readjusting the balance.

Abbreviations

ACSF: Artificial cerebrospinal fluid; AMPA: α-Amino-3-hydroxy-5-methyl-4-isoxazolepropionic acid; ASD: Autism spectrum disorder; C57BL/6: Most widely used inbred mouse strain; DL-APV: DL-2-Amino-5-phosphonopentanoic acid; E/I: Excitation/inhibition; Emx1: Empty spiracles homeobox; EPSC: Excitatory postsynaptic current; $GABA_A$: Ionotropic receptor and γ-aminobutyric acid-gated ion channel; Gabrb3: β3 subunit of the $GABA_A$ receptor; HGF: Hepatocyte growth factor; I + P: Insulin + pioglitazone; I: Insulin; IPSC: Inhibitory postsynaptic current; Met: Tyrosine-protein kinase Met or hepatocyte growth factor receptor; NBQX: 2,3-Dihydroxy-6-nitro-7-sulfamoyl-benzo(F) quinoxaline, potent AMPA receptor antagonist; NMDA: *N*-methyl-D-aspartate; PIO: Pioglitazone; PTX: Picrotoxin; sIPSC: Spontaneous inhibitory synaptic current; VB: Ventrobasal nucleus of thalamus; WT: Wild type (B6 mice)

Acknowledgements

We thank Dr. Elizabeth Powell for introducing us to the autism model mice and discussions on the cortical phenotypes of the *Met* mutant mice.

Funding

Research supported by NIH/NINDS R01 NS092216

Authors' contributions

FSL and RSE designed the study. FSL performed the experiments. FSL and RSE interpreted the results and wrote the manuscript. Both authors read and approved the final manuscript.

Competing interests

The authors declare that they have no competing interests.

References

1. Eagleson KL, Xie Z, Levitt P. The pleiotropic MET receptor network: circuit development and the neural-medical interface of autism. Biol Psychiatry. 2017;81:424–33.
2. Peng Y, Lu Z, Li G, Piechowicz M, Anderson M, Uddin Y, et al. The autism-associated MET receptor tyrosine kinase engages early neuronal growth mechanism and controls glutamatergic circuits development in the forebrain. Mol Psychiatry. 2016;21:925–35.
3. Xie Z, Li J, Baker J, Eagleson KL, Coba MP, Levitt P. Receptor tyrosine kinase MET interactome and neurodevelopmental disorder partners at the developing synapse. Biol Psychiatry. 2016;80:933–42.
4. Judson MC, Bergman MY, Campbell DB, Eagleson KL, Levitt P. Dynamic gene and protein expression patterns of the autism-associated met receptor tyrosine kinase in the developing mouse forebrain. J Comp Neurol. 2009;513:511–31.
5. Qui S, Anderson CT, Levitt P, Shepherd GM. Circuit-specific intracortical hyperconnectivity in mice with deletion of the autism-associated met receptor tyrosine kinase. J Neurosci. 2011;31:5855–64.
6. Lo FS, Erzurumlu RS, Powell EM. Insulin-independent GABAA receptor-mediated response in the barrel cortex of mice with impaired met activity. J Neurosci. 2016;36:3691–7.
7. Nelson SB, Valakh V. Excitatory/inhibitory balance and circuit homeostasis in autism spectrum disorders. Neuron. 2015;87:684–98.
8. Tatti R, Haley MS, Swanson OK, Tselha T, Maffei A. Neurophysiology and regulation of the balance between excitation and inhibition in neocortical circuits. Biol Psychiatry. 2016;81:821–31.
9. Gralle M. The neuronal insulin receptor in its environment. J Neurochem. 2017;140:359–67.
10. Werne H, LeRoith D. Insulin and insulin-like growth factor receptors in the brain: physiological and pathological aspects. Eur Neuropsychopharmacol. 2014;24:1947–53.
11. Vetiska SM, Ahmadian G, Ju W, Liu L, Wymann MP, Wang YT. GABAA receptor-associated phosphoinositide 3-kinase is required for insulin-induced recruitment of postsynaptic GABAA receptors. Neuropharmacology. 2007;52:146–55.
12. Accardi MV, Brown PM, Miraucourt LS, Orser BA, Bowie D. α6-containing GABAA receptors are the principal mediators of inhibitory synapse strengthening by insulin in cerebellar granule cells. J Neurosci. 2015;35:9676–88.
13. Kawaguchi-Suzuki M, Frye RF. Current clinical evidence on pioglitazone pharmacogenomics. Front Pharmacol. 2013;4:147.
14. Boris M, Kaiser CC, Goldblatt A, Elice MW, Edelson SM, Adams JB, Feinstein DL. Effect of pioglitazone treatment on behavioral symptoms in autistic children. J Neuroinflammation. 2007;4:3.
15. Emanuele E, Lossano C, Politi P, Barale F. Pioglitazone as a therapeutic agent in autistic spectrum disorder. Med Hypotheses. 2007;69:699.
16. Doyle CA, McDougle CJ. Pharmacotherapy to control behavioral symptoms in children with autism. Expert Opin Pharmacother. 2012;13:1615–29.
17. Read S, Wu P, Biscow M. Sustained 4-year cognitive and functional response in early Alzheimer's disease with pioglitazone. J Am Geriatr Soc. 2014;62:584–6.
18. Ghaleiha A, Rasa SM, Nikoo M, Farokhnia M, Mohammadi MR, Akhondzadeh S. A pilot double-blind placebo-controlled trial of pioglitazone as adjunctive treatment to risperidone: effects on aberrant behavior in children with autism. Psychiatry Res. 2015;229:181–7.
19. Galimberti D, Scarpini E. Pioglitazone for the treatment of Alzheimer's disease. Expert Opin Investig Drugs. 2017;26:97–101.
20. Hsu D, Marshall GA. Primary and secondary prevention trials in Alzheimer's disease looking back, moving forward. Curr Allzheimer Re. 2017;14:426–40.
21. Agmon A, Connors BW. Thalamocortical responses of mouse somatosensory (barrel) cortex in vitro. Neuroscience. 1991;41:365–79.
22. Lee LJ, Iwasato T, Itohara S, Erzurumlu RS. Exuberant thalamocortical axon arborization in cortex-specific NMDAR1 knockout mice. J Comp Neurol. 2005;485:280–92.
23. Lee CC, Sherman SM. Synaptic properties of thalamic and intracortical inputs to layer 4 of the first- and higher-order cortical areas in the auditory and somatosensory systems. J Neurophysiol. 2008;100:317–26.
24. Agmon A, Connors BW. Correlation between intrinsic firing patterns and thalamocortical synaptic responses of neurons in mouse barrel cortex. J Neurosci. 1992;12:319–29.
25. Feldmeyer D, Egger V, Lubke J, Sakmann B. Reliable synaptic connections between pairs of excitatory layer 4 neurones within a single 'barrel' of developing rat somatosensory cortex. J Physiol. 1999;521(Pt 1):169–90.
26. Beierlein M, Gibson JR, Connors BW. Two dynamically distinct inhibitory networks in layer 4 of the neocortex. J Neurophysiol. 2003;90:2987–3000.
27. Lo FS, Akkentli F, Tsytsarev V, Erzurumlu RS. Functional significance of cortical NMDA receptors in somatosensory information processing. J Neurophysiol. 2013;110:2627–36.
28. Lo FS, Blue ME, Erzurumlu RS. Enhancement of postsynaptic GABAA and extrasynaptic NMDA receptor-mediated responses in the barrel cortex of Mecp2-null mice. J Neurophysiol. 2016;115:1298–306.
29. Turrigiano G. Homeostatic synaptic plasticity: local and global mechanisms for stabilizing neuronal function. Cold Spring Harb Perspect Biol. 2012;4(1):a005736.
30. Rubenstein JL, Merzenich MM. Model of autism: increased ratio of excitation/inhibition in key neural systems. Genes Brain Behav. 2003;2:255–67.
31. Gogolla N, Leblanc JJ, Quast KB, Südhof TC, Fagiolini M, Hensch TK. Common circuit defect of excitatory-inhibitory balance in mouse models of autism. J Neurodev Disord. 2009;1:172–81.
32. Mihalas AB, Hevner RF. Control of neuronal development by T-box genes in the brain. Curr Top Dev Biol. 2017;122:279–312.
33. Tong XJ, Hu Z, Liu Y, Anderson D, Kaplan JM. A network of autism linked genes stabilizes two pools of synaptic GABA(a) receptors. elife. 2015;4:e09648.
34. Tang W, Thevathasan JV, Lin Q, Lim KB, Kuroda K, Kaibuchi K, et al. Stimulation of synaptic vesicle exocytosis by the mental disease gene DISC1 is mediated by N-type voltage-gated calcium channels. Front Synaptic Neurosci. 2016;8:15.
35. Fafalios A, Ma J, Tan X, Stoops J, Luo J, DeFrances MC, Zarnegar R. A hepatocyte growth factor receptor (met)-insulin receptor hybrid governs hepatic glucose mechanism. Nat Med. 2011;17:1577–84.
36. Zhang Y-Y, Li C, Yao G-F, Du L-J, Liu Y, et al. Deletion of macrophage mineralocorticoid receptor protects hepatic steatosis and insulin resistance through Erα/HGF/met pathway. Diabetes. 2017;66:1535–47.
37. Wei H, Ma Y, Ding C, Jin G, Liu J, Chang Q, et al. Reduced glutamate release in adult BTBR mouse model of autism spectrum disorder. Neurochem Res. 2016;41:3129–37.
38. DeLorey TM, Handforth A, Anagnostaras SG, Homanics GE, Minassianm BA, Asatourian A, et al. Mice lacking the beta3 subunit of the GABAA receptor have the epilepsy phenotype and many of the behavioral characteristics of Angelman syndrome. J Neurosci. 1998;18:8505–14.
39. Homanics GE, DeLorey TM, Firestone LL, Quinlan JJ, Handforth A, Harrison NL, et al. Mice devoid of gamma-aminobutyrate type a receptor beta3 subunit have epilepsy, cleft palate, and hypersensitive behavior. Proc Natl Acad Sci U S A. 1997;94:4143–8.
40. El Idrissi A, Ding XH, Scalia J, Trenkner E, Brown WT, Dobkin C. Decreased GABA(a) receptor expression in the seizure-prone fragile X mouse. Neurosci Lett. 2005;377:141–6.
41. Gantois I, Vandesompele J, Speleman F, Reyniers E, D'Hooge R, Severijnen LA, et al. Expression profiling suggests underexpression of the GABA(a) receptor subunit delta in the fragile X knockout mouse model. Neurobiol Dis. 2006;21:346–57.
42. Adusei DC, Pacey LK, Chen D, Hampson DR. Early developmental alterations in GABAergic protein expression in fragile X knockout mice. Neuropharmacology. 2010;59:167–71.
43. Wan Q, Xiong ZG, Man HY, Ackerley CA, Braunton J, et al. Recruitment of functional GABA(a) receptors to postsynaptic domains by insulin. Nature. 1997;388:686–90.
44. Mielke JG, Wang YT. Insulin exerts neuroprotection by counteracting the decrease in cell-surface GABA receptors following oxygen-glucose deprivation in cultured cortical neurons. J Neurochem. 2005;92:103–13.

8

Identification of mutations in the PI3K-AKT-mTOR signalling pathway in patients with macrocephaly and developmental delay and/or autism

Kit San Yeung[1†], Winnie Wan Yee Tso[1,2†], Janice Jing Kun Ip[3], Christopher Chun Yu Mak[1], Gordon Ka Chun Leung[1], Mandy Ho Yin Tsang[1], Dingge Ying[1], Steven Lim Cho Pei[1], So Lun Lee[1,2], Wanling Yang[1] and Brian Hon-Yin Chung[1,2,3*]

Abstract

Background: Macrocephaly, which is defined as a head circumference greater than or equal to + 2 standard deviations, is a feature commonly observed in children with developmental delay and/or autism spectrum disorder. Although *PTEN* is a well-known gene identified in patients with this syndromic presentation, other genes in the PI3K-AKT-mTOR signalling pathway have also recently been suggested to have important roles. The aim of this study is to characterise the mutation spectrum of this group of patients.

Methods: We performed whole-exome sequencing of 21 patients with macrocephaly and developmental delay/autism spectrum disorder. Sources of genomic DNA included blood, buccal mucosa and saliva. Germline mutations were validated by Sanger sequencing, whereas somatic mutations were validated by droplet digital PCR.

Results: We identified ten pathogenic/likely pathogenic mutations in *PTEN* ($n = 4$), *PIK3CA* ($n = 3$), *MTOR* ($n = 1$) and *PPP2R5D* ($n = 2$) in ten patients. An additional *PTEN* mutation, which was classified as variant of unknown significance, was identified in a patient with a pathogenic *PTEN* mutation, making him harbour bi-allelic germline *PTEN* mutations. Two patients harboured somatic *PIK3CA* mutations, and the level of somatic mosaicism in blood DNA was low. Patients who tested positive for mutations in the PI3K-AKT-mTOR pathway had a lower developmental quotient than the rest of the cohort (DQ = 62.8 vs. 76.1, $p = 0.021$). Their dysmorphic features were non-specific, except for macrocephaly. Among the ten patients with identified mutations, brain magnetic resonance imaging was performed in nine, all of whom showed megalencephaly.

(Continued on next page)

* Correspondence: bhychung@hku.hk
†Equal contributors
[1]Department of Paediatrics and Adolescent Medicine, The University of Hong Kong, Pok Fu Lam, Hong Kong, China
[2]Department of Paediatrics and Adolescent Medicine, The Duchess of Kent Children's Hospital, Pok Fu Lam, Hong Kong, China
Full list of author information is available at the end of the article

(Continued from previous page)

Conclusion: We identified mutations in the PI3K-AKT-mTOR signalling pathway in nearly half of our patients with macrocephaly and developmental delay/autism spectrum disorder. These patients have subtle dysmorphic features and mild developmental issues. Clinically, patients with germline mutations are difficult to distinguish from patients with somatic mutations, and therefore, sequencing of buccal or saliva DNA is important to identify somatic mosaicism. Given the high diagnostic yield and the management implications, we suggest implementing comprehensive genetic testing in the PI3K-AKT-mTOR pathway in the clinical evaluation of patients with macrocephaly and developmental delay and/or autism spectrum disorder.

Keywords: Somatic mosaicism, Macrocephaly, Megalencephaly, Developmental delay, Autism spectrum disorder, *PTEN*, *MTOR*, *PIK3CA*, *PPP2R5D*

Background

Macrocephaly is defined as a disproportionally enlarged head size with an occipitofrontal circumference greater than or equal to +2 standard deviations (SDs). On the other hand, megalencephaly is defined as hyperplasia of the brain parenchyma observed in a radiological examination together with clinical features of macrocephaly. Both conditions are associated with developmental delay (DD) and/or autism spectrum disorder (ASD). Moreover, a recent neuroimaging study has shown that brain volume overgrowth is linked to the emergence and severity of autistic social deficits [1].

ASD is a complex, behaviourally defined disorder characterised by impairments in communication and reciprocal social interaction, restrictive interests and repetitive stereotypic behaviours [2]. It is known that ASD has a strong genetic basis [3, 4], and environmental factors might also influence the development of ASD [5–7]. Previous studies have reported a genetic diagnosis in 10% to 40% of patients with ASD [8–11]. According to the American Academy of Pediatrics guidelines for ASD published in 2000, genetic testing is a standard diagnostic test for children with ASD and dysmorphic features or intellectual disability (ID).

As shown in previous studies, 14–34% of children with ASD also have macrocephaly [12–17], and a meta-analysis revealed that 15.7% have macrocephaly and 9.1% have brain overgrowth [18]. *PTEN* is a well-known gene associated with ASD and macrocephaly [19–21]. Hence, genetic testing for *PTEN* mutations is recommended as part of the clinical evaluation in this group of patients [22–24]. Recently, mutations in other genes in the PI3K-AKT-mTOR signalling pathway, including *PIK3CA*, *PIK3R2*, *MTOR*, *CCND2* and *PPP2R5D*, were also reported in patients with ASD/DD and macrocephaly [25–30]. Although most *PTEN* mutations reported in this group of patients were germline mutations [20, 31], mutations in other genes in the PI3K-AKT-mTOR signalling pathway were frequently detected with a low level of mosaicism, which are undetectable using conventional Sanger sequencing. The use of next-generation sequencing, such as whole-exome sequencing (WES) or target panel sequencing, enables the detection of the low level of mosaicism in these patients. In this study, we aim to define the mutation spectrum in a cohort of patients with ASD/DD and macrocephaly using WES.

Methods

Patient recruitment

We recruited patients from January 2013 to December 2016 at the Duchess of Kent Children's Hospital Child Assessment Center (DKCAC). Patients were initially assessed by a developmental paediatrician and relevant allied health professionals, including clinical psychologists, physiotherapists, occupational therapists and speech therapists. The developmental profile of patients less than 72 months of age was assessed using the Griffiths Mental Developmental Scales-Extended Revised (GMDS-ER). The developmental quotient (DQ) score was calculated based on the neurodevelopmental assessment to compare the developmental profiles between mutation-positive and mutation-negative patients. Because many patients were examined using more than one developmental assessment, the DQ scores from the first assessment were used. DQ scores were estimated for four patients based on their allied health assessment records and a clinical assessment by a developmental paediatrician because the patient was either too sick for the formal assessment with GMDS-ER (patient 3) or data were missing (patients 5, 15 and 19). Intellectual functioning of children ≥72 months of age was assessed using the Hong Kong Wechsler Intelligence Scale. ASD was diagnosed based on the Diagnostic and Statistical Manual of Mental Disorders—Fourth Edition (DSM-IV) criteria for ASD. Suspected cases were further assessed using the Autism Diagnostic Observation schedule (ADOS).

Developmental paediatricians at DKCAC referred patients with negative findings in the chromosomal microarray to the clinical geneticist when the patients also presented with macrocephaly (head circumference ≥ + 2 SD). These patients were recruited by the clinical geneticist, with the exception of patients presenting with obvious syndromic diseases who were assessed using targeted genetic tests and excluded from this study. Twenty-one unrelated patients were recruited in this study. Anthropometric data used for the measurements are specific to Hong Kong. Buccal swab or saliva sample was obtained in addition to the blood sample from five patients. This study was approved by the Institutional Review Board of the University of Hong Kong/Hospital Authority Hong Kong West Cluster (UW 12–211), and written consent was obtained from the patients' parents.

WES

WES was first performed at Macrogen Inc. and then at our university at a later stage of the project using either a TruSeq Exome Enrichment Kit ($n = 9$), SeqCap EZ Exome + UTR Exome Kit ($n = 9$) or TruSeq Rapid Exome Library Prep Kit ($n = 3$). The choice of the enrichment kit depended on the library preparation kit available at the time of sequencing. We aimed to obtain a minimum of 50X depth for WES performed with genomic DNA obtained from the blood and a minimum of 100X depth for WES performed with DNA derived from buccal mucosa or saliva samples. The increased sequencing depth in buccal and saliva samples served to increase the chance of detecting somatic mutations. Details of the library preparation method, sequencer used and average depth after sequence alignment of each individual is presented in Additional file 1.

Variant calling and data analysis

Raw reads were aligned to the UCSC hg19 reference human genome using BWA 0.5.7, and variant calling was performed according to the best practices of GATK 3.4. The output VCF files were than annotated using ANNOVAR. The following criteria were applied to filter the variants and generate a list of high-quality variants for subsequent analyses: variants located outside the exonic regions and splice sites, synonymous variants, population frequency ≥ 1% or total depth < 10X. Genes involved in the PI3K-AKT-mTOR signalling pathway (*PTEN, AKT1, AKT3, PIK3CA, MTOR, PIK3R2, CCND2, PPP2R5D* and *PPP2R1A*) were prioritised for analysis because of their known pathogenicity in patients with macrocephaly and DD/ASD, and other genes in the PI3K-AKT signalling pathway obtained from Kyoto Encylopedia of Genes and Genomes (KEGG; reference: hsa04151) were also analysed. Mutations identified in this pathway that are associated with diseases are expected to be rare, and activating mutations are likely to be found in the Catalogue of Somatic Mutations in Cancer (COSMIC) database [27, 32]. In addition, genes involved in epigenetic regulation have recently been reported to be an important cause of macrocephaly/overgrowth and DD/ASD, and thus, genes related to epigenetic regulation (*CHD8, DNMT3A, EED, EZH2, HIST1H1E* and *NSD1*) were also prioritised for analysis [33].

Confirmation of variants

For germline mutations, variants were confirmed by Sanger sequencing, and parental sequencing was also performed to determine whether the mutation was de novo or inherited. For somatic mosaic mutations, droplet digital PCR was used for validation, as described previously [32].

Statistical analysis

Unpaired t tests were performed to assess the significance between the DQ scores of patients with and without mutations. A p-value < 0.05 was considered statistically significant. Analyses were performed using SPSS Statistics version 19 (IBM).

Results

Twenty-one patients (17 males and 4 females, 4 to 108 months of age at the time of clinical assessment/ recruitment) with macrocephaly and DD/ID/ASD were recruited. All patients had DD at the time of recruitment, and three patients were diagnosed with ID in subsequent assessments. Among the 21 patients, ten were also diagnosed with ASD and two with suspected ASD (i.e., patients with autistic features who had not yet satisfied all the DSM-IV criteria for a diagnosis of ASD). A summary of the patients' clinical presentations is presented in Table 1. Prior to WES, the chromosomal microarray was performed on these patients, as described previously [34], and no pathogenic/likely pathogenic copy number variations were identified in these patients. WES identified ten pathogenic/likely pathogenic mutations in ten patients (Fig. 1, Table 2), corresponding to a diagnostic yield of 47.6%. All pathogenic mutations were located in genes involved in the PI3K-AKT-mTOR signalling pathway, including *PTEN* ($n = 4$), *PIK3CA* ($n = 3$), *MTOR* ($n = 1$) and *PPP2R5D* ($n = 2$). Although most variants were germline mutations, two somatic *PIK3CA* mutations were identified. No pathogenic mutations were identified in genes related to epigenetic regulation, such as *CHD8, DNMT3A, EED* and *NSD1*, as reported by Tatton-Brown K et al. [33], and the analysis of the remainder of the exome did not reveal other variants of interest.

Mutations in the *PTEN* gene were the most frequently identified mutations in our patients, with four

Table 1 Clinical presentations of all patients recruited in this study

Patient ID	Sex	First assessment (years)	Most recent assessment (years)	HC (z-score)	DQ	ASD	Developmental problem(s)	Other clinical features	MRI findings	Gene
1	M	3.0	5.2	3.6	75		Mild GDD with severe language delay	2/3/4 syndactyly	MEG, PG, VM, PWMSA	*PIK3CA*
2	M	1.5	4.1	3.2	55		Moderate GDD	Mild 2/3 syndactyly	MEG, PG, PWMSA	*PIK3CA*
3	M	0.8	1.6	5.9	50*		Moderate GDD	Recurrent respiratory infections, hypoglycaemia	MEG, PG, VM, PWMSA	*PTEN*
4	M	2.3	6.5	4.0	73	Suspected ASD	Mild GDD	NA	MEG, PG, PWMSA	*PTEN*
5	M	0.4	0.7	6.7	62*		Mild GDD	Liver haemangioma	MEG, PG, VM, PWMSA	*MTOR*
6	M	2.7	8.2	4.5	80	ASD	Mild GDD	2/3 syndactyly	NA	*PTEN*
7	M	2.0	11.6	2.6	49	ASD	Moderate GDD, mild ID	Hypertelorism, epilepsy[a]	MEG	*PPP2R5D*
8	M	1.8	5.3	2.2	54	Suspected ASD	Moderate GDD, mild ID	Hypertelorism, epilepsy[b]	MEG	*PPP2R5D*
9	M	2.0	3.5	3.5	62	ASD	Mild GDD with moderate language delay	Left lower limb hypertrophy with 2/3 syndactyly	MEG	*PIK3CA*
10	M	2.6	6.0	3.4	68		Mild GDD	Frontal bossing	MEG	*PTEN*
11	M	4.4	10.1	3.4	95	ASD	Language delay	z-scores for height: 3.0; weight: 5.6	Normal	Negative
12	M	2.3	6.3	3.3	79	ASD	Borderline delay with language delay	Left ptosis, scoliosis	Dilated cisterna magna, relative atrophy of the right cerebellar hemisphere	Negative
13	F	9.8	10.3	3.1	NA	ASD		NA	Normal	Negative
14	F	1.6	7.3	3.3	75		Borderline delay with language delay	Intra-cranial haemorrhage in the perinatal period	Aqueduct stenosis with hydrocephalus	Negative
15	F	4.0	6.0	4.2	90*	ASD	Language delay	NA	NA	Negative
16	M	2.2	23.4	3.2	71	ASD	Borderline delay	NA	NA	Negative
17	M	1.8	14.4	4.8	84	ASD	Borderline delay	Epilepsy[c]	Normal	Negative
18	F	2.4	6.2	2.2	78		Borderline delay	NA	NA	Negative
19	M	2.0	19.8	2.1	50*	ASD	Moderate GDD, moderate ID	Epilepsy[d]	NA	Negative
20	M	2.0	2.3	2.8	67		Mild GDD	NA	Dilated ventricles with external hydrocephalus	Negative
21	M	2.4	10.8	3.0	72		Mild GDD	Cleft lip and palate, nasal deformity	Normal	Negative

*Estimated DQ scores
[a]Epilepsy: onset at 4 years of age, generalised tonic-clonic seizure
[b]Epilepsy: onset at 4 days of age, generalised epileptic spasm
[c]Epilepsy: onset at 11 months, focal seizure with impaired awareness
[d]Epilepsy: onset 11 years of age, generalised tonic-clonic seizure
MEG megalencephaly, *PG* polymicrogyria, *VM* ventriculomegaly, *PWMSA* periventricular white matter signal abnormalities, *NA* not available

pathogenic variants found in four patients (19% among 21 patients). Both missense and frameshift mutations were identified. Although the *PTEN* p.(Ser170Thr) mutation detected in patient 4 has not previously been reported, a mutation in the same codon, resulting in *PTEN* p.(Ser170Arg), has been reported in multiple patients with *PTEN* cancer syndrome [35, 36], suggesting the pathogenicity of mutations in this amino acid. The mutation in patient 6 was a frameshift mutation and therefore a pathogenic mutation, because loss of

Table 2 Mutations in genes involved in the PI3K-AKT-mTOR pathway identified in the ten patients with macrocephaly and DD/ASD

Patient ID	Gene	Nucleotide change	Amino acid change	Inheritance	Mutation type	Allelic count in ExAC	No. of cases in COSMIC	Reported mutation
1	*PIK3CA*	c.G263A	p.(Arg88Gln)	De novo	Mosaic	0	137	43
2	*PIK3CA*	c.G1030A	p.(Val344Met)	Maternal	Germline	0	15	27
3	*PTEN*	c.G314T	p.(Cys105Phe)	De novo	Germline	0	6	39b
		c.G492T	p.(Lys164Asn)	Maternal	Germline	1 in 120,466	0[b]	
4	*PTEN*	c.G509C	p.(Ser170Thr)	De novo	Germline	0	0[b]	35.36[b]
5[a]	*MTOR*	c.G5395A	p.(Glu1799Lys)	De novo	Germline	0	10	28.45
6	*PTEN*	c.546delA	p.(Lys183ArgfsTer16)	De novo	Germline	0	0[b]	
7	*PPP2R5D*	c.G592A	p.(Glu198Lys)	De novo	Germline	0	1	29.46
8	*PPP2R5D*	c.G592A	p.(Glu198Lys)	De novo	Germline	0	1	29.46
9	*PIK3CA*	c.G2740A	p.(Gly914Arg)	De novo	Mosaic	0	2	25.27
10	*PTEN*	c.A203G	p.(Tyr68Cys)	De novo	Germline	0	4	37.38

The COSMIC database (June 2017) was accessed to retrieve the number of somatic mutations identified in cancer samples
[a]This patient was reported in a previous study [28] with the patient ID LR15-065
[b]Other mutations in the same codon have been reported

function mutations is known to cause disease. The *PTEN* p.(Tyr68Cys) mutation identified in patient 10 has already been reported in multiple patients with Cowden Syndrome [37, 38].

In addition, we report here a second patient with bi-allelic germline *PTEN* mutations. Two *PTEN* mutations were identified in patient 3, where p.(Cys105Phe) was a de novo mutation and p.(Lys164Asn) was maternally inherited. Based on the sequencing data, the two mutations did not occur in the same allele (Additional file 2, Fig. S1a). Exon 5 was cloned to confirm that the mutations were located on different alleles, and clonal sequencing showed that the two mutations occurred on different alleles (Additional file 2, Fig. S1b). The mutation p.(Cys105Phe) has not been reported, but a mutation in the same codon resulting in p.(Cys105Tyr) has been reported in patients with Bannayan-Riley-Ruvalcaba Syndrome [39], suggesting the pathogenicity of mutations in this amino acid. The maternally inherited p.(Lys164Asn) mutation has not been reported in a disease-specific database and has only been reported in the Exome Aggregation Consortium (ExAC) database with an allelic frequency of 1 in 120,466. Familial testing showed that this mutation was also detected in the patient's mother and elder sister, and both the mother and elder sister had macrocephaly (z-scores for the head circumference were 2.6 and 3.7, respectively). Both had unremarkable developmental issues. Active cancer surveillance was recommended, and at the age of 38, the patient's mother was diagnosed with multifocal papillary carcinoma. Based on the above evidence, although the variant p.(Lys164Asn) being pathogenic was compelling, it was still classified as a variant of unknown significance. It was because the mother did not meet the diagnostic criteria for *PTEN* hamartoma tumour syndrome, who only fulfilled one major criterion (macrocephaly) and one minor criterion (papillary carcinoma) [40]. Patient 3 who had bi-allelic mutations, however, displayed a severe clinical presentation despite one of the mutation being classified as a variant of unknown significance. In addition to megalencephaly, polymicrogyria and developmental delay, he suffered from recurrent sinopulmonary infections and colitis, resulting in persistent fever and septic shock that required care in the intensive care unit. The immune workup showed hypogammaglobulinaemia, specifically, a low level of IgG subclass 3. During a salmonella gastrointestinal infection at 19 months of age, a dihydrorhodamine test showed a suppressed oxidative burst with only half of the function compared to the control. However, a specific primary immunodeficiency syndrome was not identified. Second, this patient had suffered from recurrent hypoglycaemia since 19 months of age that required high glucose infusions; however, his insulin level was normal and an extensive endocrine workup was unremarkable. The patient died at 25 months of age due to sepsis. This case showed that patients with bi-allelic *PTEN* mutations can present with other PI3K-AKT-mTOR pathway-related features, including the recurrent respiratory infections observed in patients with *PIK3CD* mutations [41, 42] and hypoglycaemia observed in patients with *AKT2* or *AKT3* mutations [43, 44].

The *PIK3CA* mutation was the second most common mutation identified in our patients (patients 1, 2 and 9). The germline mutation in patient 2 was inherited from his mother, who had macrocephaly (z-score of head circumference was 4.6) but no history of developmental issues. In addition to the germline mutation, two somatic mutations were identified, and all mutations have been reported previously [25, 27]. WES detected a p.(Arg88Gln) mutation in patient 1, with a percentage of 4.5% (4 of 89 reads) in the blood and 27.1% (29 of 107 reads) in the buccal mucosa, whereas confirmation using droplet digital PCR showed that the percentages of p.(Arg88Gln) mutations in the blood and buccal mucosa samples were 8.6 and 22.8%, respectively. For patient 9, WES detected a p.(Gly914Arg) mutation with a percentage of 2.8% (3 of 109 reads) in the blood and 11.9% (13 of 109 reads) in the saliva. Again, droplet digital PCR confirmed the WES results, showing that the percentages of mutations were 2.6, 9.3 and 22.8% in the blood, saliva and buccal mucosa samples from patient 9, respectively. Our results confirmed previous findings that the mutation load in saliva or buccal mucosa is higher than the mutation load in the blood [25–27].

Finally, known pathogenic variants in the *MTOR* [28, 45] and *PPP2R5D* [29, 46] genes were also identified in our patients. Patient 5, who had a *MTOR* mutation, has already been reported in another publication (referred to as LR15-065 in the publication) describing a wide spectrum of patients with germline/somatic *MTOR* mutations [28]. In addition, *PPP2R5D* p.(Glu198Lys) was identified twice in two unrelated patients as de novo mutation. Both patients had a clinical presentation compatible with other patients with *PPP2R5D* mutations, including hypertelorism, frontal bossing, and a history of epilepsy.

At the time when genetic counselling was provided to patients with mutations, patients were re-examined to determine whether they had features of *PTEN* hamartoma tumour syndrome [40] such as macular pigmentation of the glans penis, mucocutaneous lesions and lipomas. For megalencephaly-capillary malformation syndrome (MCAP)/megalencephaly-polymicrogyria-polydactyly-hydrocephalus syndrome (MPPH) [47], features of syndactyly, signs of overgrowth and vascular anomalies were assessed. Most of these features were absent in our patients. Only a small minority of patients presented with additional clinical features, such as syndactyly, hypertelorism and epilepsy. Our findings demonstrated the diversity of the clinical spectrum in this group of patients (see Table 1). Overall, patients with identified mutations had only subtle dysmorphic features (Fig 1). The mean DQ scores for mutation-positive and mutation-negative patients were 62.8 and 76.1, respectively, and the difference was statistically significant ($p = 0.021$). The prevalence of ASD/autistic features was similar between the two groups. It was noted that except for the two patients with *PPP2R5D* mutations, the head circumference of other mutation-positive patients were > + 3 SD. However, patients who tested positive for mutations in the PI3K-AKT-mTOR pathway did not had a significant difference in head circumference than mutation-negative patients. We also reviewed the brain magnetic resonance imaging (MRI) findings. Of the ten patients with an identified mutation, nine underwent MRI (Fig. 2). Megalencephaly was present in all nine of these patients; in addition, polymicrogyria was also identified in five patients, periventricular white matter signal abnormalities were identified in five patients, and ventriculomegaly was identified in three patients. With the exception of brain overgrowth, mutation-positive patients had no structural brain abnormalities. In contrast, three of the seven mutation-negative patients also had brain abnormalities, such as Dandy-Walker variant ($n = 1$) or aqueduct stenosis with hydrocephalus ($n = 2$). The brain MRI findings of the remaining four patients were normal.

Discussion

In this study, we aimed to characterise the mutation spectrum of patients with macrocephaly and DD/ASD. Among the 21 patients, ten had mutations in the PI3K-AKT-mTOR signalling pathway, indicating the importance of this pathway in macrocephaly with DD/ASD (Table 2). Our overall diagnostic yield was 47.6%, and *PTEN* mutations were detected in 19% of patients ($n = 4$), similar to previous studies detecting *PTEN* mutations/deletions in patients with DD/ASD [20, 21, 48, 49]. The higher diagnostic yield in this study is because multiple genes in the PI3K-AKT-mTOR pathway in addition to *PTEN* were considered, and in selected patients, WES of reasonably high depth was performed using additional sources of DNA, including saliva or buccal mucosa samples, rather than blood samples alone. Findings from our study suggest the need to refine the recommendation of current guidelines for the genetic evaluation of patients with macrocephaly and DD/ID/ASD. The American Academy of Pediatrics guidelines do not specifically mention an evaluation of children with macrocephaly and DD/ID [50], but the ASD evaluation proposed by the Autism Consortium Clinical Genetics/DNA Diagnostics Collaboration [22], the American College of Medical Genetics and Genomics [23] and other experts [24] only suggests genetic testing for *PTEN* mutations. From a practical perspective, children with DD/ASD will be referred for genetic consultation when their developmental problem is moderate to severe or when they present with dysmorphic features. However, based on our findings, most patients with mutations present with mild to moderate developmental problems, and dysmorphism is mild and non-specific. The absence of typical features of *PTEN* hamartoma tumour syndrome (such as glans penis pigmentation, mucocutaneous lesions and lipomas) may be due to the relatively young age of the patients or to

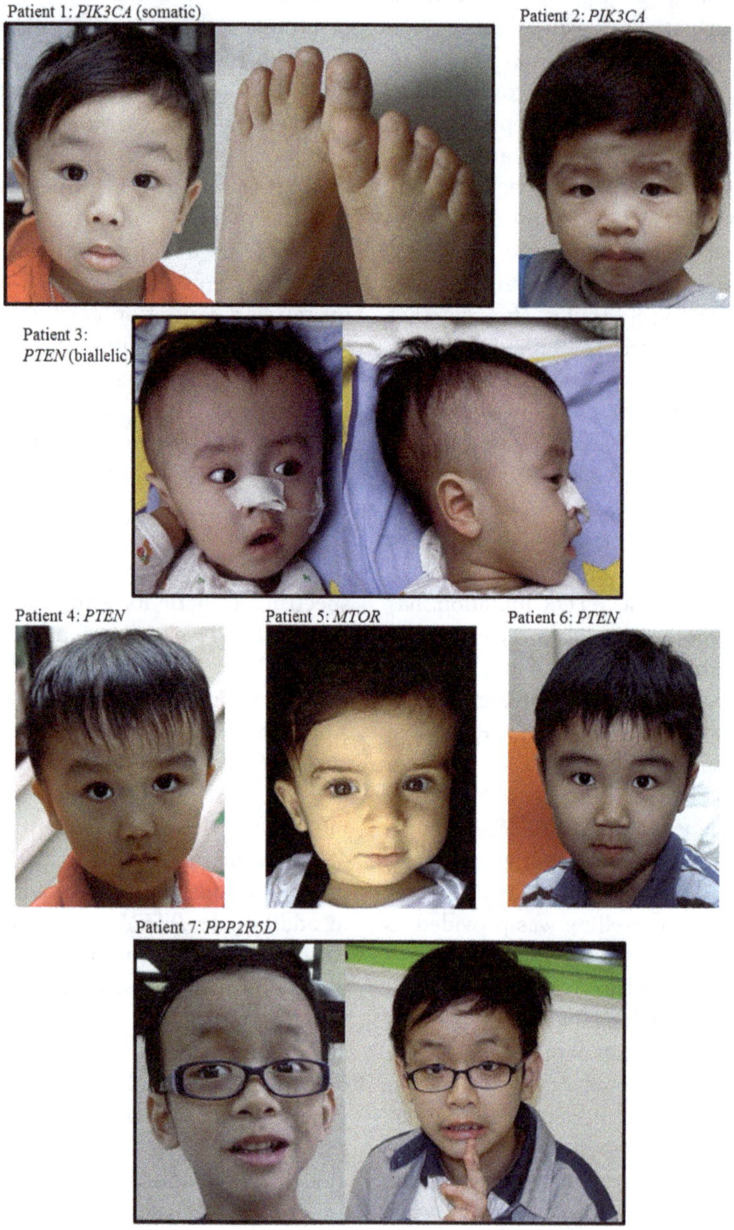

Fig. 1 Clinical photographs of patients with mutations in the PI3K-AKT-mTOR pathway. Clinical photographs of patients with mutations identified in the PI3K-AKT-mTOR pathway are shown. For patient 1, syndactyly is shown. Patient 7 presented with hypertelorism and frontal bossing

the variable presentation of these features. Thus, genetic tests should be considered for patients with DD/ASD and macrocephaly, regardless of the degree of DD/ASD and the presence/absence of dysmorphic features. A panel of genes in the PI3K-AKT-mTOR pathway, including but not limited to *PTEN*, should be tested, and a low level of mosaicism for variants should be considered when collecting samples from patients for DNA extraction and determining the methodology to use to detect mutations [25–28]. Additional sources of DNA obtained from the buccal mucosa, saliva or brain (if available) should also be used for sequencing, and next-generation sequencing with reasonably high depth and coverage of genes in the PI3K-AKT-mTOR pathway should be performed. Although our use of WES successfully identified somatic mutations in two patients, a targeted gene panel has the advantage of higher depth than WES and therefore is a better choice for testing.

The genetic diagnosis of mutations in genes involved in the PI3K-AKT-mTOR pathway is clinically important. First, monogenic mutations in the PI3K-AKT-mTOR

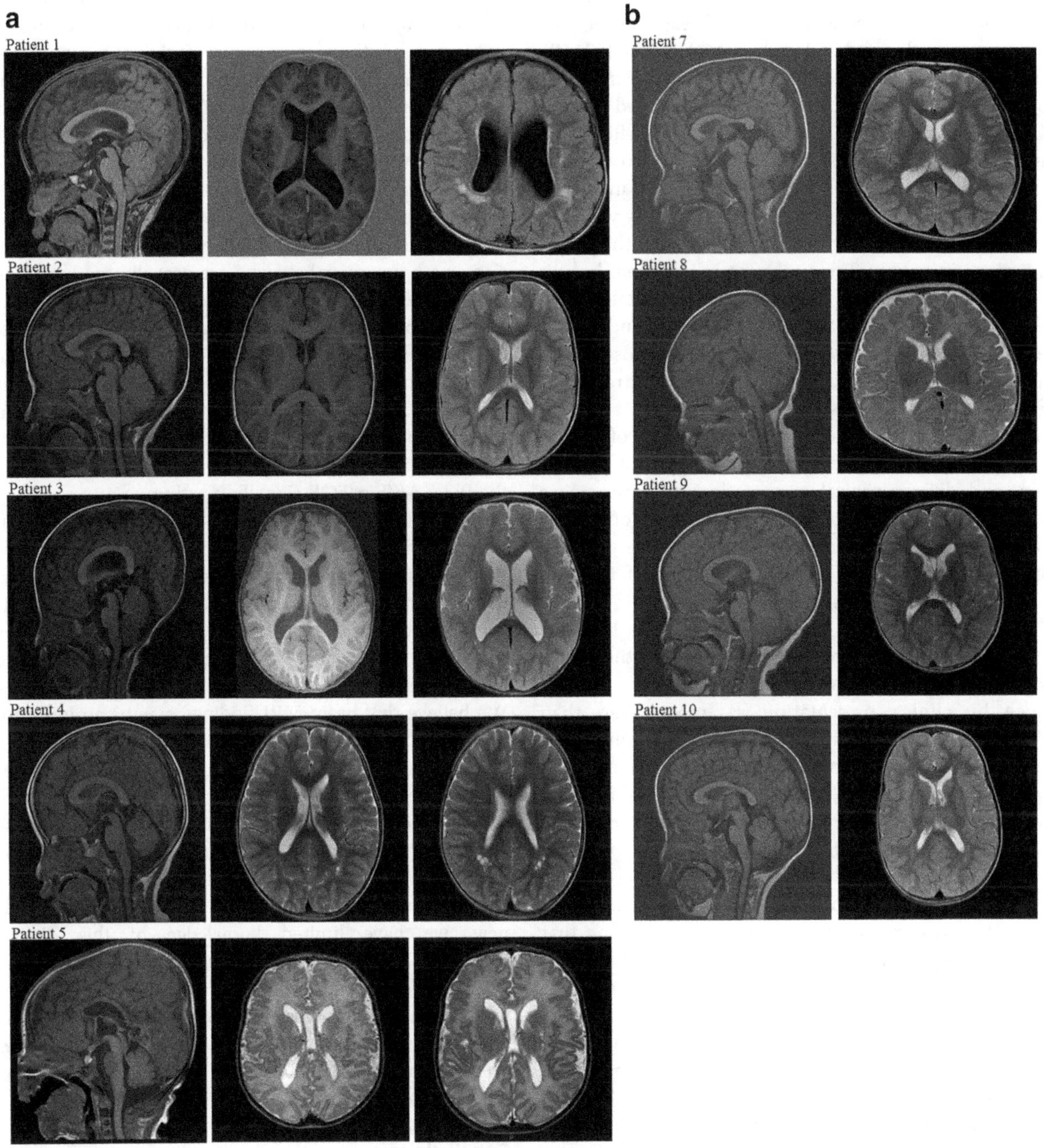

Fig. 2 MRI of patients with mutations in the PI3K-AKT-mTOR pathway. **a** MRI in patients 1–5 showing megalencephaly, polymicrogyria and periventricular white matter signal abnormalities. Ventriculomegaly was observed in patients 1, 3 and 5. **b** MRI in patients 7–10 showing megalencephaly, without other abnormalities. MRI was not available for patient 6 because the family declined the MRI

pathway are important in the pathogenesis of a subset of patients with DD/ASD. The genetic information may facilitate genetic counselling and estimate the risk of occurrence. Second, the genetic diagnosis facilitates a determination of prognosis. For example, patients with *PPP2R5D* mutations are expected to have poor language and locomotor performance, moderate to severe ID/DD and epilepsy [29, 46]. Third, Riviere et al. recommended that brain MRI should be performed on these children, with special attention to abnormal patterns of headache, changes in gait or other neurological problems [25]. Fourth, long-term cancer surveillance should be provided for these patients, because the PI3K-AKT-mTOR pathway is an important cancer-related pathway and is frequently mutated in tumours [51]. Patients with *PTEN* mutations have an increased risk of breast cancer, thyroid cancer, melanoma and endometrial cancer [52, 53], and recently, Peterman et al. found that patients with somatic *PIK3CA* mutations had an increased risk of Wilms tumour [54]. Finally, genetic counselling and family cascade testing should be provided to patients with germline mutations, because mutations may have been inherited from parents with macrocephaly yet without a remarkable history of DD/ID. One of the *PTEN* mutations in patient 3 was maternally inherited, but his mother had a clinically unremarkable presentation, except for macrocephaly. She was counselled, and after a year of cancer surveillance, she was diagnosed with early-stage thyroid cancer. This finding illustrates the importance of family cascade testing and cancer surveillance. Nevertheless, because of the complexity of genetic tests (such as the choice of tissue and depth of sequencing) and diverse clinical presentations in patients, we emphasise that genetic testing should only be offered by clinical geneticists who provide comprehensive pre- and post-test counselling to ensure the quality of the test, data interpretation and standard of care.

Here, we reported a second patient with bi-allelic germline *PTEN* mutations. Although one of the mutations was classified as variant of unknown significance, his clinical presentation was more severe than typical patients with heterozygous *PTEN* mutations and siblings with homozygous mutations, as reported by Schwerd et al. [55]. According to these authors, the homozygous p.Leu182Ser mutation is functionally hypomorphic, and thus, the patients have a recessive form of macrocephaly syndrome with a milder clinical course and lower risk of malignancy. Our patient (patient 3) serves as a contrasting example, showing that patients with bi-allelic *PTEN* mutations can present with a more severe clinical course involving multiple systems and display early lethality.

Historically, different nomenclatures have been used in this group of patients, including but not limited to macrocephaly-capillary malformation [56], MCAP [25], MPPH [25, 30], hemimegalencephaly [26], focal cortical dysplasia [28], megalencephaly [28, 57], and *PIK3CA*-related overgrowth spectrum [58]. The overlapping phenotypic presentation makes a differential diagnosis difficult, and the use of different nomenclatures is confusing to clinicians and patients. For example, MCAP and MPPH are usually associated with *PIK3CA* and *PIK3R2* mutations, respectively. However, patients 1 and 9 in our study, who had somatic *PIK3CA* mutations, did not present with somatic features observed in MCAP other than syndactyly [47], whereas patients 3, 4 and 5 who did not have *PIK3R2* mutations, presented with megalencephaly, polymicrogyria or ventriculomegaly, consistent with MPPH. Thus, a differential diagnosis is difficult, and the clinical presentation is a spectrum. A consensus on the nomenclature for this group of patients should be reached among international clinicians and scientists to facilitate communication, management, determination of prognoses, and further research and clinical trials [58]. Although the umbrella term "*PIK3CA*-related overgrowth spectrum" has been proposed to encompass patients with *PIK3CA* mutations [58], it is not sufficiently comprehensive to describe patients with macrocephaly who are complicated with DD/ID/ASD, because mutations in genes other than *PIK3CA* have also been identified in this group of patients. Since these patients share overlapping phenotypes and mutations in the same pathway, we propose the umbrella term "mTOR pathway-related macrocephaly spectrum" to encompass patients with macrocephaly and DD/ID/ASD associated with germline or somatic mutations in the PI3K-AKT-mTOR signalling pathway.

The limitation of the present study is that we only included a small number of patients, and long-term follow up was not available for all patients. In addition, the sequencing strategy was not uniform throughout the study because we made changes to improve the sequencing depth and to include DNA obtained from saliva and buccal mucosa samples, in addition to blood samples. We believe that brain MRI findings may be an indicator for genetic testing because all patients with mutations in the PI3K-AKT-mTOR pathway had features of megalencephaly and/or brain overgrowth, rather than macrocephaly alone. Nevertheless, our findings should be confirmed in larger studies, given our small sample size. Because the association between the PI3K-AKT-mTOR pathway and macrocephaly and DD/ID/ASD is relatively new, we have limited knowledge of this disease spectrum. We hope that the identification of more patients will enable the better characterisation of the clinical presentation of this group of diseases, and hence, clinicians will be able to provide better clinical management for these patients.

Conclusions

In summary, nearly 50% of children with macrocephaly and developmental delay/ASD had mutations in the PI3K-AKT-mTOR pathway, suggesting the importance of this pathway in this patient group. The presence of somatic mosaicism increases the difficulty in providing a molecular diagnosis, and therefore, DNA samples from different tissues should be sequenced. Finally, we propose the use of the umbrella term "mTOR pathway-related macrocephaly spectrum" to emphasise the overlapping clinical phenotypes and genotypes associated with this spectrum of patients.

Abbreviations

ASD: Autism spectrum disorder; COSMIC: Catalogue of Somatic Mutations in Cancer; DD: Developmental delay; DKCAC: Duchess of Kent Children's Hospital Child Assessment Center; DQ: Developmental quotient; ExAC: Exome Aggregation Consortium; GDD: Global developmental delay; ID: Intellectual disability; MCAP: Megalencephaly-capillary malformation syndrome; MPPH: Megalencephaly-polymicrogyria-polydactyly-hydrocephalus syndrome; MRI: Magnetic resonance imaging; SD: Standard deviation; WES: Whole-exome sequencing

Acknowledgements

We thank all the participating patients and their families.

Funding

This study was supported by grants from the SK Yee Medical Research Fund, The Society for the Relief of Disabled Children and HKU Seed Funding for Basic Research. The funding agencies were not involved in the design of the study; in the collection, analysis and interpretation of the data; or in the writing of the manuscript.

Authors' contributions

KSY and WWYT performed the data analysis and wrote the manuscript. KSY performed the Sanger validations. JJKI performed the MRI analysis. KSY, CCYM, GKCL, MHYT, DY and SLCP assisted with the study design, data management and WES analysis. WWYT, SLL and BHYC recruited and managed the patients and provided facilities and resources for the study. BHYC designed and supervised the study. All authors read the manuscript, revised it critically for important intellectual content and approved the final manuscript.

Competing interests

The authors declare that they have no competing interests.

Author details

[1]Department of Paediatrics and Adolescent Medicine, The University of Hong Kong, Pok Fu Lam, Hong Kong, China. [2]Department of Paediatrics and Adolescent Medicine, The Duchess of Kent Children's Hospital, Pok Fu Lam, Hong Kong, China. [3]Department of Radiology, Queen Mary Hospital, Room 103, New Clinical Building, 102 Pokfulam Road, Pok Fu Lam, Hong Kong, China.

References

1. Hazlett HC, Gu H, Munsell BC, et al. Early brain development in infants at high risk for autism spectrum disorder. Nature. 2017;542(7641):348–51.
2. Constantino JN, Charman T. Diagnosis of autism spectrum disorder: reconciling the syndrome, its diverse origins, and variation in expression. Lancet Neurol. 2016;15(3):279–91.
3. Muhle R, Trentacoste SV, Rapin I. The genetics of autism. Pediatrics. 2004; 113(5):e472–86.
4. Vorstman JAS, Parr JR, Moreno-De-Luca D, RJL A, Nurnberger JI Jr, Hallmayer JF. Autism genetics: opportunities and challenges for clinical translation. Nat Rev Genet. 2017;18(6):362–76.
5. Williams G, King J, Cunningham M, Stephan M, Kerr B, Hersh JH. Fetal valproate syndrome and autism: additional evidence of an association. Dev Med Child Neurol. 2001;43(3):202–6.
6. Isaksson J, Pettersson E, Kostrzewa E, Diaz Heijtz R, Bolte S. Brief report: association between autism spectrum disorder, gastrointestinal problems and perinatal risk factors within sibling pairs. J Autism Dev Disord. 2017; 47(8):2621–7.
7. Juul-Dam N, Townsend J, Courchesne E. Prenatal, perinatal, and neonatal factors in autism, pervasive developmental disorder-not otherwise specified, and the general population. Pediatrics. 2001;107(4):E63.
8. Herman GE, Henninger N, Ratliff-Schaub K, Pastore M, Fitzgerald S, McBride KL. Genetic testing in autism: how much is enough? Genet Med. 2007;9(5): 268–74.
9. Schaefer GB, Lutz RE. Diagnostic yield in the clinical genetic evaluation of autism spectrum disorders. Genet Med. 2006;8(9):549–56.
10. Tammimies K, Marshall CR, Walker S, et al. Molecular diagnostic yield of chromosomal microarray analysis and whole-exome sequencing in children with autism spectrum disorder. JAMA. 2015;314(9):895–903.
11. CY RK, Merico D, Bookman M, et al. Whole genome sequencing resource identifies 18 new candidate genes for autism spectrum disorder. Nat Neurosci. 2017;20(4):602–11.
12. Courchesne E, Karns CM, Davis HR, et al. Unusual brain growth patterns in early life in patients with autistic disorder: an MRI study. Neurology. 2001; 57(2):245–54.
13. Aylward EH, Minshew NJ, Field K, Sparks BF, Singh N. Effects of age on brain volume and head circumference in autism. Neurology. 2002;59(2):175–83.
14. Dementieva YA, Vance DD, Donnelly SL, et al. Accelerated head growth in early development of individuals with autism. Pediatr Neurol. 2005; 32(2):102–8.
15. Dissanayake C, Bui QM, Huggins R, Loesch DZ. Growth in stature and head circumference in high-functioning autism and Asperger disorder during the first 3 years of life. Dev Psychopathol. 2006;18(2):381–93.
16. Sacco R, Curatolo P, Manzi B, et al. Principal pathogenetic components and biological endophenotypes in autism spectrum disorders. Autism Res. 2010; 3(5):237–52.
17. Sacco R, Militerni R, Frolli A, et al. Clinical, morphological, and biochemical correlates of head circumference in autism. Biol Psychiatry. 2007;62(9):1038–47.
18. Sacco R, Gabriele S, Persico AM. Head circumference and brain size in autism spectrum disorder: a systematic review and meta-analysis. Psychiatry Res. 2015;234(2):239–51.
19. Zhou J, Parada LFPTEN. Signaling in autism spectrum disorders. Curr Opin Neurobiol. 2012;22(5):873–9.
20. Varga EA, Pastore M, Prior T, Herman GE, KL MB. The prevalence of PTEN mutations in a clinical pediatric cohort with autism spectrum disorders, developmental delay, and macrocephaly. Genet Med. 2009;11(2):111–7.
21. Butler MG, Dasouki MJ, Zhou XP, et al. Subset of individuals with autism spectrum disorders and extreme macrocephaly associated with germline PTEN tumour suppressor gene mutations. J Med Genet. 2005;42(4):318–21.
22. Shen Y, Dies KA, Holm IA, et al. Clinical genetic testing for patients with autism spectrum disorders. Pediatrics. 2010;125(4):e727–35.
23. Schaefer GB, Mendelsohn NJ, Professional P, Guidelines C. Clinical genetics evaluation in identifying the etiology of autism spectrum disorders: 2013 guideline revisions. Genet Med. 2013;15(5):399–407.
24. Anagnostou E, Zwaigenbaum L, Szatmari P, et al. Autism spectrum disorder: advances in evidence-based practice. CMAJ. 2014;186(7):509–19.
25. Riviere JB, Mirzaa GM, O'Roak BJ, et al. De novo germline and postzygotic mutations in AKT3, PIK3R2 and PIK3CA cause a spectrum of related megalencephaly syndromes. Nat Genet. 2012;44(8):934–40.
26. Lee JH, Huynh M, Silhavy JL, et al. De novo somatic mutations in components of the PI3K-AKT3-mTOR pathway cause hemimegalencephaly. Nat Genet. 2012;44(8):941–5.
27. Mirzaa G, Timms AE, Conti V, et al. PIK3CA-associated developmental disorders exhibit distinct classes of mutations with variable expression and tissue distribution. JCI Insight. 2016;1(9):e87623.
28. Mirzaa GM, Campbell CD, Solovieff N, et al. Association of MTOR mutations with developmental brain disorders, including megalencephaly, focal cortical dysplasia, and pigmentary mosaicism. JAMA neurology. 2016;73(7):836–45.
29. Houge G, Haesen D, Vissers LE, et al. B56delta-related protein phosphatase 2A dysfunction identified in patients with intellectual disability. J Clin Invest. 2015;125(8):3051–62.
30. Mirzaa GM, Parry DA, Fry AE, et al. De novo CCND2 mutations leading to stabilization of cyclin D2 cause megalencephaly-polymicrogyria-polydactyly-hydrocephalus syndrome. Nat Genet. 2014;46(5):510–5.
31. Frazier TW, Embacher R, Tilot AK, Koenig K, Mester J, Eng C. Molecular and phenotypic abnormalities in individuals with germline heterozygous PTEN mutations and autism. Mol Psychiatry. 2015;20(9):1132–8.
32. Yeung KS, Ip JJ, Chow CP, et al. Somatic PIK3CA mutations in seven patients with PIK3CA-related overgrowth spectrum. Am J Med Genet A. 2017;173(4):978–84.

33. Tatton-Brown K, Loveday C, Yost S, et al. Mutations in epigenetic regulation genes are a major cause of overgrowth with intellectual disability. Am J Hum Genet. 2017;100(5):725–36.
34. Tao VQ, Chan KY, Chu YW, et al. The clinical impact of chromosomal microarray on paediatric care in Hong Kong. PLoS One. 2014;9(10):e109629.
35. Marsh DJ, Dahia PL, Zheng Z, et al. Germline mutations in PTEN are present in Bannayan-Zonana syndrome. Nat Genet. 1997;16(4):333–4.
36. de Leon MP, Di Gregorio C, Giunti L, et al. Duodenal carcinoma in a 37-year-old man with Cowden/Bannayan syndrome. Dig Liver Dis. 2013; 45(1):75–8.
37. Lobo GP, Waite KA, Planchon SM, Romigh T, Nassif NT, Eng C. Germline and somatic cancer-associated mutations in the ATP-binding motifs of PTEN influence its subcellular localization and tumor suppressive function. Hum Mol Genet. 2009;18(15):2851–62.
38. Browning MJ, Chandra A, Carbonaro V, Okkenhaug K, Barwell J. Cowden's syndrome with immunodeficiency. J Med Genet. 2015;52(12):856–9.
39. Marsh DJ, Kum JB, Lunetta KL, et al. PTEN mutation spectrum and genotype-phenotype correlations in Bannayan-Riley-Ruvalcaba syndrome suggest a single entity with Cowden syndrome. Hum Mol Genet. 1999;8(8): 1461–72.
40. Pilarski R, Burt R, Kohlman W, Pho L, Shannon KM, Swisher E. Cowden syndrome and the PTEN hamartoma tumor syndrome: systematic review and revised diagnostic criteria. J Natl Cancer Inst. 2013;105(21):1607–16.
41. Angulo I, Vadas O, Garcon F, et al. Phosphoinositide 3-kinase delta gene mutation predisposes to respiratory infection and airway damage. Science. 2013;342(6160):866–71.
42. Lucas CL, Kuehn HS, Zhao F, et al. Dominant-activating germline mutations in the gene encoding the PI(3)K catalytic subunit p110delta result in T cell senescence and human immunodeficiency. Nat Immunol. 2014;15(1):88–97.
43. Hussain K, Challis B, Rocha N, et al. An activating mutation of AKT2 and human hypoglycemia. Science. 2011;334(6055):474.
44. Nellist M, Schot R, Hoogeveen-Westerveld M, et al. Germline activating AKT3 mutation associated with megalencephaly, polymicrogyria, epilepsy and hypoglycemia. Mol Genet Metab. 2015;114(3):467–73.
45. Baynam G, Overkov A, Davis M, et al. A germline MTOR mutation in aboriginal Australian siblings with intellectual disability, dysmorphism, macrocephaly, and small thoraces. Am J Med Genet A. 2015;167(7):1659–67.
46. Shang L, Henderson LB, Cho MT, et al. De novo missense variants in PPP2R5D are associated with intellectual disability, macrocephaly, hypotonia, and autism. Neurogenetics. 2016;17(1):43–9.
47. Mirzaa GM, Riviere JB, Dobyns WB. Megalencephaly syndromes and activating mutations in the PI3K-AKT pathway: MPPH and MCAP. Am J Med Genet C Semin Med Genet. 2013;163C(2):122–30.
48. Buxbaum JD, Cai G, Chaste P, et al. Mutation screening of the PTEN gene in patients with autism spectrum disorders and macrocephaly. Am J Med Genet B Neuropsychiatr Genet. 2007;144B(4):484–91.
49. McBride KL, Varga EA, Pastore MT, et al. Confirmation study of PTEN mutations among individuals with autism or developmental delays/mental retardation and macrocephaly. Autism Res. 2010;3(3):137–41.
50. Moeschler JB, Shevell M. Committee on G. Comprehensive evaluation of the child with intellectual disability or global developmental delays. Pediatrics. 2014;134(3):e903–18.
51. Fruman DA, Rommel C. PI3K and cancer: lessons, challenges and opportunities. Nat Rev Drug Discov. 2014;13(2):140–56.
52. Tan MH, Mester JL, Ngeow J, Rybicki LA, Orloff MS, Eng C. Lifetime cancer risks in individuals with germline PTEN mutations. Clin Cancer Res. 2012; 18(2):400–7.
53. Bubien V, Bonnet F, Brouste V, et al. High cumulative risks of cancer in patients with PTEN hamartoma tumour syndrome. J Med Genet. 2013; 50(4):255–63.
54. Peterman CM, Fevurly RD, Alomari AI, et al. Sonographic screening for Wilms tumor in children with CLOVES syndrome. Pediatric blood & cancer. 2017;64(12):e26684.
55. Schwerd T, Khaled AV, Schurmann M, et al. A recessive form of extreme macrocephaly and mild intellectual disability complements the spectrum of PTEN hamartoma tumour syndrome. Eur J Hum Genet. 2016;24(6):889–94.
56. Toriello HV, Mulliken JB. Accurately renaming macrocephaly-cutis marmorata telangiectatica congenita (M-CMTC) as macrocephaly-capillary malformation (M-CM). Am J Med Genet A. 2007;143A(24):3009.
57. Tapper WJ, Foulds N, Cross NC, et al. Megalencephaly syndromes: exome pipeline strategies for detecting low-level mosaic mutations. PLoS One. 2014;9(1):e86940.
58. Keppler-Noreuil KM, Rios JJ, Parker VE, et al. PIK3CA-related overgrowth spectrum (PROS): diagnostic and testing eligibility criteria, differential diagnosis, and evaluation. Am J Med Genet A. 2015;167A(2):287–95.

9

Analysis of the expression pattern of the schizophrenia-risk and intellectual disability gene TCF4 in the developing and adult brain suggests a role in development and plasticity of cortical and hippocampal neurons

Matthias Jung[1†], Benjamin M. Häberle[1†], Tristan Tschaikowsky[1], Marie-Theres Wittmann[1,2], Elli-Anna Balta[1], Vivien-Charlott Stadler[1], Christiane Zweier[2], Arnd Dörfler[3], Christian Johannes Gloeckner[4,5] and D. Chichung Lie[1*]

Abstract

Background: Haploinsufficiency of the class I bHLH transcription factor TCF4 causes Pitt-Hopkins syndrome (PTHS), a severe neurodevelopmental disorder, while common variants in the *TCF4* gene have been identified as susceptibility factors for schizophrenia. It remains largely unknown, which brain regions are dependent on TCF4 for their development and function.

Methods: We systematically analyzed the expression pattern of TCF4 in the developing and adult mouse brain. We used immunofluorescent staining to identify candidate regions whose development and function depend on TCF4. In addition, we determined TCF4 expression in the developing rhesus monkey brain and in the developing and adult human brain through analysis of transcriptomic datasets and compared the expression pattern between species. Finally, we morphometrically and histologically analyzed selected brain structures in *Tcf4*-haploinsufficient mice and compared our morphometric findings to neuroanatomical findings in PTHS patients.

Results: TCF4 is broadly expressed in cortical and subcortical structures in the developing and adult mouse brain. The TCF4 expression pattern was highly similar between humans, rhesus monkeys, and mice. Moreover, *Tcf4* haploinsufficiency in mice replicated structural brain anomalies observed in PTHS patients.

Conclusion: Our data suggests that TCF4 is involved in the development and function of multiple brain regions and indicates that its regulation is evolutionary conserved. Moreover, our data validate *Tcf4*-haploinsufficient mice as a model to study the neurodevelopmental basis of PTHS.

Keywords: Pitt-Hopkins syndrome, Schizophrenia, TCF4, Neurodevelopment

* Correspondence: chi.lie@fau.de
[†]Equal contributors
[1]Institute of Biochemistry, Emil Fischer Center, Friedrich-Alexander-Universität Erlangen-Nürnberg, 91054 Erlangen, Germany
Full list of author information is available at the end of the article

Background

The transcription factor 4 (TCF4, Gene ID: 6925) and its paralogues TCF3 and TCF12 form the subgroup of class I basic Helix-Loop-Helix (bHLH) transcription factors (TFs). Class I bHLH TFs are ubiquitously expressed, and their transcriptional output is dependent on their interaction partners. They are obligate partners for proneural class II bHLH TFs, which are unable to exert transcriptional function without dimerization to Class I bHLH. Class I bHLH TF are inhibited by interaction Class V bHLH factors, which do not possess a DNA-binding domain and sequester class I factors [1].

TCF4 has gained major attention following the discoveries that heterozygote loss-of-function mutations in *TCF4* cause Pitt-Hopkins syndrome (PTHS) [2, 3]—a neurodevelopmental disorder characterized by early onset developmental delay, moderate to severe intellectual disability, autistic behavior, intermittent breathing abnormalities, seizures, and distinctive facial features—and that single nucleotide polymorphisms (SNPs) in potentially regulatory regions of *TCF4* are associated with an increased risk of schizophrenia [4–6].

The extent of cognitive deficits in PTHS suggests that TCF4 dosage is critical for the development of various brain regions, but it remains largely unknown which neural populations develop in a TCF4-dependent fashion. Based on the rationale that TCF4 expression will predict regions that require TCF4 activity for their development, we performed a systematic analysis of the temporo-spatial expression pattern of TCF4 protein in mouse brain development. Moreover, we determined TCF4 expression in the adult mouse brain to identify neural systems, in which TCF4 may serve functions in maintenance and plasticity. Our analyses reveal that TCF4 is broadly expressed in cortical and subcortical structures in the development and adulthood with prominent expression in the cortex, hippocampus, and a subset of hypothalamic and amygdaloid nuclei. Comparison of the developmental and adult murine expression pattern with transcriptomic datasets from rhesus monkey and human brain revealed strong similarities in TCF4 expression between species. Moreover, we found that *Tcf4* haploinsuffiency in mice replicated structural brain anomalies that have been observed in individuals with PTHS. Thus, our data suggest that TCF4 regulation and function in brain development may be evolutionary conserved.

Results

We first determined the specificity of the Tcf4-antibody intended for immunohistochemical analysis. To this end, HEK 293T cells were transfected with a C-terminally Flag-tagged TCF4-expression construct or with a control expression construct. The anti-TCF4-antibody as well as the anti-Flag antibody detected a single 100 kDa band in cell lysates from TCF4-transfected cells. The 100 kDa band was absent from cell lysates of control-transfected cells and was reduced in cells, in which a *TCF4*-specific shRNA construct was co-transfected with the *TCF4*-expression construct (Fig. 1a). Homozygous *Tcf4*-knockout (*Tcf4*$^{lacZ/lacZ}$) is associated with high perinatal lethality, and from our breedings, we obtained only one *Tcf4*$^{lacZ/lacZ}$ mouse that survived into adulthood. We used brain tissue from this mouse to further validate specificity of the TCF4-antibody. Staining with the TCF4 antibody yielded a robust signal in tissue from wildtype mice but no signal in homozygote *Tcf4*-knockout tissue (Fig. 1b, c). Collectively, these data demonstrate the specificity of the antibody for TCF4.

Next, we systematically analyzed the expression pattern of TCF4 protein in the developing and adult mouse brain. On embryonic day 11.5 (E11.5), TCF4 was broadly expressed in the germinal regions for cortical glutamatergic neurons and GABAergic neurons. Immunoreactive intensity varied between the distinct germinal regions. It was high in the cortical and hippocampal neuroepithelium and remained intense in the expanding neocortex and in the developing hippocampal formation (Fig. 1d–h). The ganglionic eminences are the main germinal zones for GABAergic neurons. The lateral ganglionic eminence (LGE) generates GABAergic interneurons and projection neurons of the olfactory bulb, amygdala, and striatum from E12 until birth [7, 8], while the medial ganglionic eminence (MGE) generates the majority of cortical interneurons between E12 and E16.5. MGE-derived interneuron precursors migrate tangentially to their final neocortical location [9]. Notably, the expression of TCF4 in the MGE correlated with the time of cortical interneuron production [10] (Fig. 1d–f). Moreover, TCF4 expression showed a lateral to medial gradient with moderate to high levels in the most medial part of the MGE and low to absent immunoreactivity in the LGE (Fig. 1d–f).

Regionally distinct TCF4 expression levels were observed in subcortical areas. Developing hypothalamic nuclei showed moderate expression of TCF4 starting from E11.5 onwards (Fig. 1d–h); at E15.5 and postnatal day 7 (P7), TCF4 showed prominent expression in a subset of cells in the paraventricular hypothalamic nucleus and the basal peduncular hypothalamus, respectively (Fig. 2a, d). From E15.5, when the amygdaloid complex can be clearly distinguished, we found continuously high expression of TCF4 in this region (Fig. 2b–e). In the globus pallidus (GP), TCF4 expression was high at E15.5 but decreased at subsequent stages (Fig. 2b, c, e). Scattered cells with low to intermediate TCF4 expression were observed in the caudoputamen (CP) at postnatal stages (Fig. 1h; Fig. 2e, f). A summary of the developmental expression pattern and levels of TCF4 is provided in Fig. 3a.

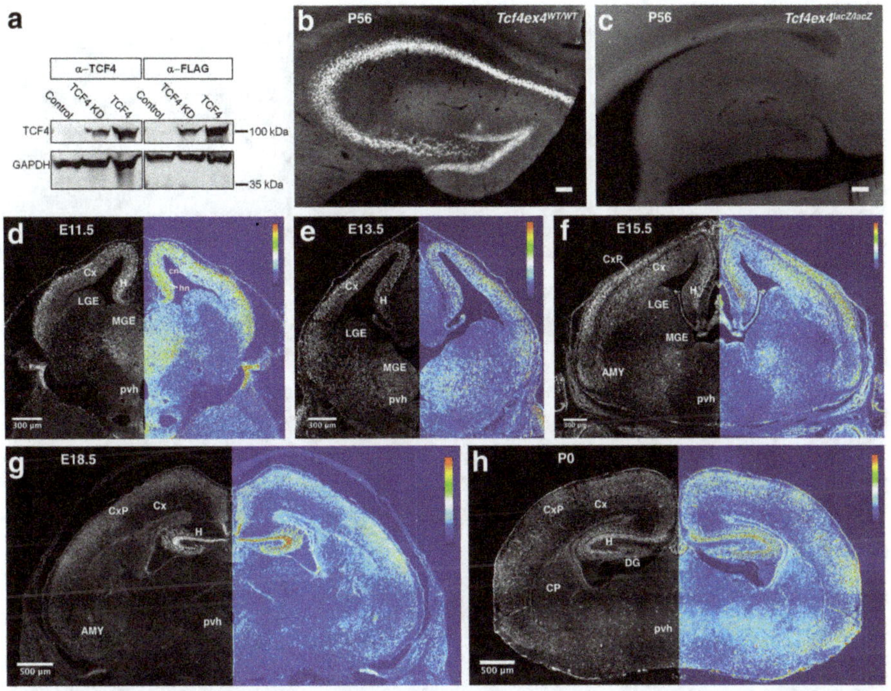

Fig. 1 TCF4 expression at different developmental stages and validation of antibody specificity. **a** Western blot analysis of HEK 293T transfected with either CAG-GFP-IRES-GFP (Control), CAG-TCF4-IRES-GFP/ CAG-shTCF4-IRES-GFP (TCF4 KD), or CAG-TCF4-IRES-GFP (TCF4). Detection using the anti-TCF4 antibody revealed a clear band in the TCF4 transfected cells, which was reduced in size in the TCF4 KD (left panel). Detection using an anti-FLAG antibody resulted in bands equal in height compared to the TCF4 staining and also showed reduction upon TCF4 KD (right panel). GAPDH was used as the loading control. **b**, **c** Immunostaining using the anti-TCF4 antibody of brain tissue of TCF4 wildtype (WT) and constitutive TCF4-KO mice. **d**–**h** Left-hand side of each image, TCF4 immunostaining. Right-hand side, heatmap converted image. Relative immunoreactivity scale is shown in the upper right corner: red and blue represent high and low immunoreactivity, respectively. Abbreviations: AMY, amygdala; cn, cortical neuroepithelium; CP, caudoputamen; Cx, cortex; CxP, cortical plate; DG, dentate gyrus; H, hippocampal formation; hn, hippocampal neuroepithelium; LGE, lateral ganglionic eminence; MGE, medial ganglionic eminence; pvh, paraventricular hypothalamus

In young adult mice (P56), the highest TCF4 immunoreactivity was found in the hippocampal formation, the cortex, the purkinje cell layer of the cerebellum, and the amygdala (Fig. 4A–D'). Of the amygdala subnuclei, cells of the lateral (LA) and basolateral (BLA) nucleus highly express TCF4. The central nucleus (CEA) also shows high TCF4 immunoreactivity; in contrast to the LA and BLA nuclei, TCF4 signal in the CEA was not nuclear but was located in fibers, whose distribution strongly resembled the distribution pattern of calcitonin gene-related peptide immunoreactive projections that arise from posterior thalamic nuclei [11]. Low to intermediate TCF4 immunoreactivity was found in structures of the diencephalon, the midbrain, and in scattered cells of the caudoputamen (Fig. 4E). The expression pattern of TCF4 in the adult mouse brain is summarized in Fig. 3d.

Next, we analyzed the expression of TCF4 in glial cells. TCF4 was expressed in the majority of astroglia and some Sox10-positive oligodendroglia (Fig. 4F–H"). Expression levels in both glial populations varied from low to high. *Iba1*-positive microglial cells did not show TCF4 immunoreactivity (Fig. 4F–I").

Given the prominent expression of TCF4 in the cortex and hippocampus, we analyzed these areas in more detail. During cortical development, radial glial cells (RGCs) in the ventricular zone (VZ) divide to self-renew and to generate either immature neurons or intermediate progenitor cells (IPCs) [12, 13]. IPCs accumulate in the subventricular zone (SVZ) where they give rise to postmitotic neurons via asymmetric cell division [13]. Neurons migrate radially into the expanding cortical plate (CP), forming the distinct cortical layers in an inside-out fashion with later-born excitatory neurons migrating to more superficial layers of the CP passing over earlier born neurons [14, 15]. At E11.5, TCF4 expression is high in the ventricular zone (VZ), which coincides with the generation of preplate (PP) neurons from neural progenitors in this region (Fig. 5A). Co-staining with the precursor marker Sox2 confirmed that TCF4 was indeed highly expressed by VZ precursors at this time point (Fig. 5G–G"). At later stages (E13.5 and thereafter), TCF4 immunoreactivity was low to moderate in the germinal zones, i.e., the VZ and SVZ, but was high in the PP and the expanding cortical plate (Fig. 5B–

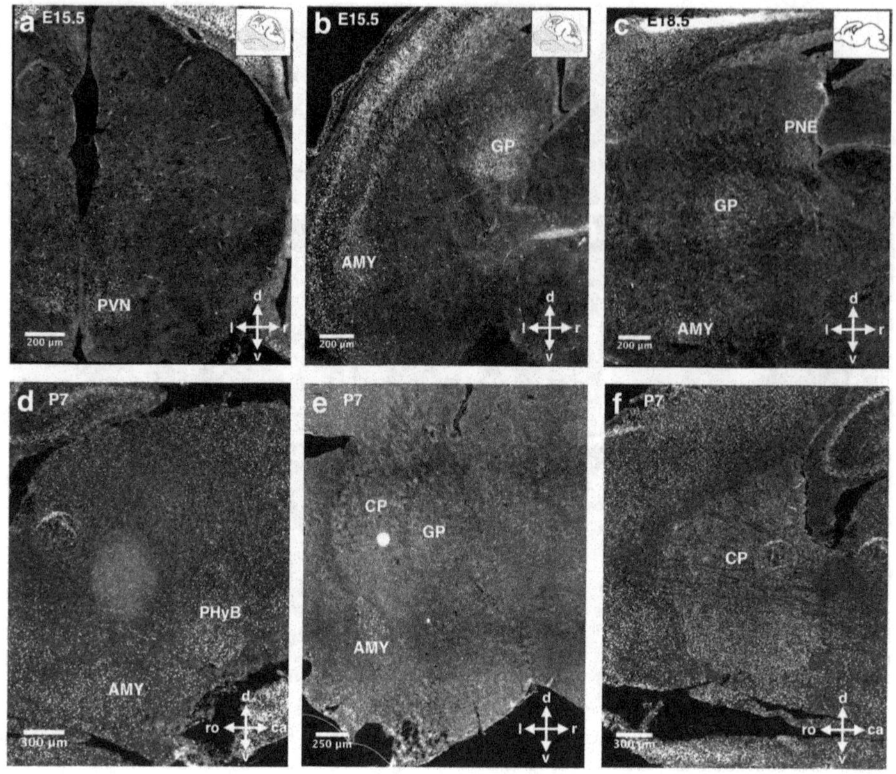

Fig. 2 TCF4 expression in subcortical areas during neuronal development. TCF4 is expressed in developing hypothalamic nuclei (**a**), the globus pallidus (**b**, **c**, **e**), the amygdala (**b**, **c**, **d**, **e**), and the pallidal neuroepithelium (**c**). TCF4 immunoreactivity is also observed in the developing caudoputamen (**e**, **f**). Abbreviations: AMY, amygdala; PHyB, basal peduncular hypothalamus; CP, caudoputamen; GP, globus pallidus; MGE, medial ganglionic eminence; PVN, paraventricular hypothalamic nucleus; PNE, pallidal neuroepithelium

D). At E13.5, the highest TCF4 expression levels co-localized with DCX, a marker for immature migrating neurons (Fig. 5H–H"); at E18.5, high TCF4 expression levels frequently co-localized with NeuN, a marker for post-migratory neurons (Fig. 5I–I"). Cells with high TCF4 expression were also observed in the postnatal and adult cortex (Fig. 5E, F, J–L"). These TCF4-expressing cells also expressed the layer V/VI neuronal marker CTIP2 or the layer II-IV neuronal marker Cux1, demonstrating that subsets of cortical neurons expressed high levels of TCF4 (Fig. 5J–K"). In addition, high TCF4 expression was observed in a subset of GAD67-positive cortical interneurons (Fig. 5L–L").

The hippocampal neuroepithelium is the germinal zone for hippocampal neurons and is subdivided into the Ammon's horn neuroepithelium (ANE) and the dentate gyrus neuroepithelium (DNE). CA1-CA3 pyramidal neuron precursors are generated in the ANE and migrate radially from the VZ to the prospective CA1-CA3 subfields where they undergo terminal differentiation and maturation. The DNE, which is also called primary matrix, generates dentate granule neuron precursors (secondary matrix) that migrate along a radial glial scaffold to the subpial zone of the hippocampus [16–19]. Reaching the hippocampal fissure, precursors accumulate and form the tertiary matrix [16]. During the first postnatal week, the secondary matrix disappears, while the tertiary matrix remains the proliferative zone generating the inner shell of the granule cell layer [16, 19]. From P14 onwards, the tertiary matrix resolves and the neurogenic niche becomes successively confined to the subgranular zone (SGZ) of the dentate gyrus (DG) [16, 20]. TCF4 is highly expressed in pyramidal and dentate granule precursors and neurons during the course of hippocampal development (Fig. 6a–f). In contrast to the adult cortex, where high TCF4 expression is observed only in a subset of neurons, TCF4 expression in the adult hippocampus remained prominent throughout the CA subfields and the dentate gyrus (Fig. 6g–o). In the dentate gyrus, TCF4 was not only strongly expressed in Calbindin-positive mature dentate granule neurons but also in Parvalbumin-positive interneurons (Fig. 7D–E"). The dentate gyrus is one of two regions of the adult mammalian brain, where stem cells generate neurons throughout life [21]. Nestin-positive radial glia-like stem cells in the subgranular zone displayed moderate TCF4 immunoreactivity (Fig. 7A–A"). Sox2-

a

Region	E11.5	E13.5	E15.5	E18.5	P0	P7	P14	P21
Neocortex								
ventricular zone	++/+++	+/+++	+/+++	+/++	+/++			
subventricular zone		+/+++	+/++	+/++	+			
intermediate zone			++/+++	+/++	+			
marginal zone			+++	+++	+++	-		
subplate			+	+	+			
preplate/cortical plate	+++	+++	+++	+++	+/+++			
layer II/III						+/++		
layer IV						+/+++		
layer V/VI					++/+++	+/+++		
Hippocampus								
ANE	+++	+++	++	+				
DNE	+++	+++	+++	+				
1ry			+++	++	+			
2ry			+++	+++	+++			
3ry				+/++	++/+++			
Dentate Gyrus					+/++	++/+++		
CA1/CA2				+++	+++	+++		
CA3				+++	+++	+++		
Basal forebrain								
Amygdaloid complex			+++	+++	+++	+++		
MGE/PNE	+/++	+/++	+/++	++/+++				
LGE	+	-	-					
Caudoputamen			-	+	+	+/++		
Globus pallidus			++/+++	++/+++	+/+++	+/++		
Thalamus		-	-	-	-	+		
Hypothalamus	+/++		++/+++	+/++	+	++/+++		
Cerebellum								
Internal granular layer						++	+++	++/+++
External granular layer						+++		
Purkinje layer							+++	+++
Molecular layer						+	+	+/++

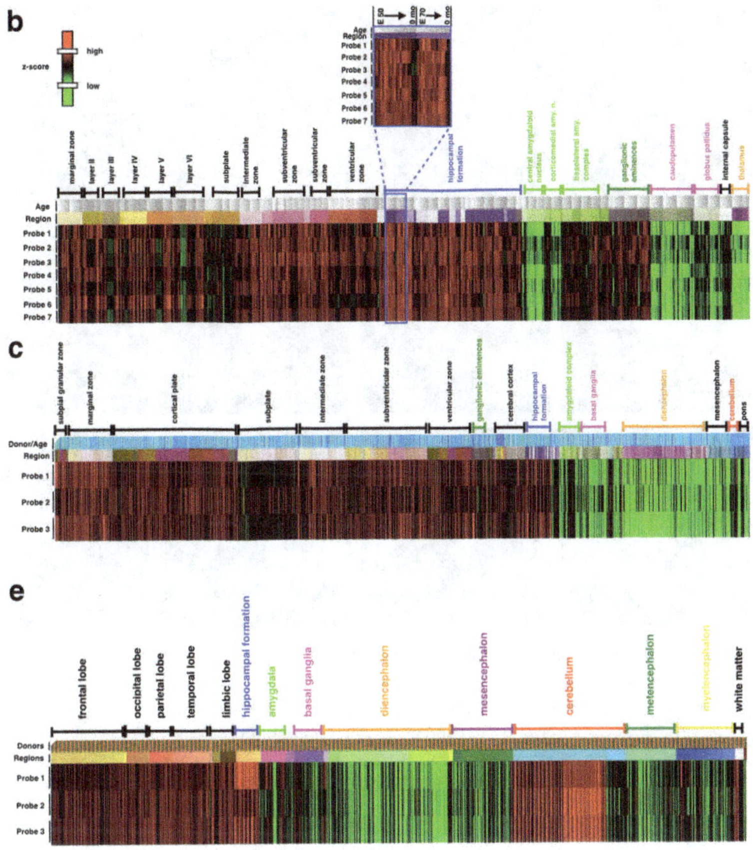

d

Region		IHC	Region		IHC
Cortex	Frontal lobe	++	Mesencephalon	Superior colliculus	++
	Visual Cortex	++		Inferior colliculus	+
	Motor Cortex	++	Cerebellum	Molecular Layer	+
	Sensory Cortex	++		Purkinje Cell Layer	+++
	Temporal lobe	++		Granule Cell Layer	+
	Piriform cortex	+++		White Matter	-
Hippocampal formation	CA 1-3 PML	+++	Metencephalon	Pons	+
	Dentate GCL	+++	Myelencephalon	Medulla	+
	Dentate MCL	+	Neurogenic areas	SGZ (Hippocampus)	+++
	Subiculum	++		RMS	+
	Indusium griseum	+++		SVZ	++
Amygdala	Lateral Nucleus	++	Olfactory bulb	Granule cell layer	++
	Basolateral Nucleus	+++		Internal plexiform layer	+
	Basomedial Nucleus	+		Mitral cell layer	++
	Medial Nucleus	+		External plexiform layer	-
	Central Nucleus	-		Glomerular layer	+
Basal ganglia	Caudoputamen	+		Accessory olfactory bulb	++
	Pallidum	++	Olfactory processing	Medial Habenula	+
	Ncl. accumbens	++		Septal Area	+
Diencephalon	Thalamus	+		Olfactory Nucleus	++
	Hypothalamus	++		Endopiriform Nucleus	++

Fig. 3 Comparison of developmental and adult TCF4 expression. **a** Tabular overview of TCF4 expression during neural development. +++, high. ++, moderate. +, low. -, not detected. Hatched cell: structure not defined at developmental stage. Empty cell: expression not determined. **b** TCF4 expression in selected brain areas during non-human primate neural development from E40–0 months. Microarray data of six probes is grouped by brain regions and arranged by ascending age per region (blow-up) (The NIH Blueprint Non-Human Primate (NHP) Atlas, http://www.blueprintnhpatlas.org). **c** TCF4 expression in selected brain areas during human neural development from post-conception week 15–21. Microarray data of three probes are grouped by brain regions and aligned by ascending age per region (BrainSpan: Atlas of the Developing Human Brain [Internet]. Funded by ARRA Awards 1RC2MH089921-01, 1RC2MH090047-01, and 1RC2MH089929-01. © 2011. Available from: http://www.brainspan.org/lcm/search?search_type=user_selections). **d** Tabular overview of TCF4 expression in the adult mouse brain (P56). **e** Brain region-specific TCF4 expression in the adult human brain [23]

positive precursors and astroglia in the SGZ showed variable levels of TCF4 expression, whereas NeuroD1-positive immature dentate granule neurons showed strong TCF4 immunoreactivity (Fig. 7B–C"). Collectively, the expression data of TCF4 strongly suggests that TCF4 is intimately linked to developmental and adult hippocampal neurogenesis. The persistence of high TCF4 expression in mature neurons of all hippocampal subfields raises the intriguing possibility that TCF4 is also involved in hippocampal plasticity.

Next, we sought to evaluate whether the TCF4 expression pattern is conserved from mice to humans. The NIH Blueprint Non-Human Primate (NHP) Atlas (2009) (http://www.blueprintnhpatlas.org) provides mRNA expression data of the developing rhesus monkey brain from E40–0 months; the BrainSpan Atlas documents mRNA expression data of human neural development for post conception weeks 15–21 [22]. *TCF4* mRNA expression data in the adult human brain was extracted from the Allen Human Brain Atlas (© 2010 Allen Institute for Brain Science. Allen Human Brain Atlas. Available from: human.brain-map.org, [23]). The neurodevelopmental expression pattern of *TCF4* was highly similar between mice, rhesus monkeys, and humans: regions with high expression during murine neural development such as the hippocampus, the cortex, the ganglionic eminences, and some nuclei of the amygdaloid complex, consistently show high *TCF4* expression in the developing brain of rhesus monkey and humans, whereas low *TCF4* expressing regions such as the caudoputamen also show low expression

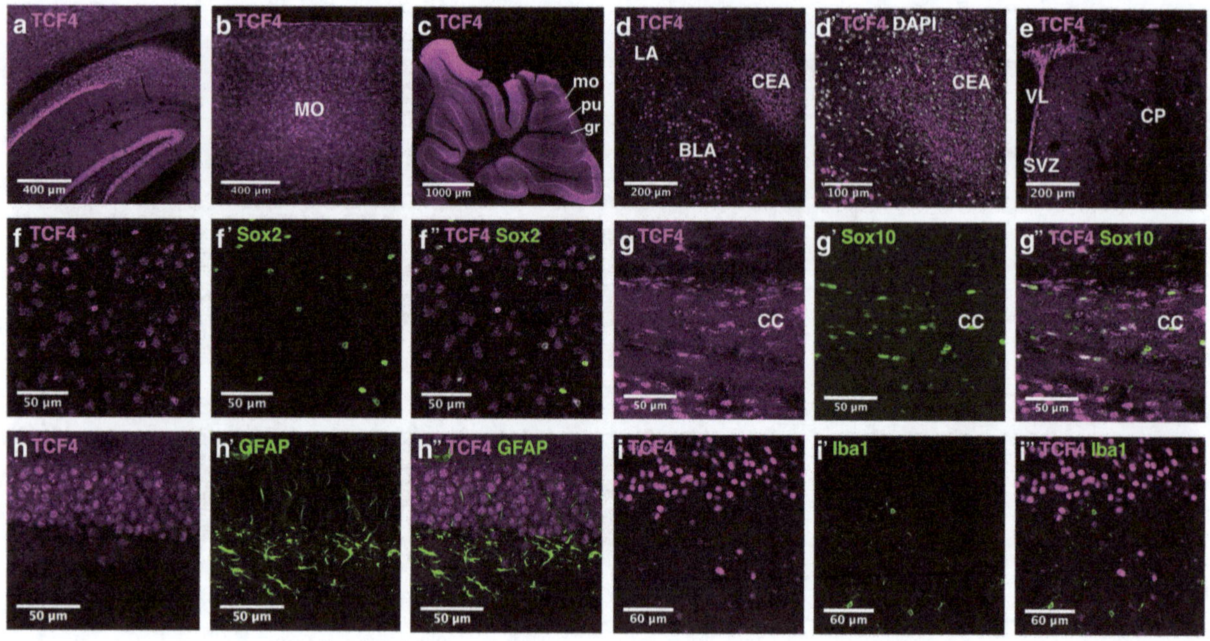

Fig. 4 TCF4 expression in regions and non-neuronal cell types of the adult brain. In the adult brain, TCF4 is expressed in the hippocampus (**A**), the cortex (**A**, **B**), the cerebellum (**C**), the amygdaloid complex (**D**–**D'**) and the caudoputamen (**E**). TCF4 immunoreactivity is observed in astrocytes (**F**–**F"**, **H**–**H"**) and oligodendrocytes (**G**–**G"**) but not in microglial cells (**I**–**I"**). Abbreviations: BLA basolateral amydala nucleus; CC, corpus callosum; CEA, central amygdala nucleus; CP, caudoputamen; gr, granule cell layer; LA, lateral amygdala. MO, somatomotor areas; mo, molecular cell layer; pu, purkinje cell layer nucleus; SVZ, subventricular zone; VZ, ventricular zone

during rhesus monkey and human brain development (Fig. 3a-c).

Striking similarities in the TCF4 expression pattern were also found during adulthood. Regions with high expression in adult mice, i.e., hippocampus, cerebellum, cortex, and nuclei of the amygdaloid complex, were also the highest *TCF4*-expressing regions in the adult human brain, while, for example, the diencephalon, metencephalon, myelencephalon, and parts of the basal ganglia showed low *TCF4* expression levels in humans and mice (Fig. 3d, e). These data indicate that the expression pattern of TCF4 is conserved from mouse to humans.

In humans, *TCF4* haploinsufficiency causes Pitt-Hopkins syndrome, a severe neurodevelopmental disorder, associated with psychomotor delay, intellectual disability, and autistic behavior. MRI-based findings of structural anomalies in PTHS are variable, ranging from normal cerebral MRIs (30–50% of cases) to enlarged ventricles, cerebellar atrophy, hippocampal hypoplasia, and hypoplasia of the corpus callosum [24–26]. We analyzed MRIs of two individuals with genetically confirmed PTHS. Consistent with previous studies reporting hypoplasia of the corpus callosum as a frequent structural anomaly in PTHS (24–45% of cases), we found general thinning of the corpus callosum and aplasia of the splenium of the corpus callosum in both individuals (Fig. 8A–D). One of the individuals also displayed a small hippocampal formation (Fig. 8E).

We next investigated whether *Tcf4* haploinsufficiency in mice reproduced structural anomalies of PTHS. To determine the influence of *Tcf4*-haploinsufficiency on cortical architecture, we analyzed the diameter of six different cortical regions along the rostral to caudal axis. Cortical thickness was significantly reduced in all analyzed areas in *Tcf4*-haploinsufficient (*Tcf4ex4*$^{lacZ/WT}$) mice compared to their wildtype littermates (WT) (Fig. 8I–P). Moreover, the dentate gyrus volume was significantly decreased in *Tcf4ex4*$^{lacZ/WT}$ mice (Fig. 8F–H). In addition, *Tcf4ex4*$^{lacZ/WT}$ mice displayed agenesis of the splenium of the corpus callosum (Fig. 8F–G'). Thus, *Tcf4* haploinsufficiency in mice results in anatomical deficits that resemble anatomical anomalies observed in PTHS.

Finally, we qualitatively compared TCF4-expression in the cortex and hippocampus at E15.5, E18.5, P7, and P56 between WT and *Tcf4*-haploinsufficient mice (Fig. 9) The cortex of *Tcf4ex4*$^{lacZ/WT}$ animals appeared markedly thinner at all time points (Fig. 9A–D'). The density of TCF4-expressing cells in the cortex of *Tcf4ex4*$^{lacZ/WT}$ mice seemed to be reduced, and TCF4-expressing cells showed a less regular distribution. Similarly, the arrangement of TCF4-expressing cells in the developing hippocampus (E15.5–P7) of *Tcf4ex4*$^{lacZ/WT}$ mice was less organized (Fig. 9E–H'). Moreover, TCF4-expressing cells

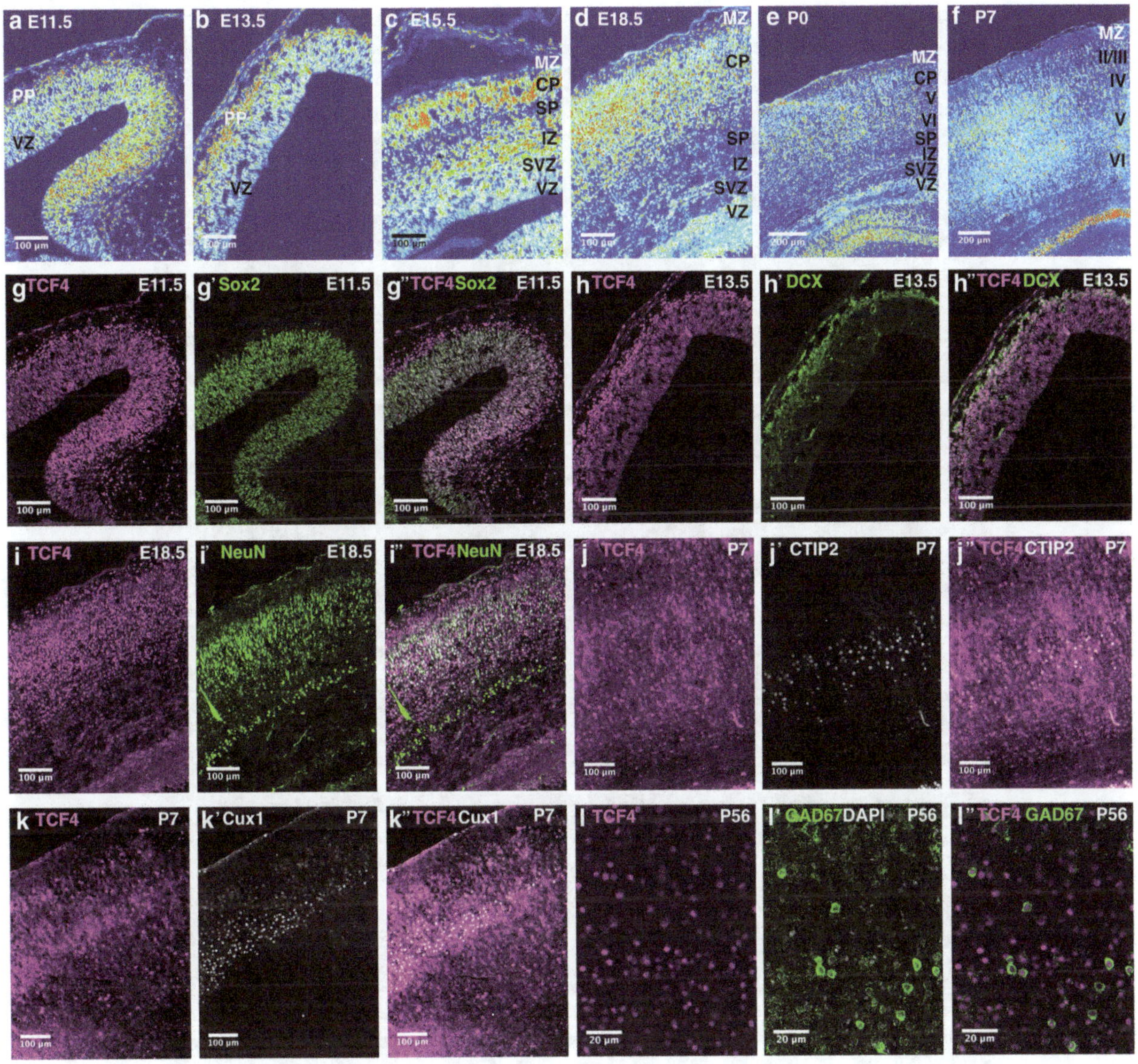

Fig. 5 TCF4 expression during corticogenesis. (**A**–**F**) Heatmap converted TCF4 immunoreactivity at different stages of cortical development. TCF4 is expressed in all layers of the neocortex with particular high intensity in the expanding cortical plate during development (**G**–**I″**). TCF4 is expressed in Sox2-positive ventricular zone cells (**G**–**G″**), DCX-positive immature neurons (**H**–**H″**), and NeuN-positive neurons (**I**–**I″**). TCF4 co-stainings with layer V/VI neuron marker CTIP2 (**J**–**J″**) or layer II/III/IV neuron marker Cux1 (K-K″) at P7. TCF4 is expressed in layers II-VI but only individual TCF4-positive cells co-localize with the layer markers. TCF4 is expressed in GAD67-positive interneurons (**L**–**L″**). Abbreviations: CP, cortical plate; IZ, intermediate zone; MZ, marginal zone; PP, preplate; SP, subplate; SVZ, subventricular zone; VZ, ventricular zone

in the CA3 subfield of adult *Tcf4*-haploinsufficient mice appeared to be less densely packed (Fig. 9H–H').

Discussion

Here, we used immunohistochemical analysis to systematically investigate the expression of the intellectual disability and schizophrenia-associated *Tcf4* gene in the developing and adult murine CNS. Consistent with recent experimental evidence linking TCF4 to precursor proliferation, neuronal positioning and development of excitability in the developing cortex [27–29], and the suggestion that TCF4 regulates neurite branching and synapse formation in prefrontal cortical neurons [30], we found TCF4 to be expressed from the early precursor stage up to the post-migratory neuronal stage in the developing cortex. We also demonstrate that TCF4 is expressed in the major germinal zones for the principal neurons of the hippocampus, for cortical interneurons, as well as in developing neurons of, for example, the cerebellum and some nuclei of the amygdaloid complex. The broad expression of TCF4 strongly suggests that

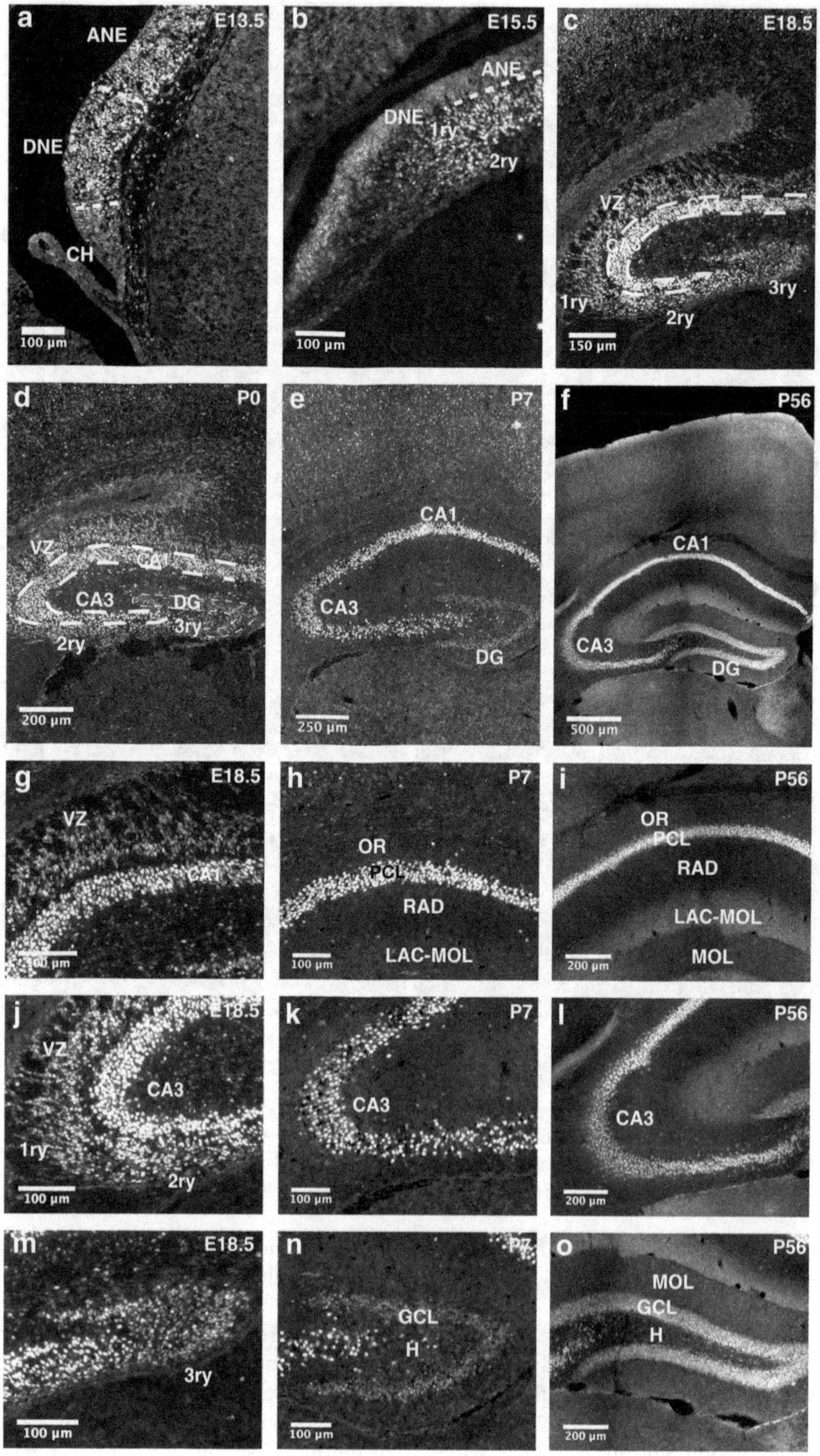

Fig. 6 (See legend on next page.)

(See figure on previous page.)
Fig. 6 TCF4 expression during hippocampal development. **a–f** Overview images of the hippocampal formation at different developmental stages. TCF4 is expressed throughout pre- and postnatal development of the hippocampus. **g–i** TCF4 expression in the CA1 region of the hippocampus. At E18.5, TCF4 is expressed in radially migrating pyramidal progenitor cells and in the forming pyramidal cell layer. Postnatally, TCF4 is expressed in the pyramidal cell layer and in scattered cells in the stratum oriens and radiatum. **j–l** At E18.5, TCF4 is expressed in dentate progenitor cells that migrate to the subpial zone (primary and secondary matrix) and in the forming pyramidal cell layer of the CA3 region. At postnatal stages P7 and P56, TCF4 is expressed in the pyramidal cell layer and in scattered cells of the strata oriens and radiatum. **m–o** At E18.5, TCF4 is expressed in dentate progenitor cells that accumulate in the hippocampal fissure (tertiary matrix). Postnatally, TCF4 is expressed in the granular cell layer of the dentate gyrus and in individual cells of the hilus. Abbreviations: 1ry, primary matrix; 2ry, secondary matrix; 3ry, tertiary matrix; ANE, ammonic neuroepithelium; CH, cortical hem; DG, dentate gyrus; DNE, dentate neuroepithelium; GCL, granular cell layer; H, hilus; LAC-MOL, stratum lacunosum-moleculare; MOL, molecular layer; OR, stratum oriens; PCL, pyramidal cell layer; RAD, stratum radiatum; SVZ, subventricular zone

TCF4 regulates early and late development of cortical and subcortical structures.

As a class I bHLH TF, the transcriptional output of TCF4 is dependent on interaction with other bHLH TFs. Through such interactions, TCF4 may act as a network hub coordinating different transcriptional modules and developmental processes. The interaction partners of TCF4 in the developing CNS have not been defined. The bHLH TFs Ascl1, Neurogenin 1 and 2, NeuroD1, and NeuroD6, have a restricted developmental expression pattern and fulfill defined stage-specific functions during hippocampal and cortical development [31–33]. It is tempting to speculate that TCF4 fulfills at least part of its functions in CNS development through interaction with these proneural class II bHLH TFs.

Recent work indicated that TCF4 activity is modulated by post-translational mechanisms such as neuronal activity-dependent phosphorylation [34]. Interestingly, we detected TCF4 immunoreactivity in fibers of the CEA, raising the possibility that TCF4 activity may be modulated by nuclear-cytoplasmatic translocation.

PTHS is associated with deficits in various functional domains including cognition, social interaction, speech, motor skills, and vegetative function, and there is some debate to which extent the PTHS phenotype may be due to post-developmental functions of TCF4 in mature neurons [35]. Indeed, it has been shown that TCF4 directly regulates plasticity of CA1 pyramidal neurons potentially through the control of activity-dependent DNA methylation [35]. Strikingly, we found that TCF4 is highly expressed not only in the hippocampus but also in a

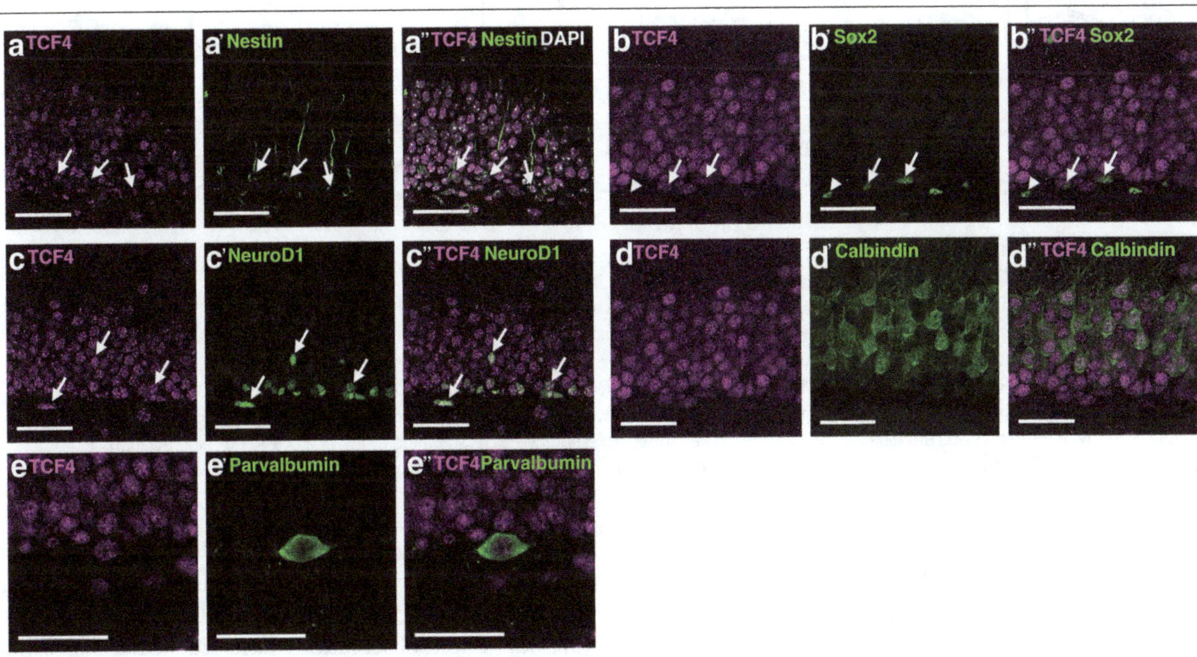

Fig. 7 TCF4 expression in different cell types in the adult dentate gyrus. **A–A''** TCF4 is expressed in Nestin-positive radial glia-like cells. **B–B''** TCF4 is partially expressed in Sox2-positive cells. **C–C''** TCF4 is expressed in NeuroD-positive immature neurons, **D–D''** TCF4 is expressed in Calbindin-positive mature neurons, and **E–E''** in Parvalbumin-positive interneurons. Arrowheads mark TCF4 negative/cell type marker positive cells. Scale bars are 40 μm

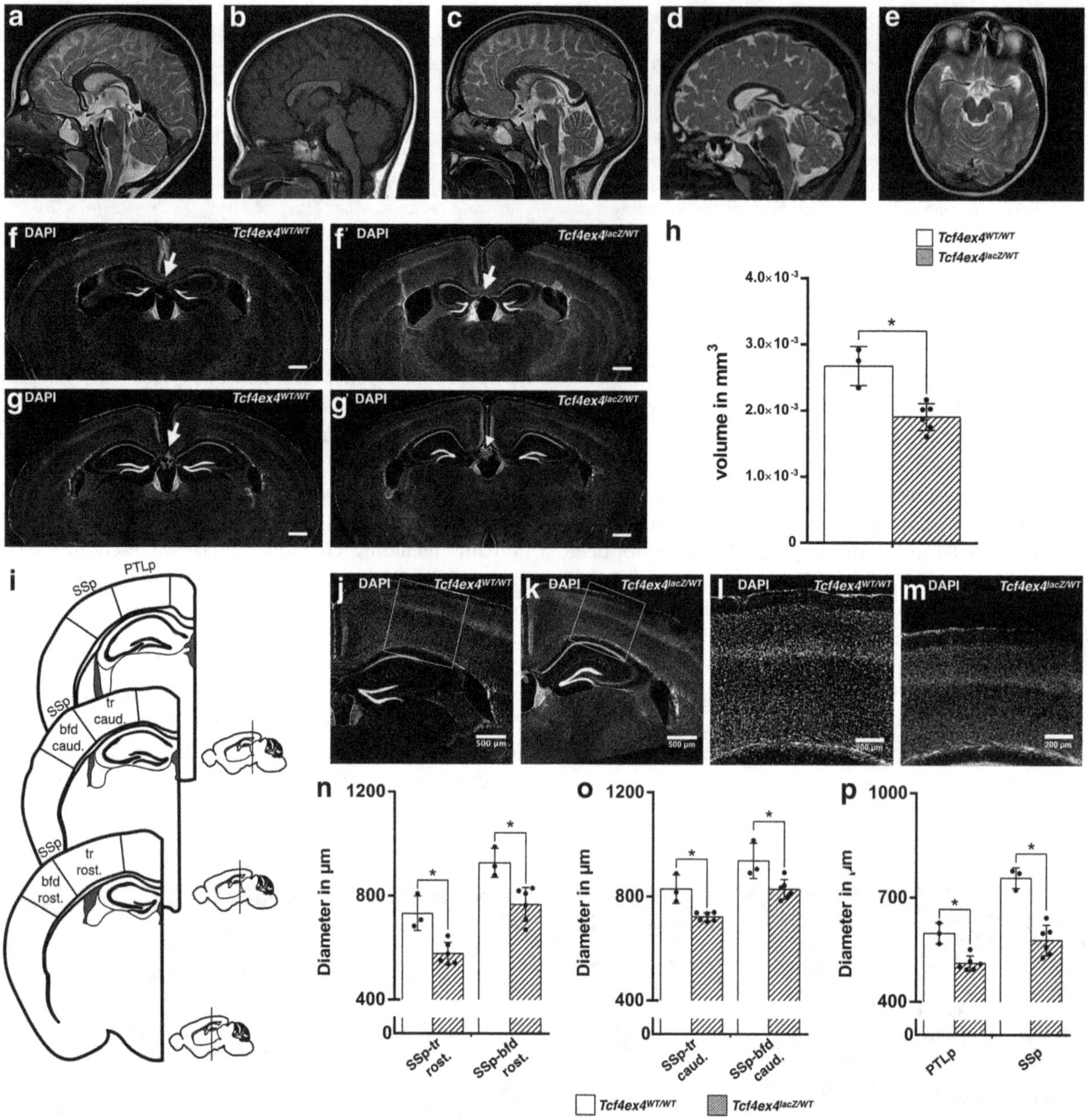

Fig. 8 PTHS-associated brain anomalies in TCF4-haploinsufficient mice. Hypoplastic corpus callosum in *Tcf4*-haploinsufficient PTHS patients at the age of 3 years (**B**) and 7 years (**D**). **A**, **C** Age-matched references. **E** Small hippocampus in PTHS patient at the age of 7 years. *Tcf4*-haploinsufficient mice (**F'**, **G'**) show agenesis of the corpus callosum and reduced hippocampal volume (**H**) compared to WT mice (**F**, **G**). Cortical diameter was determined along the rostro-caudal axis (**I**). Representative images of the cortical thickness of *Tcf4ex4*$^{WT/WT}$ mice (**J**, **L**) and *Tcf4ex4*$^{lacZ/WT}$ mice (**K**, **M**). Cortical diameter of *Tcf4ex4*$^{lacZ/WT}$ mice was significantly decreased compared to *Tcf4ex4*$^{WT/WT}$ mice in all analyzed cortical regions. The results are displayed as mean in microns ± SD. **N**–**P** Scale bars 500 μm. The DG area was measured in six representative slices spanning a distance of 240 μm. Abbreviations: PTLp, posterior parietal association area; SSp-bfd, primary somatosensory area-barrel field; SSp-tr, primary somatosensory area-trunk; Rost, rostral; Caud, caudal

number of cortical and subcortical structures during adulthood, raising the possibility that TCF4 function in mature neurons is critical for plasticity in many neural circuits.

TCF4 haploinsufficiency causes PTHS, while SNPs in regulatory regions, which may cause increased TCF4 expression [36], are associated with an elevated risk for schizophrenia. Moreover, behavioral deficits have been reported not only for *Tcf4*-haploinsufficient mice but also for transgenic mice with mild TCF4 over-expression [37, 38]. These observations have led to the suggestion that TCF4 levels have to be kept in a tight range to allow for neuronal development and function. Intriguingly, we observed cell type- and region-dependent differences in

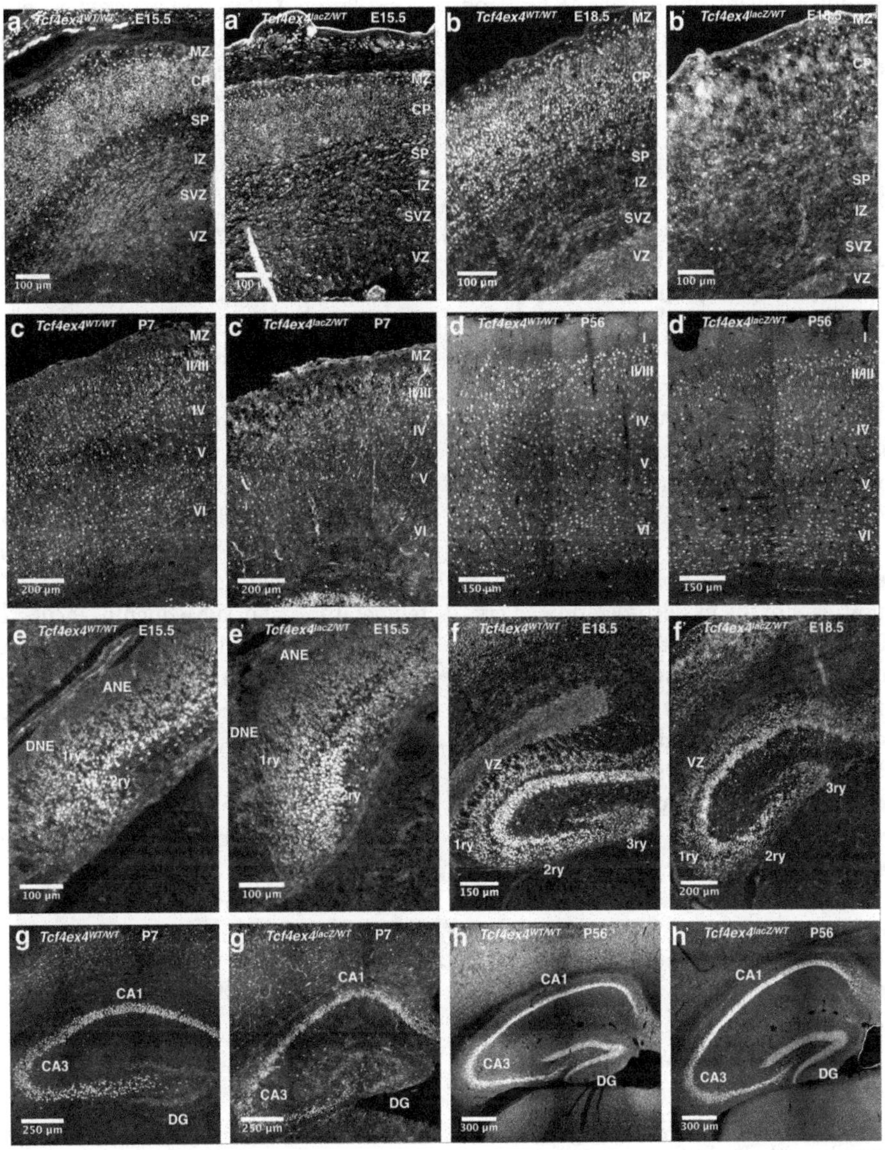

Fig. 9 Comparison of TCF4 protein expression at different stages of cortical and hippocampal development between *Tcf4ex4*$^{WT/WT}$ and *Tcf4ex4*$^{lacZ/WT}$ mice. **A**–**D′** Immunostaining using the anti-TCF4 antibody on brain tissue of *Tcf4ex4*$^{WT/WT}$ and *Tcf4ex*$^{lacZ/WT}$ animals during cortical development and in the adult. **E**–**H′** Immunostaining using the anti-TCF4 antibody on brain tissue of *Tcf4ex4*$^{WT/WT}$ and *Tcf4ex4*$^{lacZ/WT}$ animals during hippocampus formation and in the adult. Abbreviations: ANE, ammonic neuroepithelium; CP, cortical plate; DG, dentate gyrus; DNE, dentate neuroepithelium; IZ, intermediate zone; MZ, marginal zone; PP, preplate; SP, subplate; SVZ, subventricular zone; VZ, ventricular zone; 1ry, primary matrix; 2ry, secondary matrix; 3ry, tertiary matrix

TCF4 expression, raising the questions whether distinct cell populations may require different TCF4 dosages and whether there is cell type-/region-specific vulnerability to pathologically altered TCF4 expression levels.

Conclusion

A recent study reported similarities in the expression of *TCF4* mRNA in the developing prefrontal cortex of rats and humans [39]. Here, we show that the expression pattern of *TCF4* between mice and humans is highly similar across the developing and adult brain and provide evidence that *Tcf4* haploinsufficiency in mice reproduces structural anomalies that are observed in PTHS. These observations strongly suggest that the regulation and function of TCF4 is conserved between species and further validate *Tcf4*-haploinsufficient mice as a preclinical model for PTHS.

Our preliminary analysis indicated an irregular distribution of TCF4-expressing cells in the cortex and hippocampus of *Tcf4*-haploinsufficient mice strengthening the notion that TCF4 plays a role in migration and positioning of neurons [40]. A more detailed analysis of *Tcf4*-haploinsufficient mice will allow to decipher the pathophysiological mechanisms underlying PTHS on the molecular, cellular, and neural circuit level and to explore experimental strategies to ameliorate cognitive and behavioral deficits in this disorder [35, 41, 42].

Methods

Animal husbandry

All animal experiments were carried out in accordance with the European Communities Council Directive (86/609/EEC) and approved by the government of Middle-Franconia, Germany. C57Bl/6NRj mice were obtained from Janvier Labs (Le Genest-Saint-Isle, France) and group-housed under a 12 h light/dark cycle with ad libitum access to food and water. Tcf4ex4WT/lacZ mice were obtained from the Wellcome Trust Sanger Institute (Alleles produced for the EUCOMM and EUCOMMTools projects by the Wellcome Trust Sanger Institute; MGI ID: 4432303). For generation of the knockout allele, the L1L2_gt1 cassette was inserted at position 69461371 of Chromosome 18 upstream of the in silico-determined critical exon four. The L1L2_gt1 cassette harbors an FRT flanked lacZ/neomycin sequence followed by a loxP site resulting in a "knockout first" allele. An additional loxP site is inserted downstream of the targeted exon four at position 69462143 [39]. For embryonic studies, mice were bred in the afternoon and vaginal post-coitum protein plug check ("Plug check") was performed the next morning. This time point was defined as E0.5.

Tissue preparation and dissection

Timed pregnant mice were killed by cervical dislocation. E11.5 and E13.5 embryos were fixed overnight in 4% PFA. For the E15.5 time point, heads were fixed overnight in 4% PFA. For the E18.5 and P0 time points, brains were dissected and fixed overnight in 4% PFA. Tails were used for genotyping. After fixation tissue was washed repeatedly with 1× PBS and transferred to 30% sucrose in PBS overnight for dehydration. Embryonic tissues were embedded in freezing media (Jung, Nussloch) and stored at − 80 °C. Adult mice were killed using CO_2 and transcardially perfused with PBS for 5 min (20 ml/min) followed by fixation with 4% paraformaldehyde (PFA) in PBS, pH 7.4, for 5 min. The brains were post-fixed overnight in 4% PFA at 4 °C followed by dehydration at 4 °C in 30% sucrose in TBS.

Histology

Embryonic tissue was cut in 10 μm thin sections with a cryotom (Leica Microsystems, Wetzlar). Sections were transferred on laminated object slides and dried for 2 h at room temperature and stored at − 80 °C until further use. Sections were washed three times for 5 min with 1xPBS, treated with 50 mM citrate buffer at 70 °C for 3 min for antigen retrieval. Tissue was permeabilized for 10 min in 0.1% Triton-X/PBS and blocked with blocking solution (10% FCS, 1% BSA in PBS) at room temperature for 2 h in a wet chamber. Sections were incubated with primary antibodies diluted in blocking solution at 4 °C overnight (Table 1). Slides were washed six times for 10 min with 1xPBS, incubated with secondary antibodies diluted in blocking solution for 2 h at room temperature, and washed six times with 1xPBS. Nuclei were stained with DAPI (1:10.000 in 1xPBS) for 2 min. After additional washing with 1xPBS for 10 min, slides were mounted with 50 μl Mowiol (Sigma-Aldrich) and stored at 4 °C.

Adult brains were coronally cut at 40 μm thickness using a sliding microtome. Immunofluorescent stainings were performed on free-floating slices. Slices were washed three times with TBS, blocked in TBS containing 0.25% Triton X-100 and 3% normal donkey serum (TBS ++), and incubated with primary antibodies in TBS++ for 72 h at 4 °C. Tissue was washed with TBS at room temperature, blocked with TBS++ for 30 min at room temperature, and subsequently incubated with the secondary antibodies diluted in TBS++ overnight at 4 °C or for 2 h at RT. After washing in PBS, nuclei were stained with DAPI and sections were mounted on coverslips with Aqua poly mount (Polysciences).

Validation of TCF4 antibody

The *TCF4* knockdown construct was generated cloning the *TCF4* forward and reverse oligonucleotides TCF4 forward: 5′-CCGGGCTGAGTGATTTACTGGATTTCTCGAGAAATCCAGTAAATCACTCAGCTTTTT-3′; and

Table 1 Primary antibodies

Antigen	Species	Company	Dilution	Catalog number
Calbindin D-28k	Mouse	Swant	1:300	300
		Doublecortin	Guinea pig	Millipore
1:1000	ab2253			
FLAG	Mouse	Sigma	1:1000	F1804
GFAP	Mouse	Sigma	1:500	G3893
GAPDH	Mouse	Santa Cruz Biotechnologies	1:1000	SC32233
Iba	Goat	Abcam	1:500	ab5076
NeuN	Mouse	–	1:20	–
Nestin	Mouse	Millipore	1:500	MAB353
NeuroD1	Goat	Santa Cruz Biotechnologies	1:500	sc-1084
Parvalbumin	Mouse	Swant	1:500	235
Sox2	Goat	Santa Cruz Biotechnologies	1:500	sc17320
Sox10	Guinea pig	–	1:500	–
TCF4	Rabbit	Abcam	1:500	ab130014

TCF4 reverse: 5′-CGAAAAAGCTGAGTGATTTACTG GATTTCTCGAGAAATCCAGTAAATCACTCAGC-3′.

CCGG into the PWXG1 expression vector (gift from X. Zhao, University of Wisconsin, Madison). The TCF4 expression construct was generated by cloning the human *TCF4* coding sequence fused with a tandem Strep II tag and a FLAG tag on the C-terminus into the CAG-IRES-GFP expression vector [43, 44]. The resulting CAG-TCF4-IRES-GFP was either transfected alone or together with the *TCF4* knockdown construct in HEK 293T cells (ATCC, Wesel, Germany; CRL-3216), and the proteins were extracted 2 days post-transfection. Protein extract obtained from HEK 293T cells transfected with a GFP control construct (CAG-GFP-IRES-GFP) served as a control. Cells were lysed in RIPA buffer (50 mM Tris pH 8, 150 mM NaCl, 1 mM EDTA, 1% NP-40, 0.1%SDS, 0.5% S-DOC,1x protease inhibitor cocktail-EDTAfree-Roche). The extracts were separated in a 10% SDS-PAGE gel. Gels underwent wet transfer onto a nitrocellulose membrane. Membranes were blocked in 5% *w*/*v* skim milk (Sigma Aldrich) in TBS with 0.1% Tween 20 (TBS-T). Incubation with primary antibodies diluted in blocking solution was performed overnight at 4 °C and was followed by washing with TBS-T. Secondary antibodies were diluted in blocking solutions and incubated with the membranes for at least 1 h at room temperature followed by washing with TBS-T. Membranes were treated with Clarity Western Enhanced Chemiluminescence (ECL) Substrate (Bio-Rad) and visualized with ChemiDoc XRS+ System (Bio-Rad). Images were processed using ImageLab 5.2.1 Setup (Bio-Rad).

Imaging

For embryonic sections, fluorescence signal was detected with an AF6000 Modular Systems Leica fluorescent microscope and documented with a SPOT-CCD camera and the Leica software LAS AF (Version 2.6.0.7266; Leica Microsystems, Wetzlar Germany). For comparison of expression levels, settings were kept constant. For expression and co-localization analysis in the adult murine brain, fluorescence signal was detected using a Zeiss LSM 780 confocal microscope with four lasers (405, 488, 550, and 633 nm) and × 20, × 40, × 63 objective lens. Images were processed using ImageJ.

Analysis of Tcf4 expression levels

For evaluation of expression levels in the murine brain, images were taken with fixed settings. Expression was categorized into four categories, i.e., high, moderate, low, and not detected, based on intensity of TCF4-immunoreactivity. For comparison of neurodevelopmental TCF4 expression between species, mRNA expression data from selected brain areas of non-human primates and humans were extracted from the NIH Blueprint Non-Human Primate (NHP) Atlas (http://www.blueprintnhpatlas.org) and the BrainSpan Atlas (BrainSpan: Atlas of the Developing Human Brain [Internet]. Funded by ARRA Awards 1RC2MH089921-01, 1RC2MH090047-01, and 1RC2MH0 89929-01. © 2011. Available from: http://www.brainspan.org/lcm/search?search_type=user_selections), respectively. The NIH Blueprint Non-Human Primate (NHP) Atlas provides microarray-based mRNA expression data of non-human primate neural development from E40–0 months. Microarray data of TCF4 expression in select brain regions was extracted and arranged by ascending age for documentation. The BrainSpan: Atlas of the Developing Human Brain provides microarray based mRNA expression data of human neural development from post conception week 15–21. Microarray data of TCF4 expression in select brain regions was extracted and arranged by ascending age for documentation. For comparison of TCF4 expression between human and mice during adulthood, TCF4 mRNA expression data in the adult human brain was extracted from the Allen Human Brain Atlas [23]. Heatmaps for mRNA expression were manually compared to the immunoreactivity score.

Cortical thickness measurements

The diameter of the cortex was determined in six areas of the cortex, corresponding to the anatomical divisions documented in the Allen Mouse Brain Atlas [45] Posterior parietal association area (PTLp), Somatosensory area (SSp), rostral and caudal primary somatosensory area-barrel field (SSp-bfd), rostral and caudal primary somatosensory area-trunk (SSp-tr). Measurements were performed using ImageJ (version 2.0.0). Because of the variability of the pial surface, we determined the cortical thickness, as the diameter between layer II/III and the white matter. Five measurements were taken per area in each animal ($n = 3$ for $TCF4ex4^{WT/WT}$; $n = 6$ for $TCF4ex4^{LacZ/WT}$) and averaged prior to statistical analysis. Statistical significance was determined using the Mann-Whitney *U* test,$^{*}p < 0.05$.

Volume measurement of the dentate gyrus

DG volumes were calculated after measuring the DG area of six consecutive 40-μm thick coronal mouse brain slices spanning a distance of 240 μm from the rostral to caudal hippocampus. Measurements were performed using ImageJ (version 2.0.0) [46], $n = 3$ for $\text{TCF4ex4}^{WT/WT}$; $n = 6$ for $\text{TCF4ex4}^{LacZ/WT}$. Statistical significance was determined using the Mann-Whitney *U* test,$^{*}p < 0.05$.

Patients

cMRIs were obtained from two female individuals with confirmed PTHS. Individual 1 is a 5-year-old girl carrying the de novo mutation c.1880-11A>G in *TCF4* which was confirmed to lead to aberrant splicing and is therefore predicted to result in frameshifting and truncation of the protein (p.(Glu623Valfs*87)). The girl has severe ID with a walking age of 4 years 9 months and lack of speech. She has PTHS typical facial features, behavioral anomalies, sleeping difficulties, constipation, and myopia. Her head circumference is on the 10th centile, and no seizures or breathing anomalies occurred so far. Individual 2 is a 7.5-year-old girl carrying the splice site mutation c.655G>A, predicted to result in frameshifting and truncation of the protein (p.(Asp219Glyfs*37)). She could walk with 2 years 9 months and speaks single words and 2–3-word sentences. She has severe constipation, muscular hypotonia, recurrent infections, and typical facial features. Her head circumference in on the 10th centile, and no seizures or breathing anomalies occurred so far. The individuals had been recruited for a study to unravel the genetic causes for developmental disorders, which was approved by the ethics committee of the Medical Faculty of the Friedrich-Alexander-Universität Erlangen-Nürnberg. All participating families had given their informed consent.

Acknowledgements
This work was supported by grants from the German Research Foundation (LI 858/9-1 to D.C.L, INST 410/45-1 FUGG), the Bavarian Research Network "ForIPS" (D.C.L.), the BMBF Network "Cell Based Regenerative Medicine" (C.J.G. and D.C.L.), iMed—the Helmholtz Initiative on Personalized Medicine (C.J.G.), the University Hospital Erlangen (IZKF grants E12, E16, and E21 to D.C.L., E26 to C.Z.). B.M.H. and E.-A. B. are doctoral fellows of the IZKF (Interdisziplinäres Zentrum für Klinische Forschung) of the University Clinic Erlangen (Project IZKF E12 and E16). M.-T.W. is a graduate student of the research training group 2162 "Neurodevelopment and Vulnerability of the Central Nervous System" of the Deutsche Forschungsgemeinschaft (DFG GRK2162/1). C.Z. and D.C.L. are investigators of the research training group 2162 "Neurodevelopment and Vulnerability of the Central Nervous System" of the Deutsche Forschungsgemeinschaft (DFG GRK2162/1). M.J. is supported by a M.D. doctoral fellowship of the Interdisciplinary Center for Clinical Research (IZKF) Erlangen. This work was performed in (partial) fulfillment of the requirements for obtaining the degree "Dr. med.".

Authors' contributions
MJ carried out the immunohistochemical experiments, bioinformatic comparison, formal analysis and wrote the original draft of the manuscript. BMH conceptualized the experiments, performed immunohistochemical stainings, performed formal-analysis, wrote and edited the final manuscript. TT performed immunohistochemical stainings on adult mouse brain and bioinformatical comparison. M-TW performed immunohistochemical experiments on embryonic mouse brains, E-AB performed Western Blot experiments and analysis. V-CS performed Western Blot experiments. CZ recruited and examined patients, and participated in manuscript editing. AD provided MRI image resources and helped with analysis. CJG provided resources and assisted in funding acquisition. DCL conceptualized and supervised the project, performed formal analysis, provided resources and funding, wrote and edited the final manuscript. All authors read and approved the final manuscript.

Competing interests
The authors declare that they have no competing interests.

Author details
[1]Institute of Biochemistry, Emil Fischer Center, Friedrich-Alexander-Universität Erlangen-Nürnberg, 91054 Erlangen, Germany. [2]Institute of Human Genetics, Friedrich-Alexander-Universität Erlangen-Nürnberg, Erlangen, Germany. [3]Department of Neuroradiology, University Clinic Erlangen, Friedrich-Alexander-Universität Erlangen-Nürnberg, 91054 Erlangen, Germany. [4]German Center for Neurodegenerative Diseases, 72076 Tübingen, Germany. [5]Institute for Ophthalmic Research, Center for Ophthalmology, University of Tübingen, 72076 Tübingen, Germany.

References
1. Massari ME, Murre C. Helix-Loop-Helix proteins: regulators of transcription in eucaryotic organisms. Mol Cell Biol. 2000;20:429–40.
2. Amiel J, Rio M, de Pontual L, Redon R, Malan V, Boddaert N, Plouin P, Carter NP, Lyonnet S, Munnich A, Colleaux L. Mutations in TCF4, encoding a class I basic helix-loop-helix transcription factor, are responsible for Pitt-Hopkins syndrome, a severe epileptic encephalopathy associated with autonomic dysfunction. Am J Hum Genet. 2007;80:988–93.
3. Zweier C, Peippo MM, Hoyer J, Sousa S, Bottani A, Clayton-Smith J, Reardon W, Saraiva J, Cabral A, Gohring I, et al. Haploinsufficiency of TCF4 causes syndromal mental retardation with intermittent hyperventilation (Pitt-Hopkins syndrome). Am J Hum Genet. 2007;80:994–1001.
4. Schizophrenia Psychiatric Genome-Wide Association Study C. Genome-wide association study identifies five new schizophrenia loci. Nat Genet. 2011;43:969–76.
5. Stefansson H, Ophoff RA, Steinberg S, Andreassen OA, Cichon S, Rujescu D, Werge T, Pietilainen OP, Mors O, Mortensen PB, et al. Common variants conferring risk of schizophrenia. Nature. 2009;460:744–7.
6. Steinberg S, de Jong S, Irish Schizophrenia Genomics C, Andreassen OA, Werge T, Borglum AD, Mors O, Mortensen PB, Gustafsson O, Costas J, et al. Common variants at VRK2 and TCF4 conferring risk of schizophrenia. Hum Mol Genet. 2011;20:4076–81.
7. Stenman J, Toresson H, Campbell K. Identification of two distinct progenitor populations in the lateral ganglionic eminence: implications for striatal and olfactory bulb neurogenesis. J Neurosci. 2003;23:167–74.
8. Batista-Brito R, Close J, Machold R, Fishell G. The distinct temporal origins of olfactory bulb interneuron subtypes. J Neurosci. 2008;28:3966–75.
9. Brandao JA, Romcy-Pereira RN. Interplay of environmental signals and progenitor diversity on fate specification of cortical GABAergic neurons. Front Cell Neurosci. 2015;9:149.
10. Marin O, Rubenstein JL. A long, remarkable journey: tangential migration in the telencephalon. Nat Rev Neurosci. 2001;2:780–90.
11. D'Hanis W, Linke R, Yilmazer-Hanke DM. Topography of thalamic and parabrachial calcitonin gene-related peptide (CGRP) immunoreactive neurons projecting to subnuclei of the amygdala and extended amygdala. J Comp Neurol. 2007;505:268–91.
12. Noctor SC, Flint AC, Weissman TA, Dammerman RS, Kriegstein AR. Neurons derived from radial glial cells establish radial units in neocortex. Nature. 2001;409:714–20.
13. Noctor SC, Martinez-Cerdeno V, Ivic L, Kriegstein AR. Cortical neurons arise in symmetric and asymmetric division zones and migrate through specific phases. Nat Neurosci. 2004;7:136–44.
14. Angevine JB Jr, Sidman RL. Autoradiographic study of cell migration during histogenesis of cerebral cortex in the mouse. Nature. 1961;192:766–8.
15. Berry M, Rogers AW. The migration of neuroblasts in the developing cerebral cortex. J Anat. 1965;99:691–709.
16. Altman J, Bayer SA. Migration and distribution of two populations of hippocampal granule cell precursors during the perinatal and postnatal periods. J Comp Neurol. 1990;301:365–81.
17. Nakahira E, Yuasa S. Neuronal generation, migration, and differentiation in the mouse hippocampal primoridium as revealed by enhanced green fluorescent protein gene transfer by means of in utero electroporation. J Comp Neurol. 2005;483:329–40.
18. Rickmann M, Amaral DG, Cowan WM. Organization of radial glial cells during the development of the rat dentate gyrus. J Comp Neurol. 1987;264:449–79.
19. Urban N, Guillemot F. Neurogenesis in the embryonic and adult brain: same regulators, different roles. Front Cell Neurosci. 2014;8:396.
20. Nicola Z, Fabel K, Kempermann G. Development of the adult neurogenic niche in the hippocampus of mice. Front Neuroanat. 2015;9:53.

21. Ming GL, Song H. Adult neurogenesis in the mammalian brain: significant answers and significant questions. Neuron. 2011;70:687–702.
22. Miller JA, Ding SL, Sunkin SM, Smith KA, Ng L, Szafer A, Ebbert A, Riley ZL, Royall JJ, Aiona K, et al. Transcriptional landscape of the prenatal human brain. Nature. 2014;508:199–206.
23. Hawrylycz MJ, Lein ES, Guillozet-Bongaarts AL, Shen EH, Ng L, Miller JA, van de Lagemaat LN, Smith KA, Ebbert A, Riley ZL, et al. An anatomically comprehensive atlas of the adult human brain transcriptome. Nature. 2012; 489:391–9. https://doi.org/10.1038/nature11405. Available from: http://human.brain-map.org/microarray/search/show?search_type=user_selections&user_selection_mode=1
24. Marangi G, Ricciardi S, Orteschi D, Lattante S, Murdolo M, Dallapiccola B, Biscione C, Lecce R, Chiurazzi P, Romano C, et al. The Pitt-Hopkins syndrome: report of 16 new patients and clinical diagnostic criteria. Am J Med Genet A. 2011;155A:1536–45.
25. de Pontual L, Mathieu Y, Golzio C, Rio M, Malan V, Boddaert N, Soufflet C, Picard C, Durandy A, Dobbie A, et al. Mutational, functional, and expression studies of the TCF4 gene in Pitt-Hopkins syndrome. Hum Mutat. 2009;30:669–76.
26. Whalen S, Heron D, Gaillon T, Moldovan O, Rossi M, Devillard F, Giuliano F, Soares G, Mathieu-Dramard M, Afenjar A, et al. Novel comprehensive diagnostic strategy in Pitt-Hopkins syndrome: clinical score and further delineation of the TCF4 mutational spectrum. Hum Mutat. 2012;33:64–72.
27. Chen T, Wu Q, Zhang Y, Lu T, Yue W, Zhang D. Tcf4 controls neuronal migration of the cerebral cortex through regulation of Bmp7. Front Mol Neurosci. 2016;9:94.
28. Schmidt-Edelkraut U, Daniel G, Hoffmann A, Spengler D. Zac1 regulates cell cycle arrest in neuronal progenitors via Tcf4. Mol Cell Biol. 2014;34:1020–30.
29. Fischer B, Azim K, Hurtado-Chong A, Ramelli S, Fernandez M, Raineteau O. E-proteins orchestrate the progression of neural stem cell differentiation in the postnatal forebrain. Neural Dev. 2014;9:23.
30. D'Rozario M, Zhang T, Waddell EA, Zhang Y, Sahin C, Sharoni M, Hu T, Nayal M, Kutty K, Liebl F, et al. Type I bHLH proteins daughterless and Tcf4 restrict neurite branching and synapse formation by repressing neurexin in postmitotic neurons. Cell Rep. 2016;15:386–97.
31. Roybon L, Hjalt T, Stott S, Guillemot F, Li JY, Brundin P. Neurogenin2 directs granule neuroblast production and amplification while NeuroD1 specifies neuronal fate during hippocampal neurogenesis. PLoS One. 2009;4:e4779.
32. Fode C, Ma Q, Casarosa S, Ang SL, Anderson DJ, Guillemot F. A role for neural determination genes in specifying the dorsoventral identity of telencephalic neurons. Genes Dev. 2000;14:67–80.
33. Schuurmans C, Armant O, Nieto M, Stenman JM, Britz O, Klenin N, Brown C, Langevin LM, Seibt J, Tang H, et al. Sequential phases of cortical specification involve Neurogenin-dependent and -independent pathways. EMBO J. 2004;23:2892–902.
34. Sepp M, Vihma H, Nurm K, Urb M, Page SC, Roots K, Hark A, Maher BJ, Pruunsild P, Timmusk T. The intellectual disability and schizophrenia associated transcription factor TCF4 is regulated by neuronal activity and protein kinase a. J Neurosci. 2017;37:10516–27.
35. Kennedy AJ, Rahn EJ, Paulukaitis BS, Savell KE, Kordasiewicz HB, Wang J, Lewis JW, Posey J, Strange SK, Guzman-Karlsson MC, et al. Tcf4 regulates synaptic plasticity, DNA methylation, and memory function. Cell Rep. 2016; 16:2666–85.
36. Cattane N, Minelli A, Milanesi E, Maj C, Bignotti S, Bortolomasi M, Bocchio Chiavetto L, Gennarelli M. Altered gene expression in schizophrenia: findings from transcriptional signatures in fibroblasts and blood. PLoS One. 2015;10:e0116686.
37. Brzozka MM, Rossner MJ. Deficits in trace fear memory in a mouse model of the schizophrenia risk gene TCF4. Behav Brain Res. 2013;237:348–56.
38. Brzozka MM, Radyushkin K, Wichert SP, Ehrenreich H, Rossner MJ. Cognitive and sensorimotor gating impairments in transgenic mice overexpressing the schizophrenia susceptibility gene Tcf4 in the brain. Biol Psychiatry. 2010;68:33–40.
39. Rannals MD, Hamersky GR, Page SC, Campbell MN, Briley A, Gallo RA, Phan BN, Hyde TM, Kleinman JE, Shin JH, et al. Psychiatric risk gene transcription factor 4 regulates intrinsic excitability of prefrontal neurons via repression of SCN10a and KCNQ1. Neuron. 2016;90:43–55.
40. Page SC, Hamersky GR, Gallo RA, Rannals MD, Calcaterra NE, Campbell MN, Mayfield B, Briley A, Phan BN, Jaffe AE, Maher BJ. The schizophrenia- and autism-associated gene, transcription factor 4 regulates the columnar distribution of layer 2/3 prefrontal pyramidal neurons in an activity-dependent manner. Mol Psychiatry. 2018;23:304–15.
41. Grubisic V, Kennedy AJ, Sweatt JD, Parpura V. Pitt-Hopkins mouse model has altered particular gastrointestinal transits in vivo. Autism Res. 2015;8:629–33.
42. Sweatt JD. Pitt-Hopkins syndrome: intellectual disability due to loss of TCF4-regulated gene transcription. Exp Mol Med. 2013;45:e21.
43. Jessberger S, Aigner S, Clemenson GD Jr, Toni N, Lie DC, Karalay O, Overall R, Kempermann G, Gage FH. Cdk5 regulates accurate maturation of newborn granule cells in the adult hippocampus. PLoS Biol. 2008;6:e272.
44. Gloeckner CJ, Boldt K, Schumacher A, Roepman R, Ueffing M. A novel tandem affinity purification strategy for the efficient isolation and characterisation of native protein complexes. Proteomics. 2007;7:4228–34.
45. Lein ES, Hawrylycz MJ, Ao N, Ayres M, Bensinger A, Bernard A, Boe AF, Boguski MS, Brockway KS, Byrnes EJ, et al. Genome-wide atlas of gene expression in the adult mouse brain. Nature. 2007;445:168–76.
46. Schindelin J, Arganda-Carreras I, Frise E, Kaynig V, Longair M, Pietzsch T, Preibisch S, Rueden C, Saalfeld S, Schmid B, et al. Fiji: an open-source platform for biological-image analysis. Nat Methods. 2012;9:676–82.

Plasma anandamide concentrations are lower in children with autism spectrum disorder

Debra S. Karhson[1*], Karolina M. Krasinska[2], Jamie Ahloy Dallaire[3], Robin A. Libove[1], Jennifer M. Phillips[1], Allis S. Chien[2], Joseph P. Garner[1,3], Antonio Y. Hardan[1] and Karen J. Parker[1]

Abstract

Background: Autism spectrum disorder (ASD) is a neurodevelopmental disorder characterized by restricted, stereotyped behaviors and impairments in social communication. Although the underlying biological mechanisms of ASD remain poorly understood, recent preclinical research has implicated the endogenous cannabinoid (or endocannabinoid), anandamide, as a significant neuromodulator in rodent models of ASD. Despite this promising preclinical evidence, no clinical studies to date have tested whether endocannabinoids are dysregulated in individuals with ASD. Here, we addressed this critical gap in knowledge by optimizing liquid chromatography-tandem mass spectrometry methodology to quantitatively analyze anandamide concentrations in banked blood samples collected from a cohort of children with and without ASD ($N = 112$).

Findings: Anandamide concentrations significantly differentiated ASD cases ($N = 59$) from controls ($N = 53$), such that children with lower anandamide concentrations were more likely to have ASD ($p = 0.041$). In keeping with this notion, anandamide concentrations were also significantly lower in ASD compared to control children ($p = 0.034$).

Conclusions: These findings are the first empirical human data to translate preclinical rodent findings to confirm a link between plasma anandamide concentrations in children with ASD. Although preliminary, these data suggest that impaired anandamide signaling may be involved in the pathophysiology of ASD.

Keywords: Anandamide, Autism spectrum disorder, Blood biomarker, Cannabinoid

Introduction

Autism spectrum disorder (ASD) is a neurodevelopmental disorder characterized by restricted, stereotyped behaviors and impairments in social communication [1]. ASD affects approximately 1% of US children [2], yet its underlying biological mechanisms are poorly understood. Identification of ASD biomarkers therefore is a public health priority, as this would enhance diagnostic accuracy and facilitate targeted therapeutic development. One biological system of increasing interest for ASD is the endogenous cannabinoid or endocannabinoid system [3, 4]. Endocannabinoids (eCBs) are a specialized class of lipid neuromodulators that regulate synaptic transmission, and play an important role in behavioral functions with relevance to ASD (i.e., cognitive function, emotional regulation, social functioning, motivation, and reward processing) [5].

Anandamide (AEA) is one of the most studied eCBs and has been implicated in several preclinical ASD models [6]. Specifically, mice with neurexin and neuroligin genetic mutations demonstrate disrupted tonic eCB signaling at the synapse. In humans, neuroligin gene mutations are associated with ASD risk, suggesting that eCB system dysregulation may also occur in ASD patients [7]. Moreover, four additional ASD rodent models which demonstrate ASD-related behavioral impairments (i.e., FMR1 knockout, BTBR strain, valproate acid exposed, and postnatal lipopolysaccharide administered) show improvements in social functioning and anxiety-like behavior following pharmacological AEA modulation [6, 8, 9]. These collective findings suggest that heterogeneity in

* Correspondence: dkarhson@stanford.edu
[1]Department of Psychiatry and Behavioral Sciences, Stanford University, 401 Quarry Rd., Stanford, CA 94305, USA

ASD pathophysiology may have a point of convergence within the eCB system. Yet, despite the promise of these preclinical data, no studies to date have investigated AEA concentrations in humans with ASD.

One reason for this gap in knowledge is that the majority of preclinical AEA studies have used brain tissue (in part, due to AEA's high stable abundance in this matrix). Opportunities to study human brain tissue are of course rare, yet alternative matrices which are more accessible (e.g., blood) present their own challenges. These include (1) selection and refinement of appropriate lipid extraction and purification methods for AEA and (2) the low circulating abundance of AEA in blood. The present study therefore was designed to address these barriers to scientific progress regarding the role of AEA in ASD. The aims of this project were twofold: (1) optimize lipid extraction and liquid chromatography-tandem mass spectrometry (LC-MS/MS) methodology to detect AEA (350 Da) concentrations in small volumes (~ 100 µl) of human blood and (2) quantify plasma AEA concentrations in children with ASD and neurotypical control children. We hypothesized that children with ASD would have lower plasma AEA concentrations compared to control children, in keeping with preclinical ASD findings.

Methods

Participants, recruitment, and eligibility criteria

Participants were $N = 116$ children ($N = 60$ children with ASD and $N = 56$ neurotypical control children), aged 3 to 12 years. Participants had been recruited as part of a previous study to investigate blood biomarkers and genetic variants in children with ASD [10]. Participants with ASD were primarily recruited through the Autism and Developmental Disorders Research Registry and by flyers posted in the Stanford University Autism and Developmental Disorders Clinic. Unrelated control participants were recruited through advertisements posted online or hardcopy in the surrounding community.

A comprehensive diagnostic evaluation was performed in children with ASD to confirm the accuracy of their existing diagnosis based on the *Diagnostic and Statistical Manual of Mental Disorders, Fourth Edition, Text Revision* (DSM-IV-TR) criteria [11]. This diagnosis was confirmed using research diagnostic methods (i.e., the Autism Diagnostic Instrument-Revised and the Autism Diagnostic Observation Schedule [12, 13]) by assessors trained by a research-reliable clinician. Study eligibility criteria were as follows. All participants were required to be (1) pre-pubertal, (2) in good medical health, (3) willing to provide a blood sample, and (4) capable of completing behavioral testing. Participants with ASD were included if they had a full-scale IQ of 50 and above. Control participants were included if they had an IQ score of 70 and above. Cognitive functioning was determined using the Stanford Binet 5th Edition [14]. ASD participant exclusion criteria included (1) a genetic, metabolic, or infectious etiology for ASD or (2) a DSM-IV-TR diagnosis of any severe mental disorder (e.g., schizophrenia, bipolar disorder). Participants using psychotropic medications were included if medications were stable for at least 1 week before blood collection. The most common medications in use by participants with ASD were stimulants ($n = 10$), selective serotonin reuptake inhibitors ($n = 8$), norepinephrine reuptake inhibitors ($n = 5$), and antipsychotics ($n = 5$). Controls were required to (1) be free of present or past neurological disorders; (2) be free of present or past psychiatric disorders on the basis of behavioral scales, a psychiatric evaluation, and, if needed, the Kiddie-Schedule for Affective Disorders and Schizophrenia for School-Aged Children [15]; (3) have no evidence of difficulty during gestation, labor, delivery, or immediate neonatal period, or abnormal neurological or developmental milestones; and (4) have no siblings with ASD.

Sample preparation and quantification

Blood collection was performed between 10 am and 2 pm to control for any potential circadian rhythmicity in plasma AEA concentrations [16, 17]. Whole blood samples were collected into EDTA-treated vacutainer tubes and promptly centrifuged (1300×g at 4 °C for 10 min). The plasma fraction was aliquoted into polypropylene tubes and stored at − 80 °C until the morning of quantitative analysis. Plasma samples underwent lipid extraction with a modified salt-assisted liquid-liquid extraction (SALLE) [18]. During method optimization, comparison of traditional toluene liquid-liquid extraction to SALLE demonstrated that although both methods provided similar extraction yields (toluene vs SALLE, 85–90% vs 90–95%, respectively), SALLE was more reproducible, provided greater precision with decreased matrix effects, and had more efficient recovery. Commercially available stable isotope-labeled AEA-d8 (Cayman Chemicals; Ann Arbor, MI) was used as an internal standard (IS) for LC-MS/MS in creation of a calibration curve for quantitation of the analyte of interest, endogenous AEA. Plasma samples (100 µl/participant) were thawed in an ice bath (in less than 30 min), de-proteinized with 200 µl of acetonitrile containing 10 ng/ml internal standard solution mix and 50 µl of 5 M ammonium formate. Sample mixtures were then vortexed for 1 min before being spun at 13,000 rpm at 4 °C for 5 min. Organic layers from each sample were collected and transferred to autosampler vials in preparation for LC-MS/MS. Each sample was measured in triplicate. The samples could not be run as one group and, thus, were run in three sets.

The LC-MS/MS system was a TSQ Vantage triple quadrupole mass spectrometer coupled with an Accela 1250 HPLC system (Thermo Fisher Scientific, San Jose,

CA). Baseline separation was achieved with gradient elution from an Acquity BEH C18 column (150 mm × 2.1 mm, 1.7 μm particle size) (Waters, Millford, MA). Calibration curve linearity was validated in spiked plasma from 0.25–10,000 pg/μl. The lower limit of AEA quantification was 50 fg on column. The total LC-MS/MS run was 8 min in duration, and samples were maintained at 4 °C throughout. Mobile phases were 0.1% formic acid (A) and acetonitrile containing 0.1% formic acid (B). Linear gradient conditions were as follows: 0–1 min, 50% B; 1–2 min ramp to 98% B; 2–4 min, 98% B; 4–5 min ramp back to 50% B; and 5–8 min equilibration at 50% B. The heated electrospray source was operated in positive ion mode. The triple quadrupole mass spectrometer was operated in selected reaction monitoring (SRM) mode for mass/charge transitions specific to AEA (*m/z*: 348.3 > 287.4, 203.4, 269.2, 91.0) and AEA-d8 (*m/z*: 356.25 > 294.3, 252.1, 206.1). Chromatograms were processed using Xcalibur software as well as visually inspected for inconsistencies.

Calibration curves and linearity

Intrinsic to the consideration of AEA quantification is the "endogenous level challenge," which relates to the difficulty encompassed by efforts to minimize contributions of sample matrix (e.g., plasma) effects through the use of a blank matrix for preparation of calibration standards in LC-MS/MS quantitation [19, 20]. It is known that for analytes of interest, such as AEA, that will be present at basal conditions, availability of a true blank matrix is rare. Thus, several strategies have been proposed to overcome this confound. The following strategy is a variation of the "authentic analyte in authentic matrix" approach and is related to the "standard addition" approach [19, 20]. For the calibration curve, peak area ratio of spiked unlabeled to labeled analyte (AEA/D8-AEA) was determined in buffer (i.e., phosphate-buffered saline, termed PBS) and extracted "blank pooled plasma" (i.e., from non-affected, healthy adult plasma) and used to construct a linear regression equation: $y = m\ (x) + b$, where y is equal to the peak area ratio of spiked analyte/internal standard, m is equal to the slope of the calibration curve, x is equal to the concentration of analyte, and b is equal to the y-intercept of the calibration. Calibration curves were fitted using different weighting schemes (unweighted, $1/x$, or $1/x^2$) and over different ranges of spiked AEA concentrations (minimum 0.1 pg/μl; maximum between 20 and 10,000 pg/μl prepared in plasma, equivalent to 0.5 pg to 50 ng on column). As experimental samples produced calculated AEA concentrations near the lower end of this range, the curve that generated the lowest average relative error at the lower end of the spiked concentration range was retained (range 0.2–20 pg/μl, weighted by $1/x^2$). Unknown sample AEA concentrations were corrected for the endogenous presence of the analyte in plasma, estimated as the negative X-intercept of the calibration curve. The lowest limit of quantification (LLOQ) in extracted plasma was defined as signal-to-noise ratio of 10 to 1 and was 50 fg for AEA. Additionally, the triplicate measures for each participant were highly consistent, with intra-class correlation (ICC) coefficients within each sample set between 90.2 and 94.8%. High ICC coefficients provide evidentiary support for the reliability of calculated AEA concentrations [21].

Statistical analysis

Study data were managed using REDCap [22] and analyzed using JMP V.13 (SAS Institute, Cary, NC, USA). Four participants were excluded from analyses because their samples either produced highly inconsistent concentrations between replicates ($N = 1$F with ASD) or extremely elevated AEA outlier concentrations were detected (i.e., three standard deviations above mean; $N = 3$ controls: 2M, 1F). A logistic regression was performed to test whether mean AEA concentrations predicted group membership (i.e., ASD vs. control), using a generalized linear model with a binomial error distribution and logit link function. All models included the following blocking factors: age, full-scale IQ, ethnicity, gender, sample set, and sample order within set (as described below).

Results

Characteristics of participants included in the statistical analyses are provided in Table 1. Full-scale IQ and age differed between children with and without ASD. To eliminate the possibility that these (or any other variables) could exert confounding effects and generate false positive or false negative results [23, 24], we adopted the standard epidemiological approach to this problem and included these variables in the statistical models as blocking factors. Additionally, secondary analyses were performed to determine whether blocking factors were related to plasma AEA concentrations. Plasma AEA concentrations were not predicted by age ($F_{1,107} = 1.54$, $p = 0.218$) or sex ($F_{1,107} = 1.36$, $p = 0.246$) alone. We also verified that blood AEA concentrations were not significantly related to blood collection time ($F_{1,98} = 0.5595$; $p = 0.4563$), including when analysis was performed using a quadratic term ($F_{1,98} = 0.0417$ $p = 0.386$).

Plasma AEA concentrations significantly differentiated cases and controls (likelihood ratio chi-square, $\chi^2 = 4.16$, $p = 0.041$; Fig. 1a). Across the range of observed plasma AEA concentrations, the likelihood of ASD decreased over 20-fold, corresponding to nearly a fourfold decrease in risk with each twofold increase in plasma AEA concentration (range odds ratio = 0.043; unit odds ratio = 0.257; regression coefficient ± SE = − 1.359 ± 0.698). We next tested whether children with and without ASD

Table 1 Participant characteristics

Demographics	Control children	Children with ASD
N	53	59
Female	20	14
Male	33	45
Age	7.13 ± 2.96	8.25 ± 2.67*
Full-scale IQ	115.49 ± 9.51	83.24 ± 28.37*
Full-scale IQ range	92–134	50–140
N cases with IQ < 70	0	17
N cases of psychotropic medication use	0	29
Ethnicity		
Asian	6	11
Caucasian	38	35
Other	9	13

Values in the table are reported as arithmetic means ± standard deviation. The χ^2 likelihood ratio was used to examine whether the distribution of individuals in the two groups differed by sex and by ethnicity; no significant effects were found (sex, $\chi^2(1) = 2.60$, $p = 0.107$; ethnicity, $\chi^2(2) = 2.03$, $p = 0.363$). Welch's unequal variances *t* test was used to test for differences in age and full-scale IQ between groups (* = $p < 0.05$). Significant group differences were observed for both measures (age, $t(105.4) = 2.09$, $p = 0.039$; IQ, $t(72.2) = 8.23$, $p < 0.0001$) and therefore were used as blocking variables in the analysis
Abbreviations: *ASD* autism spectrum disorder, *IQ* intelligence quotient

differed in AEA concentrations. As predicted, plasma AEA concentration was significantly lower in ASD compared to control children ($F_{1,102} = 4.64$, $p = 0.034$; Fig. 1b).

Most experimental samples had calculated AEA concentrations that were higher than the LLOQ, but lower than the endogenous concentration for the AEA-spiked plasma matrix used in calibration. Therefore, to provide secondary support of the calculated AEA concentrations in patient samples, all analyses were also performed using ranks of AEA concentrations (instead of mean log-transformed concentrations) to verify that the results were robust deviations from linearity. Analyses using AEA concentration rank instead of AEA concentrations themselves produced qualitatively identical results and support the reliability of quantified AEA concentrations.

Discussion

There is a growing body of preclinical data that suggests the eCB system may be involved in ASD pathophysiology. Specifically, AEA signaling has been shown to exert a modulatory role in rodent behaviors that are relevant to ASD symptomatology and to pharmacologically rescue the social deficits observed in ASD rodent models [25, 26]. The present study is the first to translate these preclinical data to patients, by optimizing a LC-MS/MS method to quantitatively analyze AEA concentrations in small volumes of banked plasma with short sample preparation time and high sample repeatability. Two significant findings were observed: (1) plasma AEA concentrations significantly differentiated ASD cases from controls, such that children with lower AEA concentrations were more likely to have ASD, and (2) AEA concentrations were significantly lower in ASD compared to control children (Fig. 1). These results, although preliminary, corroborate preclinical evidence that AEA signaling may be impaired in patients with ASD.

Detection of biomarkers in plasma is highly advantageous for brain disorders due to the relatively non-invasive procedures required to collect blood (compared with those required to access brain-relevant tissues). Circulating eCB concentrations are thought to be in equilibrium with brain-related eCB concentrations [27], suggesting that plasma eCB concentrations may be a viable proxy for the behavioral effects generated by bioactive, brain-related

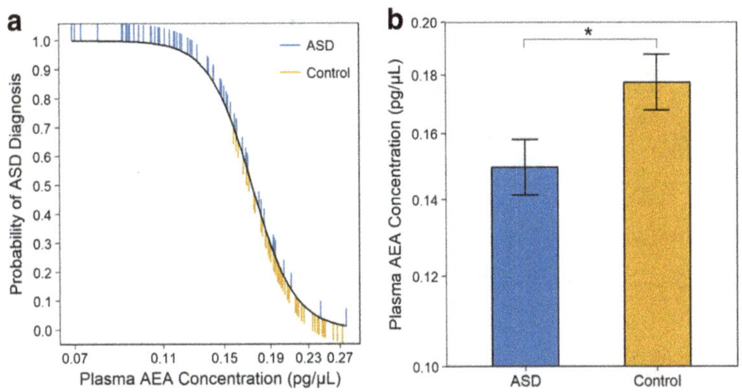

Fig. 1 Plasma AEA concentrations in children with ASD and neurotypical control children. **a** Plasma AEA concentration significantly differentiates cases from controls. Plasma AEA is plotted partialed (adjusted) for other variables in the statistical model. ASD individuals plotted above, and control individuals plotted below, the dashed lines are correctly classified. **b** Plasma AEA concentrations in children with and without ASD, back-transformed from logged values. Data are presented as LSM ± SEM. Children with ASD had lower plasma AEA concentrations (mean 0.149 pg/μl) compared to control children (mean 0.177 pg/μl)

AEA. Therefore, although plasma AEA concentrations do not perfectly classify idiopathic ASD and control participants, AEA signaling impairments nevertheless may characterize a specific subset of ASD patients or be useful for inclusion in a multidimensional biomarker panel employed to detect idiopathic ASD.

The present findings are preliminary and warrant subsequent replication in an independent study cohort. These findings must also be considered in the context of several limitations. First, our study was not powered to assess potential sex differences and relationships with between behavioral symptomology and AEA concentrations within the heterogeneous ASD population. Second, our ASD participants were taking a variety of prescription medications in contrast to the control participants, which were medication free (Table 2). Thus, it is possible that our findings were driven by medication status, particularly as inclusion criteria only required medication to be stable for 1 week prior to blood collection. We think this is unlikely in light of the aforementioned preclinical AEA data (in which "affected" mice were medication-free); nevertheless, future research is required to evaluate the impact of commonly prescribed ASD medications on plasma AEA concentrations and other eCBs. Finally, we measured a single eCB analyte using extrapolated AEA concentrations. Further optimization of the present LC-MS/MS methodology would allow for more precise AEA quantitation as well as concomitant study of additional eCBs, such as 2-arachidonoylglycerol (2-AG), which has also been implicated in preclinical ASD models with respect to pathophysiology and behavioral features. AEA concentrations have been studied in other brain disorders and have been reported to be lower in patients with temporal lobe epilepsy and post-traumatic stress disorder [28, 29]. Whether the lower plasma AEA concentrations observed in ASD patients in the present study are related to common, associated features (e.g., epilepsy, anxiety), or core symptoms, remains to be determined.

Table 2 Participant medications

Medication class	Medications prescribed	Percent use in ASD (*n*)
α2A agonist	Guanfacine, Tenex, Clonidine	6.78% (4)
Antipsychotic	Abilify, Risperdal, Seroquel	8.47% (5)
Benzodiazepine	Lorazepam	1.69% (1)
NEI	Atomoxetine	8.47% (5)
SSRI	Citalopram, Escitalopram, Paroxetine, Sertraline, Fluoxetine	13.56% (8)
Stimulant	Mehtylphenidate, Dexmethylphenidate, Amphetamine salts, Lisdexamfetamine	16.9% (10)

Approximately 55.9% of the participants with ASD analyzed were using psychotropic medications at the time of blood collection
Abbreviations: *α2A agonist*, alpha-2 adrenergic agonist, *NEI* norepinephrine reuptake inhibitor, *SSRI* selective serotonin reuptake inhibitory

Conclusion

In conclusion, this report extends preclinical findings to provide the first empirical evidence that plasma AEA concentrations are lower in individuals with ASD compared to neurotypical control individuals. Future research must now determine the relationship between plasma AEA concentrations and ASD symptom severity, particularly with regard to the core and associated features thought to be related to AEA signaling deficits in patients with ASD (i.e., phenotypic profiles with atypical cognitive and social functioning as measured by gold-standard assessments like the Autism Diagnosis Observational Schedule). In parallel, research is also needed to identify the mechanisms responsible for the lower AEA concentrations observed in ASD patients (e.g., is this reduction related to changes in AEA transporter proteins, synthesizing enzymes, catabolizing enzymes, and/or eCB receptor expression? [8, 25, 26, 30–32]). Should these follow-up studies implicate a convincing role for AEA in the pathophysiology of ASD, the eCB system may represent a promising target for therapeutic development in ASD.

Abbreviations

2-AG: 2-Arachidonoylglycerol; AEA: Anandamide; ASD: Autism spectrum disorder; DSM-IV-TR: Diagnostic and Statistical Manual of Mental Disorders, Fourth Edition, Text Revision; eCB: Endocannabinoid;
EDTA: Ethylenediaminetetraacetic acid; F: Female; FMR1: Fragile X Mental Retardation knockout mice; ICC: Intra-class correlation; IS: Internal standard; LC-MS/MS: Liquid chromatography with tandem mass spectrometry;
LLOQ: Lowest limit of quantification; M: Male; PBS: Phosphate-buffered saline; SALLE: Salt-assisted liquid-liquid extraction; SRM: Selected reaction monitoring

Acknowledgements

We gratefully acknowledge the contributions and participation of the children and their families without whom this research would not be possible.

Funding

This research was supported by the NIH (T32 MH019908; DSK), the Vincent Coates Foundation Mass Spectrometry Laboratory Seed Grant Program (DSK and KJP), the Simons Foundation/SFARI (#93231; KJP), the Teresa and Charles Michael Endowed Fund for Autism Research and Education (AYH), and the Mosbacher Family Fund for Autism Research (KJP).

Authors' contributions

DSK, KMK, ASC, AYH, JPG, and KJP designed the research study. DSK, AYH, and KJP secured funding for the research. RAL, JMP, and AYH recruited and/or performed the clinical phenotyping of participants. KJP oversaw the blood sample collection and provided the banked samples. DSK and KMK performed the biological quantification. KMK and ASC contributed the reagents and analytic tools. JAD and JPG optimized and performed the advanced statistical data analysis. All authors contributed to and approved the final manuscript.

Competing interests

The authors declare that they have no competing interests.

Author details

[1]Department of Psychiatry and Behavioral Sciences, Stanford University, 401 Quarry Rd., Stanford, CA 94305, USA. [2]Vincent Coates Foundation Mass Spectrometry Laboratory, Stanford University, 333 Campus Dr., Stanford, CA 94305, USA. [3]Department of Comparative Medicine, Stanford University, 287 Campus Dr., Stanford, CA 94305, USA.

References

1. Association AP. DSM 5. Washington: American Psychiatric Association; 2013.
2. Christensen DL, Baio J, Braun KVN, Bilder D, Charles J, Constantino JN, et al. Prevalence and characteristics of autism spectrum disorder among children aged 8 years—autism and developmental disabilities monitoring network, 11 sites, United States, 2012. MMWR Surveill Summ [Internet]. 2016 [cited 2016 Oct 21];65:1–23. Available from: http://www.cdc.gov/mmwr/volumes/65/ss/ss6503a1.htm.
3. Chakrabarti B, Persico A, Battista N, Maccarrone M. Endocannabinoid signaling in autism. Neurotherapeutics. 2015;12(4):837–47.
4. Karhson DS, Hardan AY, Parker KJ. Endocannabinoid signaling in social functioning: an RDoC perspective. Transl Psychiatry [Internet]. 2016 [cited 2016 Oct 4];6:e905. Available from: http://www.nature.com/tp/journal/v6/n9/full/tp2016169a.html.
5. Mechoulam R, Parker LA. The endocannabinoid system and the brain. Annu Rev Psychol [Internet]. 2013 [cited 2015 Jul 13];64:21–47. Available from: https://doi.org/10.1146/annurev-psych-113011-143739.
6. Zamberletti E, Gabaglio M, Parolaro D. The endocannabinoid system and autism spectrum disorders: insights from animal models. Int J Mol Sci [Internet]. 2017 [cited 2017 Sep 12];18:1916. Available from: http://www.mdpi.com/1422-0067/18/9/1916.
7. Földy C, Malenka RC, Südhof TC. Autism-associated neuroligin-3 mutations commonly disrupt tonic endocannabinoid signaling. Neuron. 2013;78:498–509.
8. Kerr DM, Gilmartin A, Roche M. Pharmacological inhibition of fatty acid amide hydrolase attenuates social behavioural deficits in male rats prenatally exposed to valproic acid. Pharmacol Res. 2016;113:228–35.
9. Kerr DM, Downey L, Conboy M, Finn DP, Roche M. Alterations in the endocannabinoid system in the rat valproic acid model of autism. Behav Brain Res. 2013;249:124–32.
10. Parker KJ, Garner JP, Libove RA, Hyde SA, Hornbeak KB, Carson DS, et al. Plasma oxytocin concentrations and OXTR polymorphisms predict social impairments in children with and without autism spectrum disorder. Proc Natl Acad Sci [Internet]. 2014 [cited 2015 Feb 12];111:12258–63. Available from: http://www.pnas.org/cgi/doi/10.1073/pnas.1402236111.
11. Bell CC. DSM-IV: diagnostic and statistical manual of mental disorders. JAMA [Internet]. 1994 [cited 2017 Oct 31];272:828–9. Available from: https://jamanetwork.com/journals/jama/fullarticle/379036.
12. Lord C, Rutter M, Le Couteur A. Autism diagnostic interview-revised: a revised version of a diagnostic interview for caregivers of individuals with possible pervasive developmental disorders. J Autism Dev Disord [Internet]. 1994 [cited 2010 Oct 12];24:659–85. Available from: http://www.ncbi.nlm.nih.gov/pubmed/7814313.
13. Lord C, Risi S, Lambrecht L, Cook EH, Leventhal BL, DiLavore PC, et al. The autism diagnostic observation schedule-generic: a standard measure of social and communication deficits associated with the spectrum of autism. J Autism Dev Disord. 2000;30:205–23.
14. Roid GH. Stanford-Binet intelligence scales. Itasca: Riverside Publishing Itasca, IL; 2003.
15. Ambrosini PJ. Historical development and present status of the schedule for affective disorders and schizophrenia for school-age children (K-SADS). J Am Acad Child Adolesc Psychiatry. 2000;39:49–58.
16. Vaughn LK, Denning G, Stuhr KL, de Wit H, Hill MN, Hillard CJ. Endocannabinoid signalling: has it got rhythm? Br J Pharmacol [Internet]. 2010 [cited 2018 Jan 31];160:530–43. Available from: https://www.ncbi.nlm.nih.gov/pmc/articles/PMC2931554/.
17. Hillard CJ. Circulating endocannabinoids: from whence do they come and where are they going? Neuropsychopharmacology [Internet]. 2018 [cited 2018 Jan 31];43:155. Available from: https://www.nature.com/articles/npp2017130.
18. Xiong X, Zhang L, Cheng L, Mao W. High-throughput salting-out assisted liquid-liquid extraction with acetonitrile for the determination of anandamide in plasma of hemodialysis patients with liquid chromatography tandem mass spectrometry. Biomed Chromatogr BMC. 2015;29:1317–24.
19. Jian W, Edom R, Weng N, Zannikos P, Zhang Z, Wang H. Validation and application of an LC-MS/MS method for quantitation of three fatty acid ethanolamides as biomarkers for fatty acid hydrolase inhibition in human plasma. J Chromatogr B Analyt Technol Biomed Life Sci. 2010;878:1687–99.
20. Liu G. Overcome the endogenous levels in biomarker quantitation using LC–MS. In: Weng N, Jian W, editors. Target biomark quant LC–MS [Internet]. John Wiley & Sons, Inc.; 2017 [cited 2017 Oct 8]. p. 107–17. Available from: http://dx.doi.org/10.1002/9781119413073.ch7.
21. McGraw KO, Wong SP. Forming inferences about some intraclass correlation coefficients. Psychol Methods. 1996;1:30–46.
22. Harris PA, Taylor R, Thielke R, Payne J, Gonzalez N, Conde JG. Research electronic data capture (REDCap)—a metadata-driven methodology and workflow process for providing translational research informatics support. J Biomed Inform. 2009;42:377–81.
23. Woodward M. Epidemiology: study design and data analysis: CRC Press; 1999.
24. Grafen A, Hails R. Modern statistics for the life sciences. Oxford: Oxford University Press; 2002.
25. Servadio M, Melancia F, Manduca A, di Masi A, Schiavi S, Cartocci V, et al. Targeting anandamide metabolism rescues core and associated autistic-like symptoms in rats prenatally exposed to valproic acid. Transl Psychiatry. 2016;6:e902.
26. Wei D, Dinh D, Lee D, Li D, Anguren A, Moreno-Sanz G, et al. Enhancement of anandamide-mediated endocannabinoid signaling corrects autism-related social impairment. Cannabis Cannabinoid Res [Internet]. 2016 [cited 2016 Mar 18];1:81–89. Available from: http://online.liebertpub.com/doi/abs/10.1089/can.2015.0008.
27. Lerner R, Post J, Loch S, Lutz B, Bindila L. Targeting brain and peripheral plasticity of the lipidome in acute kainic acid-induced epileptic seizures in mice via quantitative mass spectrometry. Biochim Biophys Acta. 1862;2017:255–67.
28. Romigi A, Bari M, Placidi F, Marciani MG, Malaponti M, Torelli F, et al. Cerebrospinal fluid levels of the endocannabinoid anandamide are reduced in patients with untreated newly diagnosed temporal lobe epilepsy. Epilepsia. 2010;51:768–72.
29. Neumeister A, Normandin MD, Pietrzak RH, Piomelli D, Zheng MQ, Gujarro-Anton A, et al. Elevated brain cannabinoid CB1 receptor availability in post-traumatic stress disorder: a positron emission tomography study. Mol Psychiatry. 2013;18:1034–40.
30. Siniscalco D, Sapone A, Giordano C, Cirillo A, de Magistris L, Rossi F, et al. Cannabinoid receptor type 2, but not type 1, is up-regulated in peripheral blood mononuclear cells of children affected by autistic disorders. J Autism Dev Disord. 2013;43:2686–95.
31. Trezza V, Vanderschuren LJMJ. Divergent effects of anandamide transporter inhibitors with different target selectivity on social play behavior in adolescent rats. J Pharmacol Exp Ther [Internet]. 2009 [cited 2015 Dec 15];328:343–50. Available from: http://www.ncbi.nlm.nih.gov/pmc/articles/PMC2605777/.
32. Fegley D, Kathuria S, Mercier R, Li C, Goutopoulos A, Makriyannis A, et al. Anandamide transport is independent of fatty-acid amide hydrolase activity and is blocked by the hydrolysis-resistant inhibitor AM1172. Proc Natl Acad Sci U S A [Internet]. 2004 [cited 2016 Jul 11];101:8756–61. Available from: http://www.pnas.org/content/101/23/8756.

11

Case-control meta-analysis of blood DNA methylation and autism spectrum disorder

Shan V. Andrews[1,2], Brooke Sheppard[1,2], Gayle C. Windham[3], Laura A. Schieve[4], Diana E. Schendel[5,6,7], Lisa A. Croen[8], Pankaj Chopra[9], Reid S. Alisch[10], Craig J. Newschaffer[11,12], Stephen T. Warren[9,13,14], Andrew P. Feinberg[15,16], M. Daniele Fallin[2,15,17*†] and Christine Ladd-Acosta[1,2*†]

Abstract

Background: Several reports have suggested a role for epigenetic mechanisms in ASD etiology. Epigenome-wide association studies (EWAS) in autism spectrum disorder (ASD) may shed light on particular biological mechanisms. However, studies of ASD cases versus controls have been limited by post-mortem timing and severely small sample sizes. Reports from in-life sampling of blood or saliva have also been very limited in sample size and/or genomic coverage. We present the largest case-control EWAS for ASD to date, combining data from population-based case-control and case-sibling pair studies.

Methods: DNA from 968 blood samples from children in the Study to Explore Early Development (SEED 1) was used to generate epigenome-wide array DNA methylation (DNAm) data at 485,512 CpG sites for 453 cases and 515 controls, using the Illumina 450K Beadchip. The Simons Simplex Collection (SSC) provided 450K array DNAm data on an additional 343 cases and their unaffected siblings. We performed EWAS meta-analysis across results from the two data sets, with adjustment for sex and surrogate variables that reflect major sources of biological variation and technical confounding such as cell type, batch, and ancestry. We compared top EWAS results to those from a previous brain-based analysis. We also tested for enrichment of ASD EWAS CpGs for being targets of meQTL associations using available SNP genotype data in the SEED sample.

Findings: In this meta-analysis of blood-based DNA from 796 cases and 858 controls, no single CpG met a Bonferroni discovery threshold of $p < 1.12 \times 10^{-7}$. Seven CpGs showed differences at $p < 1 \times 10^{-5}$ and 48 at 1×10^{-4}. Of the top 7, 5 showed brain-based ASD associations as well, often with larger effect sizes, and the top 48 overall showed modest concordance ($r = 0.31$) in direction of effect with cerebellum samples. Finally, we observed suggestive evidence for enrichment of CpG sites controlled by SNPs (meQTL targets) among the EWAS CpG hits, which was consistent across EWAS and meQTL discovery p value thresholds.

(Continued on next page)

* Correspondence: dfallin@jhu.edu; claddac1@jhu.edu
†M. Daniele Fallin and Christine Ladd-Acosta contributed equally to this work.
[2]Wendy Klag Center for Autism and Developmental Disabilities, Johns Hopkins Bloomberg School of Public Health, 615 N. Wolfe Street, W6509, Baltimore, MD 21205, USA
[1]Department of Epidemiology, Johns Hopkins Bloomberg School of Public Health, 615 N. Wolfe Street, Baltimore, MD 21205, USA
Full list of author information is available at the end of the article

(Continued from previous page)
Conclusions: No single CpG site showed a large enough DNAm difference between cases and controls to achieve epigenome-wide significance in this sample size. However, our results suggest the potential to observe disease associations from blood-based samples. Among the seven sites achieving suggestive statistical significance, we observed consistent, and stronger, effects at the same sites among brain samples. Discovery-oriented EWAS for ASD using blood samples will likely need even larger samples and unified genetic data to further understand DNAm differences in ASD.

Keywords: DNA methylation, Epigenome, Autism spectrum disorders, Peripheral blood, Study to Explore Early Development, Simons Simplex Collection

Findings

The etiology of autism spectrum disorder (ASD) may involve epigenetic mechanisms. Indirect evidence supporting this hypothesis comes from the observation that children with Rett, Fragile X, and Angelman syndromes often show impaired communication and exhibit repetitive behaviors [1–3], two core domains affected in autism. All three of these syndromes are caused by epigenetic defects [4–9]. Additional evidence stems from genetic studies of rare variation in non-syndromic forms of ASD. Although these studies have primarily identified private variants associated with ASD, there is now strong evidence that the ASD-associated variants converge upon three biological pathways, one of which is chromatin remodeling [10–12]. Finally, there is direct evidence from case-control postmortem brain studies supporting epigenetic involvement in ASD. Several candidate gene-based studies have shown altered epigenetic states associated with autism [13–18]. Genome-scale screens have identified changes in DNA methylation (DNAm) at specific CpG sites [19, 20] as well as global changes in non-CpG methylation levels [21] in postmortem cerebral tissue from individuals with ASD relative to controls. Studies of cerebral cortex tissue has revealed genomic spreading of histone H3 lysine 4 methylation and histone H3 lysine 27 acetylation marks, away from the promoter region, among a subset of individuals with ASD compared to controls [22, 23].

Examination of the affected tissue, i.e., the brain, can provide important insights into potential mechanisms of disease etiology; however, there are considerable limitations with these types of studies. They suffer from severely small sample sizes, have historically had low genomic coverage, and often lack comprehensive unified clinical, demographic, and genomic data. Importantly, they are based on autopsy-derived tissue and do not reflect epigenetic marks in a living individual, are not at optimal developmental timing, and may be influenced by life experiences and cause of death. To overcome these barriers, complementary, large population-based autism epigenetic studies using accessible tissues, such as blood, from living individuals are needed. DNAm from peripheral tissues is useful to analyze for its potential to mimic DNAm signatures from the brain. But outside of brain concordance, it can also be useful for its ability reflect consequences of ASD, provided that sample collection is performed following ASD onset. Moreover, peripheral tissue DNAm signatures related to ASD may result from environmental exposures that simultaneously contribute to ASD. To date, three genome-scale epigenetic studies of autism in accessible peripheral tissues have been performed. One study of peripheral blood from 50 monozygotic twin pairs, including 6 pairs discordant for ASD at age 15, examined DNAm at over 27,000 CpG sites in promoter regions. The authors found suggestive evidence for epigenetic alterations associated with ASD and associated traits within families [24]. Similarly, an investigation of DNAm at CpG island regions in lymphoblastoid cell lines, obtained from 7 twin pairs including 3 discordant for ASD, found ASD-related DNAm changes at the *RORA* gene [25]. Both of these studies were limited by the small number of samples examined, lack of genome-scale coverage, and specific focus on twin pairs with a lack of extension to the general population. Ectoderm cell lineage-derived buccal cells, obtained from 47 ASD cases and 48 controls born to mothers aged 35 and older, have also shown suggestive epigenetic alterations associated with ASD [26]. While suggestive, it is unclear how these buccal-based epigenetic findings relate to a population sample and in a larger number of individuals. Thus, more research in accessible tissues from larger population-based, non-familial, samples is needed.

Here, we overcome previous limitations and perform the largest epigenome-scale examination of DNAm, to date, among two large US case-control studies of autism: the Study to Explore Early Development, phase I (SEED I) and the Simons Simplex Collection (SSC). Both measured DNAm at over 450,000 loci in childhood blood samples from either population-based cases and controls (SEED I) or discordant sibling pairs (SSC). Meta-analysis across both sets included 796 ASD cases and 858 controls. In addition to CpG-specific differential DNAm, we explored the set of blood-derived differentially methylated sites for their concordance in post-mortem brain tissue and their enrichment for genetically controlled CpG sites.

Methods

Study to Explore Early Development (SEED)

The Study to Explore Early Development is a multi-site case-control study with population-based ascertainment. In SEED phase 1, a total of 3899 families were recruited across 6 study sites (California, Colorado, Georgia, Maryland, North Carolina, and Pennsylvania) and classified into 3 groups according to a child's diagnosis: an autism spectrum disorder (ASD) group, a general population control group (POP), and a (non-ASD) developmental delay group. Details regarding participant recruitment, biospecimen collection, and final outcome classification have been previously described [27, 28]. Briefly, eligible children were born in one of the catchment areas between September 1, 2003, and August 31, 2006, which corresponded to being aged 2–5 years at the time of SEED phase I enrollment, resided in the same catchment area at the time of initial contact, and were required to live with a knowledgeable caregiver who could communicate in English (or in English or Spanish in California or Colorado) [27]. Biospecimens were collected when the children were between the ages of 3 and 5 years. Children with possible ASD and DDs were ascertained through multiple sources providing services for children with developmental disorders including hospitals, individual providers, clinics, and education and intervention programs. Parents with a child with an ASD or DD diagnosis could also contact the study directly to enroll. General population controls were ascertained through random sampling of vital records in the catchment areas [27]. This provides a more diverse segment of the population than solely recruiting participants from autism clinics.

Primary caregivers completed the Social Communications Questionnaire (SCQ) [29], a screener for autism spectrum disorder, during the study invitation phone call. Children with an SCQ score below 11 and without a previous ASD diagnosis were asked to participate in a general developmental evaluation in the clinic using the Mullen Scale of Early Learning (MSEL) [30]. If the SCQ score was above 11, the child had previously received an ASD diagnosis, or a clinician suspected ASD during the clinic visit, the child additionally completed a full ASD evaluation that included the Autism Diagnostic Observation Schedule (ADOS) [31–33] and the Autism Diagnostic Interview Revised (ADI-R) [34, 35]. ASD was confirmed based on scores on the ADI-R and ADOS, as described in detail elsewhere [36]. Institutional review boards at each study site and at the Centers for Disease Control and Prevention (CDC) approved the SEED study. Informed consent was obtained from all enrolled participants. For this study, we measured methylation among a subset of SEED phase 1 individuals ($n = 980$) with genome-wide genotyping data, a complete caregiver interview, an ASD or POP classification, and a sufficient amount of DNA available for methylation measurements.

Simons Simplex Collection (SSC) A complete description of the SSC, which enrolled and collected biospecimens from children and adolescents aged 4–18 years, can be found elsewhere [37]. Briefly, a geneticist and a clinical psychologist were appointed as co-principal investigators at each site. Probands were evaluated with a battery of diagnostic measures, including the Autism Diagnostic Interview – Revised (ADI-R) [34] and the Autism Diagnostic Observation Schedule (ADOS) [31]. Other instruments provided additional measures of the core features of autism, as well as of intellectual ability (verbal and nonverbal), adaptive behavior, emotional and behavior problems, motor function, and language. A description of instruments employed can be found at https://sfari.org/ssc-instruments. A comprehensive family medical history was obtained that included the proband's prenatal and perinatal history, developmental milestones, immunizations, medications, dietary supplements, and common behavioral treatments. Emphasis was placed on common "comorbidities" including gastrointestinal complaints, sleep irregularities, and seizures. In addition, questions were asked about genetic, autoimmune, and psychiatric disorders in members of the extended family. Probands were excluded who were younger than 4 years of age or older than 18. Probands were also excluded for conditions that might compromise the validity of diagnostic instruments, such as nonverbal mental age below 18 months, severe neurological deficits, birth trauma, perinatal complications, or genetic evidence of fragile X or Down syndromes. A complete description of exclusion/inclusion criteria can be found at http://sfari.org. Measures of adaptive function, behavior-emotional problems, and symptoms of autism were examined in parents and siblings as well as probands.

Thus, the SSC represents a unique, well-described sample of able children and adolescents with relatively severe ASD, as indicated by ADI-R and ADOS Calibrated Severity Scores [38].

Reliability of data

To maximize the consistency of clinical observations across sites, each clinician was trained in administration of the ADOS and ADI-R to achieve research reliability as judged by expert clinicians. Most clinicians who had not previously received research training required 4–6 months of practice. Videotapes of interviews were exchanged to ensure that reliability requirements were met and maintained throughout the study. Error rates were very low, averaging less than 0.50 errors/1000 data points. Most errors could be corrected immediately, resulting in an unusually clean data set for a multisite study of this size. During each visit, a blood sample was collected from each study participant and DNA was extracted from blood cells, while plasma was stored for future use.

DNA methylation data quality control (QC) and processing

For the SEED samples, genomic DNA was isolated from 980 whole blood samples using the QIAsymphony midi kit (Qiagen). For each sample, 500 ng of DNA was bisulfite treated using the 96-well EZ DNA methylation kit (Zymo Research). Samples were randomized within and across plates, and across two main processing dates to minimize batch effects, and run on the Illumina HumanMethylation450 BeadChip. Background correction and dye-bias equalization was performed using the function *preprocessNoob()* [39, 40] in the *minfi* R package [41]. We included 12 cross-plate duplicates for quality control purposes; pairwise correlation metrics for the duplicate samples ranged from 0.990 to 0.997 with a mean correlation value equal to 0.995. Samples were removed if they had low overall intensity (median unmethylated or methylated signal < 11) or had a detection p value > 0.01 in more than 1% of probes ($N = 7$), or if reported sex did not match predicted sex generated via the *minfi* function *getSex()* ($N = 3$). Probes were removed if they had a detection p value > 0.01 in more than 10% of samples ($n = 702$) and then if they had been previously identified as being ambiguously mapped [42] ($n = 29{,}146$). Following QC, the analytic data included DNAm for 455,664 sites on 970 samples. We further removed two samples who were missing a final outcome classification, leaving a total of 453 cases and 515 controls used for association analyses.

For the SSC samples, 500 ng of human genomic DNA was sodium bisulfite-treated for cytosine to thymine conversion using the EZ DNA Methylation Gold kit (Zymo Research). A total of 728 samples (from 364 families) were randomized within and across plates to minimize batch effects and run on the Illumina HumanMethylation450 BeadChip. Additional details have been previously described [43]. Similar quality control procedures as used for the SEED samples were used for the SSC samples. After background correction and dye-bias equalization, samples were removed for low overall intensity (median unmethylated or methylated signal < 11) or for detection p value > 0.01 in more than 1% of probes ($N = 42$). Probes were removed if they had a detection p value > 0.01 in more than 10% of samples ($n = 483$) and then if they had been previously identified as being ambiguously mapped ($n = 29{,}213$). These steps resulted in an analytic data set with 455,816 sites on 686 samples, consisting of 343 proband-sibling pairs.

Finally, for all SEED and SSC samples, we estimated cell type proportions for six different cell types (granulocytes, monocytes, CD4 T cells, CD8 T cells, B cells, and natural killer cells) using the *estimateCellCounts()* function in the *minfi* R package. Estimation incorporated reference data from 60 samples generated from 6 healthy adult men [44].

Genotype data quality control and processing

Whole genome genotyping data was available for 943 of the 970 SEED 1 samples which passed DNAm quality control steps. After genotype measurement using the Illumina HumanOmni1-Quad BeadChip, standard quality control measures were applied, including removal of samples with < 95% SNP call rate, sex discrepancies, relatedness (Pi-hat > 0.2), or excess hetero- or homozygosity, and removal of markers with < 98.5% call rate, or that were monomorphic. Phasing was performed using SHAPEIT [45] followed by SNP imputation via the IMPUTE2 software [46], using 1000 Genomes Project samples as reference. Principal components to account for ancestry were determined via the EigenStrat program [47].

Epigenome-wide association testing and meta-analysis

For the SEED data, we used linear regression modeling of the M value (the ratio of methylated to total signal determined at every probe in every sample) [48] as a dependent variable and ASD status, sex, and surrogate variables (SVs) (described below) as independent variables. We implemented this model using the *lmFit()* function in the *limma* R package [49], separately for each of the DNAm probes that passed QC. For the SSC data, we implemented a generalized estimating equation (GEE) model using the *gee()* function in the *gee* R package [50] to account for the correlation inherent to the familial structure in the data. We used a fixed correlation structure of 0.5 for each sibling pair, and regressed M value onto ASD status, sex, and SVs.

To account for sources of technical and biological variability in our association analyses, we estimated surrogate variables (SVs) [51] in the cleaned SEED and SSC dataset to include as covariates in our downstream analyses. SVs have been shown to capture and adjust for differences related to batch effects and cell type proportions across samples in a wide variety of simulated settings [52], and to remove the effects of unwanted sources of technical and biological variation [51]. In order to explicitly address the strong confounding effect of sex resulting from the high degree of male bias in ASD diagnosis, we removed sex chromosomes, where DNAm values strongly correlate to sex, before SV estimation, and included sex along with ASD status in the model used for SV estimation. We then used a data-driven procedure individually in the SEED and SSC data to select the number of SVs to include in the association models.

First, to examine the relationship between each SV and known sources of technical and biological variation, we estimated the association between each estimated SV and cell type composition, principal components of genetic ancestry, and processing batch. We then generated a visual representation of the degree of association with these variables using a heat map (Additional file 1: Figures S1a, S2a).

We next examined the influence of iterative inclusion of SVs as adjustment variables in our association regression models. To do this, we first ran a case-control association model with adjustment for the strongest estimated SV [51], then progressively included the next strongest SV in the analysis and continued this procedure until all estimated SVs were included. For each model, we recorded the inflation factor, or lambda, calculated via the *estlambda()* function from the *GenABEL* R package [53], and visualized the relationship between number of SVs adjusted for and lambda values (Additional file 1: Figures S1b, S2b). We chose the number of SVs to include in the model by considering both the number of SVs at which the estimated lambda values began to plateau and where the known potential confounders appeared to be captured by one or more SVs. We chose to include 19 SVs in the SEED association analysis and 14 in the SSC analysis.

After completing each association analysis, we then performed a meta-analysis using the METAL software [54] on the 445,068 probes that were present in both the SEED and SSC cleaned datasets. Our approach weighted individual study effects by sample size and also took into account the direction of effect. We also computed the false discovery rate (FDR) using the Benjamini-Hochberg method [55]. We also determined statistical power for this meta-analysis a priori using an estimation method specifically designed for epigenome-wide association studies [56].

Comparison of blood epigenome-wide association studies (EWAS) hits to brain-based DNAm

We sought to compare the consistency of top EWAS results from the blood-based meta-analysis to our previous analysis of post-mortem brain samples from ASD cases and controls [19]. These data consist of DNAm from three brain regions: cerebellum, prefrontal cortex, and temporal cortex. For the CpG sites reaching suggestive levels of significance ($p < 1 \times 10^{-4}$) in the meta-analysis, we computed mean differences between cases and controls in each of these three brain regions. We then computed Pearson correlations and quadrant count ratios between the blood effect sizes and three lists of brain effect sizes. We computed quadrant count ratios as the sum of concordant effect sizes (both positive or both negative) minus the sum of discordant effect sizes, all divided by the total number of effect sizes being compared.

Methylation quantitative trait loci (meQTL) query and meQTL target enrichment test

We were interested in exploring the propensity of CpG sites that reached a level of suggestive significance in the EWAS meta-analysis to be significantly associated with nearby SNPs. We used joint DNAm and genotype data to define SNPs associated DNAm, sometimes referred to as "methylation quantitative trait loci (meQTLs)", and the CpG sites under genetic control, or "meQTL targets". We then tested for enrichment of meQTL targets in the top ranked CpG sites from the meta-analysis.

In lieu of applying our SV selection method (see "Epigenome-wide association testing and meta-analysis") to every SNP-CpG association test in the meQTL query, we conducted separate meQTL queries in each processing batch of the SEED data ($N_{\text{Batch1}} = 606$; $N_{\text{Batch2}} = 362$). In each batch, we first used a data-driven procedure we have described in detail previously [57] to select three key parameters for the meQTL query: the SNP minor allele frequency threshold for inclusion, the CpG variability threshold for inclusion, and the maximum distance between SNP and CpG site to be considered for analysis. Briefly, this procedure selects parameters to ensure 80% power to detect a 5% DNAm difference with each addition of the minor allele, at a Bonferroni-defined significance threshold. We then performed the meQTL query in each batch using the *MatrixEQTL* R package, adjusting for sex, the first five principal components to account for genetic ancestry, and the first two principal components derived from the cell composition estimates. We then defined SNP-CpG association pairs based on results that can gain 100% power in the parameter survey ("permissive"), 90% power ("intermediate"), and 80% power ("stringent"). If a SNP-CpG association pair was significant at a designated threshold in each batch, the CpG site was labeled a meQTL target under that threshold for the downstream enrichment analysis.

We tested for enrichment of meQTL targets in ASD-associated CpG sites. We examined this using two ASD EWAS meta-analysis p value thresholds ($p < 1 \times 10^{-3}$ and $p < 1 \times 10^{-4}$) and the three meQTL p value thresholds. In each enrichment test, we accounted for the two main features of CpG sites likely to affect results: the degree of variability in DNAm at that CpG and the number of SNPs in the boundary considered. To do this, we binned each CpG site by decile according to these factors. For each EWAS/meQTL threshold scenario, we compared the proportion of meQTL targets among ASD-related CpGs to a null distribution of randomly selected CpGs, equal in count to the number of ASD-associated sites, matched on the same variability and nearby SNP decile. We defined a fold enrichment statistic as the count of meQTL targets in the ASD-associated CpGs divided by the mean proportion of meQTL targets from the null set, and an enrichment p value as the number of null CpG sets with a count of meQTL targets that was equal to or exceeded the count in the ASD-associated CpG list.

Results

ASD EWAS meta-analysis in blood

We performed a meta-analysis over the 445,068 probes that were present in both the SEED (Table 1) and SSC (Additional file 2: Table S1) cleaned datasets. Figure 1a shows the range of p values and effect sizes detected in our meta-analysis. No CpG sites reached a Bonferroni level of significance, and effect sizes were modest (1.12×10^{-7}; Fig. 1a). The genomic inflation factor (λ) was 1.03, with a slight separation from expectation at the tail (Fig. 1b). A total of 48 CpG sites met or exceeded a p value $< 1 \times 10^{-4}$, and 7 CpG sites (Table 2) reached a significance level of $p < 1 \times 10^{-5}$. We have provided a full list of summary statistics for both SEED and SSC for all 445,068 probes (Additional file 3: Table S2). Based on our analytic sample size, we had 80% power to detect a 3.8% DNAm difference between cases and controls at a Bonferonni level of significance.

Consistency of blood EWAS hits in brain

We considered the consistency of signal for the 48 blood-based CpGs with suggestive significance (p value $< 1 \times 10^{-4}$), among results from three different brain regions with data available from our previous analysis of post-mortem brain samples and ASD [19]. The cerebellum exhibited a moderate degree of concordance in effect size and direction ($r = 0.31$; QCR = 0.33), although prefrontal cortex ($r = 0.02$; QCR = 0.125) and temporal cortex ($r = -0.10$; QCR = − 0.125) showed only minimal concordance (Additional file 4: Table S3, Additional file 5: Figure S3). When considering the seven CpG sites with more stringent blood-based p values $< 1 \times 10^{-5}$, the direction of effect was consistent for at least five of these seven in all three brain region results, with typically larger effect sizes (Table 3). The CpG site with the largest effect size in blood (cg09671955) displayed consistent, and larger, effect sizes in all three brain regions (Table 2, Additional file 4: Table S3).

Table 1 Demographic characteristics for SEED samples

	ASD ($N = 453$)	Control ($N = 515$)	p value
Sex	N (%)	N (%)	< 2.2E−16
M	368 (0.81)	273 (0.53)	
F	85 (0.19)	242 (0.47)	
Processing batch	N (%)	N (%)	0.5136
1	289 (0.64)	317 (0.62)	
2	164 (0.36)	198 (0.28)	
Cell composition	Mean (IQR)	Mean (IQR)	
Granulocytes	0.46 [0.38–0.52]	0.47 [0.40–0.54]	0.02
CD4T	0.21 [0.16–0.26]	0.20 [0.16–0.24]	0.09
B cell	0.12 [0.08–0.15]	0.11 [0.08–0.13]	0.01
CD8T	0.11 [0.08–0.15]	0.11 [0.08–0.13]	0.58
Monocytes	0.07 [0.05–0.09]	0.07 [0.06–0.09]	0.63
NK	0.02 [0.00–0.03]	0.02 [0.00–0.03]	0.83
Genetic ancestry	N (%)	N (%)	1.02E−06
European	214 (0.47)	324 (0.63)	
African	71 (0.16)	39 (0.08)	
Admixed or Asian	153 (0.34)	142 (0.28)	
Missing	15 (0.03)	10 (0.02)	

meQTL target enrichment test

When considering all CpGs associated with ASD at a liberal $p < 1 \times 10^{-3}$ EWAS threshold, we found meQTL target enrichment at nominal significance ($p_{enrichment} = 0.041$), but not at a significance threshold corrected for the six tests performed overall (Table 4). All other combinations of EWAS and meQTL p values tested displayed similar suggestive levels of significance ($0.089 \le p_{enrichment} \le 0.243$) and a consistent direction of effect towards enrichment. Also, tests conducted for CpGs meeting the more stringent EWAS p value threshold (1×10^{-4}) displayed a consistently greater effect size than their corresponding tests from the more liberal EWAS threshold.

Discussion

We report results from a large study investigating the relationship between ASD and DNAm. A case-control meta-analysis of peripheral blood samples from the Study to Explore Early Development and the Simons Simplex Collection revealed that none of the 455,068 CpG sites investigated were associated with ASD at a genome-wide significant threshold. However, 48 CpG sites reached suggestive significance levels at $p < 1 \times 10^{-4}$, including 7 CpGs at $p < 1 \times 10^{-5}$. Associations with ASD at these sites display moderate concordance with post-mortem brain sample results from a previous study and display suggestive evidence for enrichment of SNP-controlled CpG sites, or meQTL targets.

Blood-based DNAm signatures of ASD may reflect causal mechanisms that mimic signatures seen in the brain. However, case-control sampling, by design occurring after disease onset, can also reflect consequences of ASD or of environmental exposures. Nonetheless, given the potential involvement of epigenetic mechanisms in ASD [4–12], and the availability of blood samples from existing studies, this was an important project to pursue. In contrast to our null findings in blood samples, previous work using brain samples has shown specific DNAm to be associated with ASD [15, 19, 20]. The difference in tissue type—specifically that brain-based signatures better reflect ASD etiology—might explain the inconsistent results across these studies. Nonetheless, a previous study of ASD and DNAm in peripheral blood [24] using the earlier 27K Illumina array reported numerous differentially methylated sites. Our study,

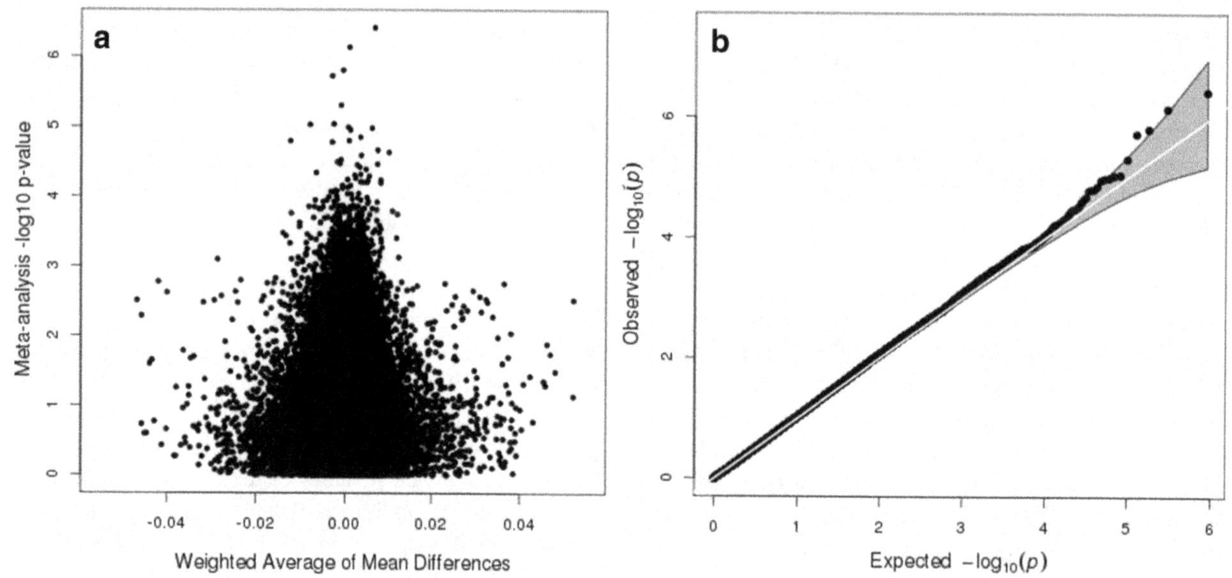

Fig. 1 Meta-analysis results of epigenome-wide association analysis for ASD in peripheral blood in SEED in SSC samples. **a** Volcano plot depicting meta-analysis *p* value (log base 10 scale) on the *y*-axis and average of mean difference values in SEED and SSC samples weighted by sample size on the *x*-axis. **b** Quantile-quantile plot ($\lambda = 1.03$)

despite a much higher sample size, did not observe associations at these same sites. However, the previous study's reported differentially methylated sites were based on a ranking that integrated both degree of statistical significance and effect size; none of their single CpG associations achieved statistical significance at a Bonferroni correction level. Also, the previous study did not explicitly account for potential confounding by cell type proportions or address potential batch effects in the analytic pipeline, as this was not yet commonplace in EWAS pipelines at the time of their report. We used a rigorous, data-driven method to account for these factors and control the genome-wide type I error rate. It is also possible that true differentially methylated positions for ASD exist in blood but have smaller effects sizes than we were powered to detect. Recent EWAS discoveries have indeed found replicable very small effect sizes, particularly in environmental health [58].

Ideally, tissue-relevant samples from earliest in utero development would provide the greatest mechanistic insights. However, this is not typically available and our study is based instead on a case-control design using blood-based samples. Recent examples of blood-based epigenetic work in brain-based disorders have shown utility, particularly when focused on integration of genetic and epigenetic variation or when inferring biological pathways rather than discovery of specific CpGs [57, 59–63]. For example, DNAm under genetic control (meQTL targets) can inform genetic associations observed for ASD. Further, consideration of aggregated sets of CpGs associated with ASD, rather than single sites, can elucidate pathways of interest [57]. In

Table 2 CpG sites identified from meta-analysis as being suggestively associated (1×10^{-5}) with ASD

Probe ID	CHR	Position	SEED *p*	SEED mean diff[a]	SSC *p*	SSC mean diff[a]	METAL *p*	FDR	Nearest gene[b]	Location
cg21151899	22	42,337,657	1.74E−06	0.78	2.75E−02	0.54	3.82E−07	0.16	*CENPM*	Intronic
cg03731974	16	86,531,598	2.59E−04	0.09	8.03E−04	0.08	7.29E−07	0.16	*FENDRR*	Intronic
cg09962502	2	96,971,189	1.89E−04	− 0.05	2.53E−03	− 0.08	1.58E−06	0.21	*SNRNP200*	Exonic
cg01798266	1	1.53E+08	2.06E−05	− 0.43	1.93E−02	− 0.13	1.90E−06	0.21	*PGLYRP4*	Exonic
cg01716316	17	40,897,182	1.28E−03	− 0.09	1.09E−03	− 0.13	4.94E−06	0.44	*EZH1*	111 bp
cg16234726	14	1.02E+08	3.41E−04	− 0.2	8.42E−03	− 0.37	9.13E−06	0.5	*DIO3*	69 Kb
cg09671955	1	1.69E+08	7.20E−03	− 0.47	2.25E−04	− 1.25	9.33E−06	0.5	*CCDC181*	65 bp

[a]Mean difference values computed as mean in cases − mean in controls
[b]Location within gene or distance to nearest gene

Table 3 Suggestively associated ($p < 1 \times 10^{-5}$) CpG sites in peripheral blood and their corresponding effect sizes in three brain regions

Probe ID	CHR	Position	SEED mean diff[a]	SSC mean diff[a]	Weighted average mean diff[b]	PFC[a,c]	TC[a,d]	CER[a,e]
cg21151899	22	42,337,657	0.78	0.54	0.68	1.60	4.07	1.64
cg03731974	16	86,531,598	0.09	0.08	0.08	0.20	− 7.18	0.74
cg09962502	2	96,971,189	− 0.05	− 0.08	− 0.06	− 2.50	− 0.43	− 1.34
cg01798266	1	1.53E+08	− 0.43	− 0.13	− 0.31	− 2.70	− 0.91	0.87
cg01716316	17	40,897,182	− 0.09	− 0.13	− 0.1	− 0.30	− 0.02	0.39
cg16234726	14	1.02E+08	− 0.2	− 0.37	− 0.27	0.50	− 0.3	− 0.03
cg09671955	1	1.69E+08	− 0.47	− 1.25	− 0.79	− 1.40	− 1.38	− 5.11

[a]Mean difference values computed as mean in cases – mean in controls
[b]Average of SEED and SSC mean difference values weighted by sample size ($N_{SEED} = 968$, $N_{SSC} = 686$)
[c]Prefrontal cortex data from Ladd-Acosta et al. [19]
[d]Temporal cortex data from Ladd-Acosta et al. [19]
[e]Cerebellum data from Ladd-Acosta et al. [19]

our own analysis, the most differential blood-based CpGs had consistent effect sizes and directions, although weaker, with brain-based results, particularly for cerebellum. Blood-based CpGs were also moderately enriched (though not to a statistically significant extent) for meQTL targets. These results suggest that blood DNAm can be reflective of DNAm in affected tissues and suggest genetic control of DNAm as a mechanism for this occurrence, at least in an ASD context. More precise evidence is needed, but given the easy accessibility of blood for DNAm measurements versus brain [61], the utility of blood-based DNAm research in ASD is worthy of additional consideration.

In summary, our results suggest a potential role of genetic factors in contributing to DNAm differences in ASD. This is consistent with a recently reported meta-analysis combining these results with an additional European case control sample. In that report, while ASD itself was not associated with DNAm at a genome-wide significance threshold, polygenic risk scores for ASD were associated with DNAm at particular CpGs [64]. In contrast, we show enrichment for meQTL targets (DNAm at least partially controlled by SNP variation) among CpGs with at least marginal association with ASD. We further characterize these ASD DNAm associations and compare to brain-based results. Together, our work and the report by Hannon et al. suggest more investigation of the relationship between genetic risk, epigenetic marks, and ASD is warranted in larger samples and across multiple tissues and designs. To this end, we have provided our full summary statistics and meta-analysis results. The need for greater sample sizes mimics the initial stages of genetic variation discovery in ASD, for which large mega-analyses are starting to pay dividends [65].

Table 4 Enrichment statistics for meQTL targets in ASD-related CpG sites

		meQTL p value threshold[b]		
		Permissive[c]	Intermediate[d]	Stringent[e]
ASD EWAS p value[a]	1×10^{-3}	1.20 (0.041)	1.11 (0.218)	1.11 (0.243)
	1×10^{-4}	1.46 (0.134)	1.71 (0.089)	1.50 (0.205)

Enrichment fold statistics and p values based on 1000 permutations are reported
[a]ASD to DNAm association p value defined from meta-analysis
[b]SNP to CpG association p value thresholds
[c]p values in each methylation processing batch that allowed for 100% power to detect a 5% methylation difference with each addition of minor allele (see "Methods")
[d]p values in each methylation processing batch that allowed for 90% power to detect same methylation difference
[e]p values in each methylation processing batch that allowed for 80% power to detect same methylation difference

Additional files

Additional file 1 Figures S1-S2. Depiction of surrogate variable selection process for SEED (S1) and SSC (S2). Panel A: Heatmap indicating degree of association with known potential technical variables or confounders with estimated surrogate variables. Panel B: Inflation factor (lambda) calculated for progressively including surrogate variables in association models. The number of surrogate variables to include in the ultimate association testing model was to determine to be that which properly controlled the inflation factor and adequately captured known technical variables or confounders. See "Methods" for additional explanation.

Additional file 2 Table S1. Demographic characteristics for samples in the SSC (S2) dataset.

Additional file 3 Table S2. Full summary statistics and meta-analysis results for all 445,608 CpG sites that were present in both the cleaned SEED and SSC datasets.

Additional file 4 Table S3. Concordance between suggestively associated ($p < 1 \times 10^{-4}$) CpG sites in peripheral blood and their corresponding effect sizes in three brain regions.

Additional file 5 Figures S3. Quadrant plots depicting concordance in effect sizes between suggestively associated ($p < 1 \times 10^{-4}$) CpG sites in peripheral blood and three brain regions. A) Prefrontal cortex B) Temporal Cortex C) Cerebellum. Points in red indicate those sites with $p < 1 \times 10^{-5}$ in peripheral blood.

Abbreviations

ASD: Autism spectrum disorder; DNAm: DNA methylation; EWAS: Epigenome-wide association study; meQTL: Methylation quantitative trait loci; SEED: Study to Explore Early Development; SNP: Single nucleotide polymorphism; SSC: Simons Simplex Collection; SV: Surrogate variable

Funding

This project was supported by Centers for Disease Control and Prevention (CDC) Cooperative Agreements announced under the following RFAs: 01086, 02199, DD11-002, DD06-003, DD04-001, and DD09-002. The findings and conclusions in this report are those of the authors and do not necessarily represent the official position of the Centers for Disease Control and Prevention. The DNA methylation assays were supported by Autism Speaks Award #7659 and the genotype assays were supported by NIEHS (R01ES019001; R01ES017646). S. Andrews was supported by the Burroughs-Wellcome Trust training grant: Maryland, Genetics, Epidemiology and Medicine (MD-GEM). The SSC was supported by Simons Foundation (SFARI) award and NIH grant MH089606, both awarded to S.T. Warren.

Authors' contributions

MDF and CL-A conceived the study. GCW, LAS, DES, LAC, MDF, and CJN led the participation and sample recruitment for SEED. STW, RSA, and PC generated the methylation data and performed initial analysis on all the SSC samples. CL-A and APF supervised methylation data collection. SVA performed quality control and preprocessing for the SEED and SSC methylation data. BS and CL-A performed quality control for the SEED genotype data. SVA performed all analyses, supervised by MDF, and CL-A. CL-A, MDF, and APF obtained funding for the DNA methylation measurements in SEED. SVA, MDF, and CL-A wrote the manuscript. All authors contributed to interpretation of results and edited and reviewed the manuscript. All authors read and approved the final manuscript.

Ethics approval and consent to participate

This study was approved by the institutional review boards at each SEED site: SEED 1 recruitment was approved by the IRBs of each recruitment site: Institutional Review Board (IRB)-C, CDC Human Research Protection Office; Kaiser Foundation Research Institute (KFRI) Kaiser Permanente Northern California IRB, Colorado Multiple IRB, Emory University IRB, Georgia Department of Public Health IRB, Maryland Department of Health and Mental Hygiene IRB, Johns Hopkins Bloomberg School of Public Health Review Board, University of North Carolina IRB and Office of Human Research Ethics, IRB of The Children's Hospital of Philadelphia, and IRB of the University of Pennsylvania. All enrolled families provided written consent for participation. This methylation substudy was approved as an amendment of the Johns Hopkins Institutional Review Board (IRB) approval. For participants from the Simons simplex collection, parents consented and children assented as required by each local institutional review board, which included a coalition of clinics located at Michigan, Yale, Emory, Columbia, Vanderbilt, McGill Washington, and Harvard Universities (Children's Hospital of Boston), and at the Universities of Washington, Illinois (Chicago), Missouri, UCLA, and the Baylor College of Medicine. To protect the privacy of participants, Global Unique Identifiers (GUIDs) were constructed from personal information using an algorithm devised in collaboration with scientists at the NIH [66]. Each clinic retained personal identifiers on site and transmitted de-identified GUIDs to a central database, as described previously [37].

Competing interests

The authors declare that they have no competing interests.

Author details

[1]Department of Epidemiology, Johns Hopkins Bloomberg School of Public Health, 615 N. Wolfe Street, Baltimore, MD 21205, USA. [2]Wendy Klag Center for Autism and Developmental Disabilities, Johns Hopkins Bloomberg School of Public Health, 615 N. Wolfe Street, W6509, Baltimore, MD 21205, USA. [3]California Department of Public Health, Environmental Health Investigations Branch, 850 Marina Bay Parkway, Richmond, CA 94804, USA. [4]National Center on Birth Defects and Developmental Disabilities, Centers for Disease Control and Prevention, MS E-86, 1600 Clifton Road, Atlanta, GA 30333, USA. [5]Deparment of Public Health, Section of Epidemiology, Aarhus University, Aarhus, Denmark. [6]Department of Economics and Business, National Centre for Register-based Research, Aarhus University, Aarhus, Denmark. [7]Lundbeck Foundation Initiative for Integrative Psychiatric Research, iPSYCH, Aarhus, Denmark. [8]Kaiser Permanente Division of Research, 2000 Broadway, Oakland, CA 94612, USA. [9]Department of Human Genetics, Emory University School of Medicine, 615 Michael Street, Atlanta, GA 30322, USA. [10]Department of Psychiatry, University of Wisconsin-Madison, 6001 Research Park Blvd, Madison, WI 53719, USA. [11]Department of Epidemiology and Biostatistics, Drexel University School of Public Health, 3215 Market Street, Philadelphia, PA 19104, USA. [12]A.J. Drexel Autism Institute, 3020 Market Street Suite 560, Philadelphia, PA 19104, USA. [13]Department of Biochemistry, Emory University School of Medicine, 615 Michael Street, Atlanta, GA 30322, USA. [14]Department of Pediatrics, Emory University School of Medicine, 615 Michael Street, Atlanta, GA 30322, USA. [15]Center for Epigenetics, Johns Hopkins School of Medicine, 855 N. Wolfe Street, Baltimore, MD 21205, USA. [16]Department of Medicine, Johns Hopkins School of Medicine, 855 N. Wolfe Street, Baltimore, MD 21205, USA. [17]Department of Mental Health, Johns Hopkins Bloomberg School of Public Health, 624 N. Broadway, HH850, Baltimore, MD 21205, USA.

References

1. Jedele KB. The overlapping spectrum of Rett and Angelman syndromes: a clinical review. Semin Pediatr Neurol. 2007;14:108–17.
2. Mount RH, Charman T, Hastings RP, Reilly S, Cass H. Features of autism in Rett syndrome and severe mental retardation. J Autism Dev Disord. 2003;33:435–42.
3. Budimirovic DB, Kaufmann WE. What can we learn about autism from studying fragile X syndrome? Dev Neurosci. 2011;33:379–94.
4. Amir RE, Van den Veyver IB, Wan M, Tran CQ, Francke U, Zoghbi HY. Rett syndrome is caused by mutations in X-linked MECP2, encoding methyl-CpG-binding protein 2. Nat Genet. 1999;23:185–8.
5. Wan M, Lee SS, Zhang X, Houwink-Manville I, Song HR, Amir RE, et al. Rett syndrome and beyond: recurrent spontaneous and familial MECP2 mutations at CpG hotspots. Am J Hum Genet. 1999;65:1520–9.
6. Sutcliffe JS, Nakao M, Christian S, Orstavik KH, Tommerup N, Ledbetter DH, et al. Deletions of a differentially methylated CpG island at the SNRPN gene define a putative imprinting control region. Nat Genet. 1994;8:52–8.
7. Kishino T, Lalande M, Wagstaff J. UBE3A/E6-AP mutations cause Angelman syndrome. Nat Genet. 1997;15:70–3.
8. Bell MV, Hirst MC, Nakahori Y, MacKinnon RN, Roche A, Flint TJ, et al. Physical mapping across the fragile X: hypermethylation and clinical expression of the fragile X syndrome. Cell. 1991;64:861–6.
9. Vincent A, Heitz D, Petit C, Kretz C, Oberlé I, Mandel JL. Abnormal pattern detected in fragile-X patients by pulsed-field gel electrophoresis. Nature. 1991;349:624–6.
10. Sanders SJ, He X, Willsey AJ, Ercan-Sencicek AG, Samocha KE, Cicek AE, et al. Insights into autism spectrum disorder genomic architecture and biology from 71 risk loci. Neuron. 2015;87:1215–33.
11. Pinto D, Delaby E, Merico D, Barbosa M, Merikangas A, Klei L, et al. Convergence of genes and cellular pathways dysregulated in autism spectrum disorders. Am J Hum Genet. 2014;94:677–94.
12. Krumm N, O'Roak BJ, Shendure J, Eichler EE. A de novo convergence of autism genetics and molecular neuroscience. Trends Neurosci. 2014;37:95–105.

13. Nagarajan RP, Hogart AR, Gwye Y, Martin MR, LaSalle JM. Reduced MeCP2 expression is frequent in autism frontal cortex and correlates with aberrant MECP2 promoter methylation. Epigenetics. 2006;1:e1–11.
14. Gregory SG, Connelly JJ, Towers AJ, Johnson J, Biscocho D, Markunas CA, et al. Genomic and epigenetic evidence for oxytocin receptor deficiency in autism. BMC Med. 2009;7:62.
15. James SJ, Shpyleva S, Melnyk S, Pavliv O, Pogribny IP. Elevated 5-hydroxymethylcytosine in the Engrailed-2 (EN-2) promoter is associated with increased gene expression and decreased MeCP2 binding in autism cerebellum. Transl Psychiatry. 2014;4:e460.
16. James SJ, Shpyleva S, Melnyk S, Pavliv O, Pogribny IP. Complex epigenetic regulation of engrailed-2 (EN-2) homeobox gene in the autism cerebellum. Transl Psychiatry. 2013;3:e232.
17. Zhu L, Wang X, Li X-L, Towers A, Cao X, Wang P, et al. Epigenetic dysregulation of SHANK3 in brain tissues from individuals with autism spectrum disorders. Hum Mol Genet. 2014;23:1563–78.
18. Mor M, Nardone S, Sams DS, Elliott E. Hypomethylation of miR-142 promoter and upregulation of microRNAs that target the oxytocin receptor gene in the autism prefrontal cortex. Mol Autism. 2015;6:46.
19. Ladd-Acosta C, Hansen KD, Briem E, Fallin MD, Kaufmann WE, Feinberg AP. Common DNA methylation alterations in multiple brain regions in autism. Mol Psychiatry. 2014;19:862–71.
20. Nardone S, Sams DS, Reuveni E, Getselter D, Oron O, Karpuj M, et al. DNA methylation analysis of the autistic brain reveals multiple dysregulated biological pathways. Transl Psychiatry. 2014;4:e433.
21. Ellis SE, Gupta S, Moes A, West AB, Arking DE. Exaggerated CpH methylation in the autism-affected brain. Mol Autism. 2017;8:6.
22. Shulha HP, Cheung I, Whittle C, Wang J, Virgil D, Lin CL, et al. Epigenetic signatures of autism: trimethylated H3K4 landscapes in prefrontal neurons. Arch Gen Psychiatry. 2012;69:314–24.
23. Sun W, Poschmann J, Cruz-Herrera Del Rosario R, Parikshak NN, Hajan HS, Kumar V, et al. Histone acetylome-wide association study of autism spectrum disorder. Cell 2016;167:1385–1397.e11.
24. Wong CCY, Meaburn EL, Ronald A, Price TS, Jeffries AR, Schalkwyk LC, et al. Methylomic analysis of monozygotic twins discordant for autism spectrum disorder and related behavioural traits. Mol Psychiatry. 2014;19:495–503.
25. Nguyen A, Rauch TA, Pfeifer GP, Hu VW. Global methylation profiling of lymphoblastoid cell lines reveals epigenetic contributions to autism spectrum disorders and a novel autism candidate gene, RORA, whose protein product is reduced in autistic brain. FASEB J Off Publ Fed Am Soc Exp Biol. 2010;24:3036–51.
26. Berko ER, Suzuki M, Beren F, Lemetre C, Alaimo CM, Calder RB, et al. Mosaic epigenetic dysregulation of ectodermal cells in autism spectrum disorder. PLoS Genet. 2014;10:e1004402.
27. Schendel DE, Diguiseppi C, Croen LA, Fallin MD, Reed PL, Schieve LA, et al. The Study to Explore Early Development (SEED): a multisite epidemiologic study of autism by the Centers for Autism and Developmental Disabilities Research and Epidemiology (CADDRE) network. J Autism Dev Disord. 2012; 42:2121–40.
28. Wiggins LD, Levy SE, Daniels J, Schieve L, Croen LA, DiGuiseppi C, et al. Autism spectrum disorder symptoms among children enrolled in the Study to Explore Early Development (SEED). J Autism Dev Disord. 2015; 45:3183–94.
29. Rutter M, Bailey A, Lord C. The social communication questionnaire: manual. Western Psychological Services. West Psychol Serv. 2003;
30. Mullen EM. Mullen Scales of Early Learning. Am Guid Serv Inc. 1995;
31. Lord C, Risi S, Lambrecht L, Cook EH, Leventhal BL, DiLavore PC, et al. The autism diagnostic observation schedule-generic: a standard measure of social and communication deficits associated with the spectrum of autism. J Autism Dev Disord. 2000;30:205–23.
32. Gotham K, Risi S, Pickles A, Lord C. The Autism Diagnostic Observation Schedule: revised algorithms for improved diagnostic validity. J Autism Dev Disord. 2007;37:613–27.
33. Lord C, Rutter M, DeLavore P, Risi S. Autism Diagnostic Observation Schedule-WPS (ADOS-WPS). West Psychol Serv. 1999;
34. Lord C, Rutter M, Le Couteur A. Autism Diagnostic Interview-Revised: a revised version of a diagnostic interview for caregivers of individuals with possible pervasive developmental disorders. J Autism Dev Disord. 1994;24:659–85.
35. Rutter M, Le Couteur A, Lord C. ADI-R: Autism diagnostic interview-revised: manual. Western Psychological Services. West Psychol Serv. 2003;
36. Wiggins LD, Piazza V, Robins DL. Comparison of a broad-based screen versus disorder-specific screen in detecting young children with an autism spectrum disorder. Autism Int J Res Pract. 2014;18:76–84.
37. Fischbach GD, Lord C. The Simons Simplex Collection: a resource for identification of autism genetic risk factors. Neuron. 2010;68:192–5.
38. Gotham K, Pickles A, Lord C. Standardizing ADOS scores for a measure of severity in autism spectrum disorders. J Autism Dev Disord. 2009;39:693–705.
39. Fortin J-P, Labbe A, Lemire M, Zanke BW, Hudson TJ, Fertig EJ, et al. Functional normalization of 450k methylation array data improves replication in large cancer studies. Genome Biol. 2014;15(12):503.
40. Triche TJ, Weisenberger DJ, Van Den Berg D, Laird PW, Siegmund KD. Low-level processing of Illumina Infinium DNA Methylation BeadArrays. Nucleic Acids Res. 2013;41:e90.
41. Aryee MJ, Jaffe AE, Corrada-Bravo H, Ladd-Acosta C, Feinberg AP, Hansen KD, et al. Minfi: a flexible and comprehensive Bioconductor package for the analysis of Infinium DNA methylation microarrays. Bioinforma Oxf Engl. 2014;30:1363–9.
42. Chen Y, Lemire M, Choufani S, Butcher DT, Grafodatskaya D, Zanke BW, et al. Discovery of cross-reactive probes and polymorphic CpGs in the Illumina Infinium HumanMethylation450 microarray. Epigenetics. 2013;8:203–9.
43. Alisch RS, Barwick BG, Chopra P, Myrick LK, Satten GA, Conneely KN, et al. Age-associated DNA methylation in pediatric populations. Genome Res. 2012;22:623–32.
44. Reinius LE, Acevedo N, Joerink M, Pershagen G, Dahlén S-E, Greco D, et al. Differential DNA methylation in purified human blood cells: implications for cell lineage and studies on disease susceptibility. PLoS One. 2012;7:e41361.
45. Delaneau O, Zagury J-F, Marchini J. Improved whole-chromosome phasing for disease and population genetic studies. Nat Methods. 2013;10:5–6.
46. Howie B, Fuchsberger C, Stephens M, Marchini J, Abecasis GR. Fast and accurate genotype imputation in genome-wide association studies through pre-phasing. Nat Genet. 2012;44:955–9.
47. Price AL, Patterson NJ, Plenge RM, Weinblatt ME, Shadick NA, Reich D. Principal components analysis corrects for stratification in genome-wide association studies. Nat Genet. 2006;38:904–9.
48. Du P, Zhang X, Huang C-C, Jafari N, Kibbe WA, Hou L, et al. Comparison of Beta-value and M-value methods for quantifying methylation levels by microarray analysis. BMC Bioinformatics. 2010;11:587.
49. limma. Bioconductor. http://bioconductor.org/packages/limma/. Accessed 21 Sep 2016.
50. Author VJCP to R by TL (versions 3 13 and 4 4) and BR (version 4 13) N that maintainers are not available to give advice on using a package they did not. gee: Generalized Estimation Equation Solver. 2015. https://CRAN.R-project.org/package=gee. Accessed 19 Jun 2018.
51. Leek JT, Storey JD. Capturing heterogeneity in gene expression studies by surrogate variable analysis. PLoS Genet. 2007;3:1724–35.
52. McGregor K, Bernatsky S, Colmegna I, Hudson M, Pastinen T, Labbe A, et al. An evaluation of methods correcting for cell-type heterogeneity in DNA methylation studies. Genome Biol. 2016;17:84.
53. GenABEL.pdf. http://www.genabel.org/packages/GenABEL. Accessed 15 Mar 2017.
54. Willer CJ, Li Y, Abecasis GR. METAL: fast and efficient meta-analysis of genomewide association scans. Bioinforma Oxf Engl. 2010;26:2190–1.
55. Benjamini Y, Hochberg Y. Controlling the False Discovery Rate: A Practical and Powerful Approach to Multiple Testing. J R Stat Soc Ser B Methodol. 1995;57:289–300.
56. Tsai P-C, Bell JT. Power and sample size estimation for epigenome-wide association scans to detect differential DNA methylation. Int J Epidemiol. 2015;
57. Andrews SV, Ellis SE, Bakulski KM, Sheppard B, Croen LA, Hertz-Picciotto I, et al. Cross-tissue integration of genetic and epigenetic data offers insight into autism spectrum disorder. Nat Commun. 2017;8:1011.
58. Breton CV, Marsit CJ, Faustman E, Nadeau K, Goodrich JM, Dolinoy DC, et al. Small-magnitude effect sizes in epigenetic end points are important in children's environmental health studies: the children's environmental health and disease prevention research center's epigenetics working group. Environ Health Perspect. 2017;125:511–26.
59. Hannon E, Lunnon K, Schalkwyk L, Mill J. Interindividual methylomic variation across blood, cortex, and cerebellum: implications for epigenetic studies of neurological and neuropsychiatric phenotypes. Epigenetics. 2015; 10:1024–32.
60. Davies MN, Volta M, Pidsley R, Lunnon K, Dixit A, Lovestone S, et al. Functional annotation of the human brain methylome identifies tissue-

specific epigenetic variation across brain and blood. Genome Biol. 2012;13:R43.
61. Bakulski KM, Halladay A, Hu VW, Mill J, Fallin MD. Epigenetic research in neuropsychiatric disorders: the "tissue issue". Curr Behav Neurosci Rep. 2016;3:264–74.
62. Montano C, Taub MA, Jaffe A, Briem E, Feinberg JI, Trygvadottir R, et al. Association of DNA methylation differences with schizophrenia in an epigenome-wide association study. JAMA Psychiatry. 2016;73:506–14.
63. Edgar RD, Jones MJ, Meaney MJ, Turecki G, Kobor MS. BECon: a tool for interpreting DNA methylation findings from blood in the context of brain. Transl Psychiatry. 2017;7:e1187.
64. Hannon E, Schendel D, Ladd-Acosta C, Grove J, iPSYCH-Broad ASD Group, Hansen CS, et al. Elevated polygenic burden for autism is associated with differential DNA methylation at birth. Genome Med. 2018;10:19.
65. Autism Spectrum Disorders Working Group of The Psychiatric Genomics Consortium. Meta-analysis of GWAS of over 16,000 individuals with autism spectrum disorder highlights a novel locus at 10q24.32 and a significant overlap with schizophrenia. Mol Autism. 2017;8:21.
66. Johnson SB, Whitney G, McAuliffe M, Wang H, McCreedy E, Rozenblit L, et al. Using global unique identifiers to link autism collections. J Am Med Inform Assoc JAMIA. 2010;17:689–95.

12

A pilot dose finding study of pioglitazone in autistic children

Lucia Capano[1*], Annie Dupuis[2], Jessica Brian[1], Deepali Mankad[1], Lisa Genore[3], Rianne Hastie Adams[3], Sharon Smile[1], Toni Lui[3], Dina Odrobina[3], Jane A. Foster[4] and Evdokia Anagnostou[1]

Abstract

Background: Pioglitazone is a promising compound for treatment of core autism spectrum disorder (ASD) symptoms as it targets multiple relevant pathways, including immune system alterations.

Objective: This pilot study aimed to elucidate the maximum tolerated dose, safety, preliminary evidence of efficacy, and appropriate outcome measures in autistic children ages 5–12 years old.

Methods: We conducted a 16-week prospective cohort, single blind, single arm, 2-week placebo run-in, dose-finding study of pioglitazone. Twenty-five participants completed treatment. A modified dose finding method was used to determine safety and dose response among three dose levels: 0.25 mg/kg, 0.5 mg/kg, and 0.75 mg/kg once daily.

Results: Maximum tolerated dose: there were no serious adverse events (SAEs) and as such the maximum tolerated dose within the range tested was 0.75 mg/Kg once daily.
Safety: overall, pioglitazone was well tolerated. Two participants discontinued intervention due to perceived non-efficacy and one due to the inability to tolerate interim blood work. Three participants experienced mild neutropenia.
Early evidence of efficacy: statistically significant improvement was observed in social withdrawal, repetitive behaviors, and externalizing behaviors as measured by the Aberrant Behavior Checklist (ABC), Child Yale-Brown Obsessive Compulsive Scale (CY-BOCS), and Repetitive Behavior Scale–Revised (RBS-R). Forty-six percent of those enrolled were deemed to be global responders.

Conclusions and relevance: Pioglitazone is well-tolerated and shows a potential signal in measures of social withdrawal, repetitive, and externalizing behaviors. Randomized controlled trials using the confirmed dose are warranted.

Keywords: Pioglitazone, Autism spectrum disorder, Cytokines, Treatment, Clinical trial, Efficacy, Safety profile, Inflammation, Drug therapy, Physiological effects of drugs, Maximum tolerated dose (MTD)

Introduction

Autism spectrum disorder (ASD) is a complex neurodevelopmental condition with life-long impact on patients, affecting almost 1 in 59 children [1, 2]. The core symptoms of ASD involve varying degrees of difficulty in social communication, repetitive behavior, and restricted interests [1]. Autistic individuals[1] also experience frequent physical and mental health comorbidity. Risperidone and aripiprazole are the only medications approved for use in ASD for the treatment of irritability and aggression. There are no pharmaceutical treatment options for the core symptoms of ASD, and perhaps more importantly, none that impact the developmental trajectory of autistic children. Part of the challenge in the development of new treatments is identifying the biological basis of the pathophysiology underlying the clinical heterogeneity in ASD.

The pathophysiology underlying ASD is under investigation. The disorder is known to have strong genetic influences and some environmental risk factors. Clinical heterogeneity in autism makes it difficult to match individuals with effective treatments. Literature evidence supports a role for immune signaling and inflammation in ASD [3–10] but current approaches have not

* Correspondence: lcapano@hollandbloorview.ca
[1]Holland Bloorview Kids Rehabilitation Hospital, University of Toronto, 150 Kilgour Road, Toronto, ON M4G 1R8, Canada

examined or identified individual differences in biology that underlie the striking clinical heterogeneity. Of note, whether immune differences are primary to the pathophysiology or a later epiphenomenon has not been clarified. In an effort to advance our understanding of the role of the immune system in ASD, we assessed baseline and treatment-related changes in peripheral cytokines in an exploratory fashion, as part of a maximum tolerated dose (MTD) study with pioglitazone (NCT01205282).

Evidence of abnormal central nervous system immune signaling and inflammation in ASD

Evidence of immune system alterations within the brains of autistic individuals comes from examination of post-mortem brain tissue, cerebrospinal fluid (CSF), and positron emission tomography (PET) studies. Post-mortem tissue analysis has demonstrated activated microglia and astrocytes in several areas of cerebral cortex, cingulate gyrus, white matter, and cerebellum [11–13]. Recently, elevated microglial activation was demonstrated in vivo using PET [14]. The ages of individuals in these studies varies from early childhood to adulthood suggesting that such neuroinflammation may affect the presentation of autism across the life span. In comparison to controls, autistic individuals have elevated levels of glial fibrillary acidic protein (GFAP), confirming astroglial activation (reviewed in [15]). Increased expression and release of cytokines and chemokines, the mediators of inflammatory reactions in the CNS, have also been observed. Elevated levels of proinflammatory chemokines reported in ASD include macrophage chemoattractant protein-1 (MCP-1), thymus activation-regulated chemokine (TARC), proinflammatory cytokines interleukin-6 (IL-6), interleukin-10 (IL-10), macrophage chemoattractant protein-3 (MCP-3), eotaxin, eotaxin 2, macrophage derived chemokine (MDC), chemokine-β8 (Ckβ8.1), neutrophil activating peptide-2 (NAP-2), monokine induced by interferon-ϒ (MIG), and B-lymphocyte chemoattractant (BLC) [11]. Studies comparing CSF in autistic children versus controls have shown elevated pro-inflammatory cytokines tumor necrosis factor-α (TNF-α), IL-6 and granulocyte-macrophage colony stimulating factor (GM-CSF), Th1 cytokine (IFN-ϒ), and chemokine (IL-8) (reviewed in [15]). Other studies have found that patients with ASD produce lower levels of anti-inflammatory cytokines IL-10 and TGF-1β [16, 17].

Evidence of abnormal peripheral immune system signaling and inflammation in ASD

Studies comparing cytokine levels from the peripheral immune system (from blood samples) to CNS (via CSF) do not find a clear relationship, suggesting that blood samples may not provide a clear indication of CNS immune activity [4]. However, cross-talk between peripheral cytokines and the CNS are known to impact behavior [18, 19]. Elevated levels of pro-inflammatory cytokines and reduced levels of anti-inflammatory cytokines have been observed in autistic children compared to controls [20–22]. A recent meta-analysis of studies of peripheral cytokine levels in ASD compared to controls demonstrated higher concentrations of interleukin (IL)-1β, IL-6, IL-8, interferon-gamma, eotaxin, and MCP-1, while concentrations of transforming growth factor-β1 (TGF-1β—anti-inflammatory cytokine) were significantly lower [20, 21]. In a study of 65 autistic children compared to healthy controls, level of IL-8 in the blood was found to be significantly higher, while IL-10 was significantly lower [23]. However, in a longitudinal study of 104 autistic children compared to controls, there was no difference in levels of traditional markers of active inflammation such as IL-6, TNF-α, and IL-1β [4].

Evidence is accumulating that demonstrates a link between elevated cytokine levels and behavior. Ashwood et al. [24] found that increased IL-6 level in autistic children was associated with increased stereotypy scores on the Aberrant Behavior Checklist (ABC). Tsilioni et al. [25] observed that both IL-6 and TNF-α were decreased significantly in autistic children when they took luteolin a natural flavonoid, and children with high levels of both IL-6 and TNF-α at baseline had significant improvement of all subscales of the Vineland adaptive behavior scale following this treatment. Reduced TGF-1β was seen in ASD versus controls and correlated with lower adaptive behavior and worse behavioral symptoms [16]. Similarly, another study found that levels of TGF-β1 and IL-23 were significantly decreased in the plasma of autistic children in comparison to healthy controls with a negative correlation between TGF-β1, IL-23, and IL-17 with the severity of autism [26]. Additionally, IL-17A was found to be significantly higher in the serum of autistic children than healthy controls, and higher levels correlated with severity of autism [7].

Pioglitazone pharmacodynamics and studies in ASD

Overall, the studies discussed above demonstrate that alterations in both peripheral and CNS cytokines are observed in ASD and identifying drug treatments that normalize some of these immune markers may be a fruitful avenue of research. Pioglitazone is an agonist of peroxisome proliferator activated receptor (PPAR)-ϒ, and is part of a drug class called thiazolidinediones (TZDs). PPAR-ϒ is a nuclear hormone receptor which modulates insulin sensitivity but is also shown to have anti-inflammatory effects [27]. The anti-inflammatory functions of PPAR-ϒ have received much attention since its agonists have been shown to exert a broad spectrum of protective effects in several animal models of neurologic and cardiovascular diseases [28, 29]. To date, pioglitazone has been shown in vitro and in early in vivo studies to have a variety of effects of interest in the pathophysiology of autism. Those include inhibition of expression of inflammatory cytokines (IL-1b, IL-6, and IL-8) [29], and reduction in TNF-α [30], but also affects on mitochondrial function and NMDA glutamate receptor activity [31, 32], which may also be important in ASD pathophysiology [33–35].

Studies of pioglitazone in autistic individuals include one case series and a pilot double-blind placebo-controlled study of pioglitazone as adjunctive treatment to risperidone [36, 37]. The authors of the case series reported on 25 children (mean age 7.9 ± 0.7 years) with autism who were treated with 30–60 mg of pioglitazone a day, over 3–4 months. They reported improvements in four of five scales of the ABC and no side effects other than mild elevation in liver enzymes, a well-known phenomenon with this medication. A drawback of this study was the choice of pioglitazone dose. The FDA-approved maximum adult dose is 45 mg. Lower doses have been used in the trials of type II diabetes and studies for use of pioglitazone in central nervous system diseases such as multiple sclerosis. Additionally, only the ABC was piloted as an outcome measure. Other outcome measures may prove to be more sensitive. Ghaleiha et al. [37] randomized autistic children receiving risperidone to pioglitazone or placebo adjunct treatment. Forty-four patients aged 4–12 years with a score of more than 12 on the Aberrant Behavior Checklist-Community (ABC-C) were included in a 10-week study. They found a significant reduction in irritability, lethargy/social withdrawal, and hyperactivity/non-compliance, but not for stereotypic behavior and inappropriate speech subscales in the pioglitazone group compared with the placebo group. Vomiting and headache were the most frequent reported side effects. Of the two studies conducted on pioglitazone in ASD to date, one used doses above the recommended maximum for adults, while the other used pioglitazone as adjunct therapy. Therefore, both the safety and efficacy of pioglitazone in ASD requires further study.

In this study, we conducted a weight-based evaluation of maximum tolerated dose using a modified dose finding method, where maximum dose was based on the FDA and Health Canada approved adult maximum. We used several outcome measures sensitive to changes in behavior, to help guide the design of a larger multisite placebo-controlled trial. In an exploratory fashion, we measured levels of cytokines (IL-1β, IL-6, TNF-α, and IL-10) pre and post treatment as potential predictors of response to drug. The design was a phase II, 16-week, single-blind, single arm, placebo run-in, modified MTD study of pioglitazone in autistic children.

Methods

Participants

Eligible participants were 5–12 years old with a Diagnostic and Statistical Manual of Mental Disorders 4th edition, text revision (DSM-IV-TR [38]) diagnosis of autistic disorder or Asperger syndrome (autism spectrum disorder) supported by the Autism Diagnostic Observational Schedule, First or Second Edition (ADOS [39] or ADOS-2 [40, 41]) and the Autism Diagnostic Interview-Revised (ADI-R [42]). The Diagnostic and Statistical Manual of Mental Disorders 5th edition (DSM-5) was published after participant enrollment had begun; therefore, the protocol was not revised for use of DSM-5 for diagnosis. Eligibility for inclusion also required a Clinical Global Impression-Severity (CGI-S [43]) score ≥ 4 to ensure participants were experiencing functional impairment at least moderate in severity that could benefit from medication treatment. The CGI-S is a standardized measure commonly used in mental health research, for ranking illness severity (therefore for autism this would include both core and associated symptoms). All participants had normal physical examination and laboratory test results at screening visit. Participants receiving non-pharmacologic educational, behavioral, or dietary interventions at study entry were required to be stable on such interventions (continuous participation during the preceding 3 months) and to not electively initiate new or modify ongoing interventions for the duration of the study. Participants were excluded if they had a primary psychiatric diagnosis other than ASD, a current neurological disease including a movement disorder, tuberous sclerosis, fragile X or any other known genetic syndrome, or any medical condition that might interfere with the conduct of the study, confound interpretation of the study results, or endanger a participant's well-being. Hence, patients with evidence or history of malignancy or any significant hematological, endocrine, cardiovascular (including any rhythm disorder), respiratory, renal, hepatic, or gastrointestinal disease were excluded. However, patients with stable epilepsy (defined as no seizures for 6 months) and on stable doses of antiepileptic medications (no changes in the 3 months preceding screening) were allowed to participate. Prior studies of pioglitazone have shown that individuals taking this medication had a slightly higher incidence of bladder cancer and the risk seemed to be higher in smokers. Therefore, participants were not allowed to participate if they had a family history of bladder cancer, a caregiver who smoked, or a personal history of bladder infection. Participants taking any psychoactive medication or insulin were excluded as were any female participants who were sexually active, taking the birth control pill for any reason, or pregnant. Participants were excluded if unable to tolerate venipuncture procedures for blood sampling.

The informed consent process was conducted in accordance with the Tri Council Policy Statement, the Declaration of Helsinki, and the International Council for Harmonization of Technical Requirements for Pharmaceuticals for Human Use (ICH)–Good Clinical Practice (GCP) guidelines and institutional policy. This study was approved by the Holland Bloorview Research Ethics Board.

Study design

This phase II pilot study was designed as a 16-week, modified maximum tolerated dose study of pioglitazone in autistic children conducted at Holland Bloorview Kids Rehabilitation Hospital in Toronto, Canada. Participants were enrolled consecutively over 2 years. Our national pharmaceutical regulatory body, Health Canada, required that a maximum tolerated dose (MTD) study be conducted prior to additional clinical trials of pioglitazone for autistic children. Such studies are normally open label; however, in an effort to improve our confidence in evaluating preliminary efficacy and safety, we employed a 2-week placebo run-in and single-blind design. Parents were blinded to the timing of the 2-week placebo period. The consent process disclosed that at some point during the study, participants would get placebo, but not when. The study involved 2 weeks of placebo run-in and 14 weeks of active treatment. The placebo was identical in composition to the active drug except for the active ingredient. Compliance with the study dosing schedule was monitored with a medication diary that was provided to parents/guardians that they completed daily. Parents were the primary efficacy raters and were blinded to treatment as described above. Clinicians were not blinded, and were solely responsible for safety assessments and outcome ratings (using CGI-S, Clinician Global Impression scale-Improvement (CGI-I) [43] and the Child Yale-Brown Obsessive Compulsive Scale (CY-BOCS; [44], modified by [45]).

Participants were required to attend approximately seven study visits—screening, baseline, 2, 4, 8, 12, and 16 weeks from baseline. A modified dose finding method was used to determine safety and dose response among three dose levels (0.25 mg/kg once daily, 0.5 mg/kg once daily, and 0.75 mg/kg once daily). The dose was based on the FDA-approved maximum adult dose of 45 mg. Taking 60 kg as an average adult weight, the per kilogram maximum dose is 0.75 mg/kg. Standard toxicity protocols are based on serious adverse events (SAEs) to determine the MTD. We defined toxicity as the presence of SAEs or severe side effects deemed by the treating clinician and investigators to be likely or probably related to study drug. The most recent monograph of pioglitazone lists heart failure, hepatic insufficiency, and allergic reactions as significant side effects of pioglitazone. Five participants were studied at the first dosing level (0.25 mg/kg), and five were studied at the second dosing level (0.5 mg/kg). No serious adverse events presented at 0.25 or 0.5 mg/kg, therefore the remaining 18 participants were studied at the final dosing level of 0.75 mg/kg.

Assessments

Screening/diagnostic assessments

At the screening visit, confirmation of DSM-IV diagnosis of autism or Asperger syndrome was obtained by medical history, either ADOS or ADOS-2 and ADI-R. Additionally, a comprehensive medical history and physical exam as well as a Safety Monitoring Uniform Report Form (SMURF) and Clinician's Global Impression (CGI)-severity (Global & Social [43]) were completed by a study physician. An estimate of intellectual ability was obtained using the Stanford Binet 5th Edition. The Stanford Binet 5th Edition was chosen to provide an estimate of intellectual ability because it provides a full-scale intelligence quotient and is able to assess the full age range of our study sample.

Outcome assessments

Treatment outcome measures were selected to elucidate a comprehensive set of behaviors. This included measures of global behavioral disturbance, social function, repetitive behaviors, and anxiety. The Aberrant Behavior Checklist (ABC) community version [46] and the CGI-improvement (CGI-I)-global were used to assess global behavioral disturbance. The ABC was designed to objectively identify five behavior subscales through observation by the primary caregiver. Items are rated on a four-point Likert scale, with higher scores indicating more severe problems. We used three subscales: irritability, hyperactivity, and social withdrawal. The CGI-I global is a well validated clinician-rated measure that employs a seven point scale (1 = very much improved to 7 = very much worse) to determine the patient's response to treatment. The Social Responsiveness Scale (SRS) [47] and the Clinical Global Impressions Improvement Scale (CGI-I)-Social [43] were used to measure social function. The SRS is a 65-item caregiver rating scale of social behaviors specific to ASD and provides a total score that quantifies ASD severity. The CGI-I social allows clinicians to provide an impression of improvement (1 = very much improved to 7 = very much worse) on a seven-point Likert Scale. The Child Yale-Brown Obsessive Compulsive Scale (CY-BOCS; [44], modified by [45]) and the Repetitive Behavior Scale-Revised (RBS-R) [48] were used to measure repetitive behaviors. The CY-BOCS is a clinician-rated questionnaire measuring the time spent, distress, interference, resistance, and control in relation to obsessions and compulsions based on a five-point scale. The RBS-R was developed to capture the breadth of repetitive behaviors specific to autism and is a 43-item parent report measure. Lastly, the Behavioral Assessment System for Children 2nd Edition (BASC-2) [49] anxiety scale and the Child and Adolescent Symptom Inventory (CASI) [50] anxiety component were used to measure symptoms of anxiety. These outcome measures were completed at the baseline visit, week 8 and week 16. Research bloodwork included

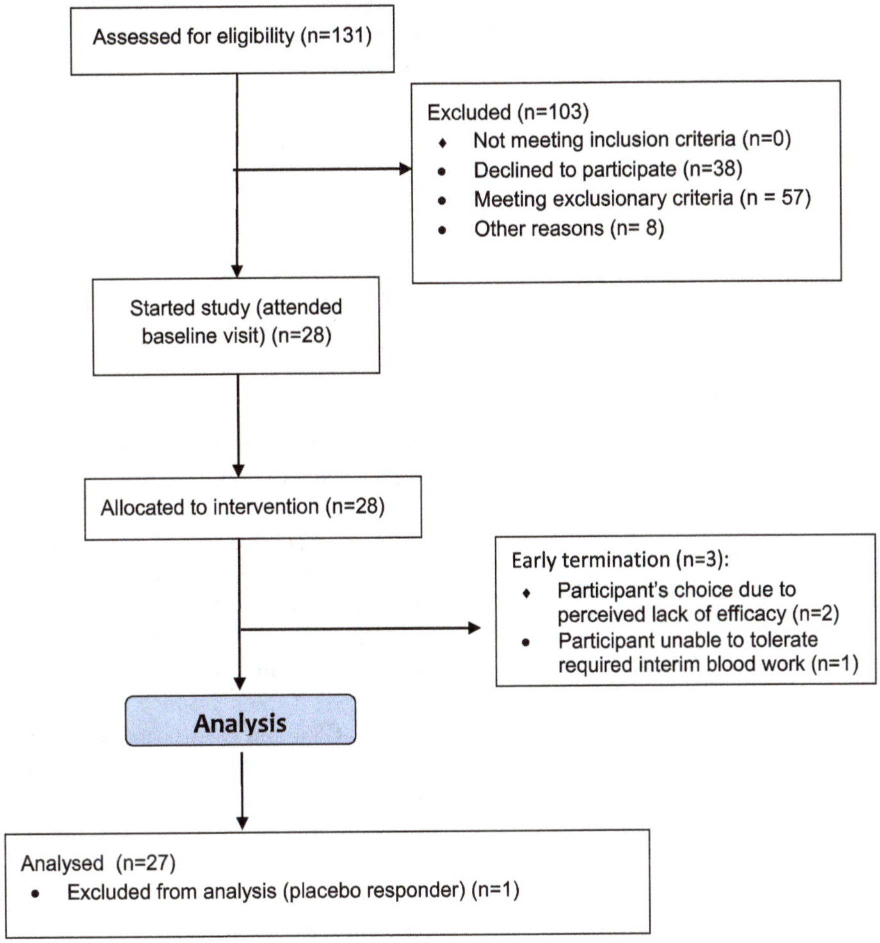

Fig. 1 CONSORT 2010 flow diagram

cytokines (IL-1β IL-6, IL-10, and TNF-α) and was performed at screening and week 16. Cytokine levels, including IL1-β, IL-10, and TNF-α in plasma; IL-6 in serum, were measured by ELISA using standard manufacturer's protocol. ELISA kits were selected based on range of sensitivity by manufacturer and previous reports. Samples were run in duplicate using human TNF-α quantikine HS ELISA (R&D systems), human IL-6 quantikine HS ELISA (R&D systems), human IL1-β ELISA (Ray Biotech), and human IL-10 ELISA (Ray Biotech). Cytokine levels (pg/ml) were detectable in all IL-6 samples and all but one TNF-α and IL1-β samples, and all but two IL-10 samples. Specifically, one baseline sample was below detectable levels for TNF-α, IL10, and IL1-β and one baseline sample was below detectable for IL-10. These samples were treated as missing values and not included in the analysis.

Safety assessments

Safety was assessed using the Clinical Global Impressions Improvement Scale (CGI-I)-Global and the Safety Monitoring Uniform Report Form (SMURF). If a participant

Table 1 Sample characteristics

Age in years [mean (SD)]	6.3 (2.4)
Male:Female	13:1
IQ [Mean (SD)]	69.9 (26.5)
ADOS score [mean (SD)]	17.1 (5.7)
Concomitant IBI (%)	10.7
Concomitant ABA (%)	21.4
Concomitant social skills group (%)	21.4
Diagnosis	# patients with comorbidity (/28)
Anxiety NYD	4
Specific phobia	2
ADHD	3
OCD	1

Abbreviations: IBI intensive behavioral therapy, *ABA* applied behavior analysis, *NYD* not yet diagnosed, *ADHD* attention deficit/hyperactivity disorder, *OCD* obsessive compulsive disorder

Table 2 Adverse events

Event	# Participants
Eye disorders	
Eye redness	1
Oral/gastrointestinal disorders	
Vomiting	3
Abdominal pain	2
Constipation	1
Diarrhea	1
Mouth sore/dry lips	2
Tooth problem	6
General disorders	
Increased energy/behavioral activation	3
Fatigue	1
Increased sweating	1
Immune system disorders	
Neutropenia	3
Infections	
Fever	1
Gastroenteritis	3
Upper respiratory tract infection	11
Injury	
Skin bruise	1
Skin burn	1
Insect bite	2
Appetite	
Decreased appetite	2
Increased appetite	1
Musculoskeletal	
Muscle pain/cramps	2
Nervous system disorder	
Concentration difficulty	1
Headache	1
Psychiatric disorders	
Disinhibition/silliness	2
Increased impulsivity	1
Emotional lability	2
Increased aggression/irritation/anger	5
Insomnia (initial/mid-cycle)	6
Negative thoughts	1
Self-injurious behavior	2
Genitourinary	
Diurnal/nocturnal enuresis	3
Increased urinary frequency	1
Genital discomfort	1

Table 2 Adverse events *(Continued)*

Event	# Participants
Respiratory	
Cough	1
Nasal congestion	2
Sleep apnea	1
Throat clearing	1
Skin	
Skin rash	2
Skin scratching/picking	3

had scored 6 or greater for two or more weeks, they would have been discontinued from the study. At each study visit, the treating physician completed the SMURF [51], assessed vital signs, height, and weight. Funduscopic exam was performed at weeks 8 and 16. Clinical laboratory tests for safety included bloodwork [complete blood count (CBC), electrolytes, blood urea nitrogen (BUN), creatinine, alanine aminotransferase (ALT), aspartate aminotransferase (AST), insulin, fasting glucose, and creatine kinase (CK)] and electrocardiogram performed at screening and weeks 4, 8, and 16. Urinalysis for micro- and macroscopic hematuria was performed at screening and week 16. A urine pregnancy test was performed at screening in any menstruating girl.

Statistical analysis

All analyses compared baseline visit to the week 16 visit, and controlled for participant's age. One subject demonstrated a placebo response and was removed from the analyses. We used repeated measures ANOVA to model the outcomes at each of the study visits, with a planned contrast statement to assess the change from baseline to week 16. CGI scores at weeks 8 and 16 were classified as responders if they scored 1 or 2 on the measure. The percentage of responders is presented with exact 95% confidence limits.

Change in cytokine levels (pg/ml) from baseline to week 16 was highly skewed and, therefore, was assessed using the Wilcoxon signed rank test. We used Spearman correlation coefficients to examine the degree of association between baseline cytokine levels and their change from baseline to the end of the study with the change in outcome measures. Only cytokines and outcomes that showed a significant difference over the course of the study were included in this analysis.

Results

Participant attrition and baseline characteristics

Potential participants were screened over the phone (131). Twenty-eight participants started treatment and

25 participants completed the study (see Fig. 1). Baseline characteristics are summarized in Table 1. Refer to Additional file 1: Table S1 for a list of educational and dietary interventions being received by participants.

Maximum tolerated dose and overall safety

There were no serious adverse events (SAEs) in any of the doses within the range tested (0.25 mg/kg, 0.5 mg/kg, and 0.75 mg/kg) and as such the maximum tolerated dose was determined to be 0.75 mg/kg once daily.

Overall, pioglitazone was well tolerated (see Table 2). Two participants discontinued intervention due to perceived non-efficacy and one due to the inability to tolerate interim blood work during the study. Adverse events (AEs) were of mild to moderate severity. Thirty-nine percent of the sample experienced upper respiratory tract infection (URTI). Three participants experienced mild neutropenia [see Additional file 1: Table S2 (a–c) for complete blood count results for each of these participants]. In one participant this was a pre-existing condition, in another it resolved while staying on medication, and in the third it only presented during the final visit and spontaneously recovered. As such, it was deemed to be unlikely related to the study intervention. BMI did not change significantly during the study [mean change 0.12; 95% confidence interval (− 0.03; 0.28) $p = 0.1$].

Preliminary evidence of efficacy

One participant had a response to placebo at week 2 and was removed from the statistical analyses. Results from the remaining participants showed statistically significant

Table 3 Change in outcome measures with treatment

	Estimate (95%CL)			Estimate (95%CL) *p* value	Effect size[d] pooled sd
	Baseline	Week 8	Week 16	Week 16–baseline	
n	27	25	25		
Social function					
ABC social withdrawal	10.1 (6.6; 13.7)	7.5 (4.8; 10.3)	6.7 (3.8; 9.6)	− 3.4 (− 5.3; 1.6) 0.0005*	− 0.43 7.96
SRS total[a]	88.4 (73.6; 103.2)	88.2 (78.9; 97.5)	85.8 (75.2; 96.4)	− 2.6 (− 17.2; 12.0) 0.7	− 0.09 29.29
Externalizing behaviors					
ABC irritability	13.8 (10.2; 17.4)	11.2 (8.3; 14.0)	10.0 (6.9; 13.0)	− 3.8 (− 6.3; − 1.3) 0.004*	− 0.46 8.27
ABC hyperactivity	21.7 (17.6; 25.7)	18.7 (14.9; 22.4)	16.5 (13.2; 19.7)	− 5.2 (− 7.8; − 2.6) 0.0003*	− 0.58 8.96
Anxiety					
BASC-2 anxiety[b]	8.9 (5.5; 12.2)	8.1 (5.3; 10.8)	8.2 (5.2; 11.3)	− 0.6 (− 2.8; 1.5) 0.6	− 0.08 7.76
CASI-4 generalized anxiety[c]	6.6 (5.1; 8.0)	5.4 (4.3; 6.6)	5.2 (4.0; 6.3)	− 1.4 (− 2.5; − 0.3) 0.02	− 0.44 3.16
CASI-4 social phobia[c]	2.4 (1.6; 3.3)	2.2 (1.4; 3.0)	1.6 (1.1; 2.1)	− 0.8 (− 1.5; − 0.2) 0.01	− 0.50 1.66
CASI-4 separation anxiety[c]	2.4 (1.3; 3.5)	1.8 (1.1; 2.6)	1.6 (0.8; 2.4)	− 0.8 (− 1.6; 0.1) 0.08	− 0.33 2.32
Repetitive behaviors					
RBSR total	33.0 (25.7; 40.3)	27.5 (20.6; 34.3)	24.5 (17.4; 31.5)	− 8.5 (− 13.3; − 3.7) 0.0009*	− 0.48 17.62
CY-BOCS[a]	12.6 (11.1; 14.2)	10.7 (9.4; 12.1)	9.4 (8.0; 10.9)	− 3.2 (− 4.4; − 2.0) < .0001*	− 0.90 3.54
Clinical global impression	% Responders: score of 1 or 2 (95%CL)				
	Week 8			Week 16	
n	25			27	
CGI social	20.3 (9.4; 38.2)			34.1 (18.6; 54.0)	
CGI global	26.0 (11.7; 48.1)			45.8 (27.8; 65.0)	

Score (95%CL) at each visit is estimated from a repeated measures linear model controlling for age; a planned contrast is used to estimate the change from baseline to week 16 from the model; model excludes one participant with a placebo response at week 2

[a] $n = 26$ at baseline and week 16

[b] $n = 24$ at week 8

[c] $n = 26$ at week 16; * = remains significant using Bonferroni adjusted level for significance of $p = 0.005$

[d] Week 16–baseline/pooled standard deviation where the pooled standard deviation is derived from the baseline and week 16 standard deviations obtained from the repeated measures model

changes in scores on global function, social function, irritability, hyperactivity, repetitive behaviors, and anxiety, although not on all measures (see Table 3, Additional file 1: Table S3, Figs. 2, 3, and 4). The outcome measures that remained statistically significant after using Bonferroni adjusted level for significance ($p = 0.05/10 = p \leq 0.005$) were ABC social withdrawal, irritability and hyperactivity, as well as CYBOCS and RBS-R total score. Effect size calculated using the pooled standard deviation ranged from medium to large (0.43 to 0.9) on these measures (see Table 3).

Cytokine levels

Cytokine levels in serum (IL-6) and plasma (TNF-α, IL-10, IL1-β) were measured at screening and week 16 visits. Two participants were removed from these analyses. The first was the placebo responder noted in the last section, and the second was an outlier in that cytokine levels were significantly higher than the rest of the cohort. One participant provided the second sample at week 8 due to early withdrawal from the study, and it was analyzed as a week 16 per a last observation carried forward approach in keeping with the intent-to-treat principle. Figure 5 shows the change in each cytokine value with pioglitazone treatment. Additional file 2: Figure S3 shows cytokine concentrations as measured pre and post-treatment with pioglitazone. Significant changes with treatment occurred with both IL-6 and IL-10 (mean change (Wilcoxon sign rank p value) IL6: − 1.6 ($p = 0.0006$); IL-10: 13.6 ($p = 0.03$)) (Table 4). IL-1β and TNF-α did not change significantly with treatment. We then looked at the association between the two cytokines showing significant change with continuous outcome measures that also showed a significant change with treatment: ABC-social withdrawal, irritability, and hyperactivity, CY-BOCS, and CASI-generalized anxiety and social phobia. Baseline IL-6 levels were significantly positively correlated (0.5, $p = 0.01$) with the change in CYBOCS scores over the course of the study, but change in IL-6 levels did not correlate with change for any of the outcome measures. Baseline IL-10 levels were not significantly correlated with the change in any of the outcome measures. Change in IL-10 levels with treatment was significantly positively correlated with change in ABC social withdrawal scores (0.44, $p = 0.05$) and showed a trend (0.41, $p = 0.06$) toward a positive correlation with change in CASI-social phobia score.

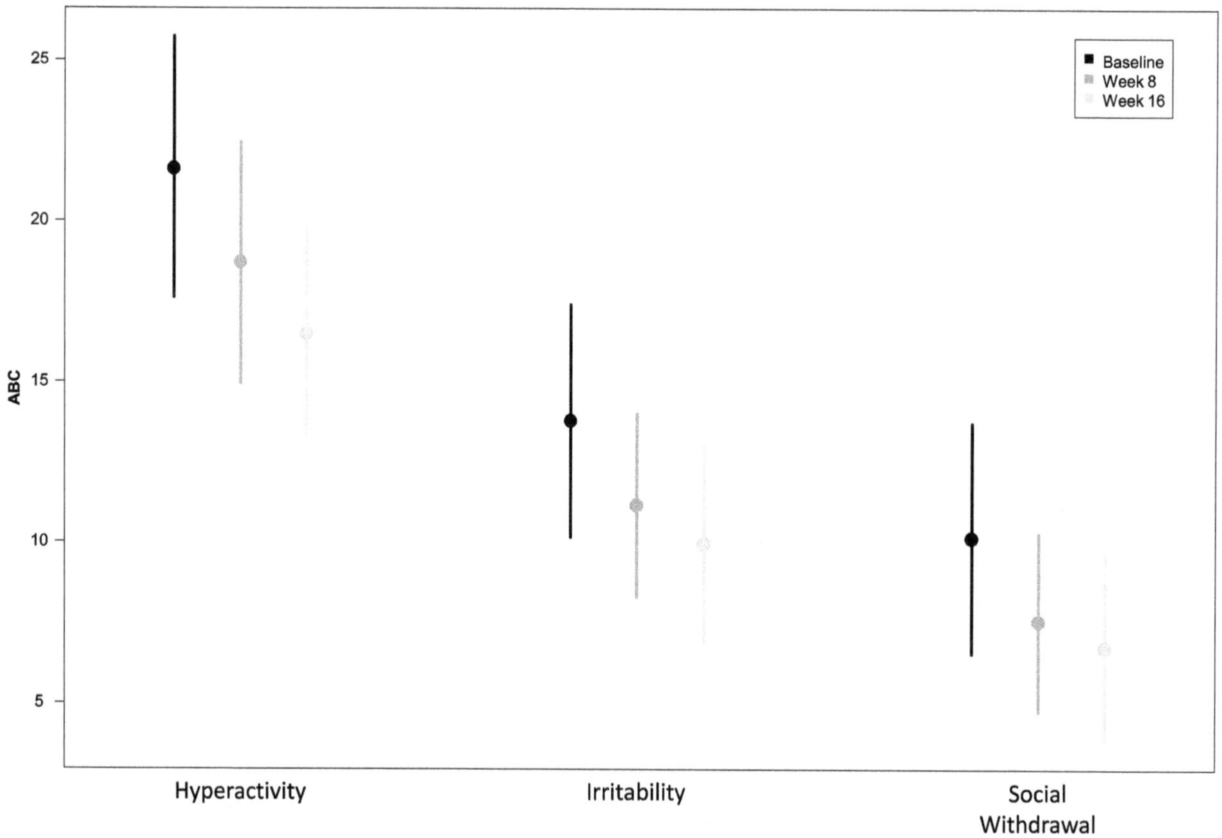

Fig. 2 Change in ABC subscales with treatment

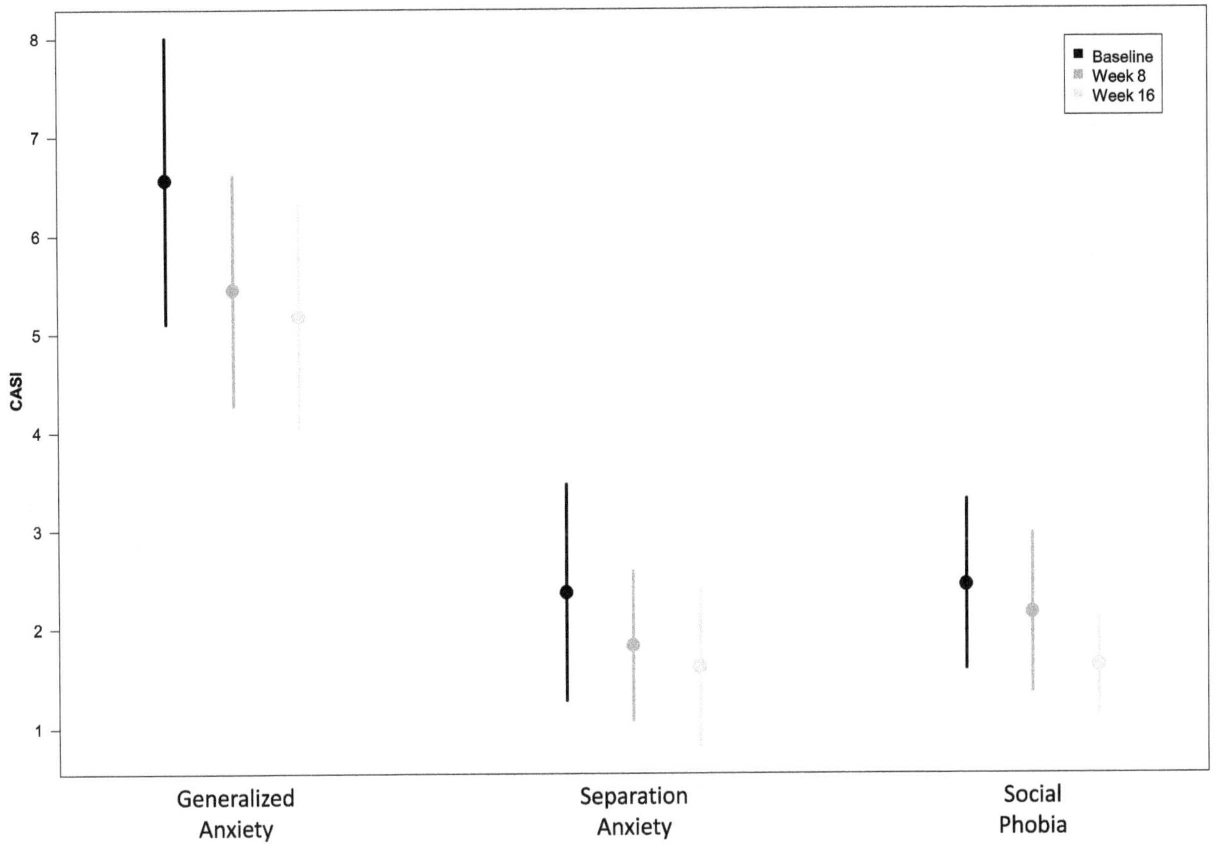

Fig. 3 Change in anxiety with treatment

Discussion

This study had three main objectives: Firstly, to identify the maximum tolerated dose of pioglitazone in autistic children within the range approved by Health Canada and the FDA. Secondly, to evaluate which of a number of outcome measures could best capture the therapeutic effect of pioglitazone in this population. Finally, to evaluate whether a biomarker, cytokine, levels in a peripheral blood sample significantly predict the effect of pioglitazone on outcome measures. The maximum tolerated dose of pioglitazone identified was 0.75 mg/kg in autistic children. No serious adverse events occurred at any of the three doses tested. None of the three participants with early termination dropped out due to adverse effects related to study drug, but rather related to perceived non-efficacy and an inability to tolerate study safety bloodwork. The most recent monograph of pioglitazone lists heart failure, hepatic insufficiency, and allergic reactions as significant side effects of pioglitazone. None of these side effects were observed in our study nor were they observed in either of the two previously published studies of pioglitazone in autistic children [36, 37]. Boris et al. [36] observed two incidents of slightly elevated white blood cell and glucose levels and three incidents of slightly elevated liver enzymes (ALT and AST), all resolved without intervention. Ghaleiha et al. [37] found that the most common adverse events were headache and vomiting, but the incidence was not statistically different between the pioglitazone group and the control group. A few studies have examined the safety and efficacy of pioglitazone and the related drug rosiglitazone (also a thiazolidinedione) in children and adolescents with diabetes and obesity and similarly found these drugs to be well tolerated [52–54]. Reported adverse events included transient elevation of liver enzymes, weight gain, edema, and hypoglycemia (only in rosiglitazone combined with metformin [52]). None of our participants experienced these adverse events. Three participants in our study experienced mild neutropenia, which was determined to be unlikely related given the time frame and course. Two cases of reversible neutropenia have been reported in adults with diabetes treated with pioglitazone [55, 56] and a retrospective study of 50 diabetic adults treated with pioglitazone showed a significant reduction in hemoglobin, hematocrit, platelets, and white blood cell count, compared to placebo suggesting a possible mild bone marrow suppressive effect of the drug

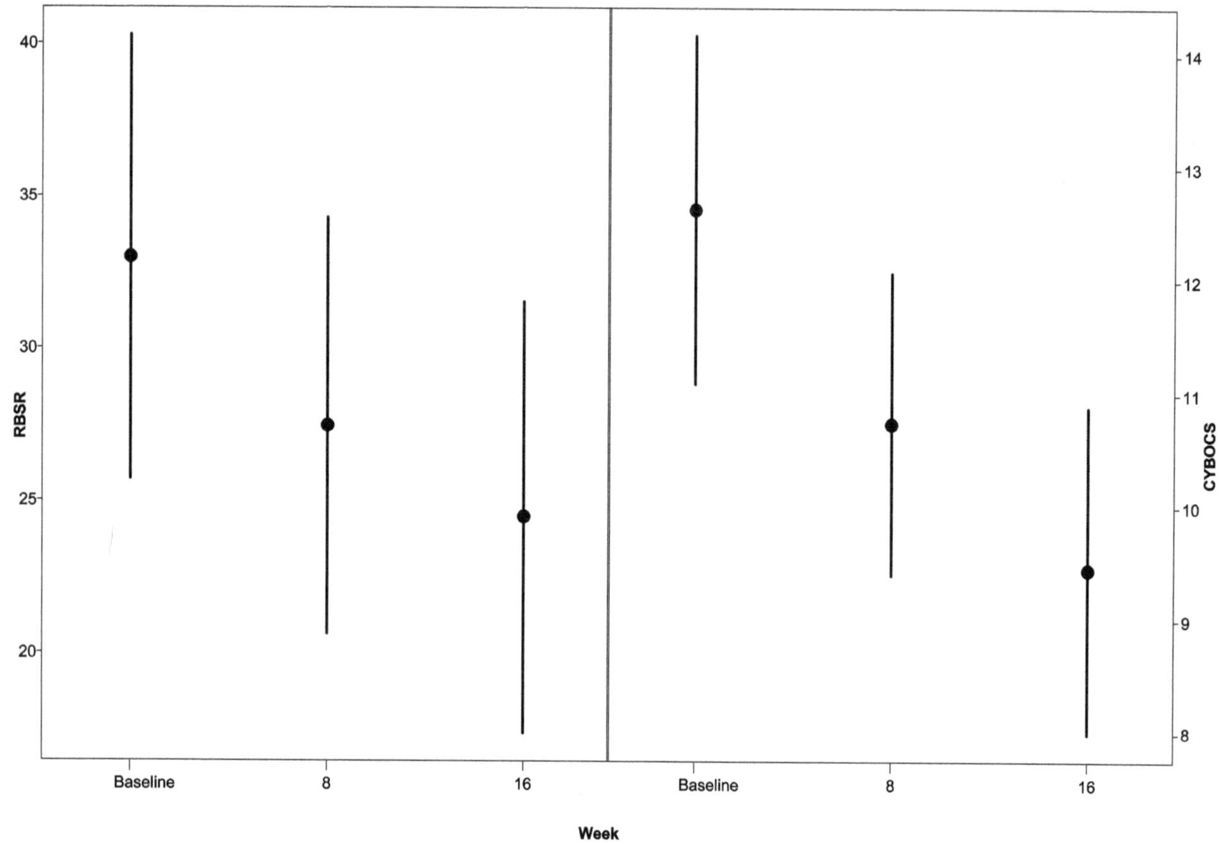

Fig. 4 Change in repetitive behavior with treatment

[57]. Therefore, future studies should carefully monitor complete blood counts of patients taking pioglitazone. Thirty-nine percent of our participants experienced upper respiratory tract infection (URTI). URTI occurs very commonly in children, and because we did not have a placebo-arm for comparison, it was unclear if pioglitazone further predisposes children to URTI. URTI is noted in the product monograph for pioglitazone as a common occurrence (occurring in > 1% to < 10% of adult patients). Placebo-controlled trials of pioglitazone in adolescents did not list URTI as a common adverse event [52–54]. Future placebo-controlled trials in children should monitor closely for a significant risk of URTI.

We used a number of outcome measures to evaluate the potential efficacy of pioglitazone in autistic children. Consistent with the prior two studies of pioglitazone in ASD, we found significant improvement in irritability, hyperactivity, and social withdrawal within the dose range approved by regulatory agencies, as measured by the ABC. In addition, we identified significant improvement in repetitive behaviors and anxiety as measured by the CY-BOCS, RBS-R, and CASI-4 anxiety scales. The ABC social withdrawal, irritability, and hyperactivity as well as CY-BOCS and RBS-R total score remained significant after correction for multiple comparisons. Improvement in repetitive behavior as measured by the CY-BOCS had a large effect size, while changes in the ABC social withdrawal, irritability, hyperactivity, and RBS-R (for repetitive behavior) had a medium effect size. Using the standard deviations of scores on the ABC social withdrawal, irritability and hyperactivity subscales taken from Brown et al. [58], and the standard deviations of the total scores of the RBS-R and CYBOCS taken from Lam and Aman [48] and Scahill et al. [59], respectively, we found that the ABC social withdrawal, irritability, and hyperactivity subscale scores as well as RBS-R total score were just shy of − 0.5 SD (with mean change of − 0.42 to − 0.49 SDs). The CYPBOCS showed a mean change of − 1.14 SD. This along with effect sizes calculated from our data suggest that pioglitazone has the largest signal for reduction of repetitive behavior as measured by the CYBOCS. Using the CGI-global and social, clinicians rated 46% of participants as significantly improved in global functioning and 34% significantly improved in social functioning. These findings require confirmation in a larger, randomized, double-blind, placebo-

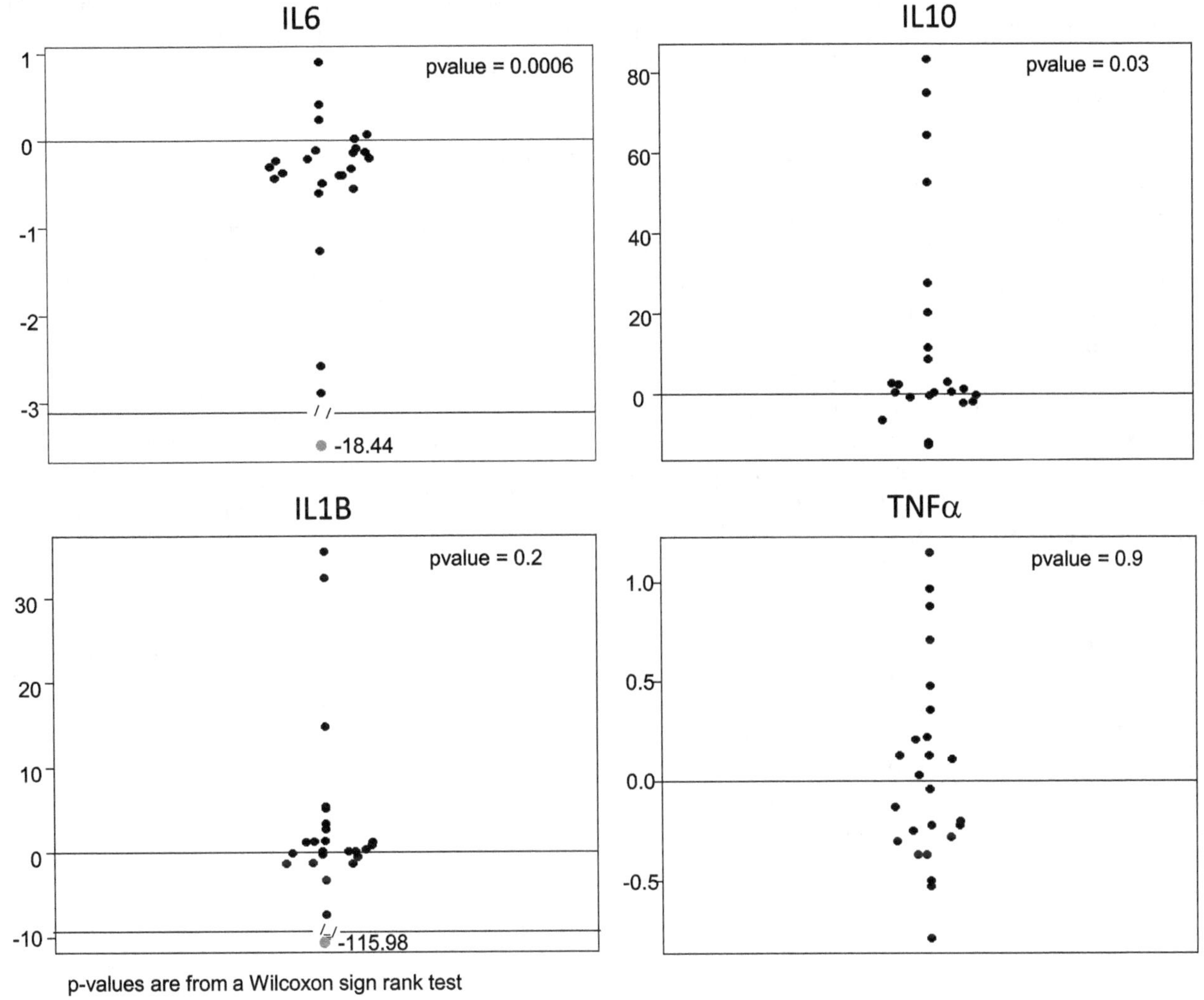

Fig. 5 Change in cytokine value with treatment

controlled study, but do provide preliminary evidence that pioglitazone may improve both core ASD symptoms and frequently associated symptoms.

The direction of change in cytokines in our study (decreasing IL-6 and increasing IL-10) is consistent with the known effect of PPAR-gamma agonists like pioglitazone [60]. It was expected that IL-1β and TNF-α would also decrease with treatment. This was not observed in our study and may relate to the small sample size. One study did not find that thiazolidinediones were able to suppress TNF-α and IL-6 in macrophages [61]. While baseline IL-6 levels were correlated with worse CYBOCS scores as expected, reduction of IL-6 with treatment was not correlated with outcome measures. Change in IL-10 with treatment was correlated with outcome measures but contrary to our expectations. This was contrary to expectation given studies such as one examining children with 22q11 deletion syndrome (at high risk of autism) that found that level of IL-1β in the blood, and the ratio of IL-6:IL10 in serum was significantly associated with social scores on the ADI-R [62]. This again may relate to the small sample size in our study. Alternatively, peripheral cytokine levels do not directly reflect cytokine levels in the CNS, nor do

Table 4 Cytokine levels measured at baseline and post-treatment

	Baseline		Post-treatment ($n = 26$)		p value
	Mean	s.d.	Mean	s.d.	
IL6 (pg/ml)	1.37	1.29	0.760	0.43	0.0006
IL1β (pg/ml)	13.5	34.8	14.4	20.3	> 0.05
TNF-α (pg/ml)	0.69	0.37	0.782	0.49	> 0.05
IL10 (pg/ml)	31.2	53.9	42.8	72.5	0.03

they reflect immune activation and inflammation in the CNS [4]. Pioglitazone is able to cross the blood-brain barrier and PPAR-ϒ is expressed in the following areas of CNS: mostly microglia and astrocytes, less so in hippocampal dentate gyrus, basal ganglia, thalamus, and piriform cortex [63–65]. Pioglitazone is able to inhibit the secretion of TNF-α, IL-1β, and IL-6 and enhance IL-10 secretion in mouse astrocytes [66]. Moreover, pioglitazone can affect mitochondrial biogenesis and reduce currents through the NMDA glutamate receptor, two alternative mechanisms that may be important in autism [31–35]. Such alternative mechanisms could explain the improvement seen on outcome measures during treatment with pioglitazone in our study, but without a direct correlate with peripheral cytokine levels. Given that IL-6 and IL-10 both changed as expected with pioglitazone treatment, it may be worth repeating these analyses in a larger study.

Limitations

This study had some important limitations to consider. Firstly, this study was primarily designed as a pilot maximum tolerated dose (MTD) study. The study used a single arm with no placebo control group with which to compare change in behavioral outcome measures and cytokine levels. Additionally, the sample size may be too small to detect cytokine change with treatment and to find an association with behavior outcome measures. A typically developing control group may help identify a subgroup of autistic children having abnormal cytokine levels and may more accurately demonstrate a relationship with outcome measures.

In summary, we identified 0.75 mg/kg of pioglitazone to be the maximum tolerated dose within the range allowed by Health Canada and the FDA using a MTD design. Pioglitazone was well tolerated with no serious adverse events identified. Pioglitazone demonstrated efficacy in improving both core (social withdrawal and repetitive behaviors) and associated (irritability, hyperactivity, and anxiety) autism symptoms and did significantly decrease the pro-inflammatory cytokine IL-6 and increase the anti-inflammatory cytokine IL-10. These findings indicate the need for a larger randomized controlled trial with potential emphasis on pioglitazone's efficacy in reducing repetitive behavior as measured by the CYBOCS, to replicate these promising findings.

Endnotes

[1]We acknowledge that there is no consensus within the community about whether to use identity-first (i.e. autistic individual) language, or person-first language (i.e. person with autism). We are choosing to use the term autistic individual in this paper, but respect both perspectives.

Abbreviations

ABC: Aberrant Behavior Checklist; ADI-R: Autism Diagnostic Interview-Revised; ADOS: Autism Diagnostic Observational Schedule; ASD: Autism spectrum disorder; BASC-2: Behavioral Assessment System for Children 2nd Edition; BLC: B-lymphocyte chemoattractant; CASI: Child and Adolescent Symptom Inventory; CGI-I: Clinician Global Impression scale-Improvement; CGI-S: Clinician Global Impression scale-Severity; Ckβ8.1: Chemokine-β8; CNS: Central nervous system; CSF: Cerebrospinal fluid; CY-BOCS: Child Yale-Brown Obsessive Compulsive Scale; DSM-5: Diagnostic and Statistical Manual of Mental Disorders 5th edition; DSM-IV-TR: Diagnostic and Statistical Manual of Mental Disorders 4th edition, text revision; ELIZA: Enzyme-linked immunosorbent assay; GCP: Good clinical practice; GFAP: Glial fibrillary acidic protein; GM-CSF: Granulocyte-macrophage colony stimulating factory; ICH: International Council for Harmonization; IFN-ϒ: Interferon-ϒ; IL: Interleukin; MCP: Macrophage chemoattractant protein; MDC: Macrophage-derived chemokine; MIG: Monokine induced by interferon-ϒ; MTD: Maximum tolerated dose; NAP-2: Neutrophil activating peptide-2; NMDA: N-methyl-D-aspartate; PET: Positron emission tomography; PPAR-ϒ: Peroxisome proliferator activated receptor - gamma; RBS-R: Repetitive Behavior Scale-Revised; SAE: Serious adverse event; SMURF: Safety Monitoring Uniform Report Form; SRS: Social Responsiveness Scale; TARC: Thymus activation-regulated chemokine; TGF-1β: Transforming growth factor-β1; TNF-α: Tumor necrosis factor-α; TZDs: Thiazolidinediones; URTI: Upper respiratory tract infection

Acknowledgements

None

Funding

Physician Services Incorporated, University of Toronto Dean's Fund.

Authors' contributions

LC: Contributed to acquisition of data, data analysis and interpretation, and complete drafting of the manuscript. AD: Contributed to data analysis and interpretation. JB: Contributed to project conception and design, data acquisition, and manuscript preparation. DM: Contributed to acquisition of data and manuscript preparation. LG: Contributed to acquisition of data and manuscript preparation. RHA: Contributed to acquisition of data and manuscript preparation. SS: Contributed to acquisition of data and manuscript preparation. TL: Contributed to acquisition of data and manuscript preparation. DO: Contributed to acquisition of data and manuscript preparation. JAF: Contributed to conception and design, data acquisition, data analysis and interpretation, and manuscript preparation. EA: Project conception and design, acquisition of data, data analysis and interpretation, manuscript preparation, and final approval of version to be published. All authors read and approved the final manuscript.

Competing interests

Dr. Evdokia Anagnostou has received consultation fees from Roche and Takeda; industry funding from SynapDx and Sanofi-Aventis; royalties from APPI and Springer International Publishing; editorial honorarium from Wiley; and other funding from the Canadian Institutes of Health Research, the Ontario Brain Institute, the Department of Defense, the National Institutes of Health (NIH), Brain Canada, Autism Speaks, the National Centers of Excellence, and Physician Services Incorporated.

Dr. Jane A. Foster has had work supported by Ontario Brain Institute (OBI) Grant Nos. NSERC (RGPIN-312435-12) and NSERC RTI (EQPEQ407645-2011) as well as an infrastructure grant from the Canada Foundation for Innovation and the Ontario Innovation Trust.
The remaining authors have no potential competing interests to disclose.

Author details

[1]Holland Bloorview Kids Rehabilitation Hospital, University of Toronto, 150 Kilgour Road, Toronto, ON M4G 1R8, Canada. [2]Sick Kids, University of Toronto, 555 University Avenue, Toronto, ON M5G 1X8, Canada. [3]Holland Bloorview Kids Rehabilitation Hospital, 150 Kilgour Road, Toronto, ON M4G 1R8, Canada. [4]St. Joseph's Health Care, McMaster University, 50 Charlton Avenue East, Hamilton, ON L8N 4A6, Canada.

References

1. Association AP. Diagnostic and statistical manual of mental disorders (DSM-5®). Arlington: American Psychiatric Publishing; 2013.
2. Baio J, Wiggins L, Christensen DL, Maenner MJ, Daniels J, Warren Z, Kurzius-Spencer M, Zahorodny W, Robinson Rosenberg C, White T, et al. Prevalence of autism spectrum disorder among children aged 8 years—autism and developmental disabilities monitoring network, 11 Sites, United States, 2014. MMWR Surveill Summ. 2018;67(6):1–23.
3. Nadeem A, Ahmad SF, Attia SM, Bakheet SA, Al-Harbi NO, Al-Ayadhi LY. Activation of IL-17 receptor leads to increased oxidative inflammation in peripheral monocytes of autistic children. Brain Behav Immun. 2018;67:335–44.
4. Pardo CA, Farmer CA, Thurm A, Shebl FM, Ilieva J, Kalra S, Swedo S. Serum and cerebrospinal fluid immune mediators in children with autistic disorder: a longitudinal study. Mol Autism. 2017;8:1.
5. Jyonouchi H, Geng L, Streck DL, Dermody JJ, Toruner GA. MicroRNA expression changes in association with changes in interleukin-1ss/interleukin10 ratios produced by monocytes in autism spectrum disorders: their association with neuropsychiatric symptoms and comorbid conditions (observational study). J Neuroinflammation. 2017;14(1):229.
6. Ahmad SF, Nadeem A, Ansari MA, Bakheet SA, Al-Ayadhi LY, Attia SM. Upregulation of IL-9 and JAK-STAT signaling pathway in children with autism. Prog Neuro-Psychopharmacol Biol Psychiatry. 2017;79(Pt B):472–80.
7. Al-Ayadhi LY, Mostafa GA. Elevated serum levels of interleukin-17A in children with autism. J Neuroinflammation. 2012;9:158.
8. Garay PA, McAllister AK. Novel roles for immune molecules in neural development: implications for neurodevelopmental disorders. Front Synaptic Neurosci. 2010;2:136.
9. Ashwood P, Wakefield AJ. Immune activation of peripheral blood and mucosal CD3+ lymphocyte cytokine profiles in children with autism and gastrointestinal symptoms. J Neuroimmunol. 2006;173(1–2):126–34.
10. Prata J, Santos SG, Almeida MI, Coelho R, Barbosa MA. Bridging autism spectrum disorders and schizophrenia through inflammation and biomarkers—pre-clinical and clinical investigations. J Neuroinflammation. 2017;14(1):179.
11. Pardo CA, Vargas DL, Zimmerman AW. Immunity, neuroglia and neuroinflammation in autism. Int Rev Psychiatry. 2005;17(6):485–95.
12. Vargas DL, Nascimbene C, Krishnan C, Zimmerman AW, Pardo CA. Neuroglial activation and neuroinflammation in the brain of patients with autism. Ann Neurol. 2005;57(1):67–81. Erratum appears in Ann Neurol. 2005 Feb;57(2):304
13. Zimmerman AW, Jyonouchi H, Comi AM, Connors SL, Milstien S, Varsou A, Heyes MP. Cerebrospinal fluid and serum markers of inflammation in autism. Pediatr Neurol. 2005;33(3):195–201.
14. Suzuki K, Sugihara G, Ouchi Y, Nakamura K, Futatsubashi M, Takebayashi K, Yoshihara Y, Omata K, Matsumoto K, Tsuchiya KJ. Microglial activation in young adults with autism spectrum disorder. JAMA Psychiatry. 2013;70(1):49–58.
15. Rodriguez JI, Kern JK. Evidence of microglial activation in autism and its possible role in brain underconnectivity. Neuron Glia Biol. 2011;7(2–4):205–13.
16. Ashwood P, Enstrom A, Krakowiak P, Hertz-Picciotto I, Hansen RL, Croen LA, Ozonoff S, Pessah IN, Van de Water J. Decreased transforming growth factor beta1 in autism: a potential link between immune dysregulation and impairment in clinical behavioral outcomes. J Neuroimmunol. 2008;204(1–2):149–53.
17. Ashwood P, Anthony A, Torrente F, Wakefield AJ. Spontaneous mucosal lymphocyte cytokine profiles in children with autism and gastrointestinal symptoms: mucosal immune activation and reduced counter regulatory interleukin-10. J Clin Immunol. 2004;24(6):664–73.
18. D'Mello C, Swain MG. Immune-to-brain communication pathways in inflammation-associated sickness and depression. Curr Top Behav Neurosci. 2017;31:73–94.
19. McCusker RH, Kelley KW. Immune-neural connections: how the immune system's response to infectious agents influences behavior. J Exp Biol. 2013;216(Pt 1):84–98.
20. Masi A, Quintana DS, Glozier N, Lloyd AR, Hickie IB, Guastella AJ. Cytokine aberrations in autism spectrum disorder: a systematic review and meta-analysis. Mol Psychiatry. 2015;20(4):440–6.
21. Masi A, Glozier N, Dale R, Guastella AJ. The immune system, cytokines, and biomarkers in autism spectrum disorder. Neurosci Bull. 2017;33(2):194–204.
22. Goines P, Van de Water J. The immune system's role in the biology of autism. Curr Opin Neurol. 2010;23(2):111–7.
23. Bryn V, Aass HC, Skjeldal OH, Isaksen J, Saugstad OD, Ormstad H. Cytokine profile in autism spectrum disorders in children. J Mol Neurosci. 2017;61(1):1–7.
24. Ashwood P, Krakowiak P, Hertz-Picciotto I, Hansen R, Pessah I, Van de Water J. Elevated plasma cytokines in autism spectrum disorders provide evidence of immune dysfunction and are associated with impaired behavioral outcome. Brain Behav Immun. 2011;25(1):40–5.
25. Tsilioni I, Taliou A, Francis K, Theoharides TC. Children with autism spectrum disorders, who improved with a luteolin-containing dietary formulation, show reduced serum levels of TNF and IL-6. Transl Psychiatry. 2015;5:e647.
26. Hashim H, Abdelrahman H, Mohammed D, Karam R. Association between plasma levels of transforming growth factor-β1, IL-23 and IL-17 and the severity of autism in Egyptian children. Res Autism Spectr Disord. 2013;7(1):199–204.
27. Landreth GE, Heneka MT. Anti-inflammatory actions of peroxisome proliferator-activated receptor gamma agonists in Alzheimer's disease. Neurobiol Aging. 2001;22(6):937–44.
28. Liu HR, Tao L, Gao E, Lopez BL, Christopher TA, Willette RN, Ohlstein EH, Yue TL, Ma XL. Anti-apoptotic effects of rosiglitazone in hypercholesterolemic rabbits subjected to myocardial ischemia and reperfusion. Cardiovasc Res. 2004;62(1):135–44.
29. Schutz B, Reimann J, Dumitrescu-Ozimek L, Kappes-Horn K, Landreth GE, Schurmann B, Zimmer A, Heneka MT. The oral antidiabetic pioglitazone protects from neurodegeneration and amyotrophic lateral sclerosis-like symptoms in superoxide dismutase-G93A transgenic mice. J Neurosci. 2005;25(34):7805–12.
30. Wu ZH, Zhao SP, Chu LX, Ye HJ. Pioglitazone reduces tumor necrosis factor-alpha serum concentration and mRNA expression of adipose tissue in hypercholesterolemic rabbits. Int J Cardiol. 2010;138(2):151–6.
31. Almasi-Nasrabadi M, Javadi-Paydar M, Mahdavian S, Babaei R, Sharifian M, Norouzi A, Dehpour AR. Involvement of NMDA receptors in the beneficial effects of pioglitazone on scopolamine-induced memory impairment in mice. Behav Brain Res. 2012;231(1):138–45.
32. Ghosh S, Patel N, Rahn D, McAllister J, Sadeghi S, Horwitz G, Berry D, Wang KX, Swerdlow RH. The thiazolidinedione pioglitazone alters mitochondrial function in human neuron-like cells. Mol Pharmacol. 2007;71(6):1695–702.
33. Siddiqui MF, Elwell C, Johnson MH. Mitochondrial dysfunction in autism spectrum disorders. Autism Open Access. 2016;6(5):27.
34. Lee EJ, Choi SY, Kim E. NMDA receptor dysfunction in autism spectrum disorders. Curr Opin Pharmacol. 2015;20:8–13.
35. Rossignol DA, Frye RE. Mitochondrial dysfunction in autism spectrum disorders: a systematic review and meta-analysis. Mol Psychiatry. 2012;17(3):290–314.
36. Boris M, Kaiser CC, Goldblatt A, Elice MW, Edelson SM, Adams JB, Feinstein DL. Effect of pioglitazone treatment on behavioral symptoms in autistic children. J Neuroinflammation. 2007;4:3.
37. Ghaleiha A, Rasa SM, Nikoo M, Farokhnia M, Mohammadi MR, Akhondzadeh S. A pilot double-blind placebo-controlled trial of pioglitazone as adjunctive treatment to risperidone: effects on aberrant behavior in children with autism. 2015;229(1-2):181–87.
38. Association AP. DSM-IV-TR: diagnostic and statistical manual of mental disorders, text revision. Washington, DC: American Psychiatric Association; 2000. p. 75.

39. Lord C, Rutter M, Goode S, Heemsbergen J, Jordan H, Mawhood L, Schopler E. Autism diagnostic observation schedule: a standardized observation of communicative and social behavior. J Autism Dev Disord. 1989;19(2):185–212.
40. Gotham K, Risi S, Pickles A, Lord C. The autism diagnostic observation schedule: revised algorithms for improved diagnostic validity. J Autism Dev Disord. 2007;37(4):613–27.
41. Lord C, Rutter M, DiLavore PC, Risi S, Gotham K, Guthrie W, Bishop SL. Autism diagnostic observation schedule, second edition (ADOS-2) manual (part I): modules 1 - 4. Torrance: Western Psychological Services; 2012.
42. Lord C, Rutter M, Le Couteur A. Autism diagnostic interview-revised: a revised version of a diagnostic interview for caregivers of individuals with possible pervasive developmental disorders. J Autism Dev Disord. 1994; 24(5):659–85.
43. Guy W. ECDEU assessment manual for psychopharmacology, revised. Rockville: US Dept. of Health, Education, and Welfare. Public Health Service, Alcohol, Drug Abuse, and Mental Health Administration, National Institute of Mental Health, Psychopharmacology Research Branch, Division of Extramural Research Programs; 1976.
44. Goodman WK, Price LH, Rasmussen SA, Mazure C, Fleischmann RL, Hill CL, Heninger GR, Charney DS. The Yale-Brown obsessive compulsive scale: I. Development, use, and reliability. Arch Gen Psychiatry. 1989;46(11):1006–11.
45. Scahill L, Riddle MA, McSwiggin-Hardin M, Ort SI, King RA, Goodman WK, Cicchetti D, Leckman JF. Children's Yale-Brown obsessive compulsive scale: reliability and validity. J Am Acad Child Adolesc Psychiatry. 1997;36(6):844–52.
46. Aman MG, Singh NN, Stewart AW, Field CJ. The aberrant behavior checklist: a behavior rating scale for the assessment of treatment effects. Am J Ment Defic. 1985;89(5):485–91.
47. Constantino JN, Gruber CP. Social responsiveness scale (SRS). Torrance: Western Psychological Services; 2012.
48. Lam KS, Aman MG. The repetitive behavior scale-revised: independent validation in individuals with autism spectrum disorders. J Autism Dev Disord. 2007;37(5):855–66.
49. Reynolds CR, Kamphaus R. BASC-2: behavior assessment system for children. 2nd ed. Upper Saddle River: Pearson Education, Inc.; 2006.
50. Sukhodolsky DG, Scahill L, Gadow KD, Arnold LE, Aman MG, McDougle CJ, McCracken JT, Tierney E, Williams White S, Lecavalier L. Parent-rated anxiety symptoms in children with pervasive developmental disorders: frequency and association with core autism symptoms and cognitive functioning. J Abnorm Child Psychol. 2008;36(1):117–28.
51. Greenhill LL, Vitiello B, Fisher P, Levine J, Davies M, Abikoff H, Chrisman AK, Chuang S, Findling RL, March J, et al. Comparison of increasingly detailed elicitation methods for the assessment of adverse events in pediatric psychopharmacology. J Am Acad Child Adolesc Psychiatry. 2004;43(12): 1488–96.
52. Group TS, Zeitler P, Hirst K, Pyle L, Linder B, Copeland K, Arslanian S, Cuttler L, Nathan DM, Tollefsen S, et al. A clinical trial to maintain glycemic control in youth with type 2 diabetes. N Engl J Med. 2012;366(24):2247–56.
53. Tafuri KS, Godil MA, Lane AH, Wilson TA. Effect of pioglitazone on the course of new-onset type 1 diabetes mellitus. J Clin Res Pediatr Endocrinol. 2013;5(4):236–9.
54. Zdravkovic V, Hamilton JK, Daneman D, Cummings EA. Pioglitazone as adjunctive therapy in adolescents with type 1 diabetes. J Pediatr. 2006; 149(6):845–9.
55. Digman C, Klein AK, Pittas AG. Leukopenia and thrombocytopenia caused by thiazolidinediones. Ann Intern Med. 2005;143(6):465–6.
56. Karakurt F, Kargili A, Kasapoglu B. Pioglitazone induced reversible pancytopenia. Exp Clin Endocrinol Diabetes. 2010;118(2):96–7.
57. Berria R, Glass L, Mahankali A, Miyazaki Y, Monroy A, De Filippis E, Cusi K, Cersosimo E, Defronzo RA, Gastaldelli A. Reduction in hematocrit and hemoglobin following pioglitazone treatment is not hemodilutional in type II diabetes mellitus. Clin Pharmacol Ther. 2007;82(3):275–81.
58. Brown EC, Aman MG, Havercamp SM. Factor analysis and norms for parent ratings on the aberrant behavior checklist-community for young people in special education. Res Dev Disabil. 2002;23(1):45–60.
59. Scahill L, Sukhodolsky DG, Anderberg E, Dimitropoulos A, Dziura J, Aman MG, McCracken J, Tierney E, Hallett V, Katz K, et al. Sensitivity of the modified Children's Yale-Brown obsessive compulsive scale to detect change: results from two multi-site trials. Autism. 2016;20(2):145–52.
60. Jiang C, Ting AT, Seed B. PPAR-gamma agonists inhibit production of monocyte inflammatory cytokines. Nature. 1998;391(6662):82–6.
61. Thieringer R, Fenyk-Melody JE, Le Grand CB, Shelton BA, Detmers PA, Somers EP, Carbin L, Moller DE, Wright SD, Berger J. Activation of peroxisome proliferator-activated receptor gamma does not inhibit IL-6 or TNF-alpha responses of macrophages to lipopolysaccharide in vitro or in vivo. J Immunol. 2000;164(2):1046–54.
62. Ross HE, Guo Y, Coleman K, Ousley O, Miller AH. Association of IL-12p70 and IL-6:IL-10 ratio with autism-related behaviors in 22q11.2 deletion syndrome: a preliminary report. Brain Behav Immun. 2013;31:76–81.
63. Braissant O, Foufelle F, Scotto C, Dauca M, Wahli W. Differential expression of peroxisome proliferator-activated receptors (PPARs): tissue distribution of PPAR-alpha, -beta, and -gamma in the adult rat. Endocrinology. 1996;137(1): 354–66.
64. Moreno S, Farioli-Vecchioli S, Ceru MP. Immunolocalization of peroxisome proliferator-activated receptors and retinoid X receptors in the adult rat CNS. Neuroscience. 2004;123(1):131–45.
65. Bernardo A, Levi G, Minghetti L. Role of the peroxisome proliferator-activated receptor-gamma (PPAR-gamma) and its natural ligand 15-deoxy-Delta12, 14-prostaglandin J2 in the regulation of microglial functions. Eur J Neurosci. 2000;12(7):2215–23.
66. Qiu D, Li XN. Pioglitazone inhibits the secretion of proinflammatory cytokines and chemokines in astrocytes stimulated with lipopolysaccharide. Int J Clin Pharmacol Ther. 2015;53(9):746–52.

13

Autism-associated CHD8 deficiency impairs axon development and migration of cortical neurons

Qiong Xu[1,3†], Yuan-yuan Liu[2†], Xiaoming Wang[3], Guo-he Tan[2], Hui-ping Li[1], Samuel W. Hulbert[4], Chun-yang Li[1], Chun-chun Hu[1], Zhi-qi Xiong[5,6], Xiu Xu[1*] and Yong-hui Jiang[3,4,7,8*]

Abstract

Background: Mutations in *CHD8*, chromodomain helicase DNA-binding protein 8, are among the most replicated and common findings in genetic studies of autism spectrum disorder (ASD). The CHD8 protein is believed to act as a transcriptional regulator by remodeling chromatin structure and recruiting histone H1 to target genes. The mechanism by which deficiency of CHD8 causes ASD has not been fully elucidated.

Methods: We examined the expression of *CHD8* in human and mouse brains using both immunohistochemistry and RNA in situ hybridization. We performed in utero electroporation, neuronal culture, and biochemical analysis using RNAi to examine the functional consequences of *CHD8* deficiency.

Results: We discovered that CHD8 is expressed highly in neurons and at low levels in glia cells in both humans and mice. Specifically, CHD8 is localized predominately in the nucleus of both MAP2 and parvalbumin-positive neurons. In the developing mouse brain, expression of *Chd8* peaks from E16 to E18 and then decreases significantly at P14 to adulthood. Knockdown of *Chd8* results in reduced axon and dendritic growth, disruption of axon projections to the contralateral cortex, and delayed neuronal migration at E18.5 which recovers by P3 and P7.

Conclusion: Our findings indicate an important role for CHD8 in dendritic and axon development and neuronal migration and thus offer novel insights to further dissect the underlying molecular and circuit mechanisms of ASD caused by CHD8 deficiency.

Keywords: CHD8, Autism spectrum disorder (ASD), Chromatin remodeling, Neurite growth, Neurodevelopment

Background

Autism spectrum disorder (ASD) is a group of clinically and molecularly heterogeneous neurodevelopmental conditions characterized by social communication deficits and restricted, repetitive behaviors [1, 2]. Genetic etiology has been implicated in approximately 20% of ASD patients. More than 70 genes or genomic loci have been confirmed as causative, and hundreds are considered strong candidates [3–12]. Of these, mutations in *CHD8* are among the most replicated and commonly identified genetic findings [6, 7, 13, 14].

CHD8 is a member of the chromodomain helicase DNA-binding protein family, which functions as an ATP-dependent chromatin remodeling factor and plays important roles in chromatin dynamics, transcription, and cell survival [15]. CHD8 is initially identified as a negative regulator of the Wnt–catenin signaling pathway through promoting the association of β-catenin and histone H1 and forming a trimeric complex on chromatin [16–18]. Accordingly, Wnt–β-catenin signaling was downregulated in *Chd8* mutant mice [18]. Homozygous deletion of *Chd8* in mice results in early embryonic lethality as a consequence of massive apoptosis in some lines of mutant mice [19, 20]. Haploinsufficiency of *CHD8* causes abnormal activation of RE-1 silencing

* Correspondence: xuxiu@fudan.edu.cn; yong-hui.jiang@duke.edu
†Qiong Xu and Yuan-yuan Liu contributed equally to this work.
[1]Department of Child Health Care, Children's Hospital of Fudan University, Shanghai 201102, China
[3]Department of Pediatrics, Duke University School of Medicine, Durham 27710, NC, USA

transcription factor (REST), which suppresses the transcription of many neuronal genes. Moreover, CHD8 interacts physically with REST in the mouse brain [21]. Knockdown of *Chd8* by RNAi during cortical development results in defective neural progenitor proliferation, differentiation, and enhanced migration [18, 22]. Deficiency of *Chd8* in mice also alters synaptic transmission in striatal circuitry and results in functional over-connectivity in cortical networks [23]. Interestingly, a recent report also shows sexually dimorphic phenotypes related to abnormal neuronal excitation, enhanced inhibitory synaptic transmission and neuronal firing, and gene dysregulation in a new line of *Chd8* mutant mice [24]. Conditional knockout of *Chd8* in oligodendrocytes results in defective myelination in mice [25]. However, whether CHD8 deficiency affects axonal growth has not been studied.

Here, we report that CHD8 is specifically expressed in both excitatory and inhibitory neurons and to a lesser extent in GFAP+ astrocytes of cerebral cortex in human and mouse brains. Similar to a previous report, we found that the expression of *Chd8* peaks during embryonic development and decreases to relatively low levels postnatally in mouse brains [22]. *Chd8* deficiency in neocortex by RNAi using in utero electroporation resulted in delayed migration of cortical neurons and impaired dendritic and axonal growth. Our findings provide additional insights into the molecular and circuitry mechanisms underlying ASD caused by CHD8 deficiency. Defective axonal development may support a mechanism underlying the abnormal long distance connectivity reported in neuroimaging studies of ASD in humans.

Methods

Immunostaining of human brain sections

For light microscopic immunohistochemistry (IHC), human brain sections (30 μm) were incubated in 0.01 M phosphate-buffered saline (PBS) supplemented with 3% hydrogen peroxide for 10 min to block endogenous peroxidase and then in a blocking buffer containing 5% BSA/10% normal goat serum/0.25% Triton X-100 for 60 min at room temperature to prevent nonspecific staining. Following this, IHC was conducted on these free-floating sections and staining was visualized with a standard ABC Elite kit (Vector Labs).

For confocal microscopic double-labeling immunofluorescence, brain sections were incubated in the blocking buffer for 60 min at room temperature and then in a solution containing primary antibodies from different species simultaneously for one night at 4 °C. After washing, sections were incubated with appropriate secondary antibodies from Alexa Fluor series (Invitrogen, USA) for 45 min at 37 °C and then counterstained with Hoechst 33342 (1:5000; #C10022, Beyotime) for 15 min at room temperature to identify cellular nuclei. After mounting the sections, we observed them under a fluorescent confocal microscope (A1R Nikon).

Primary antibodies used were as follows: anti-CHD8 (1: 500; catalog #A301-225A; Bethyl Laboratories, Inc.), anti-GFAP (1:1000, catalog #MAB3402, Millipore), anti-MAP2 (1:2000, catalog #M9942, Sigma), anti-parvalbumin (Pvalb) (1:500, catalog #MAB1572, Millipore), and anti-DCX antibodies (1:200, catalog #Sc-8066, Santa Cruz).

For Nissl staining, Neuro Trace 500/525 green fluorescent Nissl stain (N21480) was bought from Thermo Fisher Scientific and used according to the manufacture's instruction.

Confocal microscopic double-labeling immunofluorescence of mouse brain slices

Mice were sacrificed by cervical dislocation at postnatal day 3 (P3) or P7. Their brains were removed and fixed in 4% (wt/vol) paraformaldehyde (PFA) overnight. After sequential dehydration in 15% and 30% sucrose at 4 °C, 50-μm coronal brain sections were cut with a cryostat, fixed in 4% PFA for 20 min at 4 °C, washed three times with PBS, blocked with 5% BSA and 0.3% Triton X-100 in PBS for 1 h at room temperature, and then incubated with rabbit anti-GFP (1:1000, catalog #A11122, Invitrogen) primary antibody overnight at 4 °C. The rinsed sections were then incubated with Alexa 488-conjugated goat anti-rabbit secondary antibody (1:3000; catalog #A-11122; Invitrogen) for 2 h at 37 °C. For endogenous CHD8 and NeuN immunostaining, sections were incubated with anti-CHD8 antibody (1: 500; catalog #A301-225A; Bethyl Laboratories, Inc.) and anti-NeuN antibody (1:500; catalog # MAB377; Millipore).

Cultured neurons were fixed with 4%PFA and then immunostained with primary antibodies against GFAP (1:1000, catalog #MAB3402, Millipore), MAP2 (1:2000, catalog #M9942, Sigma), and Tau1 (1:3000, catalog #MAB3420, Millipore) overnight at 4 °C. After washing, sections were then incubated with Alexa 488-conjugated goat anti-rabbit secondary antibody (1:3000, catalog #A-11122, Invitrogen) and Alexa 568-conjugated goat anti-mouse secondary antibody (1:2000, catalog #A-11004, Invitrogen) for 2 h at 37 °C.

RNA extraction and real-time PCR

Forebrain tissues from embryonic or postnatal mice (C57BL/6) at different developmental stages (E16, E18, P0, P7, P14, P21, and adult) were used for RNA extraction. Mice were anesthetized with sodium pentobarbital and sacrificed via cervical dislocation, and brain tissues were quickly removed, dissected on ice, and homogenized with TRIzol Reagent (Invitrogen) at 4 °C. RNA was extracted according to the recommendations of the manufacturer, the final RNA pellet was suspended in diethylpyrocarbonate (DEPC)-treated water, and 2 μg of total mRNA was further subjected to reverse transcription using oligo (dT) primers and Moloney murine leukemia virus (M-MLV) transcriptase (Invitrogen). Real-time PCR was done with a LightCycler 480 Real-Time PCR System (Roche) according to the manufacturer's instructions. Starting RNA levels were quantified by using GAPDH as the external standard. Primer sets were chosen from Primerbank, and gene sequences are available from the GenBank database. The primer sequences to examine the mRNA expression of mouse *Chd8* were as follows: forward, 5′-AAGCCCAGGTAACTCAAC-3′; reverse, 5′-TTCACATCGTCGGCGTCT-3′; GAPDH: forward, 5′-GGTTGTCTCCTGCGACTTCA-3′; reverse, 5′-CCACCACCCTGTTGCTGTAG-3′. The primers were synthesized by Invitrogen.

RNA in situ hybridization

RNA in situ hybridization on the mouse brain sections was performed with digoxigenin (DIG)-labeled RNA probes. Full-length cDNA of *Chd8* was amplified with specific PCR primers and cloned into a pGEM-T easy vector (Promega) to generate an antisense probe for *Chd8*. The DIG-labeled antisense probes were synthesized by in vitro transcription using SP6 RNA polymerase. Mice of different developmental stages were perfused with 4% PFA, and fixed brains were sectioned into 20-μm slices using a cryostat. RNA in situ hybridization was performed as described previously [26]. Brain sections were hybridized for 18 h at 60 °C. The hybridization signal was detected with anti-DIG–alkaline phosphatase Fab fragments (Roche) and nitro blue tetrazolium chloride (NBT) plus 5-bromo-4-chlor-indolyl-phosphate (BCIP) as color reaction substrates.

Human *CHD8* cloning and mouse shRNA construct preparation

Human *CHD8* cDNA (*CHD8*, variant 1 - HaloTag® human ORF in pFN21A) was purchased by Promega (catalog: FHC12740). PCR products were cloned into the pCAGGS-IRES-EGFP vector [27]. Oligonucleotides targeting different sequences of mouse *Chd8* cDNA and a scrambled control oligonucleotide were designed, synthesized, and cloned into pSuper-basic (Oligoengine). The 21-bp target sequences were as follows: shRNA#1, 5′-GCT GGT GGA CTT GGT ATT AAT-3′; shRNA#2, 5′-GCT GCT GAT ACC TGT ATT ATC-3′; shRNA#3, 5′-GCT ACA AGA GAG AAC AAA TGA-3′; and shRNA-scramble, 5′-TTC TCC GAA CGT GTC ACG T-3′. All constructs were verified by DNA sequencing.

Western blot analysis

For the analysis of the expression of CHD8 in the developing mouse cortex, cortices were dissected and homogenized as previously described [28]. For knockdown and rescue experiments, electroporated cortical neurons were cultured for 3–7 days and lysed in 1× protein loading buffer (50 mM Tris-HCl, pH 6.8, 2% SDS, 10% glycerol, 1% 2-ME, and 0.1% bromophenol blue). All protein samples were separated by 10% SDS-polyacrylamide gel electrophoresis (Bio-Rad) and blotted onto PVDF membrane (Millipore). Membranes were blocked with 5% non-fat milk in 0.05% Tween 20 at room temperature for 1 h and probed with rabbit anti-CHD8 (Bethyl Laboratories, Inc.), HRP-coupled mouse anti-actin (Santa Cruz Biotechnology) antibodies. The secondary antibody used for CHD8 was goat anti-rabbit IgG coupled to HRP (Santa Cruz biotechnology). Bands were visualized by enhanced chemiluminescence (TIANGEN). Band intensities were measured with ImageJ Software.

Primary neuron culture and electroporation

Primary cortical neurons were prepared from brains of P0 C57 mice as described previously [28]. Before plating, neurons suspended in transfection medium (200 μl) were mixed with 1 μg pCAG-EGFP and 3 μg shRNA for immunocytochemistry. Then, neurons were transferred into a 2.0-mm electroporation cuvette (Fisher) and transfected by electroporation using the Amaxa Nucleofector apparatus.

In utero electroporation

In utero electroporation was performed as described previously with a few modifications [27]. Briefly, pregnant mice at E14.5 were anesthetized with 0.7% sodium pentobarbital at a dose of 10 μl/g and subjected to abdominal incision to expose the uterus. For different experiments, a mixture of GFP, RNAi, and/or rescue constructs was prepared. Plasmids (about 1 μl) with 0.05% Fast Green (Sigma) were injected into the lateral ventricle of embryos through a glass micropipette. Electrical pulses were then delivered to embryos by gently clasping their heads with forcep-shaped electrodes connected to an ECM-830 square-pulse generator (BTX). Five 50-ms pulses of 30 V were applied at 1-s intervals. Uterine horns were repositioned in the abdominal cavity, and the abdominal wall and the skin were sutured. Postsurgery animals were maintained in a warm animal room (25 °C) with plenty of water and food. At different developmental stages, mice were perfused transcardially with 0.9% saline followed by 4% PFA in 0.1 M phosphate buffer (PB; pH 7.4), and the brains were removed and fixed in 4% PFA for another 24 h. Fixed brains were cryoprotected with 30% sucrose and then sectioned using a cryostat.

Image acquisition and quantification

Images were obtained with a Nikon A1R inverted confocal microscope with × 20 (numerical aperture, 0.7) objectives. Each image was a composite constructed from a series of images taken throughout the *z* aspect of the neuron. Images of isolated cells or cortical neurons in regions with a low density of GFP transfected cells were chosen for illustration, and three-dimensional (3D) reconstructions were made to trace dendritic or axonal arbors for measurement of total dendritic or axonal length. Neurolucida software (MBF Bioscience) was used to generate tracings to measure neurite lengths. Sholl analysis, a quantitative analysis by counting the number of neurite intersections of concentric circles of gradually increased radius centered at the cell body, was performed with Neurolucida Explorer (MBF Bioscience). Image acquisition and data analysis were performed in a double-blind manner.

Statistical analysis

For all statistical analyses, experimenters were blinded for genotypes of mice and the treatments of the animals or cells. Data are presented as mean ± SEM. The paired or unpaired Student's *t* test, one-way ANOVA with Dunnett's post hoc tests or Bonferroni's tests, or two-way ANOVA with Bonferroni post hoc tests were used for data analyses by SPSS 13.0 software. Statistical significance was defined as $P < 0.05$.

Animals

Except in utero electroporation, for which ICR mice were used, all other experiments were performed in C57BL/6 J mice. Pregnant mice undergoing in utero electroporation were individually housed in plastic cages, and when they delivered, they were housed with their pups.

Human brain tissues

Frozen postmortem brain tissues of Brodmann 19 region from a 6-year-old child was obtained from the NIH human brain tissue bank at the University of Maryland (http://www.medschool.umaryland.edu/btbank/). The postmortem time was 19 h.

Results

CHD8 is predominantly expressed in neurons of human cerebral cortex

To probe the function of CHD8 and its pathophysiology underlying ASD, we first examined the expression pattern of CHD8 in a human brain sample. We performed immunohistological analysis using postmortem brain tissue (Brodmann 19) of a 6-year-old child. Strong staining of CHD8 was revealed in cerebral cortex (Fig. 1a). CHD8 was highly expressed in Neuro Trace Nissl stain-positive neurons but to a lesser extent in GFAP-positive glia cells (Fig. 1b, c). Consistent with the known function of CHD8 as a chromatin regulator, immunofluorescent staining showed that CHD8 was predominantly localized in the nucleus (Fig. 1b, f). Co-staining of CHD8 and neuronal markers showed that CHD8 was expressed in both MAP2-positive excitatory neurons (Fig. 1d) and parvalbumin (Pvalb)-positive interneurons (Fig. 1e). Moreover, CHD8 was expressed in Doublecortin (DCX)-positive neuronal precursor cells and immature neurons (Fig. 1f), which is consistent with the early onset of clinical manifestations in patients with *CHD8* mutations.

Chd8 is highly expressed in the developing mouse brain

Next, we examined the expression pattern of *Chd8* in the mouse brain at different developmental stages. Quantitative real-time mRNA expression analysis (qRT-PCR) (Fig. 2a) revealed that *Chd8* was detectable in neocortex from E16 to adulthood. The peak of the expression is at E18 and then markedly decreases at P7 and gradually declines to very low levels at adulthood. This expression pattern in neocortex was also confirmed at the protein level by western blot analysis (Fig. 2b, c). To examine the temporal and spatial expression pattern of *Chd8* in the developing brain, we performed RNA in situ hybridization on mouse brain sections. *Chd8* mRNA was most abundant in embryonic brain and then gradually reduced after birth, consistent with the results from the qRT-PCR and western blot analyses. Specifically, *Chd8* mRNA was present in the sub-plate (SP) and proliferative zones of the cortical wall (the ventricular zone [VZ] and the subventricular zone [SVZ]) at E16 and P0 and in the cortical plate (CP) of the cerebral cortex, hippocampus, striatum, cerebellum, and olfactory bulb from P3 to P7, a developmental period with extensive outgrowth and elaboration of dendrites and axons (Fig. 2d, e). The cellular and subcellular localizations of CHD8 in developing mouse brains and cultured neurons were also examined by immunostaining with neuronal cell markers. Consistent with the results in human cerebral cortex, mouse CHD8 was expressed in the neuronal nucleus, with a pattern similar to that of NeuN in neocortex and hippocampus in P3 mouse (Fig. 3a–c). CHD8 expression in neurons and glia cells was also confirmed by western blot analysis of cultured DIV3 neurons and glia cells of mice (Fig. 3d). However, the expression of CHD8 in glia cells was significantly lower than that in neurons. Taken together, the expression analyses of both human and mouse brains imply important roles for CHD8 during the development of cerebral cortex.

CHD8 regulates neuronal morphogenesis in vitro

Altered short- and long-distance functional connectivity has been reported frequently in brains of human ASD patients by neuroimaging studies [29, 30]. Impaired dendritic development has been reported in numerous mouse models of ASD [31–33]. However, few studies have examined axonal development in ASD animal models. We

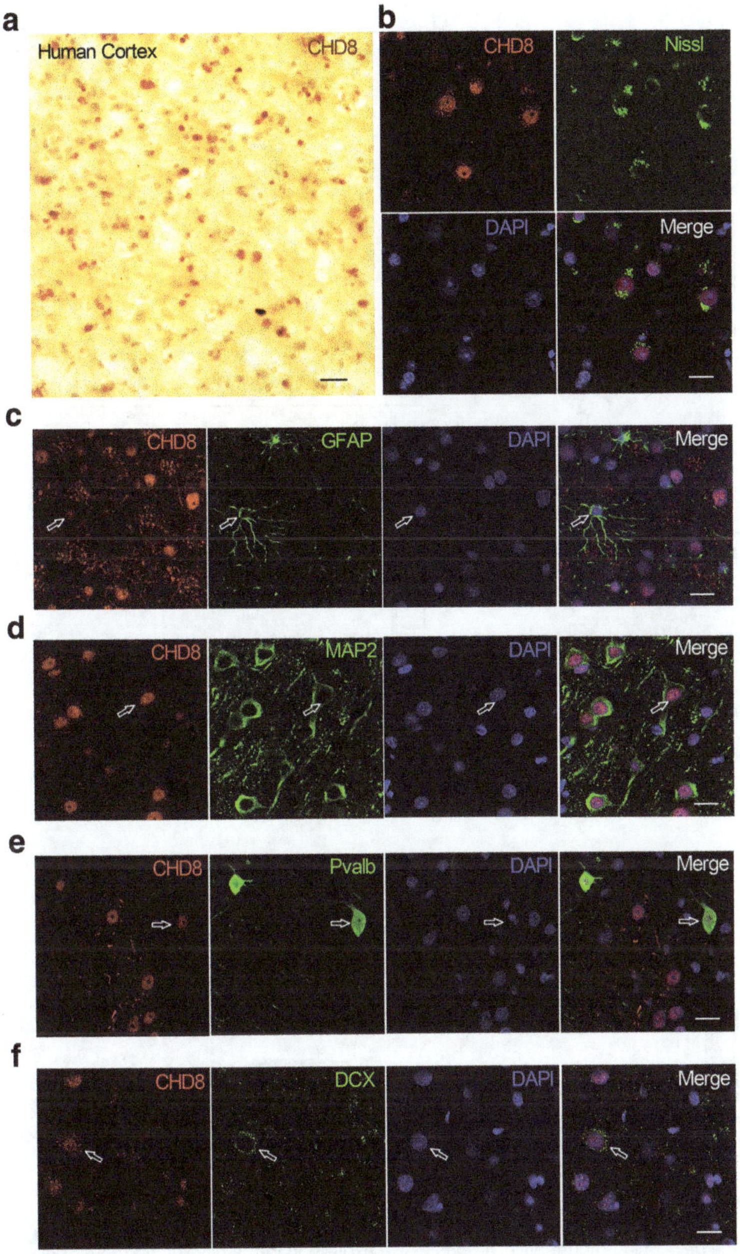

Fig. 1 Expression of CHD8 in human cerebral cortex. **a** Immunohistochemical staining revealed the expression pattern of CHD8 in human cerebral cortex from Brodmann 19 region. **b** Human CHD8 is expressed in neurons. The sections were immunostained with CHD8 antibody and counterstained with NeuroTrace 500/525 green fluorescent Nissl (Thermo Fisher Scientific). **c** CHD8 is expressed in GFAP+ astrocytes (open arrows: astrocytes). **d** CHD8 is expressed in MAP2-positive neurons (open arrows for MAP2 positive neurons). **e** CHD8 is expressed in pavalbumin (Pvalb)-positive interneurons (open arrows for Pvab-positive interneuron). **f** CHD8 is expressed in DCX-positive neurons (open arrows for DCX+ neuron) (scale bar, 20 μm)

therefore examined whether *Chd8* deficiency affects the development of both dendritic morphology and callosal axon growth during development using a shRNA approach. We designed three shRNA constructs that were targeting to *Chd8* and tested the efficiency in both cultured neurons and in vivo in mouse brains. Compared with the scramble shRNA construct, all shRNAs resulted in a significant decrease in the expression of CHD8 protein in cultured neurons, and among them, shRNA#1 had the highest efficiency (Fig. 4a). The efficacy of the shRNA constructs was confirmed in vivo in mouse brain (Fig. 4b). We also validated the rescued constructs against shRNA-mediated knockdown of mouse *Chd8* in transfected neurons in vitro (Additional file 1: Figure S1). To examine axonal growth, we co-transfected dissociated DIV0 mouse cortical neurons with plasmids encoding

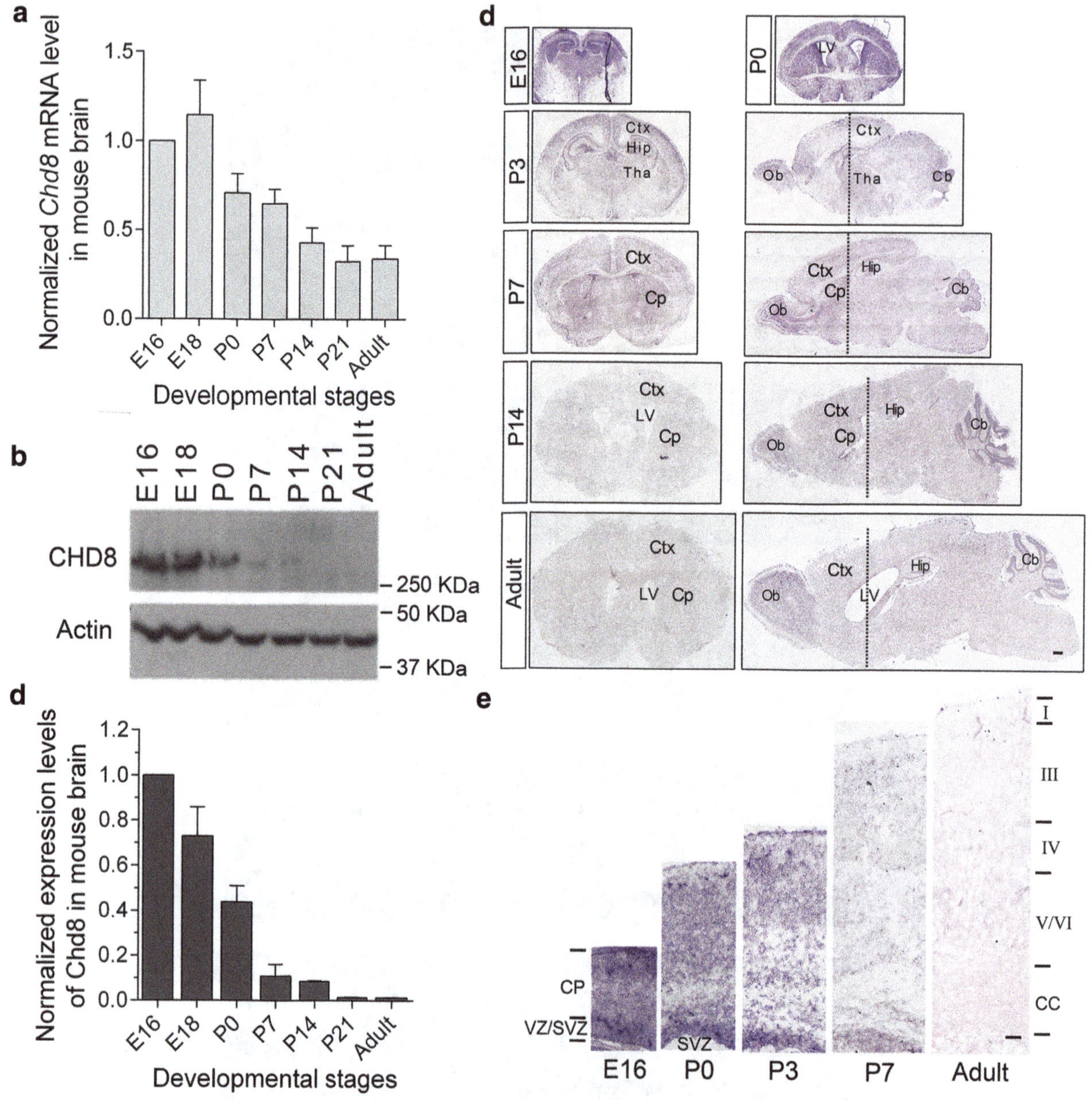

Fig. 2 Expression of *Chd8* in the developing mouse brain. **a** *Chd8* mRNA expression in the developing mouse brain ($n = 5$ at each time point) by real-time RT-PCR. The level was normalized to the E16 mice. Error bars represent SEM. **b** Western blot analysis of CHD8 protein using whole brain lysates at the different developmental stages of mouse brains. **c** Quantification of CHD8 protein levels in developing mouse brain ($n = 6$ at each time point) by western blot analysis that is normalized to E16 level. **d** *Chd8* RNA in situ hybridization of sagittal and coronal sections from mouse brains at the stages indicated. Abbreviations: cortex (Ctx), lateral ventricle (LV), hippocampus (Hip), thalamus (Tha), olfactory bulb (Ob), cerebellum (Cb). Scale bar, 600 μm. **e** RNA in situ hybridization shows the *Chd8* expression pattern in coronal sections of the cerebral cortex at the stages indicated. Scale bar, 500 μm. High levels of *Chd8* mRNA are detected in the cortex at perinatal stages. Abbreviations: cortical plate (CP), ventricular zone (VZ), subventricular zone (SVZ), corpus callosum (CC). Roman numerals (I–VI) indicate layers of the cerebral cortex (scale bar, 100 μm)

GFP and shRNA constructs by electroporation and then plated them to allow the neurons to grow in culture medium for 3 days (DIV3). We used Tau1 as an axon-specific marker. We found that depleting CHD8 significantly decreased total axon growth (Fig. 4c, d). However, co-expression of human CHD8 protein (hCHD8) that is shRNA#2-resistant was able to rescue the total axon length defects caused by shRNA#2 construct (Fig. 4c–e; Additional file 1: Figure S1). We next examined the effects of *Chd8* knockdown on dendritic outgrowth and branching in vitro. Control neurons were transfected at DIV0 with GFP plus a non-targeting shRNA construct

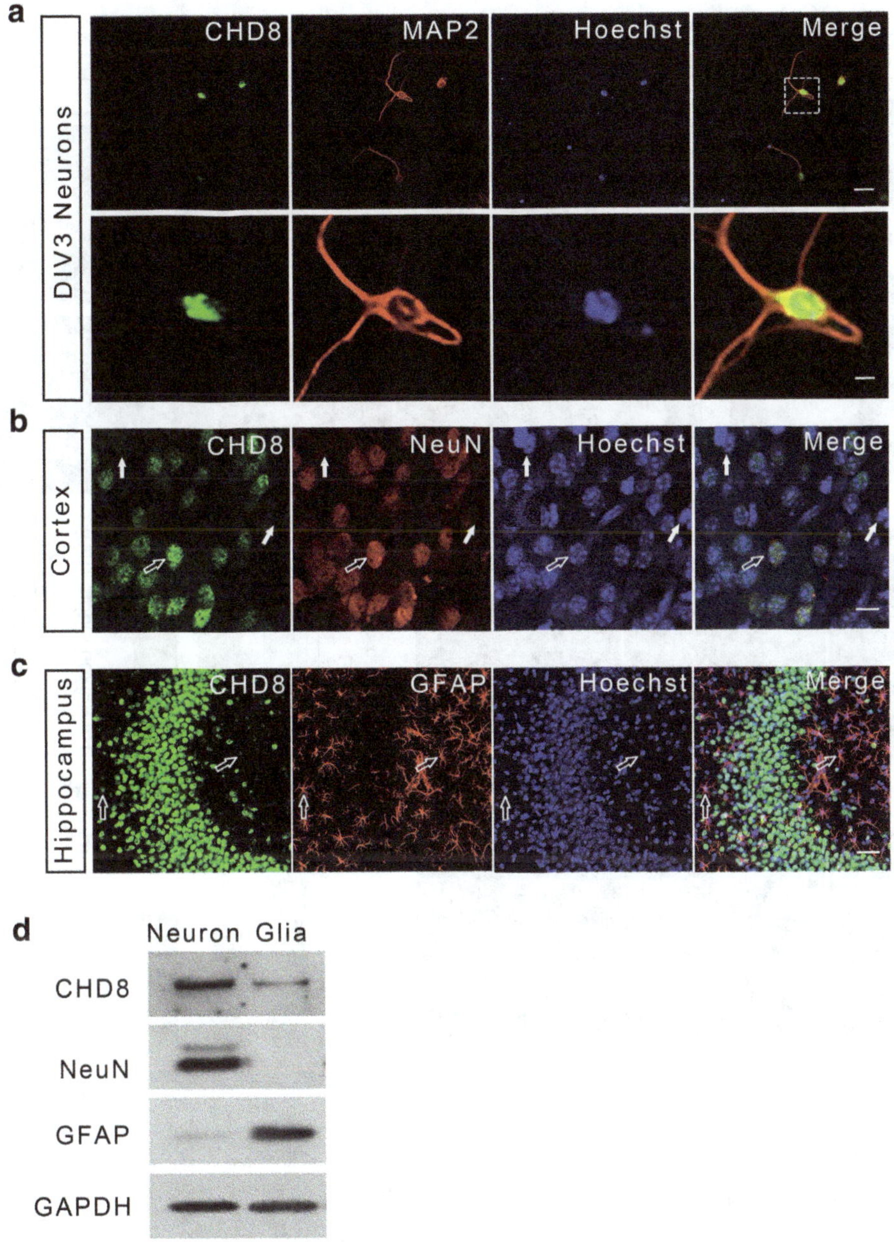

Fig. 3 Cell type-specific expression pattern of CHD8 in mouse brains. **a** Endogenous mouse CHD8 is selectively enriched in the nucleus of cultured DIV3 cortical neurons. Cells were immunolabeled with CHD8 (green), the somatodendritic marker MAP2 (red), and with counterstaining of nuclear marker Hoechst (blue). Scale bar, 2 μm. **b** Double-immunofluorescent staining shows that CHD8 is highly expressed in NeuN-positive neurons. Scale bar, 5 μm. The open arrows indicate both CHD8 and NeuN-positive neurons, while the filled arrows indicate neither CHD8 nor NeuN-positive non-neuronal cells. **c** Double-immunofluorescent staining shows that CHD8 is weakly expressed in GFAP-positive astrocytes. The open arrows indicate GFAP-positive astrocytes with weak CHD8 expression. Scale bar, 25 μm. **d** Representative western blot shows that CHD8 is predominately expressed in neurons but also in cultured glia cells

(shRNA-scr). Seven days later, we analyzed the data after staining cells with the somatodendritic marker MAP2 (Fig. 4f). The total and mean dendrite length were significantly reduced in neurons expressing both shRNA#1 and shRNA#2 constructs compared to those expressing shRNA-scr (Fig. 4g). It is worth noting that the intersections were more affected by shRNA#1 construct than by shRNA#2 construct (Fig. 4h). This appears to be consistent with the more significant reduction of *Chd8* after shRNA#1 treatment than that of shRNA#2. The effects of shRNA#2 were rescued by co-transfecting shRNA2-resistant hCHD8 (Fig. 4i, j). These results indicate CHD8 is required for both axonal and dendritic development.

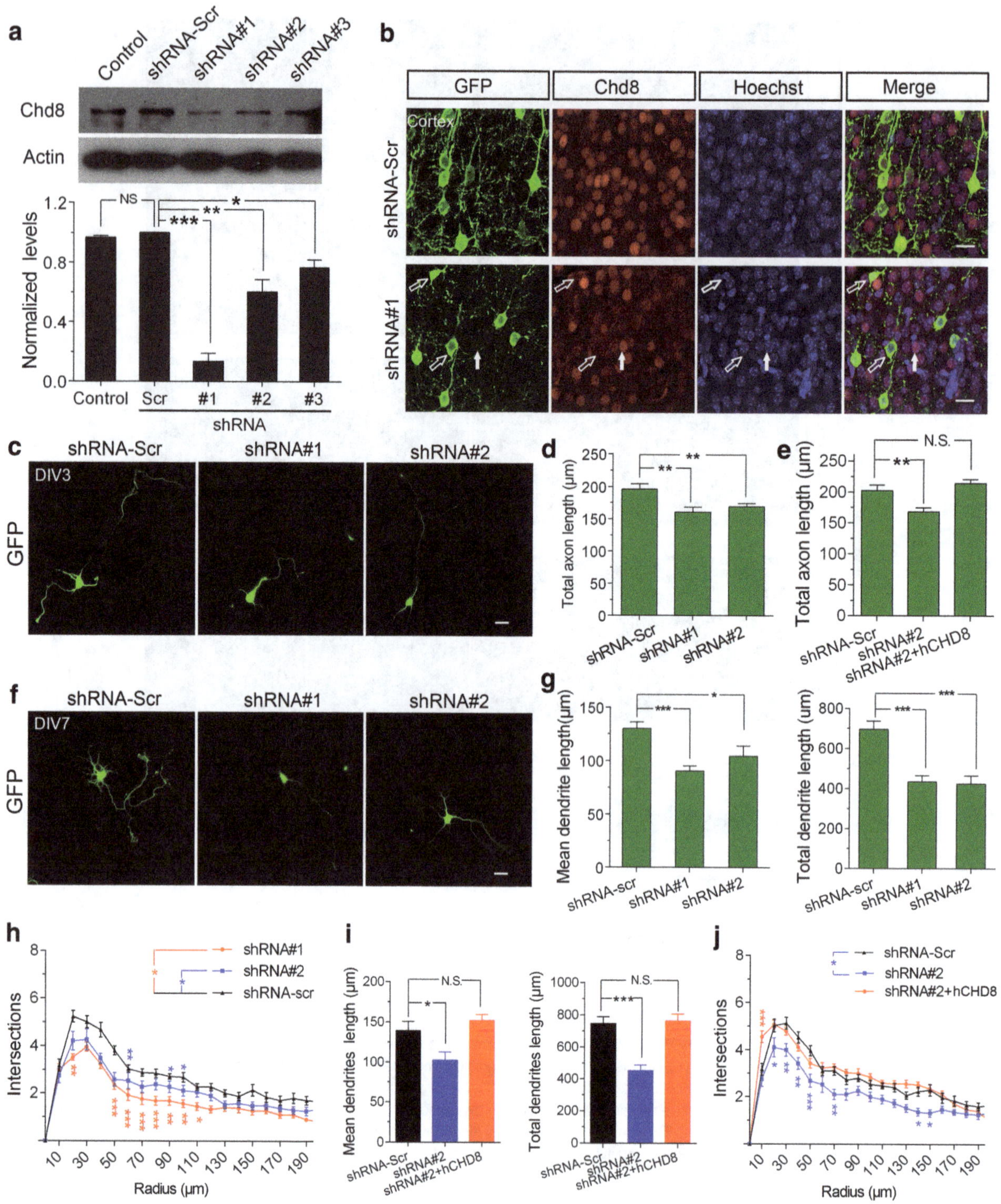

Fig. 4 (See legend on next page.)

(See figure on previous page.)

Fig. 4 CHD8 regulates neurite growth in vitro. **a** shRNA-mediated knockdown of mouse *Chd8* in transfected cultured neurons. Upper, representative western blots; lower, quantification of western blot analysis. shRNA#1, 0.14 ± 0.095; shRNA#2, 0.60 ± 0.14; shRNA#1, 0.77 ± 0.089. For ANOVA, $P = 0.587$. For post hoc Dunnets' test, $^{**}P = 0.004$ for shRNA#1 vs shRNA-scr; $^{*}P = 0.041$ for shRNA#2 vs shRNA-scr; $^{*}P = 0.046$ for shRNA#3 vs shRNA-scr. All data were shown in mean ± SEM and were collected from three to six independent experiments. **b** Immunostaining showing shRNA-mediated knockdown of *Chd8* in transfected neurons in mouse brains. Immunohistochemical staining of endogenous CHD8 in coronal sections from a P0 mouse brain electroporated with shRNA#1 and GFP at E14.5. The open arrows indicate successfully transfected cells, and the filled arrows indicate normal cells. Scale bar, 10 μm. **c** Representative images of DIV3 cultured neurons transfected with GFP and the plasmids indicated. Constructs were transfected at DIV0, cultured for 3 days in vitro, and then immunolabeled with anti-GFP. Scale bar, 100 μm. **d** Quantification of the total axon length of neurons transfected with *Chd8* shRNA constructs. $n = 126, 133, 124$ neurons per group, respectively. Total axon length: shRNA-scr, 196.0 ± 8.42 μm; shRNA#1, 160.4 ± 7.56 μm. For ANOVA, $P = 0.01$. For post hoc Dunnets' test, $^{**}P = 0.0032$ for shRNA#1 vs shRNA-scr; shRNA#2, 168.8 ± 6.98, $^{**}P = 0.0052$ for shRNA#2 vs shRNA-scr. **e** Defective axon growth in *Chd8* shRNA#2 construct was rescued in neurons by co-transfected with shRNA#2-resistant hCHD8 constructs ($n = 50$ neurons per group). Total axon length: shRNA-scr, 202.6 ± 9.13 μm; shRNA#2, 168.2 ± 6.68 μm. For ANOVA, $P = 0.07$. For post hoc Dunnets' test, $^{**}P = 0.004$ for shRNA#2 vs shRNA-scr; shRNA#2 + hCHD8, 214.4 ± 6.15, $P = 0.32$ for shRNA#2 + hCHD8 vs shRNA-scr. **f** Representative images of DIV7 cultured neurons transfected with GFP and *Chd8* shRNA constructs as indicated. **g** Quantification of dendritic length in neurons transfected with *Chd8* shRNA constructs as indicated. $n = 80$–100 neurons per group. Mean dendritic length: shRNA-scr, 130.1 ± 6.3 μm; shRNA#1, 90.7 ± 4.61 μm. For ANOVA, $P < 0.001$. For post hoc Dunnets' test, $^{***}P < 0.0001$ for shRNA#1 vs shRNA-scr; shRNA#2, 104.5 ± 9.53, $^{*}P = 0.032$ for shRNA#2 vs shRNA-scr. Total dendritic length: shRNA-scr, 694.9 ± 42.5 μm; shRNA#1 is 435.9 ± 30.6 μm. For ANOVA, $P = 0.0007$. For post hoc Dunnets' test, $^{***}P = 0.0001$ for shRNA#1 vs shRNA-scr; shRNA#2 is 425.3 ± 39.2 μm, $^{***}P = 0.0003$ for shRNA#2 vs shRNA-scr. **h** Quantification of dendritic complexity as measured by Sholl analysis ($n = 50$–80 neurons per group). For ANOVA, $P = 0.0015$. For Bonferroni post-tests, $^{*}P < 0.05$; $^{**}P < 0.01$; $^{**}P < 0.001$. **i** Co-expression of the human CHD8 rescued the defective dendritic growth by the shRNA-#2 in DIV7 neurons. $n = 100$–120 neurons in each group. Data represent mean ± SEM. For ANOVA, $P = 0.0127$ (left panel); $P = 0.0013$ (right panel). For post hoc Dunnett's test, $^{*}P < 0.05$; $^{**}P < 0.01$; $^{***}P < 0.001$. **j** Quantification of dendritic complexity as measured by Sholl analysis ($n = 50$–80 neurons per group). For ANOVA, $P < 0.001$. For Bonferroni post-tests, $^{*}P < 0.05$; $^{**}P < 0.01$; $^{***}P < 0.001$

CHD8 is essential for neurite development in vivo

To test whether *Chd8* deficiency has effects on mouse brains in vivo, we used the shRNA#2 construct for this experiment because of the feasibility of conducting rescue experiments as demonstrated in vitro. At P3, mouse pups electroporated with scrambled shRNA had callosal axons originating from the electroporated neurons that crossed the midline and formed and arborized dense projections to the contralateral side of cerebral cortex, and the axon bundles were restricted to the corpus callosum (CC) (Fig. 5a–c, j, k). In contrast, in mice transfected with the *Chd8* shRNA#2 construct, the axon terminals were barely visible in the contralateral cerebral cortex, indicating significantly retarded axon growth and elongation (Fig. 5d–f, j, k). Co-transfection of the shRNA#2-resistant *hCHD8* construct successfully rescued these defects (Fig. 5g–k). These findings suggest that reduced expression of *Chd8* in callosal projection neurons impairs axon growth and branching in vivo.

To assess the impact of *Chd8* knockdown on the development of neuronal dendrites, we performed morphological analysis of the layer II/III pyramidal neurons of somatosensory cortex 1 (S1). The layer II/III pyramidal neurons of S1 constitute the main excitatory neuronal subtypes in the neocortex and typically having an apical dendrite that branches out in an apical tuft that terminates in layer I [31]. Most scrambled shRNA-transfected neurons displayed a typical polarized dendritic arbor (Fig. 6a, b). In contrast, the *Chd8* shRNA significantly decreased the secondary branches and the total number and mean length of dendritic branches in neurons (Fig. 6c, d). The complexity of dendrites was also significantly decreased by *Chd8* shRNA constructs, revealed by Sholl analysis (Fig. 6e). These results indicated that CHD8 plays an essential role in neuronal morphogenesis in the mouse cerebral cortex.

CHD8 deficiency impairs the migration of cortical neurons

Because of the expression of CHD8 in DCX-positive neural precursors, we examined whether its deficiency affected the radial migration of cortical neurons. The shRNA and EGFP constructs were co-electroporated into the developing mouse cortex at E14.5 using in utero electroporation (IUE) as previously described [27], and the distribution of EGFP-labeled cells in neocortex was examined at E18.5. While the majority of the EGFP-positive cells (76.8 ± 0.6%) migrated to the upper cortical plate (CP) when scrambled shRNA was co-expressed, only a small percentage of EGFP cells were observed in the upper CP when the *Chd8* shRNA constructs were co-expressed (shRNA#1, 10.1 ± 1.2%; shRNA#2, 14.4 ± 0.9%;) and the majority of labeled cells remained in the VZ/SVZ (Fig. 7a, b). Interestingly, the number of EGFP-positive cells that reached the upper CP was comparable between shRNA construct and scrambled controls at P3 and P7 (Fig. 7c–f). Accordingly, there are a comparable number of neurons that remained in the white matter (WM) and layers IV–VI. Together, these results indicate that deficiency of *Chd8* could cause a delay in radial migration of cortical neurons during early embryonic development, but this normalizes during postnatal development.

Discussion

Genetic studies have provided strong evidence supporting an etiological role for genes encoding the proteins of epigenetic machinery in ASD [10, 34]. *CHD8* is one of the most prominent and repeatedly reported genes in

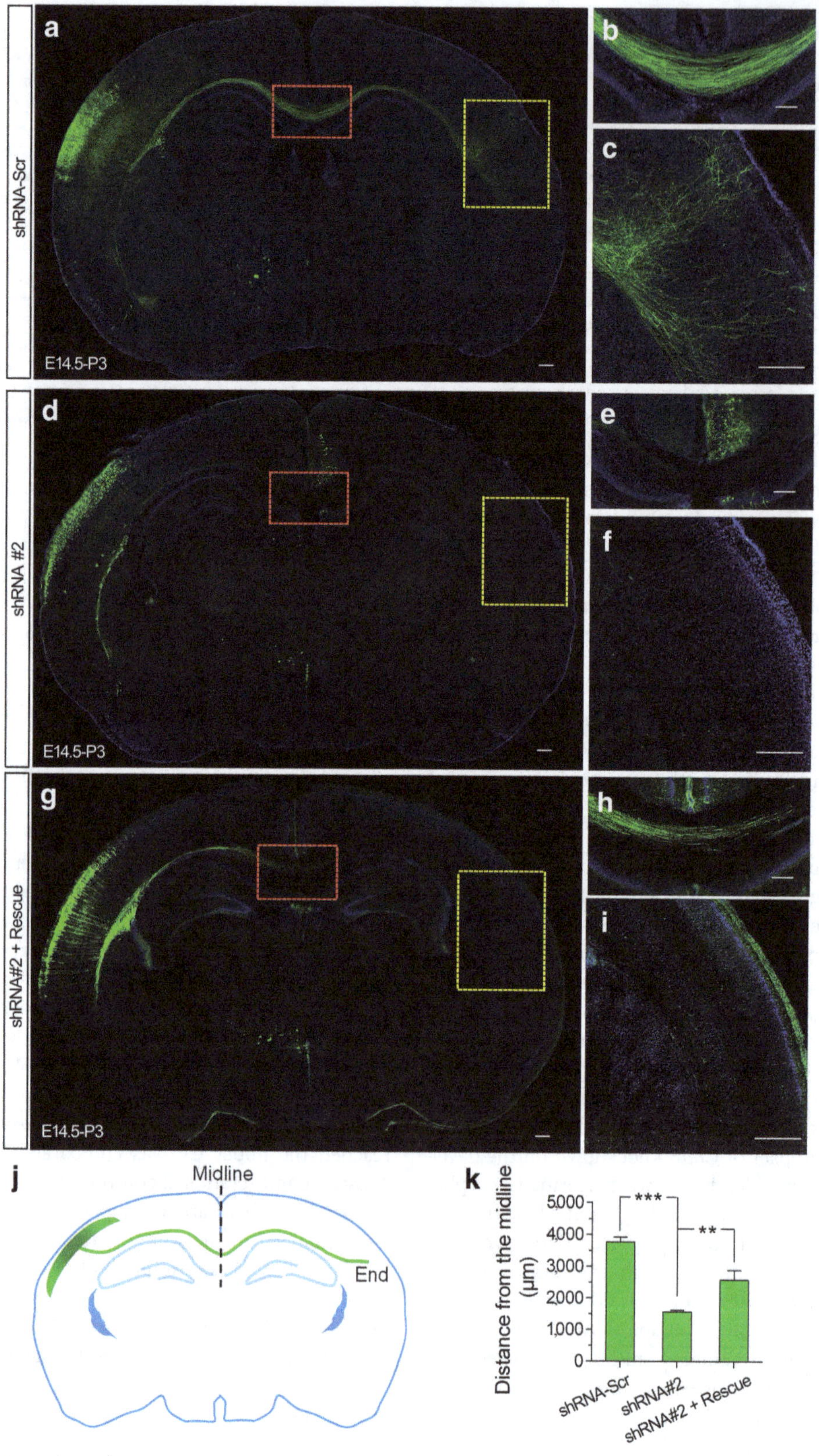

Fig. 5 (See legend on next page.)

(See figure on previous page.)
Fig. 5 CHD8 regulates the axon growth in vivo. **a–i** Representative images of coronal slices of P3 mouse brains that were transfected with GFP together with indicated constructs by in utero electroporation at E14.5. High-magnification images are shown in the right. Brain slices at the level of Bregma − 1.58 mm were stained with Hoechst and GFP antibodies to visualize the callosal. Scale bar, 150 μm (**a**, **d**, **g**), 200 μm (**b**, **e**, **h**), or 400 μm (**c**, **f**, **i**). **j** A schematic for quantitative analysis of callosal axon length. The adjacent axon lengths were measured from the midline to end. **k** Quantitative analysis of callosal axon length *Chd8* ShRNA#2 construct showed significantly shorter axonal length than scramble control. The co-expression of human hCHD8 rescued the phenotypes caused by knockdown of *Chd8* by shRNA#2 construct. Distance from the midline: shRNA-scr, 3763 ± 154.3 μm; shRNA#2, 1563 ± 47.95 μm. $^{***}P < 0.0001$ shRNA#2 vs shRNA-scr; shRNA#-h*CHD8*, 2575 ± 307.2 μm. $^{**}P = 0.0021$ shRNA#2-h*CHD8* vs shRNA-scr. Results are shown as mean ± SEM. $n = 4$ in each group. For ANOVA, $P = 0.0016$. For Bonferroni post-tests, $^{**}P < 0.01$; $^{***}P < 0.001$

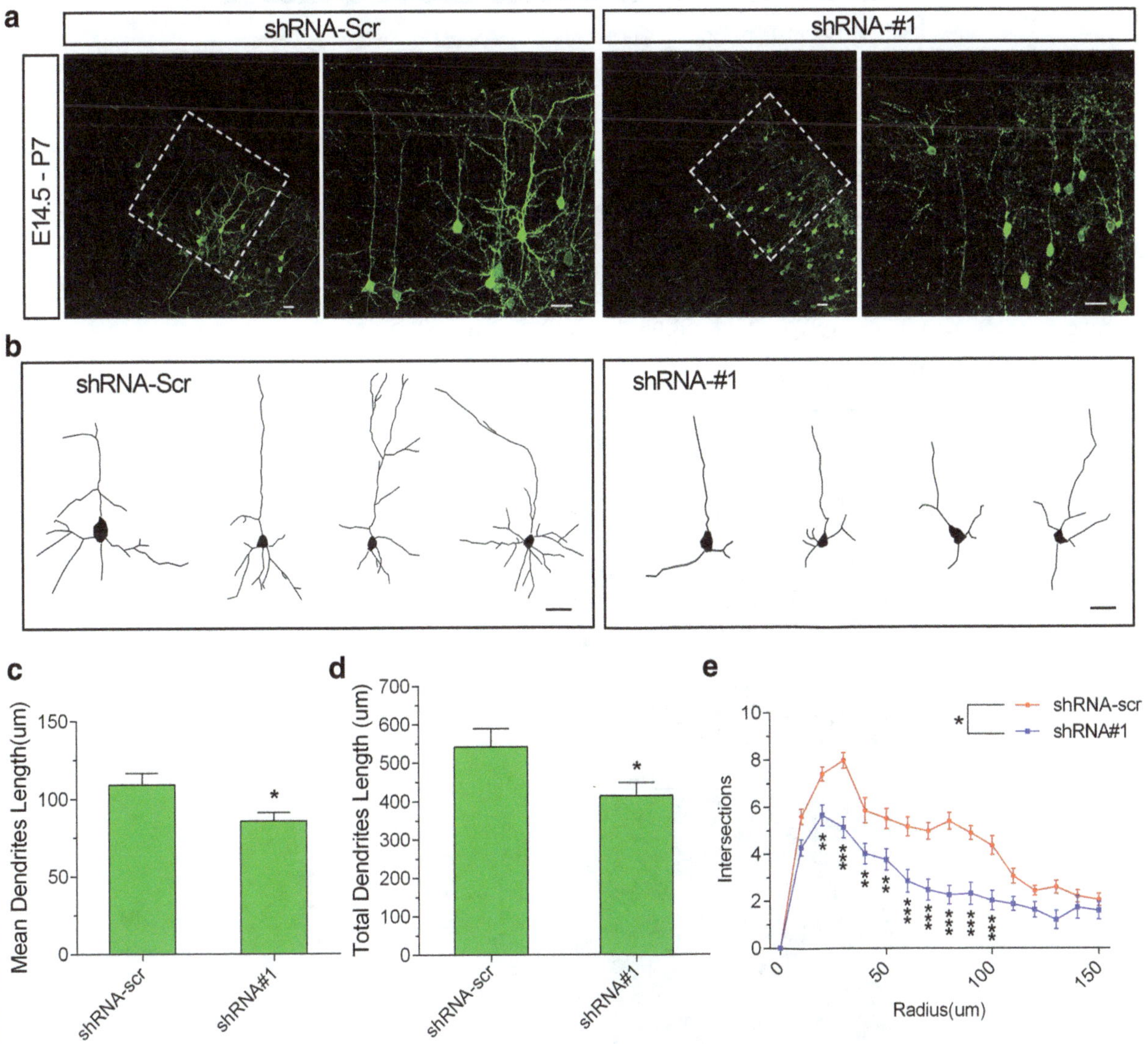

Fig. 6 CHD8 is required for dendrite growth in vivo. **a** Representative images of coronal slices of P7 mouse brains that were transfected with GFP together with indicated constructs by in utero electroporation at E14.5. Transfected cells were visualized by staining coronal slices with GFP antibody. In each image pair, the right image is from the boxed region of the left image. Scale bar, 100 μm. **b** Neurolucida tracings of representative layer II/III pyramidal neurons, from experiment shown in **a**. Scale bar, 50 μm. **c–e** Quantitative analysis of dendrite length and dendrite complexity measured from Neurolucida tracings. Mean dendritic length: shRNA-scr, 109.2 ± 7.5 μm; shRNA#1, 85.9 ± 5.59 μm, $^{*}P = 0.015$, shRNA#1 vs shRNA-scr. Total dendritic length: shRNA-scr, 541.6 ± 47.52 μm; shRNA#1, 415.233.89 μm, $^{*}P = 0.0332$, shRNA#1 vs shRNA-scr. Greater than 70 neurons were examined in each group from at least three independent experiments. Results are presented as the mean ± SEM. $^{*}P < 0.05$; $^{**}P < 0.01$; $^{***}P < 0.001$; one-way ANOVA post Dunnett's test

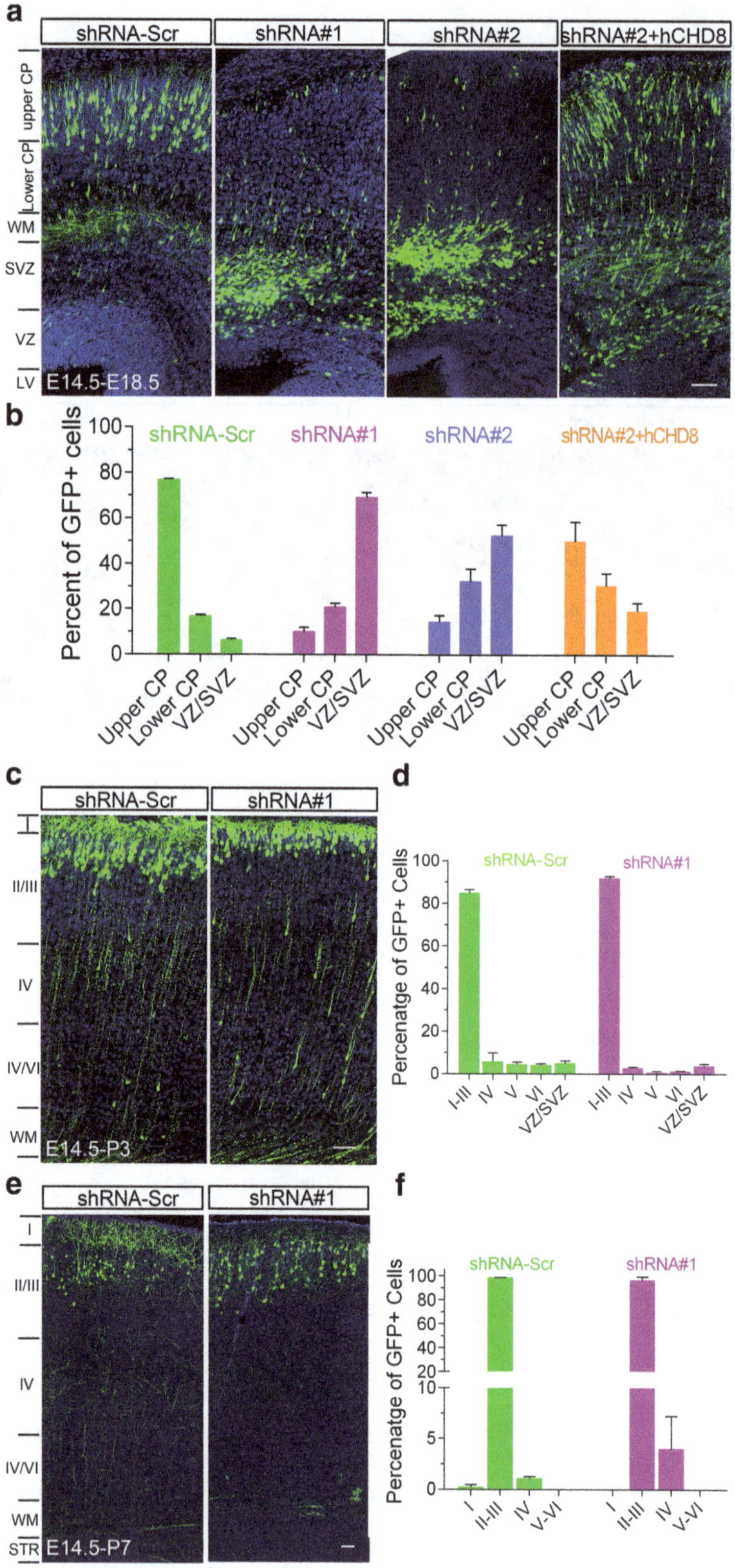

Fig. 7 (See legend on next page.)

(See figure on previous page.)
Fig. 7 *Chd8* knockdown delays neuronal migration in vivo. **a** Representative images of coronal slices of E18.5 mouse brains that were transfected with GFP together with indicated *Chd8* constructs by in utero electroporation at E14.5. At E18.5, cortical neurons transfected with *Chd8*-shRNA constructs were misplaced in the VZ/SVZ instead of CP. Transfected cells were visualized by staining coronal slices with GFP antibody. Scale bar, 200 μm. **b** Quantitative analysis of the distribution of cortical neurons transfected with different constructs across three different zones in the somatosensory cortex: upper cp, lower cp, VZ/SVZ. Results are mean ± SEM from 6 to 12 sections (one per mouse) for each experiment. **c, d** By P3, cortical neurons migrated normally from the SVZ into the cortex in both control and Chd8 RNAi-transfected brains. Scale bar, 120 μm. **e, f** At P7, most transfected neurons were located in the layers II/III in both control and *Chd8* shRNA-transfected brains. Scale bar, 200 μm

this class [13]. In contrast to the well-characterized synaptic genes that are also strongly implicated in ASD, the molecular pathogenesis of ASD caused by deficiency of epigenetic machinery proteins such as *CHD8* remains to be thoroughly investigated. Through studies of *Chd8* deficiency in cultured rodent neurons or mutant mice by different experimental approaches, several groups have provided initial evidence supporting a causal link between a deficiency of CHD8 and neural cell proliferation, synaptic function, myelination, and ASD-like behaviors. The major findings from these studies and the current study are summarized in Table 1 [18, 20–25, 35, 36]. The results among these studies are not always consistent; in some cases, opposite findings are reported. For example, the decreased proliferation of neural progenitor cells is associated with *Chd8* deficiency using RNAi by in utero electroporation but the increased proliferation was reported in mice with germline mutation. Interestingly, a recent study of a new line of *Chd8* mutant mice reports sexually dimorphic phenotypes at molecular, synaptic function, and behavioral levels [24]. Another report also finds that *Chd8* deficiency, selectively in oligodendrocytes but not in neurons, results in myelination defects in mice. Similarly, different ASD-related behavioral phenotypes are also observed among different lines of *Chd8* mutant mice. Unfortunately, behavioral phenotypes have not been examined in oligodendrocyte-specific *Chd8* deficiency mice. Whether these discrepancies are due to different *Chd8* mutations in these lines of mutant mice or other experimental procedure-related issues are not immediately clear. Future studies of performing the experiments in parallel in different lines *Chd8* mutant mice are warranted.

In this study, we have shown that CHD8 is expressed at high level in both NeuN-positive mature neurons and parvalbumin-positive interneurons and to a lesser extent in GFAP-positive astrocytes in human cerebral cortex. A previous study has found that the peak expression of CHD8 is between 13 and 19 weeks in the dorsolateral prefrontal cortex and 10–13 weeks of medial prefrontal cortex in humans [18]. In the developing mouse brain, we find that *Chd8/CHD8* expression peaks around embryonic days 16–18 and decreases to much lower levels by P21 by both mRNA and protein analyses. This finding is largely consistent with the reports of the development-specific expression of CHD8 in previous studies [18, 20, 22]. However, there are differences in the experimental designs among these studies. In our study, the *Chd8* expression study by real-time RT-PCR, RNA in situ hybridization, and western blot are performed in tissues from E16 day embryos to adult brains. In study by Nishiyama et al., the expression is examined by western blot and whole mount in situ in cells or tissues from embryonic stem (ES) cells as well as from E7.5 day embryos to adult mice [20]. The expression is high in ES and early embryonic stage, but a definitive peak is not seen. In other study by Platt et al. [22], real-time RT-PCR, western blot, and RNA in situ hybridization are used to examine the *Chd8* expression in brain tissues from E10 day embryos to adult mice. The highest expression is seen around E10–11 day embryos. In the study that the expression is examined in brain tissues from E12 to P2, the highest expression is at E12 [18]. With the caveats in the experimental designs, it is possible that the peak expression of *Chd8* is before E7 day because homozygous *Chd8* mutant are arrested before gastrulation because of massive apoptosis [20].

Consistent with previous report [18], we have also shown the evidence supporting the role of CHD8 in dendrite development of pyramidal neurons. The loss of CHD8 inhibits dendritic outgrowth and branch formation. In contrast to other reports, we have shown for the first time from both in vitro and in vivo studies that deficiency of CHD8 in developing mouse neurons inhibits axon growth and branch formation and results in a disruption of callosal axon projections to the contralateral cortex. The effect of CHD8 deficiency on the growth of axons is consistent with the report of dysregulation of genes implicated in axonal development in IPSC-derived neurons from human CHD8 patients [36, 37]. Together, our data demonstrate that CHD8 is important for normal dendritic and axonal development and that dysregulation of the process may contribute abnormal neuronal connectivity.

The peak expression in early and middle fetal development suggests a functional role of CHD8 in cortical development. Indeed, we found that *Chd8* knockdown results in a significant delayed migration of newborn cortical neurons examined at E18.5. This is opposite to the enhanced migration reported by Durak et al. using the similar approach but at different time points during the fetal development [18]. We performed in utero electroporation for *Chd8* knockdown at E14.5 and analyzed

Table 1 Summary of the findings from the current study and relevant literature

Reference(s)	Endogenous CHD8 expression data relating to the current study	Model system(s) and method(s) used for disrupting CHD8 expression	Findings caused by disrupting CHD8 expression relating to the current study
Current study	• Human (Brodmann region 19): CHD8 expressed in astrocytes (GFAP+) and in neurons (MAP2+, PV+, DCX+) by immunohistochemical stains • Mice (whole brain lysates): CHD8 expression peaks at E16-E18, decreases substantially postnatally by qPCR and western blotting • Mice (P3 brain sections and cultured neurons): CHD8 expression shows nuclear localization in MAP2+ neurons by immunostaining • Mice (cultured neurons and glia): CHD8 is expressed in cultured neurons and to a lesser extent in cultured glia by western blotting	• Mice (in vitro)—cultured neurons transfected with *Chd8* shRNA constructs • Mice (in vivo)—in utero electroporation at E14.5 with *Chd8* shRNA constructs	• Decreased axon length (both in vitro and in vivo) • Reduced dendritic complexity (both in vitro and in vivo) • Delayed neuronal migration (higher percentage of GFP+ cells in VZ/SVZ instead of CP) at E18.5 (in vivo), which normalized by P3
Durak et al. [18]	Mice (brain lysates): expression peaks at E12, then decreases during embryonic development to P2 by qPCR Human (DFC and MFC): expression peaks during early-mid fetal development and decreases from late fetal development to childhood by qPCR	Mice—in utero electroporation at E13 (for neuronal proliferation/ migration studies) or E15 (for dendritic arborization studies) with *Chd8* shRNA constructs	• Increased neuronal migration (more GFP+ cells in CP instead of VZ/SVZ) at E16, accompanied by reduced proliferation, increased cell cycle exit, reduced mitotic activity, and premature Tuj1 expression • Decreased dendritic arborization in upper cortical neurons from 5-month-old mice • CHD8 mediates cortical neurogenesis via transcriptional regulation of cell cycle and Wnt signaling
Nishiyama et al. [20] and Katayama et al. [21]	Mice (whole embryos): CHD8 was expressed in ES cells (~E3.5), E8.5 embryos, E12.5 embryos, E16.5 embryos, and to a lesser extent in newborn pups by western blotting	Mice—two lines of germline haploinsufficient mice were generated (replacing 9 exons with loxP-neo cassette, or Δexons 11–13, disrupting only the long protein isoform)	• Homozygous mutants show massive apoptosis at E7.5 and lethality • At E14.5, haploinsufficient mice showed increased expression of early-fetal genes and decreased expression of mid-fetal genes
Platt et al. [22]	Mice (whole brains): expression profile from E10-P0, adult. Expression is highest at E10 and decreases over development by western blotting Mice (adult brain sections, somatosensory cortex): CHD8 shows nuclear localization and co-expresses with NeuN, PV, CNP1, and GFAP by immunostaining	Mice—germline haploinsufficient mice were generated by CRISPR/Cas9 introducing a 7 nucleotide deletion in exon 1, which disrupted the expression of both CHD8 isoforms	• Normal lamination and specification of neuronal cell types at P21 • No difference in number of cortical progenitor cells or cell cycle length at E15.5
Zhao et al. [25]	Mice (P14 white matter tracts): CHD8 is expressed in oligodendrocytes and to a lesser extent in GFAP+ astrocytes by immunostaining Human (cerebellum): CHD8 expression in Sox10+ oligodendrocytes by immunostaining Mice (P14 cortical sections): CHD8 is expressed in NeuN+ neurons but not clearly in GFAP+ astroctyes or Iba1+ microglia by immunostaining	Conditional *Chd8* knockout mice (loxP sites surrounding exon 4) crossed with oligodendrocyte-specific Cre line	• Homozygous conditional knockout mice show lethality by P21 and myelination defects • Homozygous conditional knockout mice show reduced proliferation of oligodendrocyte precursor cells in P1 spinal cord • Dual requirement of CHD8 for chromatin landscape establishment and histone methyltransferase recruitment to promote CNS myelination and repair
Gompers et al. [35]	Expression analysis was not reported for different cell types or developmental time points	Mice—germline *Chd8* haploinsufficient mice were generated (deletion of exon 5)	• Increased proliferation of neuronal progenitors at E14.5 • No gross lamination errors by P0 and P7

Table 1 Summary of the findings from the current study and relevant literature *(Continued)*

Reference(s)	Endogenous CHD8 expression data relating to the current study	Model system(s) and method(s) used for disrupting CHD8 expression	Findings caused by disrupting CHD8 expression relating to the current study
Wang et al. [36] CRISPR/Cas9-mediated heterozygous knockout of the autism gene *CHD8* and characterization of its transcriptional networks in neurodevelopment	N/A	CRISPR/Cas9-mediated heterozygous knockout of *CHD8* in iPSCs	• Genes involved in cell cycle, neuronal differentiation, and in neuronal projection development are dysregulated
Suetterlin et al. [23]	N/A	*Chd8*+/− mice (loxP sites on exon 3) crossed β-actinCre line	• *Chd8* heterozygous mice display increased total brain volume and showed volumetric increased of several brain regions, including cortical areas, hippocampus and parts of the cerebellum by high-solution MRI • CHD8 controls the expression of ASD-associated axon guidance genes in the early postnatal neocortex
Jung et al. [24]	In both males and females, CHD8 protein was more abundant in the brain relative to other tissues, at embryonic stages relative to postnatal stages, and in non-crude synaptosomal fractions	*Chd8*+/N2373 K mice carrying a heterozygous Chd8 frame-shift mutation	• Distinct c-fos signals in male and female $Chd8^{+/N2373K}$ brains under baseline and maternal-separation conditions • Opposite changes in inhibitory synaptic transmission in the male and female $Chd8^{+/N2373K}$ hippocampus

the cell migration at E18.5 while Durak et al. performed the in utero electroporation at E14 and analyzed at E16. Whether the different timing of CHD8 deficiency is responsible for the observed phenotypic differences remains to be determined. Because transcriptional regulation implicated in cortical development is dynamic and epigenetically modulated [38], it is also conceivable that CHD8 may have different roles at the different stages of fetal brain development. Interestingly, the delayed neuronal migration associated with knockdown of *Chd8* in our study is recovered at P3 and P7. This may suggest a catch-up period of the CHD8-deficient neurons after E18.5 days. Taken together, our findings support that CHD8 plays a critical role in migration of mitotic neurons as well as both dendritic and axonal growth in neocortex.

Human patients with *CHD8* mutations present with typical autistic behaviors and comorbidities including social deficits and communication difficulties, repetitive behaviors and interests, and cognitive delays [8, 13]. However, the findings from existing studies in model organisms have not provided a clear mechanistic link between genetic defects and clinical presentations [13, 21, 22, 25, 35, 39]. One of the notable features in some of the patients with *CHD8* mutations is relatively enlarged brain (macrocephaly) [13]. This feature is consistent with the findings of enlarged brains in a sub-set of idiopathic ASD cases during early postnatal brain development. Germline mutations of *Chd8* in zebrafish and mice have recapitulated the feature of enlarged brain size [13, 21, 22, 25, 35]. Accordingly, increased proliferation of neuronal progenitor cells and dysregulation of expression cell cycle genes are associated with germline line *Chd8* mutation [35]. Whether this is the underlying mechanism for macrocephaly associated with *CHD8* mutations and whether it is generalizable to the macrocephaly in other idiopathic ASD cases remain to be investigated. Notably, massive apoptosis is observed in E5.5 embryos carrying germline *Chd8* homozygous mutation [20] and somatic knockdown of *Chd8* by RNAi using in utero electroporation results in a decrease proliferation of neural progenitors [18]. These observations may indicate a different role of CHD8 at different developmental stages. More importantly, a critical question for future investigation is whether the cellular defects and enlarged brain size are responsible for ASD-like behaviors observed in *Chd8* heterozygous mutant animals.

In summary, CHD8 protein is highly enriched in neurons of developing neocortex in both human and mice and plays a critical role in regulating neuronal migration as well as growth of neurites. Our findings suggest that *CHD8* mutations in humans may also result in defects of neuronal migration and morphogenesis defects during a crucial stage of brain development and this impaired process may contribute to the pathophysiology of ASD.

Abbreviations

ASD: Autism spectrum disorder; CC: Corpus callosum; CHD8: Chromodomain helicase DNA-binding protein 8; CP: Cortical plate; hCHD8: Human CHD8 protein; IHC: Immunohistochemistry; IUE: In utero electroporation; qRT-PCR: Quantitative real-time RNA; SP: Sub-plate; SVZ: Subventricular zone; VZ: The ventricular zone

Funding

This work was supported by the National Science Foundation of China [81701496 to QX, 81371270 to XX]; Shanghai Municipal Science and Technology Commission [15411967900 to QX]; and the National Institute of Health [MH098114, HD087795, MH104316 to YHJ].

Authors' contributions

QX and YHJ conceived the project. QX and YYL did major experiments and analyzed the data. QX, YYL, XMW, GHT, XX, SWH, and YHJ interpreted the data and wrote the manuscript. All authors read and approved the final manuscript.

Competing interests

The authors declare that they have no competing interests.

Author details

[1]Department of Child Health Care, Children's Hospital of Fudan University, Shanghai 201102, China. [2]Guangxi Key Laboratory of Regenerative Medicine & Guangxi Collaborative Innovation Center for Biomedicine, School of Preclinical Medicine, Guangxi Medical University, Nanning 530021, Guangxi, China. [3]Department of Pediatrics, Duke University School of Medicine, Durham 27710, NC, USA. [4]Department of Neurobiology, Duke University School of Medicine, Durham 27710, NC, USA. [5]Institute of Neuroscience & State Key Laboratory of Neuroscience, CAS Center for Excellence in Brain Science and Intelligence Technology, Shanghai Institutes for Biological Sciences, Chinese Academy of Sciences, Shanghai 200031, China. [6]University of Chinese Academy of Sciences, Beijing 100049, China. [7]Program in Genetics and Genomics, Duke University School of Medicine, Durham 27710, NC, USA. [8]Cellular Molecular Biology, Duke University School of Medicine, Durham 27710, NC, USA.

References

1. Miles JH. Autism spectrum disorders--a genetics review. Genet Med. 2011; 13(4):278–94.
2. Watts TJ. The pathogenesis of autism. Clin Med Pathol. 2008;1:99–103.
3. O'Roak BJ, et al. Exome sequencing in sporadic autism spectrum disorders identifies severe de novo mutations. Nat Genet. 2011;43(6):585–9.
4. Iossifov I, et al. De novo gene disruptions in children on the autistic spectrum. Neuron. 2012;74(2):285–99.
5. Michaelson JJ, et al. Whole-genome sequencing in autism identifies hot spots for de novo germline mutation. Cell. 2012;151(7):1431–42.
6. Neale BM, et al. Patterns and rates of exonic de novo mutations in autism spectrum disorders. Nature. 2012;485(7397):242–5.
7. Sanders SJ, et al. De novo mutations revealed by whole-exome sequencing are strongly associated with autism. Nature. 2012;485(7397):237–41.
8. O'Roak BJ, et al. Sporadic autism exomes reveal a highly interconnected protein network of de novo mutations. Nature. 2012;485(7397):246–50.
9. Jiang YH, et al. Detection of clinically relevant genetic variants in autism spectrum disorder by whole-genome sequencing. Am J Hum Genet. 2013; 93(2):249–63.
10. De Rubeis S, et al. Synaptic, transcriptional and chromatin genes disrupted in autism. Nature. 2014;515(7526):209–15.
11. Iossifov I, et al. The contribution of de novo coding mutations to autism spectrum disorder. Nature. 2014;515(7526):216–21.
12. Krumm N, et al. Excess of rare, inherited truncating mutations in autism. Nat Genet. 2015;47(6):582–8.
13. Bernier R, et al. Disruptive CHD8 mutations define a subtype of autism early in development. Cell. 2014;158(2):263–76.
14. O'Roak BJ, et al. Multiplex targeted sequencing identifies recurrently mutated genes in autism spectrum disorders. Science. 2012;338(6114): 1619–22.
15. Marfella CG, Imbalzano AN. The Chd family of chromatin remodelers. Mutat Res. 2007;618(1–2):30–40.
16. Okerlund ND, Cheyette BN. Synaptic Wnt signaling - a contributor to major psychiatric disorders? J Neurodev Disord. 2011;3(2):162–74.
17. Sakamoto I, et al. A novel beta-catenin-binding protein inhibits beta-catenin-dependent Tcf activation and axis formation. J Biol Chem. 2000; 275(42):32871–8.
18. Durak O, et al. Chd8 mediates cortical neurogenesis via transcriptional regulation of cell cycle and Wnt signaling. Nat Neurosci. 2016;19(11):1477–88.
19. Nishiyama M, et al. CHD8 suppresses p53-mediated apoptosis through histone H1 recruitment during early embryogenesis. Nat Cell Biol. 2009; 11(2):172–82.
20. Nishiyama M, et al. Early embryonic death in mice lacking the beta-catenin-binding protein Duplin. Mol Cell Biol. 2004;24(19):8386–94.
21. Katayama Y, et al. CHD8 haploinsufficiency results in autistic-like phenotypes in mice. Nature. 2016;537(7622):675–9.
22. Platt RJ, et al. Chd8 mutation leads to autistic-like behaviors and impaired striatal circuits. Cell Rep. 2017;19(2):335–50.
23. Suetterlin P, et al. Altered neocortical gene expression, brain overgrowth and functional over-connectivity in Chd8 haploinsufficient mice. Cereb Cortex. 2018;28(6):2192–206.
24. Jung H, et al. Sexually dimorphic behavior, neuronal activity, and gene expression in Chd8-mutant mice. Nat Neurosci. 2018;21(9):1218–28.
25. Zhao C, et al. Dual requirement of CHD8 for chromatin landscape establishment and histone methyltransferase recruitment to promote CNS myelination and repair. Dev Cell. 2018;45(6):753–68 e8.
26. Guo SL, et al. Serum inducible kinase is a positive regulator of cortical dendrite development and is required for BDNF-promoted dendritic arborization. Cell Res. 2012;22(2):387–98.
27. Miao S, et al. The Angelman syndrome protein Ube3a is required for polarized dendrite morphogenesis in pyramidal neurons. J Neurosci. 2013; 33(1):327–33.
28. Li S, et al. TORC1 regulates activity-dependent CREB-target gene transcription and dendritic growth of developing cortical neurons. J Neurosci. 2009;29(8):2334–43.
29. Anagnostou E, Taylor MJ. Review of neuroimaging in autism spectrum disorders: what have we learned and where we go from here. Mol Autism. 2011;2(1):4.
30. Di Martino A, et al. The autism brain imaging data exchange: towards a large-scale evaluation of the intrinsic brain architecture in autism. Mol Psychiatry. 2014;19(6):659–67.
31. Penzes P, et al. Dendritic spine pathology in neuropsychiatric disorders. Nat Neurosci. 2011;14(3):285–93.

32. Hulbert SW, Jiang YH. Cellular and circuitry bases of autism: lessons learned from the temporospatial manipulation of autism genes in the brain. Neurosci Bull. 2017;33(2):205–18.
33. Hulbert JC, Henson RN, Anderson MC. Inducing amnesia through systemic suppression. Nat Commun. 2016;7:11003.
34. Jeremy Willsey A, State MW. Autism spectrum disorders: from genes to neurobiology. Curr Opin Neurobiol. 2015;30C:92–9.
35. Gompers AL, et al. Germline Chd8 haploinsufficiency alters brain development in mouse. Nat Neurosci. 2017;20(8):1062–73.
36. Wang P, et al. CRISPR/Cas9-mediated heterozygous knockout of the autism gene CHD8 and characterization of its transcriptional networks in neurodevelopment. Mol Autism. 2015;6:55.
37. Sugathan A, et al. CHD8 regulates neurodevelopmental pathways associated with autism spectrum disorder in neural progenitors. Proc Natl Acad Sci U S A. 2014;111(42):E4468–77.
38. de la Torre-Ubieta L, et al. The dynamic landscape of open chromatin during human cortical neurogenesis. Cell. 2018;172(1–2):289–304 e18.
39. Wang P, et al. CRISPR/Cas9-mediated heterozygous knockout of the autism gene CHD8 and characterization of its transcriptional networks in cerebral organoids derived from iPS cells. Mol Autism. 2017;8:11.

14

The valproic acid rat model of autism presents with gut bacterial dysbiosis similar to that in human autism

Fang Liu[1], Kayla Horton-Sparks[2], Vanessa Hull[2], Robert W. Li[3*] and Verónica Martínez-Cerdeño[2,4,5*]

Abstract

Background: Gut microbiota has the capacity to impact the regular function of the brain, which can in turn affect the composition of microbiota. Autism spectrum disorder (ASD) patients suffer from gastrointestinal problems and experience changes in gut microbiota; however, it is not yet clear whether the change in the microbiota associated with ASD is a cause or a consequence of the disease.

Methods: We have investigated the species richness and microbial composition in a valproic acid (VPA)-induced rat model autism. Fecal samples from the rectum were collected at necropsy, microbial total DNA was extracted, 16 rRNA genes sequenced using Illumina, and the global microbial co-occurrence network was constructed using a random matrix theory-based pipeline. Collected rat microbiome data were compared to available data derived from cases of autism.

Results: We found that VPA administration during pregnancy reduced fecal microbial richness, changed the gut microbial composition, and altered the metabolite potential of the fecal microbial community in a pattern similar to that seen in patients with ASD. However, the global network property and network composition as well as microbial co-occurrence patterns were largely preserved in the offspring of rats exposed to prenatal administration of VPA.

Conclusions: Our data on the microbiota of the VPA rat model of autism indicate that this model, in addition to behaviorally and anatomically mimicking the autistic brain as previously shown, also mimics the microbiome features of autism, making it one of the best-suited rodent models for the study of autism and ASD.

Introduction

The gut and brain form the gut-brain axis through bidirectional nervous, endocrine, and immune communication. A change in one of these systems will most certainly have effects on the other systems. Disorders in the composition and quantity of gut microbiota can affect both the enteric nervous system and the central nervous system [1]. Specifically, microbiota has the capacity to impact the regular function of the brain, which can in turn affect the composition of microbiota via specific substances. Specific molecules and metabolic pathways in microbiota have been shown to be linked to neural development and neurodegenerative disorders, including Parkinson's disease, Alzheimer's disease, Huntington's disease, schizophrenia, and multiple sclerosis [1–3].

Valproic acid (VPA) is a medication used for epilepsy and mood swings. Children prenatally exposed to VPA have an increased chance of being diagnosed with autism [4–7]. In addition, VPA exposure leads to accelerated or early brain growth which also occurs in some cases of autism [8]. Most importantly, VPA causes an alteration in the excitation/inhibition the cerebral cortex. Specifically, rats exposed to VPA in utero present with an increased glutamatergic and a decreased GABAergic component in the cortex [9]. The VPA rat model of autism experiences behavioral, immune, and microbiota changes similar to those described in patients with autism. We recently discovered that specific GABAergic

* Correspondence: Robert.Li@ARS.USDA.GOV; vmartinezcerdeno@ucdavis.edu
[3]United States Department of Agriculture, Agriculture Research Service (USDA-ARS), Animal Genomics and Improvement Laboratory, Beltsville, MD, USA
[2]Institute for Pediatric Regenerative Medicine and Shriners Hospitals for Children Northern California, 2504 Stockton Blvd, Sacramento, CA 95817, USA

interneuron types, the parvalbumin (PV)+ Chandelier (Ch) and PV+ Baskets cells (Bsk) cells, are decreased in the prefrontal cortex in autism [10, 11]. We also demonstrated that when VPA is administered via intraperitoneal injection to pregnant rats at a specific day of prenatal development with a specific dose (E (embryonic day) 12.5, 400 mg/kg), the offspring of these rats ("400-E12 VPA rats") experienced a decrease in the number of PV+ Ch and PV+ Bsk cells in their adult cerebral cortex similar to what we found in humans with autism (under revision). In addition, the 400-E12 VPA rats also experienced behavioral changes similar to those exhibited by patients with autism (under revision).

ASD patients suffer from gastrointestinal problems and experience changes in the gut microbiota, including shifts in levels of *Firmicutes, Bacteroidetes, and Proteobacteria* with the abundance of *Lactobacillares* and *Clostridia* [12, 13]. Other gut commensals found to be altered in autism belong to the genera such as *Bifidobacterium, Lactobacillus, Prevotella,* and *Ruminococcus* [14]. Microbiome changes have been also described in several mouse models for autism, with one publication in a VPA mouse indicating a decreased abundance for *Bacteroidetes* in VPA exposed offspring [15]. It is not yet clear whether the changes in the microbiome associated to specific disease states are a cause or a consequence of the disease. Recent studies indicate that gut microbiota transplantation can transfer behavioral phenotypes, suggesting that the gut microbiota may be a modifiable factor modulating the development or pathogenesis of neuropsychiatric conditions. In this study, we investigated changes in microbial richness and microbiome composition in rats in response to VPA prenatal administration (400 mg/kg at E12) and found VPA-induced alterations similar to those seen in autism.

Results

VPA reduces fecal microbial richness of the offspring

A single IP injection of VPA during pregnancy in rats had a significant effect on fecal microbial richness in their offspring ($P < 0.05$, the Welch t test). In the control rats, Chao1 value was 1005.62 ± 120.00 ($N = 11$). VPA injection significantly reduced Chao1 to 925.98 ± 76.62 ($N = 10$, $P < 0.05$). However, other microbial diversity indicators, such as Pielou's evenness, PD whole tree, and Shannon and Simpson indices, remained unchanged by VPA.

In utero VPA exposure also had a profound impact on fecal microbial structure. At the operational taxonomic unit (OTU) level, mean Bray-Curtis similarity values (%) within either the control or VPA groups were 63.57 ± 4.04, a significantly higher than mean similarity between the control and VPA groups (59.52 ± 3.24; $P = 1.78 \times 10^{-12}$). A cluster analysis using the group average approach of the resemblance values suggested individual microbial communities from the control and VPA groups were able to form two distinct clusters, respectively (Fig. 1). Together, our findings suggest that the effect of VPA may be long-lasting and could have a significant impact on the fecal microbial community structure in rats prenatally exposed to the toxin.

VPA affects the gut microbial composition

Compared to the control group, VPA treatment significantly altered the abundance of 13 higher level taxa based on linear discriminating analysis (LDA) scores (the absolute $\log_{10}$ LDA score, or LDA, > 2.0 and $P < 0.05$ based on the Kruskal-Wallis test), including one class (α-Proteobacteria, Fig. 2a), four families (Fig. 2b, c), and six genera (Fig. 3a, b). For example, the abundance of α-Proteobacteria was significantly increased by VPA treatment (Fig. 2a; LDA > 3.4 and $P < 0.05$). The abundance of three families, Eubacteriaceae (Fig. 2b), Rikenellaceae, and Staphylococcaceae was also significantly increased by VPA (LDA > 2.0 and $P < 0.05$). On the other hand, the abundance of Enterobacteriaceae (Fig. 2c) was significantly repressed by VPA (LDA = 2.0229 and $P = 0.0014$). At the genus level, a significantly higher abundance level of the genus *Anaerotruncus* (Fig. 3a) was observed in the control group than in the VPA group while the VPA significantly increased the abundance of *Allobaculum, Anaerofustis, Proteus,* and *Staphylococcus* (LDA > 2.0 and $P < 0.01$; Fig. 3b).

The abundance of at least 100 OTU was significantly impacted by VPA treatment (LDA > 2.0 and $P < 0.05$ based on the Kruskal-Wallis test), representing approximately 10% of all OTU in a given gut microbial community (Additional file 1). Together, the relative abundance of these OTU accounted for approximately 15% of the fecal microbial community. Intriguingly, 93 of the 100 OTU significantly impacted by VPA belonged to the class Clostridia. Select OTU with significantly altered relative abundance by VPA were listed in Table 1. Compared to untreated controls, VPA repressed the abundance of 61 OTU while increasing that of 39 OTU. For example, 2 OTU assigned to a named species, *Ruminococcus flavefaciens*, ID_1110988 (Fig. 3c) and ID_562599, were significantly increased by VPA (Fig. 3c). Moreover, VPA had a profound impact on some of the most predominant OTU. Two OTU, ID_4296216 and ID_264734, belonging to the genus *Ruminococcus* and the family S24-7, respectively, were significantly increased by VPA; and both had relative abundance greater than 1.0%. OTU ID_272080 (Clostridiales, Fig. 3d) and ID_177930 (Lachnospiraceae) were also among the most abundant.

Differences in microbial composition between the sexes were investigated by comparing male and female

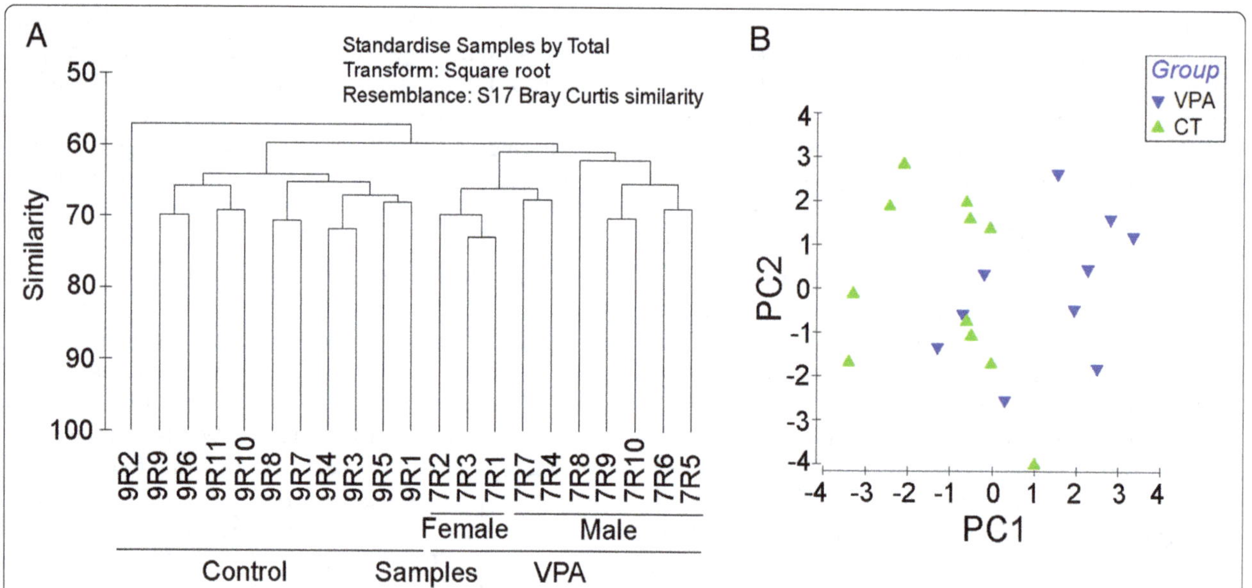

Fig. 1 β-diversity in the gut microbial community of rats with or without prenatal valproic acid (VPA) exposure. **a** Clustering analysis based on Bray-Curtis similarity. Bray-Curtis similarity matrix based on square-root-transformed abundance at an OTU level. **b** Principal component analysis (PCA) based on Bray-Curtis similarity generated using the Vegan package in the R program. Control: rats without prenatal VPA exposure ($N = 11$). VPA: rats with VAP exposure ($N = 10$)

rats prenatally exposed to VPA with same-sex control rats. While uneven sample size in the male and female comparison may be a concern, the drastic sex-dependent changes induced by VPA were evident (Fig. 4a, b). At the phylum level, the abundance of Bacteroidetes was significantly increased by VPA in males only (LDA = 4.69; $P < 0.05$) while the abundance of Actinobacteria was significantly increased by VPA in females only (LDA = 3.50; $P < 0.05$), as compared to controls of the same sex. VPA significantly repressed the abundance of the class Coriobacteriia while it increased the two classes Bacteroidia and α-Proteobacteria in males only (LDA > 2.0 and $P < 0.05$). The abundance of several genera was significantly increased by VPA only in females, including *Allobaculum*, *Bifidobacterium*, *Odoribacter*, and *Staphylococcus* (LDA > 2.6 and $P < 0.05$). Intriguingly, the abundance of the genus *Candidatus* Arthromitus, a group of the segmented filamentous bacteria (SFB), was also significantly increased by VPA in female rats (LDA = 3.774 and $P = 0.015$) but not males. There is strong evidence demonstrating that these gut epithelium-associated bacteria possess strong abilities to modulate host immune responses.

At the species (OTU) level, VPA prenatal exposure induced significant changes in the relative abundance of 66 and 72 OTU in male and female rats, respectively. Among them, the abundance of 61 OTU was also significantly impacted by VPA exposure regardless of gender. A total of 9 OTU displayed significant directional changes by VPA in both male and female rats (Table 2). For example, the relative abundance of an OTU (GreenGene ID_1110312) assigned to the order Clostridiales and an OTU (GreenGene ID_1110988) assigned to *Ruminococcus flavefaciens* was significantly higher in both male and female rats with

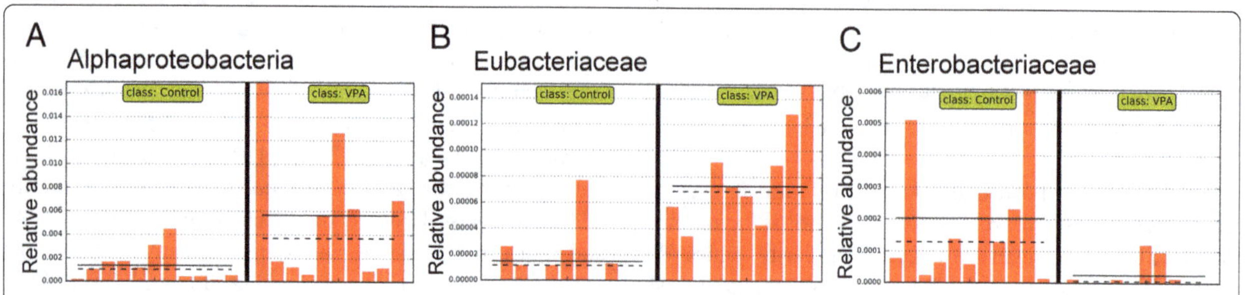

Fig. 2 Microbial taxa displaying significant differences in relative abundance between rats with and without VPA exposure. **a** The Class Alpha-Proteobacteria. **b** The family Eubacteriaceae. **c** The family Enterobacteriaceae. Straight line, group mean abundance; dotted line, median. Control: rats without prenatal VPA exposure ($N = 11$). VPA, rats with VPA exposure ($N = 10$)

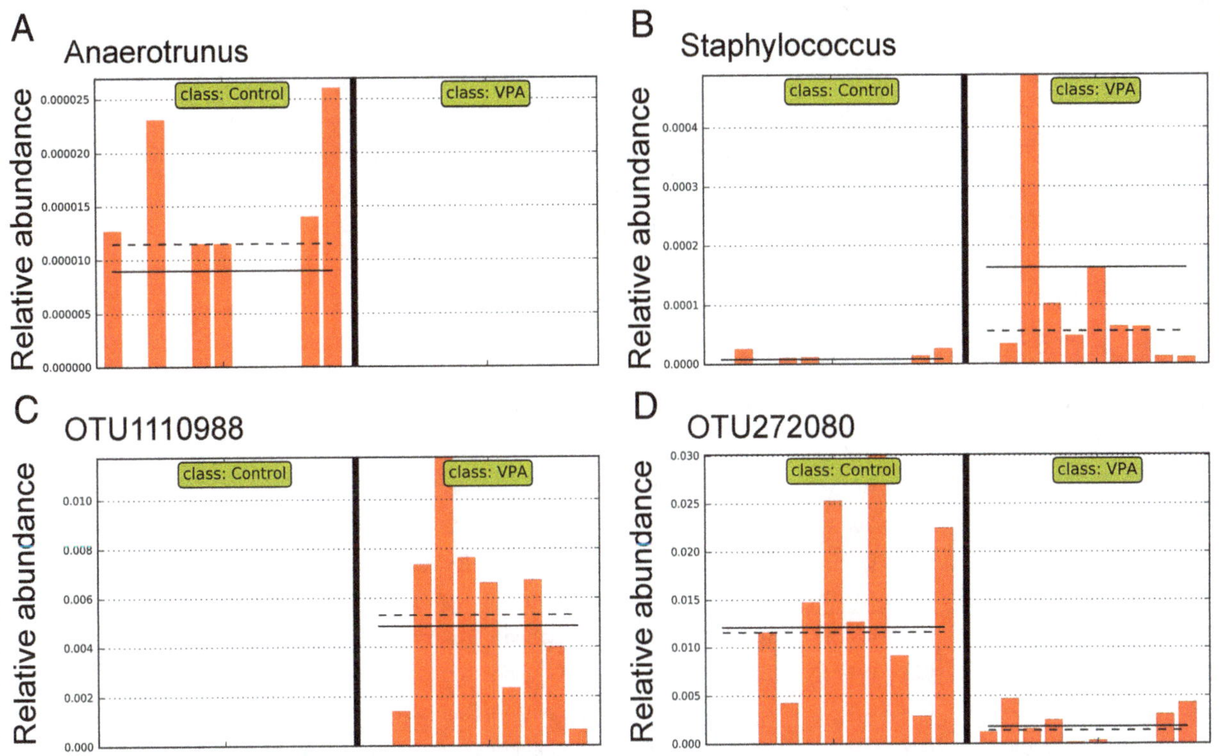

Fig. 3 Select microbial genera and species with significant differences in relative abundance between rats with and without prenatal VPA exposure. **a** *Anaerotrunus*. **b** *Staphylococcus*. **c** OTU assigned to *Ruminococcus flavefaciens* (GreenGene ID# 1110988). **d** An OTU belonging to the family Lachnospiraceae (GreenGene ID# 272080). Straight line; group mean abundance; dotted line, median. Control: rats without prenatal VPA exposure ($N = 11$). VPA: rats with VPA exposure ($N = 10$)

prenatal VPA exposure (LDA > 3.40; $P < 0.001$) while 7 other OTU were significantly reduced in fecal microbial communities of both male and female rats with VPA exposure (LDA > 2.0 and $P < 0.05$).

VPA alters the metabolite potential of the fecal microbial community

Among the 5264 predicted KEGG proteins from the rat fecal microbiome, 4331 proteins were supported by at least 10 hits. Several proteins belonging to ABC transporters, such as multiple sugar transport system permease protein (K02025) and ATP-binding cassette, subfamily B, bacterial (K06147), and RNA polymerase sigma-70 factor, ECF subfamily (K03088) were among the most abundant. Compared to the control, VPA injection repressed the abundance of 11 KEGG proteins, including putative ABC transport system ATP-binding protein (K02003), multiple sugar transport system substrate-binding protein (K02027), LacI family transcriptional regulator (K02529), methyl-accepting chemotaxis protein (K03406), two proteins related to two-component system, K07718 and K07720, and four proteins in the peptide/nickel transport system (K02031, K02032, K02033, K02034; ATP-binding and permease proteins, respectively).

VPA injection appeared to have a profound impact on gut microbial metabolic pathways. A total of 29 pathways were significantly impacted by VPA (LDA score > 2.0; $P < 0.05$), resulting in a significantly elevated hit count for 21 pathways while repressing 8 pathways (Table 3). For example, the normalized hit counts assigned to bacterial secretion system, DNA replication, DNA repairs and recombination proteins, histidine metabolism, and lipid biosynthesis were significantly increased by VPA. On the other hand, ABC transporters, the most abundant pathways in numerous biological systems, and two-component system, bacterial chemotaxis and bacterial motility proteins, were significantly repressed by VPA.

Microbial co-occurrence patterns and network structure remain unchanged by VPA

As Table 4 shows, the global network properties as well as network composition and microbial co-occurrence patterns in fecal microbial communities of the offspring between the control and VPA-treated rats were largely indistinguishable. Both global networks were highly modular with a modularity between 0.84 and 0.86. Both networks shared 230 nodes (OTU) or 57.1% of all members. The number of large modules with ≥ 10 members

Table 1 Select OTUs significantly impacted by prenatal VPA injection

OTU_ID	Control	VPA	LDA	Annotation
513,445	0.31 ± 0.19	0.56 ± 0.29	3.0954	Bacteroidetes; Bacteroidia; Bacteroidales; Bacteroidaceae; Bacteroides
264,734	0.74 ± 0.54	1.51 ± 1.25	3.6429	Bacteroidetes; Bacteroidia; Bacteroidales; S24-7
581,474	0.00 ± 0.00	0.23 ± 0.33	3.0596	Firmicutes; Bacilli; Lactobacillales; Lactobacillaceae; Lactobacillus
272,080	1.21 ± 1.03	0.18 ± 0.18	3.7107	Firmicutes; Clostridia; Clostridiales
661,055	0.01 ± 0.01	0.54 ± 1.09	3.4725	Firmicutes; Clostridia; Clostridiales
1,110,312	0.17 ± 0.07	0.72 ± 0.51	3.4043	Firmicutes; Clostridia; Clostridiales
276,770	0.51 ± 0.40	0.03 ± 0.07	3.3477	Firmicutes; Clostridia; Clostridiales
631,564	0.44 ± 0.57	0.01 ± 0.01	3.2945	Firmicutes; Clostridia; Clostridiales
276,777	0.45 ± 0.46	0.12 ± 0.20	3.2476	Firmicutes; Clostridia; Clostridiales
460,611	0.48 ± 0.41	0.18 ± 0.31	3.1188	Firmicutes; Clostridia; Clostridiales
461,487	0.26 ± 0.16	0.52 ± 0.27	3.1123	Firmicutes; Clostridia; Clostridiales
290,338	0.35 ± 0.47	0.15 ± 0.25	3.0820	Firmicutes; Clostridia; Clostridiales
408,877	0.25 ± 0.35	0.03 ± 0.02	3.0675	Firmicutes; Clostridia; Clostridiales
348,404	0.10 ± 0.08	0.31 ± 0.19	3.0249	Firmicutes; Clostridia; Clostridiales
422,727	0.32 ± 0.19	0.12 ± 0.13	3.0146	Firmicutes; Clostridia; Clostridiales
277,208	0.02 ± 0.03	0.22 ± 0.22	3.0105	Firmicutes; Clostridia; Clostridiales
421,893	0.04 ± 0.14	0.27 ± 0.48	3.0056	Firmicutes; Clostridia; Clostridiales
310,760	0.12 ± 0.24	0.84 ± 0.78	3.5307	Firmicutes; Clostridia; Clostridiales; Lachnospiraceae
350,447	0.57 ± 0.46	0.17 ± 0.18	3.2725	Firmicutes; Clostridia; Clostridiales; Lachnospiraceae
177,930	0.83 ± 0.27	0.57 ± 0.30	3.1974	Firmicutes; Clostridia; Clostridiales; Lachnospiraceae
383,971	0.50 ± 0.34	0.21 ± 0.18	3.1159	Firmicutes; Clostridia; Clostridiales; Lachnospiraceae; [Ruminococcus]; gnavus
401,384	0.55 ± 0.29	0.27 ± 0.09	3.1489	Firmicutes; Clostridia; Clostridiales; Ruminococcaceae; Oscillospira
461,795	0.04 ± 0.04	0.27 ± 0.27	3.1198	Firmicutes; Clostridia; Clostridiales; Ruminococcaceae; Oscillospira
4,296,216	1.07 ± 0.71	2.40 ± 1.66	3.8102	Firmicutes; Clostridia; Clostridiales; Ruminococcaceae; Ruminococcus
268,043	0.54 ± 0.52	0.16 ± 0.16	3.2365	Firmicutes; Clostridia; Clostridiales; Ruminococcaceae; Ruminococcus
1,110,988	0.00 ± 0.00	0.48 ± 0.38	3.4032	Firmicutes; Clostridia; Clostridiales; Ruminococcaceae; Ruminococcus; flavefaciens

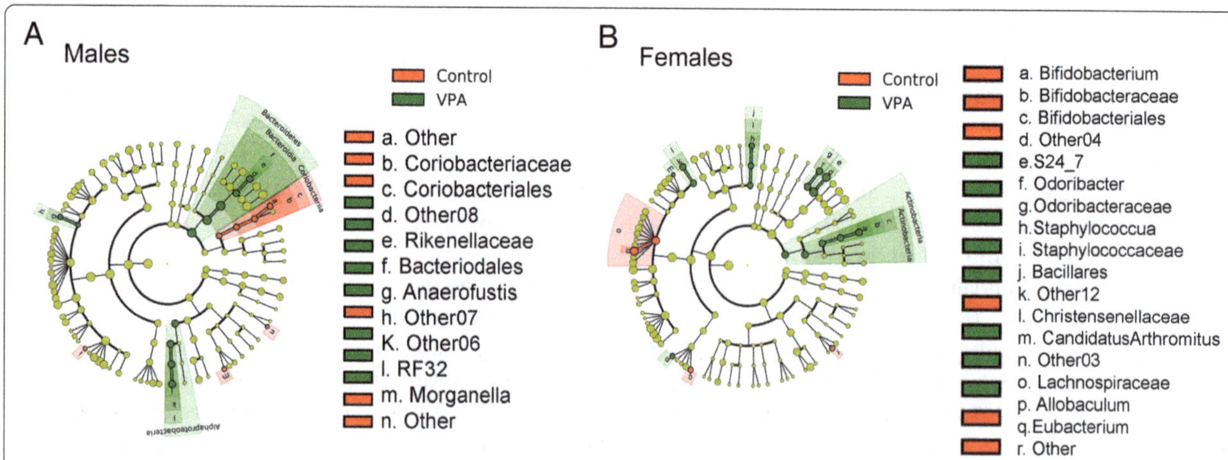

Fig. 4 Graphical representation of the taxa with significantly different abundance in the gut microbial community of rats induced by prenatal VPA exposure. **a** Male rats with prenatal VPA exposure (VPA) comparing to male rats without prenatal VPA exposure (Control). **b** Female rats with prenatal VPA exposure (VPA) comparing to female rats without prenatal VPA exposure (Control). The statistical significance cutoff: absolute linear discriminant analysis (LDA) score $\log_{10} \geq 2.0$

Table 2 Nine OTUs displayed a significant difference in relative abundance between control and VPA groups regardless of sex. The numbers denote relative abundance (mean ± SD)

OTU_ID	Control	VPA	LDA value	Annotation
50,208	0.0316 ± 0.0313	0.0000 ± 0.0000	2.1609	Clostridiales
227,788	0.0845 ± 0.0743	0.0000 ± 0.0000	2.6365	Clostridiales
321,960	0.0477 ± 0.0235	0.0000 ± 0.0000	2.3910	Clostridiales; Ruminococcaceae
352,799	0.1134 ± 0.1965	0.0091 ± 0.0059	2.7102	Clostridiales; Lachnospiraceae
450,576	0.0502 ± 0.0400	0.0000 ± 0.0000	2.4470	Clostridiales; Ruminococcaceae
839,137	0.0493 ± 0.0325	0.0215 ± 0.0146	2.1805	Clostridiales; Lachnospiraceae
1,107,799	0.0524 ± 0.0431	0.0073 ± 0.0102	2.3709	Clostridiales
1,110,312	0.1708 ± 0.0684	0.7212 ± 0.5143	3.4043	Clostridiales
1,110,988	0.0001 ± 0.0004	0.4848 ± 0.3770	3.4032	Clostridiales; Ruminococcaceae; Ruminococcus; flavefaciens

Table 3 The microbial pathways significantly impacted by VPA

Pathways	Control	VPA	LDA score	*P* value
ABC transporters	3.29 ± 0.39	3.04 ± 0.24	3.0834	0.0486
Amino acid-related enzymes	1.41 ± 0.01	1.43 ± 0.02	2.0357	0.0039
Bacterial chemotaxis	0.57 ± 0.12	0.47 ± 0.07	2.6664	0.0346
Bacterial motility proteins	1.23 ± 0.27	1.01 ± 0.15	3.0238	0.0411
Bacterial secretion system	0.48 ± 0.02	0.50 ± 0.03	2.1010	0.0167
Carbon fixation pathways in prokaryotes	0.95 ± 0.09	1.03 ± 0.07	2.5883	0.0201
Chaperones and folding catalysts	0.96 ± 0.06	1.01 ± 0.04	2.3375	0.0411
Chromosome	1.51 ± 0.03	1.53 ± 0.02	2.1418	0.0137
Citrate cycle	0.54 ± 0.08	0.62 ± 0.07	2.5479	0.0167
DNA repair and recombination proteins	2.68 ± 0.06	2.75 ± 0.05	2.5379	0.0167
DNA replication	0.62 ± 0.02	0.64 ± 0.02	2.0466	0.0112
DNA replication proteins	1.17 ± 0.03	1.20 ± 0.03	2.2293	0.0346
Flagellar assembly	0.61 ± 0.15	0.48 ± 0.09	2.7850	0.0486
Glycine, serine and threonine metabolism	0.80 ± 0.02	0.82 ± 0.02	2.0011	0.0290
Histidine metabolism	0.63 ± 0.04	0.66 ± 0.02	2.1867	0.0242
Homologous recombination	0.89 ± 0.03	0.93 ± 0.02	2.2693	0.0112
Lipid biosynthesis proteins	0.59 ± 0.03	0.61 ± 0.02	2.0892	0.0486
Oxidative phosphorylation	1.01 ± 0.08	1.08 ± 0.08	2.5044	0.0411
Peptidases	1.90 ± 0.04	1.93 ± 0.03	2.1605	0.0486
Porphyrin and chlorophyll metabolism	0.95 ± 0.04	0.89 ± 0.05	2.4393	0.0201
Protein export	0.55 ± 0.02	0.57 ± 0.02	2.1048	0.0167
Protein kinases	0.34 ± 0.03	0.31 ± 0.02	2.1524	0.0242
Pyrimidine metabolism	1.79 ± 0.03	1.82 ± 0.02	2.2223	0.0242
Riboflavin metabolism	0.19 ± 0.03	0.21 ± 0.02	2.0135	0.0486
Ribosome	2.13 ± 0.07	2.21 ± 0.07	2.6423	0.0167
Terpenoid backbone biosynthesis	0.51 ± 0.02	0.53 ± 0.02	2.0739	0.0201
Transporters	7.52 ± 1.02	6.79 ± 0.66	3.5543	0.0290
Two-component system	1.59 ± 0.13	1.49 ± 0.06	2.6900	0.0290

Table 4 Select topological properties of global networks of fecal microbial communities of the offspring of rats with prenatal administration of PBS (Control) and VPA

Network property	Control	VPA
Total nodes	403	411
Total links	487	488
Modularity	0.856	0.843
Number of modules	55	60
Number of modules with ≥ 10 members	12	12
Average degree (avgK)	2.417	2.375
Average clustering coefficient (avgCC)	0.138	0.087
Average path distance (GD)	9.579	7.169
Geodesic efficiency (*E*)	0.148	0.185
Harmonic geodesic distance (HD)	6.772	5.398
Maximal degree	13	16
Centralization of degree (CD)	0.026	0.033
Maximal eigenvector centrality	0.268	0.374
Centralization of eigenvector centrality (CE)	0.249	0.359
Density (*D*)	0.006	0.006
Transitivity (Trans)	0.187	0.117
Connectedness (Con)	0.464	0.340

in the two networks was identical [12]. Moreover, the relative proportion (%) of OTU node distributions at the phylum level was stable between the two networks (Fig. 5). For example, the most dominant phylum in both networks were Firmicutes, accounting for 89.6% and 87.6% of all OTU in the control and VPA networks, respectively, which was similar to the percentage of the OTU assigned to Firmicutes in the microbial communities prior to network inference (88.3 and 87.5%, in the control and VPA groups, respectively). Moreover, the percentage of OTU nodes assigned to Actinobacteria was 0.50 and 0.49% in the control and VPA networks, respectively. Some minor yet notable differences existed, nevertheless. The percentage of OTU nodes assigned to Proteobacteria was 0.99% and 0.49% in the control and VPA networks, respectively. Of note, one OTU (GreenGeneID_1136443) assigned to *Mucispirillum schaedleri*, the sole species in the phylum Deferribacteres, was present in every sample collected in a relatively high abundance but did not interact with any other OTU in the communities. As a result, this species was not a member of either network.

The Z-P scatter plots allowed us to dissect the topological roles of OTU nodes in the network and infer their possible ecological function in the fecal microbial community. As Fig. 6 shows, > 98% of the OTU nodes in both networks were peripherals with most of their links lying inside their own modules, based on the Olesen classification [16]. These OTU likely acted as specialists in the microbial community. A total of six OTU, all assigned to the order Clostridiales, may function as generalists in the fecal microbial community of control rats, including one OTU (GreenGene ID_545038), assigned to the family Peptostreptococcaceae, acted as a connector species, linking modules together while other five OTU were module hubs and may play an important role for the coherence of its own module. The relative abundance of the two of the five OTU, GreenGene_ID_461487 and _1109864, was also significantly altered by VPA administration. In the VPA network, the OTU acted as connectors and module hubs were completely different. While all three connectors were from the order Clostridiales, two of them belonged to the

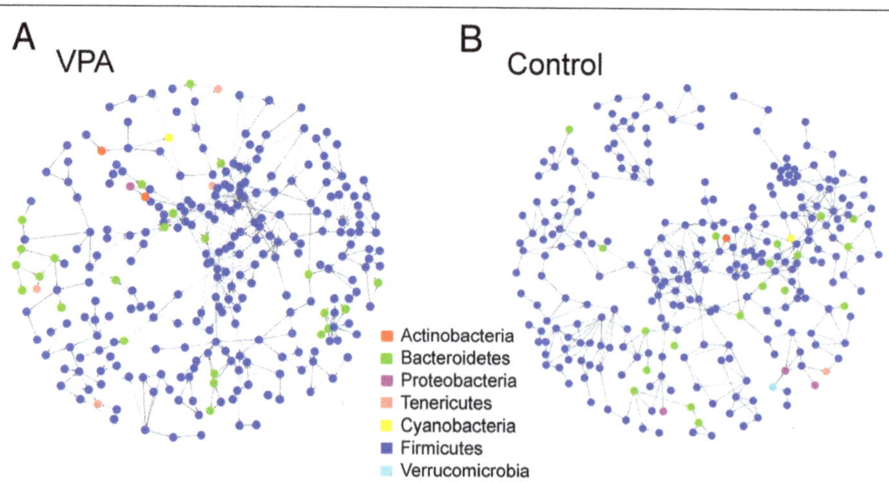

Fig. 5 Visualization of microbial co-occurrence networks identified using the fast greedy modularity optimization method in the rats with and without prenatal VPA exposure. **a** The rats with prenatal VPA exposure (VPA). **b** Control rats without prenatal VPA exposure. Nodes represent an OTU. Edge (links) with solid lines, positive connection; dashed lines, negative connection. The color of the nodes indicates the phylum to which the OTU belong

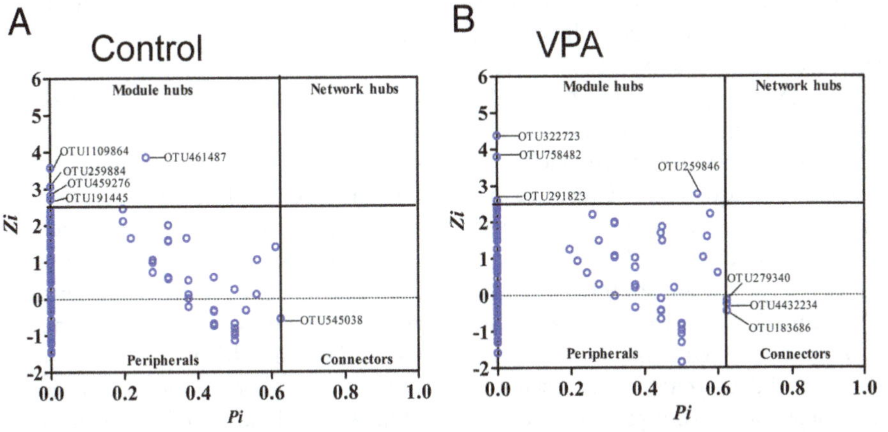

Fig. 6 The scatter plot showing the distribution of OTU based on their topological roles in the network in the gut microbial community of rats with and without prenatal VPA exposure. **a** Control. **b** VPA. Each dot represents an OTU. Z, within-module connectivity. P, Among-module connectivity

family Ruminococcaceae (GreenGene ID_183686 and _4432234). On the other hand, one of the four module hubs, GreenGene ID_322723, was from the genus *Lactobacillus* while other three OTU were from the order Clostridiales in the VPA network. Overall, we demonstrated that prenatal administration of VPA reduces fecal microbial richness, changes the gut microbial composition, and alters the metabolite potential of the fecal microbial community in rats. However, the global network property and network composition as well as microbial co-occurrence patterns are largely preserved in these animals.

Materials and methods

VPA administration

Intraperitoneal administration of VPA (valproic acid sodium salt, Sigma P4543) was delivered to pregnant Sprague Dawley rats (8 weeks old) at E12.5 ($n = 3$). Pregnant control dams of the same age were injected with sterile saline also at E12.5 ($n = 5$). The pups of these dams were the subjects of this study. We collected stool and tissue samples from 10 VPA offspring and 11 control offspring equally distributed among groups.

Fecal total DNA extraction

Fecal samples from the rectum were collected from 8-week-old rats at necropsy and snap-frozen in liquid nitrogen and stored at − 80 °C freezers until total DNA was extracted. Microbial total DNA was extracted from fecal samples using a QIAamp PowerFecal DNA Kit (Qiagen, Germantown, MD, USA). DNA integrity and concentration were quantified using a BioAnalyzer 2100 (Agilent, Palo Alto, CA, USA).

Illumina sequencing of 16S rRNA genes

The 16S rRNA gene sequencing was performed as previously described [17, 18]. The hypervariable V3–V4 regions of the 16S rRNA gene were directly amplified from 20 ng of input total DNA using Illumina platform-compatible PAGE-purified adaptor oligos that contain important features including sequencing primers, sample-specific barcodes, and 16S PCR primers (forward primer, 341/357F, CCTACGGGNGGCWGCAG; reverse primer, 805R: GACTACHVGGGTATCTAATCC). The PCR reaction included 1.25 units of AccuPrime TaqDNA Polymerase High Fidelity (Invitrogen, Carlsbad, CA, USA) in a 25-μl reaction buffer containing 200 nM primers, 200 nM dNTP, 60 mM Tris-SO4, 18 mM $(NH4)_2SO4$, 2.0 mM MgSO4, 1% glycerol, and 100 ng/uL bovine serum albumin (New England BioLabs, Ipswich, MA, USA). PCR was performed using the following cycling profile: initial denaturing at 95 °C for 2 min followed by 20 cycles of 95 °C 30 s, 60 °C 30 s, and 72 °C 60 s. Amplicons were purified using Agencourt AMPure XP bead kits (Beckman Coulter Genomics, Danvers, MA, USA) and quantified using a BioAnalyzer DNA 7500 chip kit and a QuantiFluor fluorometer. The purified amplicons from individual samples were pooled in equal molar ratios. The purified amplicon pool was further spiked with approximately 25% of whole-genome shotgun libraries prepared using an Illumina TruSeq DNA sample prep kit with a compatible adaptor barcode to enhance sequence diversity during the first few cycles of sequencing for better cluster differentiation. The concentration of the pooled final library pool was quantified using a BioAnalyzer high-sensitivity DNA chip kit (Agilent). The library pool was sequenced using an Illumina MiSeq Reagent Kit v3 on an Illumina MiSeq sequencer as described previously. The mean number of 2 × 250 bp pair-end sequences obtained was 347,849.14 (± 90,627.63, SD, $N = 21$) per sample.

Sequence data analysis

The sequence data were preprocessed using MiSeq Control Software (MCS) v2.4.1. Raw sequences were first analyzed using FastQC version 0.11.2 to check basic statistics, such as GC%, per base quality score distribution, and sequences flagged as poor quality. The four maximally degenerate bases (NNNN) at the most 5′ end of the read pair, which were designed to maximize the diversity during the first four bases of the sequencing run for better identification of unique clusters and improve base-calling accuracy, were then removed. The presence of forward and reverse PCR primers at the 5′ and 3′ ends of each sequence read was scanned; the reads without primers were discarded. Chimeric reads were also removed. The processed pair-end reads were then merged using PandaSeq v2.8 to generate representative complete nucleotide sequences (contigs) using default parameters. The overlapping regions of the pair-end read were first aligned and scored, and reads with low score alignments and high rate of mismatches were discarded. After these quality control steps and filtering procedures, greater than 91% of the input raw sequences (mean 347,849 reads per sample) retained for subsequent analysis.

The QIIME pipeline (v.1.9.1) with the default reference v. 0.1.3 was used to analyze the 16S rRNA gene sequences. Both "closed reference" and "open reference" protocols in the pipeline were used for OTU picking as previously described [18]. The rarefaction depth was set to 100,000 quality reads per sample. The default QIIME parameters were used, except for that the OTU abundance threshold (lowered to 0.0001%). The GreenGene database (v13.8) was used for taxonomy assignment (greengenes.lbl.gov). PyNAST (v1.2.2) was used for sequence alignment. PICRUSt (v1.0.0), a software package designed to predict metagenome functional contents from marker gene surveys (Langille et al., 2013), was used with default parameters to predict gene contents and metagenomic functional information based on the OTU table generated using the closed-reference protocol in QIIME. Briefly, the OTU table was first normalized by dividing each OTU by the known/predicted 16S copy number by using the PICRUSt workflow: normalize_by_copy_number.py. The gene contents or the abundance of KEGG Orthology (KO) were predicted from the normalized OTU table using the workflow: predict_metagenomes.py. The predicted metagenome function was further analyzed by collapsing thousands of KEGG Orthologs into higher functional categories (pathways) (categorize_by_function.py). In addition, specific OTU contributing to a given function or pathway was identified by using the workflow: metagenome_contributions.py, as described previously [17]. The linear discriminant analysis effect size (LEfSe) algorithm was used to identify OTU relative abundance values and KEGG gene families and pathways that display significant differences between two biological conditions [19] with a default cutoff (the absolute $\log_{10}$ LDA score or LDA > 2.0 and P values < 0.05 based on the Kruskal-Wallis test by ranks).

Network construction and visualization

The global microbial co-occurrence network was constructed using a random matrix theory (RMT)-based pipeline [20, 21]. The OTU detected in < 50% of all samples were excluded due to a drastic effect of OTU sparsity on the precision and sensitivity of network inference [22]. A similarity matrix, which measures the degree of concordance between the abundance profiles of individual OTU across different samples, was then obtained by using Pearson correlation analysis of the abundance data [20]. A threshold cutoff value (0.88) was automatically determined by calculating the transition from Gaussian orthogonal ensemble to Poisson distribution of the nearest-neighbor spacing distribution of eigenvalues, in the pipeline and then applied to generate an adjacent matrix for network inference [21]. The fast-greedy modularity optimization procedure was used for module separation. The within-module degree (Z) and among-module connectivity (P) were then calculated and plotted to generate a scatter plot for each network to gain insights into the topological roles of individual nodes in the network according to the Olesen classification [21]. The network structure was finally visualized using Cytoscape v3.6.1.

Discussion

The gut and brain form the gut-brain axis through bidirectional nervous, endocrine, and immune communications. Mammalian species often contain similar microbiome richness at the level of phylum, but diversity and richness of species are highly variable among individuals [23]. This variability is determined by many factors, including genetics, environment, diet, disease, stress, and age [24]. When microbiota composition is altered due to any of these factors, the function of the intestinal mucosal barrier is reduced; and bacterial products such as amyloids and lipopolysaccharides leak, increasing the permeability of the blood brain barrier, which, in turn, affects the central nervous system [25].

Humans with autism and mice models of autism have shown significant alterations in their microbiota composition. Children with autism present with more GI symptoms than typically developing children, and the severity of their GI symptoms is correlated to the severity of their behavioral symptoms [26, 27]. These children also demonstrate bacterial dysbiosis, which has been suggested to play a role in autism's etiology [28]. While different studies have found changes in specific bacteria are often associated to dysbiosis in autism, it is generally accepted that the gut microbial community of patients with autism displays a higher relative abundance of Lactobacillacease and

Clostridia and a reduced incidence of the *Prevotella* and other fermenters [29–35].

Studies in mice have allowed to better understand the role of the microbiota in autism [36]. The lack of microbiota produces changes in behavior. For example, germ-free mice lack a preference for spending time with another mouse over spending time in an empty chamber and deviate from the experimental expectation that they would spend more time exploring a space containing a new mouse rather than a familiar mouse [37, 38]. Germ-free mice also show a differential gene expression associated with neuronal structure and function in the amygdala [39]. Germ-free rats present with a social deficit phenotype in the reciprocal social interaction test [40]. Antibiotic treatment in wildtype and mouse models of autism also affects social behavior [15, 41, 42]. On the other hand, the use of probiotics ameliorates behavioral deficits [38, 42]. Together, these data point out a role of microbiota in regulating behavior. The nature of microbiota has been studied in several mouse models for autism. The inbred mouse, BTBR, that presents with the full spectrum of ASD-like behavior, shows an overall decrease in bacterial diversity characterized by an increase in the relative abundance of the genus *Akkermansia* and a decrease in abundance of *Bifidobacterium and Clostridiales* [43–45]. In addition, BTBR mice have impaired intestinal integrity and a deficit in the intestinal tight junction proteins *Ocln* and *Tjp1* [46]. Environmental mice models of autism have also produced information about the importance of microbiota in this condition. In the maternal immune activation (MIA) mouse model, the species richness did not differ significantly between control and MIA offspring, but the offspring displayed decreased intestinal barrier integrity, altered gut microbiota, and increased abundance of the families Lachnospiraceae, Porphyromonadaceae, and Prevotellaceae [47]. In the maternal high-fat diet (MHFD) mouse model for autism, the diversity of the microbiota was decreased compared to the control group, with marked decreased in *Lactobacillus*, *Parabacteroides*, *Helicobacter*, and *B. uniformis*. In this study, we demonstrated that species richness in the fecal microbial community in the autistic-like rat model, the 400-E12 VPA rat, was significantly reduced. Using next-generation sequencing technology in a murine autism model, it was reported that the microbiome composition in mice in utero exposed to VPA presented with a decreased of *Bacteroids* [15]. Other gut commensals found to be altered in the VPA mice were *Deltaproteobacteris* and *Erysipelotrichales*. These changes in VPA mouse microbiota composition were coincident with changes in behaviors linked to autism [15].

Our 400-E12 VPA rats showed a decrease in microbial diversity (species richness). Specifically, significant increases in the abundance of *α-Proteobacteria*, *Eubateriaceae*, *Rikenellaceae*, and *Staphylococcaceae*. On the other hand, Enterobacteriaceae was significantly decreased by VPA exposure in utero. At the genus level, we found a significantly higher abundance of the genus *Anaerotruncus* in the control group and a significantly increased abundance of the genera *Allobaculum*, *Anaerofustis*, *Proteus*, and *Staphylococcus* in the VPA group.

This is the first time the microbial species richness and microbiome composition have been studied in a rat model for autism, the 400-E12 VPA rat. The decrease in microbial diversity in this rat model was consistent with the observations in human autism and most of the mouse models of autism studied to date. The gut microbial composition was largely similar to that of humans with autism and murine autism-like models. The enteric bacteria, especially the class Clostridia, are known to play an important role in children with autism (Frye et al. 2015). In our study, Clostridia is the most dominant class in the rat fecal microbial community, accounting for more than 60% of all sequence reads, followed by the class Bacteroidia with more than 30% of the sequences. Among the 100 OTU significantly impacted by prenatal VPA administration, the vast majority of them, 94, belonged to Clostridia, suggesting that ecological manipulation via antibiotics or pre- or pro-biotic approaches targeting this class of gut bacteria may prove effective in alleviating autism symptoms. A significant reduction in microbial species richness, such as Chao1, in the 400-E12 VPA rats was consistent with the observation in BTBR $T^{+}Itpr3^{tf}/J$ mouse model of autism [44]. However, biodiversity encompasses both species richness and evenness as well as interactions among species in the ecosystem [16]. While a marked reduction in species richness was evident in the rats with prenatal VPA exposure, species evenness in the rat gut microbial community did not appear to be impacted. Furthermore, the microbial co-occurrence patterns and microbial interactions in the community appeared to be preserved in the rats with prenatal VPA exposure.

Moreover, our findings provide further evidence of sex-specific alterations of gut microbiome by prenatal VPA administration in rodents [15]. For example, in male rats, the abundance of the family Coriobacteriaceae as well as the class Coriobacteriia was significantly repressed by VPA. An OTU (GreenGene ID_1113282), belonging to Mollicutes, was significantly increased by VPA. On the other hand, a twofold increase in the relative abundance of the phylum Proteobacteria, from 1.03% in the control rats to 2.17% in the male rats with VPA exposure, was observed. The VPA-induced increase became more evident in the class α-Proteobacteria, from 0.14% in the control male rats to 0.56% in the male rats with prenatal VPA exposure. The Proteobacteria are known to be a marker for an unstable microbial community and a risk factor of human disease [48, 49]. An elevated Proteobacteria level is frequently associated with metabolic disorders and intestinal inflammation. The pathological relevance of elevated Proteobacteria abundance in autism warrants further investigation. In contrast to male rats, prenatal VPA exposure induced a distinguishingly different set of microbial taxa in female rats. The abundance of the genus Staphylococcus and the family S24-7 was significantly increased by prenatal VPA exposure only in female rats. A significant elevation of Candidatus Arthromitus, which harbors commensal SFB, by VPA was observed only in female rats. Numerous studies have established solid links between SFB colonization and human disease [50]. As a potent inducer of IgA production and T_H17 immune responses as well as innate immunity, SFB may play a role in the pathogenesis of autism. Indeed, a recent study shows that pregnant mice colonized with SFB were more likely to produce offspring with maternal immune activation (MIA)-associated abnormalities [41].

The composition of the microbiota is of great importance to the function of the brain. Bacteria can regulate brain function through several mechanisms. Some bacteria, such as *Bifidobacterium* and *Lactobacillus*, that inhabit in the gut, have the capacity to produce anti-inflammatory cytokines, while other, such as *Clostridium* and *Ruminococcus* [51], can produce pro-inflammatory cytokines. Metabolic products of the gut microbiota, such as short-chain fatty acids, have also been implicated in autism. Gut microbiota has been suggested to regulate many nervous functions including neurogenesis, differentiation, myelination, formation and integrity of the blood-brain barrier, neurotrophin and neurotransmitter release, apoptosis, gap junction modification, and synaptic pruning [52]. Moreover, several microRNAs participate in signaling networks through the intervention of the gut microbiota [53]. In addition, gut microbiota release inflammatory cytokines that can act as epigenetic regulators and regulate gene expression being a factor for example in cancer risk and diabetes-associated autoantigens [54–56]. Here, we demonstrated that VPA also alters the metabolite potential of the microbial community in rats. VPA prenatal administration significantly elevated 21 bacterial pathways while repressing 8 pathways. Among them, there was an increase in activation of the bacterial secretion system, DNA replication, DNA repairs, and recombination proteins and a decrease in ABC bacterial transporter pathways. These data indicate a potentially higher activity of those pathways related to bacterial survival and function.

In conclusion, our data on the gut microbial community of the 400-E12 rats in response to prenatal VPA exposure indicate that this model, in addition to demonstrating behavioral and anatomical similarities to autism, also mimics the microbiota features of autism, making it one of the best-suited rodent models for the study of autism.

Abbreviations

ASD: Autism spectrum disorder; Bsk: Baskets cells; Ch: Chandelier; LDA: Linear discriminating analysis; MHFD: Maternal high-fat diet; MIA: Maternal immune activation; OTU: Operational taxonomic unit; PV: Parvalbumin; RMT: Random matrix theory; SFB: Segmented filamentous bacteria; VPA: Valproic acid

Acknowledgements

Mention of trade names or commercial products in this publication is solely for the purpose of providing specific information and does not imply recommendation or endorsement by the US Department of Agriculture (USDA). The USDA is an equal opportunity provider and employer.

Funding

This work was supported by the National Institute for Mental Health (MH094681) and the Shriners Hospitals.

Authors' contributions

FL performed the experiments and analyzed the data. KH collected the samples. VH participated in the writing of the manuscript. RWL and VMC designed the study, analyzed the data, and wrote the manuscript. All authors read and approved the final manuscript.

Competing interests

The authors declare that they have no competing interests.

Author details

[1]College of Food Science and Engineering, Ocean University of China, Qingdao, China. [2]Institute for Pediatric Regenerative Medicine and Shriners Hospitals for Children Northern California, 2504 Stockton Blvd, Sacramento, CA 95817, USA. [3]United States Department of Agriculture, Agriculture Research Service (USDA-ARS), Animal Genomics and Improvement Laboratory, Beltsville, MD, USA. [4]Department of Pathology and Laboratory Medicine, UC Davis School of Medicine, Sacramento, CA, USA. [5]MIND Institute, Sacramento, CA, USA.

References

1. Zhu X, Han Y, Du J, Liu R, Jin K, Yi W. Microbiota-gut-brain axis and the central nervous system. Oncotarget. 2017;8(32):53829–38.
2. Luan H, Wang X, Cai Z. Mass spectrometry-based metabolomics: targeting the crosstalk between gut microbiota and brain in neurodegenerative disorders. Mass Spectrom Rev. 2017.
3. Quigley EMM. Microbiota-brain-gut axis and neurodegenerative diseases. Current neurology and neuroscience reports. 2017;17(12):94.
4. Rodier PM, Ingram JL, Tisdale B, Nelson S, Romano J. Embryological origin for autism: developmental anomalies of the cranial nerve motor nuclei. J Comp Neurol. 1996;370(2):247–61.
5. Williams G, King J, Cunningham M, Stephan M, Kerr B, Hersh JH. Fetal valproate syndrome and autism: additional evidence of an association. Dev Med Child Neurol. 2001;43(3):202–6.

6. Bescoby-Chambers N, Forster P, Bates G. Foetal valproate syndrome and autism: additional evidence of an association. Dev Med Child Neurol. 2001; 43(12):847.
7. Christensen J, Gronborg TK, Sorensen MJ, Schendel D, Parner ET, Pedersen LH, et al. Prenatal valproate exposure and risk of autism spectrum disorders and childhood autism. JAMA. 2013;309(16):1696–703.
8. Chomiak T, Turner N, Hu B. What we have learned about autism spectrum disorder from valproic acid. Pathol Res Int 2013;2013:712758.
9. Fukuchi M, Nii T, Ishimaru N, Minamino A, Hara D, Takasaki I, et al. Valproic acid induces up- or down-regulation of gene expression responsible for the neuronal excitation and inhibition in rat cortical neurons through its epigenetic actions. Neurosci Res. 2009;65(1):35–43.
10. Hashemi E, Ariza J, Rogers H, Noctor SC, Martinez-Cerdeno V. The number of parvalbumin-expressing interneurons is decreased in the medial prefrontal cortex in autism. Cereb Cortex. 2016.
11. Ariza J, Rogers H, Hashemi E, Noctor S, Martínez-Cerdeño V. The number of chandelier and basket cells are differentially decreased in prefrontal cortex in autism. Cereb Cortex. 2016; In press.
12. Finegold SM. State of the art; microbiology in health and disease. Intestinal bacterial flora in autism. Anaerobe. 2011;17(6):367–8.
13. Tomova A, Husarova V, Lakatosova S, Bakos J, Vlkova B, Babinska K, et al. Gastrointestinal microbiota in children with autism in Slovakia. Physiol Behav. 2015;138:179–87.
14. Mangiola F, Ianiro G, Franceschi F, Fagiuoli S, Gasbarrini G, Gasbarrini A. Gut microbiota in autism and mood disorders. World J Gastroenterol. 2016;22(1): 361–8.
15. de Theije CG, Wopereis H, Ramadan M, van Eijndthoven T, Lambert J, Knol J, et al. Altered gut microbiota and activity in a murine model of autism spectrum disorders. Brain Behav Immun. 2014;37:197–206.
16. Olesen JM, Bascompte J, Dupont YL, Jordano P. The modularity of pollination networks. Proc Natl Acad Sci U S A. 2007;104(50):19891–6.
17. Liu F, Zhang N, Li Z, Wang X, Shi H, Xue C, et al. Chondroitin sulfate disaccharides modified the structure and function of the murine gut microbiome under healthy and stressed conditions. Sci Rep. 2017;7(1):6783.
18. Li RW, Li W, Sun J, Yu P, Baldwin RL, Urban JF. The effect of helminth infection on the microbial composition and structure of the caprine abomasal microbiome. Sci Rep. 2016;6:20606.
19. Segata N, Izard J, Waldron L, Gevers D, Miropolsky L, Garrett WS, et al. Metagenomic biomarker discovery and explanation. Genome Biol. 2011; 12(6):R60.
20. Zhou J, Deng Y, Luo F, He Z, Yang Y. Phylogenetic molecular ecological network of soil microbial communities in response to elevated CO2. MBio. 2011;2(4).
21. Deng Y, Jiang YH, Yang Y, He Z, Luo F, Zhou J. Molecular ecological network analyses. BMC Bioinformatics. 2012;13:113.
22. Weiss S, Van Treuren W, Lozupone C, Faust K, Friedman J, Deng Y, et al. Correlation detection strategies in microbial data sets vary widely in sensitivity and precision. ISME J. 2016;10(7):1669–81.
23. Tremaroli V, Backhed F. Functional interactions between the gut microbiota and host metabolism. Nature. 2012;489(7415):242–9.
24. Shukla SD, Budden KF, Neal R, Hansbro PM. Microbiome effects on immunity, health and disease in the lung. Clin Transl Immunology. 2017; 6(3):e133.
25. Feng Q, Chen WD, Wang YD. Gut microbiota: an integral moderator in health and disease. Front Microbiol. 2018;9:151.
26. McElhanon BO, McCracken C, Karpen S, Sharp WG. Gastrointestinal symptoms in autism spectrum disorder: a meta-analysis. Pediatrics. 2014; 133(5):872–83.
27. Adams JB, Audhya T, McDonough-Means S, Rubin RA, Quig D, Geis E, et al. Effect of a vitamin/mineral supplement on children and adults with autism. BMC Pediatr. 2011;11:111.
28. Slattery J, MacFabe DF, Kahler SG, Frye RE. Enteric ecosystem disruption in autism spectrum disorder: can the microbiota and macrobiota be restored? Curr Pharm Des. 2016;22(40):6107–21.
29. Krajmalnik-Brown R, Lozupone C, Kang DW, Adams JB. Gut bacteria in children with autism spectrum disorders: challenges and promise of studying how a complex community influences a complex disease. Microb Ecol Health Dis. 2015;26:26914.
30. Kang DW, Park JG, Ilhan ZE, Wallstrom G, Labaer J, Adams JB, et al. Reduced incidence of Prevotella and other fermenters in intestinal microflora of autistic children. PLoS One. 2013;8(7):e68322.
31. Pulikkan J, Maji A, Dhakan DB, Saxena R, Mohan B, Anto MM, et al. Gut microbial dysbiosis in Indian children with autism spectrum disorders. Microb Ecol. 2018.
32. Adams JB, Johansen LJ, Powell LD, Quig D, Rubin RA. Gastrointestinal flora and gastrointestinal status in children with autism--comparisons to typical children and correlation with autism severity. BMC Gastroenterol. 2011;11:22.
33. Finegold SM. Desulfovibrio species are potentially important in regressive autism. Med Hypotheses. 2011;77(2):270–4.
34. Parracho HM, Bingham MO, Gibson GR, McCartney AL. Differences between the gut microflora of children with autistic spectrum disorders and that of healthy children. J Med Microbiol. 2005;54(Pt 10):987–91.
35. Williams BL, Hornig M, Parekh T, Lipkin WI. Application of novel PCR-based methods for detection, quantitation, and phylogenetic characterization of Sutterella species in intestinal biopsy samples from children with autism and gastrointestinal disturbances. MBio. 2012;3(1).
36. Needham BD, Tang W, Wu WL. Searching for the gut microbial contributing factors to social behavior in rodent models of autism spectrum disorder. Developmental neurobiology. 2018;78(5):474–99.
37. Desbonnet L, Clarke G, Shanahan F, Dinan TG, Cryan JF. Microbiota is essential for social development in the mouse. Mol Psychiatry. 2014;19(2): 146–8.
38. Buffington SA, Di Prisco GV, Auchtung TA, Ajami NJ, Petrosino JF, Costa-Mattioli M. Microbial reconstitution reverses maternal diet-induced social and synaptic deficits in offspring. Cell. 2016;165(7):1762–75.
39. Stilling RM, Ryan FJ, Hoban AE, Shanahan F, Clarke G, Claesson MJ, et al. Microbes & neurodevelopment--absence of microbiota during early life increases activity-related transcriptional pathways in the amygdala. Brain Behav Immun. 2015;50:209–20.
40. Crumeyrolle-Arias M, Jaglin M, Bruneau A, Vancassel S, Cardona A, Dauge V, et al. Absence of the gut microbiota enhances anxiety-like behavior and neuroendocrine response to acute stress in rats. Psychoneuroendocrinology. 2014;42:207–17.
41. Kim YG, Sakamoto K, Seo SU, Pickard JM, Gillilland MG 3rd, Pudlo NA, et al. Neonatal acquisition of Clostridia species protects against colonization by bacterial pathogens. Science. 2017;356(6335):315–9.
42. Leclercq S, de Timary P, Delzenne NM, Starkel P. The link between inflammation, bugs, the intestine and the brain in alcohol dependence. Transl Psychiatry. 2017;7(2):e1048.
43. Newell C, Bomhof MR, Reimer RA, Hittel DS, Rho JM, Shearer J. Ketogenic diet modifies the gut microbiota in a murine model of autism spectrum disorder. Mol Autism. 2016;7(1):37.
44. Golubeva AV, Joyce SA, Moloney G, Burokas A, Sherwin E, Arboleya S, et al. Microbiota-related changes in bile acid & tryptophan metabolism are associated with gastrointestinal dysfunction in a mouse model of autism. EBioMedicine. 2017;24:166–78.
45. Klein MS, Newell C, Bomhof MR, Reimer RA, Hittel DS, Rho JM, et al. Metabolomic modeling to monitor host responsiveness to gut microbiota manipulation in the BTBR(T+tf/j) mouse. J Proteome Res. 2016;15(4):1143–50.
46. Coretti L, Cristiano C, Florio E, Scala G, Lama A, Keller S, et al. Sex-related alterations of gut microbiota composition in the BTBR mouse model of autism spectrum disorder. Sci Rep. 2017;7:45356.
47. Hsiao EY, McBride SW, Hsien S, Sharon G, Hyde ER, McCue T, et al. Microbiota modulate behavioral and physiological abnormalities associated with neurodevelopmental disorders. Cell. 2013;155(7):1451–63.
48. Carvalho FA, Koren O, Goodrich JK, Johansson ME, Nalbantoglu I, Aitken JD, et al. Transient inability to manage proteobacteria promotes chronic gut inflammation in TLR5-deficient mice. Cell Host Microbe. 2012;12(2):139–52.
49. Shin NR, Whon TW, Bae JW. Proteobacteria: microbial signature of dysbiosis in gut microbiota. Trends Biotechnol. 2015;33(9):496–503.
50. Ericsson AC, Hagan CE, Davis DJ, Franklin CL. Segmented filamentous bacteria: commensal microbes with potential effects on research. Comp Med. 2014;64(2):90–8.
51. Heberling CA, Dhurjati PS, Sasser M. Hypothesis for a systems connectivity model of autism spectrum disorder pathogenesis: links to gut bacteria, oxidative stress, and intestinal permeability. Med Hypotheses. 2013;80(3): 264–70.
52. Sharon G, Sampson TR, Geschwind DH, Mazmanian SK. The central nervous system and the gut microbiome. Cell. 2016;167(4):915–32.

53. Belcheva A. MicroRNAs at the epicenter of intestinal homeostasis. BioEssays. 2017;39(3).
54. Hullar MA, Fu BC. Diet, the gut microbiome, and epigenetics. Cancer J. 2014;20(3):170–5.
55. Steinbrenner H, Nguyen TB, Wohlrab U, Scherbaum WA, Seissler J. Effect of proinflammatory cytokines on gene expression of the diabetes-associated autoantigen IA-2 in INS-1 cells. Endocrinology. 2002;143(10):3839–45.
56. Nankova BB, Agarwal R, MacFabe DF, La Gamma EF. Enteric bacterial metabolites propionic and butyric acid modulate gene expression, including CREB-dependent catecholaminergic neurotransmission, in PC12 cells--possible relevance to autism spectrum disorders. PLoS One. 2014;9(8): e103740.

15

Development and evaluation of a speech-generating AAC mobile app for minimally verbal children with autism spectrum disorder in Mainland China

Sainan An[1,2], Xiaoping Feng[3], Yue Dai[3], Hongli Bo[4], Xiuqing Wang[4], Mu Li[5], John Zhuohao Woo[6], Xingmei Liang[6], Cheng Guo[7], Charles Xingchao Liu[7] and Liping Wei[8*]

Abstract

Background: Mobile touchscreen devices are currently being used as speech-generating devices (SGDs) and have been shown to promote the communication skills, particularly the requesting skills of children with autism spectrum disorders (ASD) who have limited spoken language. However, no augmentative and alternative communication (AAC) mobile app has been developed and evaluated in the Chinese language in Mainland China.

Methods: We developed an AAC mobile app, which is the first in Mainland China, to our knowledge, named Yuudee (Chinese name 小雨滴 (xiaoyudi)). Yuudee was developed using the Objective-C and Java programming languages. A five-phase training protocol for making requests using Yuudee was developed based on the Picture Exchange Communication System. We trained ten minimally verbal children with ASD to make requests using Yuudee and evaluated the effectiveness of the training.

Results: Yuudee has a built-in library of over 400 pictures with corresponding spoken phrases that are divided into 39 categories ranging from making simple requests to expressing emotions. An additional important feature of Yuudee is its customization functions that allow a parent or trainer to easily select pictures and phrases to display, create new pictures and phrases, and change the layouts and orders of the pictures to fit the personal needs of each child. Yuudee is freely available in an iOS version from the iTunes App Store (https://itunes.apple.com/cn/app/xiao-yu-di/id794832934?mt=8) and in an Android version from Google Play (https://play.google.com/store/apps/details?id=com.supersuperstar.yuudee.vue) and domestic Chinese Android App stores. Three consecutive unprompted successful responses, which were defined as an initial training success, were achieved in at least three of the five phases for all ten of the evaluated children. The accuracy rate of a given phase was calculated for each child who achieved three consecutive unprompted successful responses in the phase. Seven children achieved at least 50% accuracy in at least two of the five phases. The other three children achieved at least 50% accuracy in only one phase. Two children achieved at least 50% accuracy in all of the phases in which they were trained.

Conclusions: Our data suggest that Yuudee is a useful tool for helping minimally verbal children with ASD make requests.

Keywords: Augmentative and alternative communication, App, Development, Training effectiveness, Mainland China

* Correspondence: weilp@mail.cbi.pku.edu.cn
[8]Center for Bioinformatics, State Key Laboratory of Protein and Plant Gene Research, School of Life Sciences, Peking University, No. 5, YiHeYuan Road, HaiDian District, Beijing 100871, China
Full list of author information is available at the end of the article

Background

Autism spectrum disorder (ASD) is a complex neurodevelopmental disorder characterized by deficits in social communication and social interaction and by restricted, repetitive patterns of behavior, interests, or activities [1]. The spoken language abilities of children with ASD are variable and range from high-level speech to the absence of spoken language. Approximately 30% of children with ASD are minimally verbal [2, 3]. They use a small repertoire of spoken words or fixed phrases or use stereotyped or scripted spoken language in a noncommunicative manner [4, 5].

Augmentative and alternative communication (AAC) systems, including gestures, sign language, the Picture Exchange Communication System (PECS), and speech-generating devices (SGDs), have been developed to improve the communicative capacity of children with limited functional spoken language. PECS and SGDs are commonly used for children with ASD. PECS is a visual-based system that aims to teach children how to communicate with others by exchanging pictures [6, 7]. PECS includes six phases that target communication skills ranging from making simple requests to making comments. Each phase of PECS is taught systematically using specific strategies and procedures that were developed based on the principles of applied behavior analysis [8]. Studies have demonstrated that PECS training can promote functional communication skills (e.g., requesting and commenting skills) and social communication skills in children with ASD [9–15]. Children with ASD who were trained to use PECS showed improvements in their verbal skills in some studies [14, 16]. In a randomized controlled study, PECS was more effective than Responsive Education and Prelinguistic Milieu Teaching for increasing the number of nonimitative spoken communication acts and the number of different nonimitative words used in the posttreatment period [17], although these differences were not found in a later follow-up period.

SGDs generate recorded or synthesized speech outputs when displayed pictures are activated by a user. Using SGDs can promote the communication skills of children with ASD, particularly their requesting skills [13, 18–20]. A review of 23 studies found that 78% of these studies provided conclusive evidence that using SGDs could improve the communication skills of children with ASD, although it should be noted that most of the studies targeted requesting skills only [21]. Using SGDs has been demonstrated to promote the functional speech of children with ASD in a study that used a blended, adaptive treatment design and targeted minimally verbal children aged 5–8 years [22]. Children who received SGDs at the beginning of the adaptive intervention gained significantly more spontaneous communicative language than children who received SGDs later or did not receive SGDs at all [22, 23].

In recent years, mobile touchscreen devices (e.g., iPads, iPhones, and Android phones) are increasingly being used as SGDs. Many AAC Apps (e.g., Proloquo2Go) that run on these mobile touchscreen devices have been developed [24, 25]. SGDs that consist of mobile touchscreen devices and AAC Apps have potential advantages such as the capacity to include many pictures, their portability, and their relatively low cost [26]. Studies have shown that using mobile devices with AAC Apps can improve the abilities of children with ASD to make single- or multiple-step requests [27–30] and to give social communication responses (e.g., "thank you") after making requests [31]. Mobile touchscreen devices with AAC Apps are emerging as promising alternatives of traditional SGDs and PECS. Several studies have adapted and modified the detailed and empirically validated training procedures of PECS for use in SGD training with mobile devices [29, 32].

Sun et al. [33] systematically reviewed the literature regarding estimates of the prevalence of ASD or childhood autism in Mainland China, Hong Kong, and Taiwan. Their meta-analysis concluded that the prevalence of ASD in three areas was 26.6/10,000, which is approximately an order of magnitude lower than the estimated prevalence of 224/10,000 in the USA [34]. It should be noted that there is a lack of large-scale epidemiological investigations on ASD in Mainland China that use comparable methods to those used in studies from other developed countries. The percentage of minimally verbal children with ASD in Mainland China has not been reported. We are currently conducting a project called the Autism Genetic Research Project in Mainland China (presented in detail in the Section 2). Although this project is conducted at autism intervention centers instead of at the population level, it may still shed light on the percentage of minimally verbal children in Mainland China. Among 4–6-year-old children with ASD who participated in this project (sample size around 550), 50% were minimally verbal according to the definition by Thurm et al. [35]. Extrapolating this based on the aforementioned estimate of Sun et al., one could assume that there may be about 50,000 minimally verbal children with ASD aged 4–6 years in Mainland China.

No AAC Apps for minimally verbal children with ASD have been developed and evaluated in Mainland China. Considering the potentially large number of minimally verbal children with ASD in Mainland China and given the demonstrated benefits of AAC Apps in improving communication skills, we developed a freely available AAC mobile App named Yuudee that features a large built-in picture library and a set of customization functions. We evaluated the effectiveness of training for making requests using Yuudee in ten minimally verbal children with ASD. The phases of Yuudee training were designed based on both the training phases of PECS and the functionalities of Yuudee. Our analysis revealed that the use of Yuudee with our PECS-derived training procedures was effective in improving the requesting skills of minimally verbal children with ASD.

Methods

Development of Yuudee

Considering the likely overlap of certain basic communication needs across minimally verbal children with ASD, a built-in picture library was developed. In addition, Yuudee was designed to be easily customized. The pictures displayed for the child can be edited according to the specific communication needs of the child. The characteristics of children with ASD were considered during the development of Yuudee; for example, given that fine motor impairments are common in children with ASD [36], the number of pictures displayed on the screen can be changed from one to nine according to the fine motor skills of a given child.

To make Yuudee easily available to more families, both an iOS version and an Android version were developed. The iOS version of Yuudee was developed using the Objective-C programming language. The Android version of Yuudee was developed using the Java programming language. The relationships between the pictures, texts, voices, and category information were specified. When installing Yuudee, pictures and voices included in the built-in picture library are copied into the device. The coordinates of the pictures on the screen are calculated according to the setting for the number of pictures on the screen. In the iOS version of Yuudee, pictures included within a particular courseware or a given category are arranged in a horizontally oriented UIScrollView. Users can navigate between pages by scrolling the UIScrollView. In the Android version of Yuudee, the horizontal paging is fulfilled by customizing the ScrollLayout control.

In the iOS version of Yuudee, the AVFoundation framework is used for picture selection and voice recording when inputting a new picture. The UIImagepickerController is used to select pictures from the photo library or to take new photos using the built-in digital camera. In the Android version of Yuudee, the framework for creating new pictures was developed using self-developed tools. In both versions, the touch events on the pictures are captured. When a touch event is detected, the dynamic effect of the picture is played using UIView animation (the iPad Version) or the Android Animation application programming interface (the Android version) according to the setting of the picture. Three 100*100 pixel regions at the upper left, upper right, and bottom right corners of the screen are monitored for touch events. When touch events simultaneously occur in all of these three regions, Yuudee enters the edit mode where pictures that are accessible to children can be edited. The position of the pictures can be changed after a 'long touch' event on a picture is detected.

Participants

Ten 3–6-year-old children who met our inclusion criteria were included in the present study. The inclusion criteria were (1) exceeding the cutoff for ASD of the Autism Diagnostic Observation Schedule (ADOS) and Autism Diagnostic Interview-Revised (ADI-R) [37, 38], which were conducted by certified practitioners; (2) having been diagnosed with ASD based on criteria in the Diagnostic and Statistical Manual of Mental Disorders, Fourth Edition-Text Revision by experienced child psychiatrists; (3) 'minimally verbal' based on item A1 'Overall level of non-echoed spoken language' of the ADOS (Children whose A1 codes indicated no speech, single words, or occasional phrases were identified as minimally verbal children [35]); (4) having not been diagnosed with or suspected of having epilepsy; and (5) having never previously used any other speech-generating devices or PECS. All ten of the children were diagnosed as having autism by child psychiatrists and were assessed by the ADOS module 1. The Vineland Adaptive Behavior Scales (Chinese version) were used to evaluate the everyday personal and social skills of these children [39]. Descriptive characteristics of each child are presented in Table 1; age equivalent scores and standard scores on the Vineland Adaptive Behavior Scales (Chinese version) are listed in this table.

Because all the enrolled children also participated in our Autism Genetic Research Project, the identifiers used in the present study were the same as those in that project. The ongoing Autism Genetic Research Project is collecting phenotypic data and DNA samples from children with ASD and their parents to study the genetics of ASD in China. The families affected by ASD were recruited from intervention centers.

Preferred reinforcers

Parents were asked to list the items and activities that were particularly favorable to their child before Yuudee training. The identification of individualized reinforcers is important to keep children motivated during the training. Pictures with recorded speech corresponding to the items and/or activities on each personalized list were generated before Yuudee training if no such pictures were present in the built-in library. The parent-selected reinforcers varied greatly across the children. Only a few reinforcers (e.g., biscuits and candies) were common among these

Table 1 Descriptive characteristics of each minimally verbal child with ASD

ID	Gender	Age (yr:mo)	A1 score	Age equivalent score (yr:mo)		Standard score			
				Expressive language	Receptive language	Communication	Daily living skills	Socialization	Motor skills
AU069603	M	5:3	8	1:10	2:10	55	55	57	76
AU112103	M	4:10	8	1:8	3:0	58	55	59	88
AU112003	M	4:9	8	1:4	2:10	57	58	55	103
AU110003	M	5:2	3	2:2	4:2	58	59	57	72
AU112603	M	5:11	3	2:8	4:2	60	62	56	83
AU113203	F	4:1	8	1:6	3:10	63	64	59	100
AU110203	M	6:4	3	2:8	4:6	62	52	54	92
AU113703	M	3:7	1	NA	NA	NA	NA	NA	NA
AU112303	M	4:9	3	2:10	3:10	67	53	54	73
AU131703	M	4:11	3	1:8	2:6	58	56	57	82

A1 scores were from the Autism Diagnostic Observation Schedule
NA not available, *M* male, *F* Female

children. For most of the reinforcers, digital photos taken of real objects were used during training as only a few common reinforcers were represented by pictures in the built-in picture library.

Training design

The training for making requests with Yuudee was conducted in a classroom. Yuudee training consisted of eight 30-min sessions. One or two sessions were conducted per week for 5 weeks. iPad mini or iPad devices running Yuudee were used in this study. Each child was trained by two trainers (a communication partner and a physical prompter). Training was divided into five phases based on the phases of PECS and the functionalities of Yuudee (presented in detail below). The training procedures of each phase were adapted from the training procedures of PECS.

Reinforcer assessment

At the beginning of each session, two potential reinforcers were put on the table between the child and the communication partner. The one chosen by the child was then used as the reinforcer. In the middle of each session, the procedure for choosing a reinforcer from two options was repeated to determine whether the reinforcer used in the remaining time of the session should be changed. Based on these choices, we assumed that children were motivated to obtain the preferred objects during training.

Training phases and procedures

Phase I consisted of making requests by touching a single picture on the screen; this corresponds to the first phase of PECS. This phase aimed to help children to establish the ability to initiate a request by touching a picture on the screen. At the beginning of this phase, the communication partner showed the reinforcer to the child to gain his/her attention. If the child reached toward the reinforcer, the physical prompter immediately disrupted his/her reach by picking up the child's right hand and then physically directing the child to touch the picture on the screen. When the recorded speech was broadcast by the device, the communication partner immediately spoke the name of the reinforcer and gave the reinforcer to the child. If the child did not initiate the request, full physical prompts were provided to help the child to touch the single picture on the screen. The number of full physical prompts offered was gradually reduced throughout the course of a single training phase.

Phase II consisted of discriminating between the pictures present on a single screen page; this phase corresponds to the third phase of PECS. Phase II of this study differs from the third phase of PECS in two ways: (1) the child and the communication partner continued to sit across a table, and (2) the discrimination was only made between highly preferred and non-preferred/unrelated items. This phase started by displaying two pictures on the screen. The communication partner showed both items to the child. If the child spontaneously touched one picture, the communication partner gave the corresponding item to the child. Prompts were provided to help the child to touch the target picture on the screen if the child did not initiate the request. When the child was able to select the target picture from two pictures, the number of pictures on a single screen was gradually increased. At most, nine pictures were displayed on a single screen page. Note that during this phase, the position of the target picture was changed frequently to avoid a situation where the child simply touched the same region of the screen repeatedly.

Phase III involved switching between multiple screen pages. Many pictures can be displayed by distributing them across multiple screen pages. In this phase, the pictures were put on two or more screen pages. An exemplary trial with full physical prompts was conducted to show the child how to switch between the screen pages. At the beginning of each trial, the screen page with the target picture was not the one displayed to the child. If the child did not spontaneously initiate the request, full physical prompts were provided to help the child to switch between different screen pages, to find the page with the target picture, and to touch the target picture. Prompts were gradually faded during this phase.

Phase IV corresponds to the second phase of PECS, with the aim of increasing the child's spontaneity. This phase was further divided into phases IVA and IVB. In phase IVA, the distance between the child and the communication partner was gradually increased (eventually to as far as across the room). In phase IVB, there were distances between both the child and the communication partner and the child and the device. In both IVA and IVB, the communication partner moved around the room. To acquire the desired item, the child was required to travel to the communication partner and to touch the target picture in front of the communication partner. During phase IVB, the position of the iPad was frequently changed to enhance their consciousness of being required to initially go to take the iPad.

Phase V aimed to enable children to independently open the App. In this phase, the Yuudee icon was displayed on the screen. To enter Yuudee, the child needed to touch the Yuudee icon. In an exemplary trial, the physical prompter held the right hand of the child, guided the child to touch the Yuudee icon, and then guided the child to touch the target picture. In the following trials, full physical prompts were provided if the child did not initiate the request or touched the icon for another application.

Note that the second training phase that the children experienced was phase IV. Phase IV was typically conducted as a part of every session for each child but only after the training of the other phases (i.e., after each of phase I, phase II, phase III, and phase V). Phase III (switching between multiple screen pages) is an extension of phase II (picture discrimination) and allows children to select preferred items from an increasing number of options. Therefore, phase III occurred just after phase II.

During phases I, II, III, and V, the communication partner and the child sat across a table. The iPad mini or iPad was placed on the table between them. The physical prompter sat behind the child to provide physical assistance. As in PECS training, no verbal prompts were used during the training for making requests with Yuudee. During phases I and II, the reinforcers were always in view. During other phases, reinforcers could sometimes be placed below the level of the table and outside the children's view. At the beginning of phase I, reinforcers were presented to the children by the communication partners for several (3–5) trials. During phase IV, the communication partners interacted with the reinforcers to get children's attention when the children were not actively engaged in the training process. For example, the communication partners ate a preferred food or played with a preferred toy.

Evaluation of training effectiveness

We recorded whether prompts were provided, which types of prompts were provided, and whether the child touched the target picture in each trial. An unprompted successful response was defined as spontaneously initiating a request and successfully touching the target picture without prompts to obtain the favored item in a trial. Using phase IVB as an example, an unprompted successful response was recorded if a child spontaneously traveled to take the iPad and then traveled to the trainer and touched the picture that corresponded to the reinforcer in front of the trainer without using prompts.

The training effectiveness of a given phase was measured in two steps. We initially evaluated whether the child achieved three consecutive unprompted successful responses in this phase. The achievement of three consecutive unprompted successful responses was regarded as the beginning of acquiring competence for a given phase. If a child achieved three consecutive unprompted successful responses in a given phase, then we calculated the accuracy rate (the proportion of unprompted successful responses) among the trials conducted after this initial achievement of three consecutive unprompted successful responses in this phase. In this study, we considered a threshold of at least 50% accuracy as 'accurate' because the training consisted of only eight 30-min sessions and five training phases were evaluated.

Inter-observer agreement

To assess the reliability of the data collection, two independent observers collected performance data on all sessions for all ten of the children. The inter-observer agreement (IOA) for each session was calculated. The IOA ranged from 94.28 to 100%, and the mean IOA was 98.81%.

Procedural integrity

To assess whether the procedures were correctly implemented in the proper sequence, training procedure checklists were created for each phase (Additional file 1: Table S1). Data on procedural integrity were collected for 50% of the sessions of each child. The procedural integrity values ranged from 91.34 to 100% with a mean of 99.20%.

Results

Features of Yuudee

The built-in library of Yuudee includes over 400 line drawings. Each picture is associated with corresponding text (usually a Chinese phrase) that was recorded by a Mandarin-speaking boy. These pictures have been organized into 39 categories, including categories about 'communication functions' ranging from making simple requests to expressing emotions, categories about cognition (e.g., colors, numbers, and shapes), and a category containing social stories (Fig. 1b). When a picture from a communication function category is touched, three pictures that represent three consecutive actions are displayed in order with a short time interval between each picture. Therefore, upon the selection of a picture, Yuudee presents an attractive dynamic display of the user-selected picture; this differs from the static displays that are typical of many other currently available AAC Apps.

Yuudee has two modes: the Usage Mode for children (Fig. 1c) and the Edit Mode for parents and trainers (Fig. 1d). The default mode is the Usage Mode when opening Yuudee. In the Usage Mode, pictures and

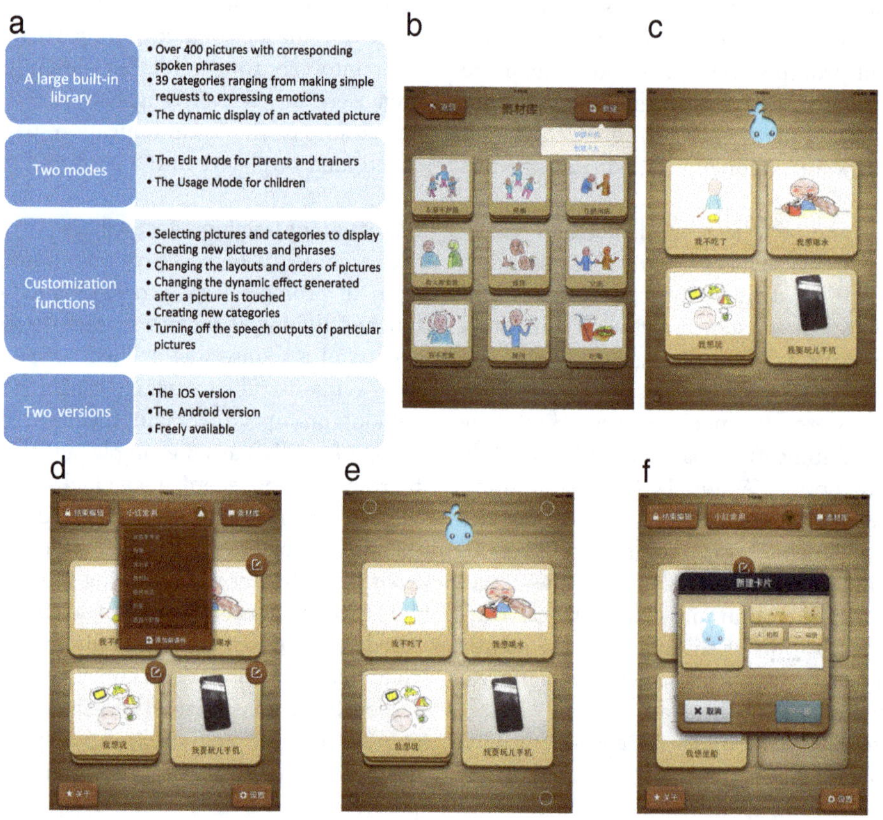

Fig. 1 Yuudee features. **a** Summary of Yuudee features. **b** The built-in picture library. **c** The Usage Mode of Yuudee. Pictures or categories that are selected from the built-in library or are made by parents or trainers according to the specific communication needs of the child are displayed on the screen. **d** The Edit Mode of Yuudee. In the Edit Mode, parents or trainers can edit the content that is accessible to the child using the customization functions of Yuudee. **e** The three-point touch gesture used to enter the Edit Mode. **f** The interface used for inputting a new picture

categories selected and edited by parents or trainers are displayed on the screen. To enter the Edit Mode, parents or trainers need to simultaneously touch three points on the upper left, upper right, and bottom right corners of the screen (Fig. 1e); this was designed to prevent children from inadvertently entering the Edit Mode.

Yuudee can be flexibly customized to suit the personal communication needs of the child as well as the particular operator level at which the child can effectively use Yuudee. Parents or trainers initially edit the content to be displayed to the child by either selecting an existing courseware unit or creating a new courseware unit. In a particular courseware unit, parents or trainers can add and delete pictures or categories. Pictures can be added by selecting built-in pictures or by creating new pictures using three steps: (1) selecting digital photos from the photo library or taking new photos using the built-in digital camera, (2) inputting text, and (3) recording speech (Fig. 1f). The number of pictures displayed on the screen can be changed from 1 to 9 using the layout setting of the pictures, thereby accommodating the fine motor skills of the child and allowing expanded options as the training phases progress. There are three types of layouts: "1 × 1," "2 × 2," and "3 × 3." The orders of the pictures displayed on the screen can be changed; this makes it possible, for example, to test whether the child is able to choose the right picture wherever it is on the screen during training. Parents or trainers can set the dynamic effect that is generated after a picture is touched; there are two types of dynamic effects: "Magnification" and "Magnification and rotation." New categories can be added to the picture library. The speech output that is generated after a picture is touched can be turned off.

There are two versions of Yuudee: one for Apple iOS and another for the Android platform. Parents can find Yuudee by searching for its Chinese name "xiaoyudi" or "小雨滴" in the iTunes App Store or in Google Play and domestic Chinese Android App stores. They can then freely install Yuudee. Yuudee runs on iPads and Android phones. Parents can choose between the two versions of Yuudee according to the touchscreen devices they have.

Download statistics of Yuudee

The iOS version of Yuudee was released in April 2014. According to the data from April 2015 to November 2016, the iOS version of Yuudee was downloaded 1995 times from the iTunes App Store with an average of approximately 100 downloads per month. The Android version of Yuudee was released in April 2015. By November 2016, the Android version of Yuudee was downloaded 35,000 times from Google play and another eight domestic Android App stores. Thus, Yuudee was downloaded more than 37,000 times by November 2016.

Evaluation of Yuudee training

For each training phase (I–V), we checked whether children were able to achieve three consecutive unprompted successful responses. In phase I, eight of the ten trained children successfully made three consecutive unprompted successful requests after an average of 36.38 trials (Fig. 2). In phase II, all ten of the trained children achieved three consecutive unprompted successful responses after an average of 9.2 trials (Fig. 2). In phase III, eight of the nine trained children made three consecutive unprompted successful requests after an average of 45.5

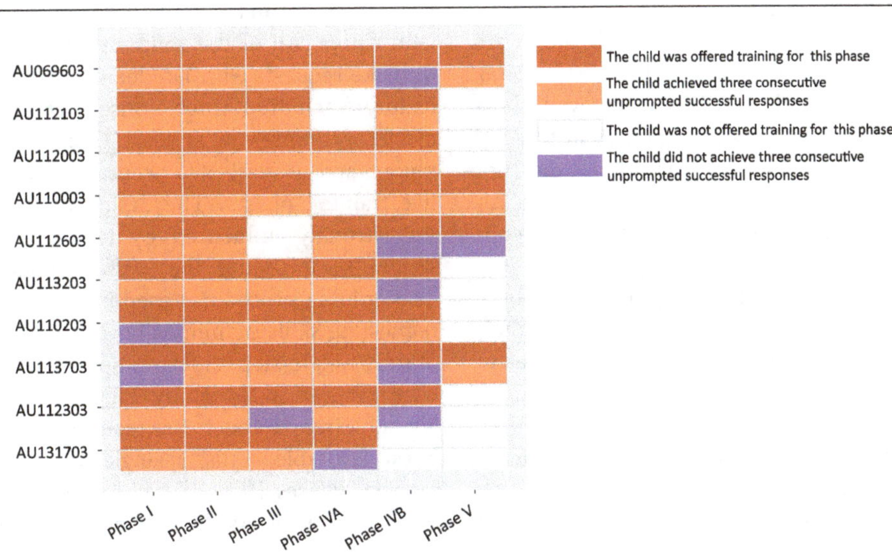

Fig. 2 The status of the achievement of three consecutive unprompted successful responses in each phase for each child. Ten minimally verbal children with ASD participated in the training for making requests using Yuudee

trials (Fig. 2). A total of 44 trials were conducted with AU112303 who failed to achieve three consecutive unprompted successful responses in phase III. In phase IVA, seven of the eight trained children made three consecutive unprompted successful requests after an average of 33.71 trials (Fig. 2). A total of 41 trials were conducted with AU131703 who failed to achieve three consecutive unprompted successful responses in phase IVA. In phase IVB, four of the nine trained children achieved three consecutive unprompted successful responses after an average of 15.5 trials (Fig. 2). A total of 19–65 trials were conducted with the five children who failed to achieve three consecutive unprompted successful responses in phase IVB. The numbers of children trained in phase IVA and phase IVB were different because some trainers skipped phase IVA and directly conducted phase IVB. Among the four children who were trained in phase V, three of them made three consecutive unprompted successful requests after an average of 4.33 trials (Fig. 2). A total of 21 trials were conducted with AU112603 who failed to achieve three consecutive unprompted successful responses in phase V. It is noteworthy that the number of trials conducted before the achievement of three consecutive unprompted successful responses was highly variable among these children. For example, while 3 trials were conducted before AU113203 achieved three consecutive unprompted successful responses in phase I, a total of 78 trials were conducted before AU112103 achieved this same level.

All ten of the children achieved three consecutive unprompted successful responses in at least three of the five phases (Fig. 2). Three children (AU112103, AU112003, and AU110003) achieved three consecutive unprompted successful responses in all of the phases in which they were trained. Two children (AU069603 and AU113203) made three consecutive unprompted successful requests in all of the phases in which they were trained with the exception of phase IVB. AU112603, AU110203, AU112303, and AU131703 achieved three consecutive unprompted successful responses in three of the five phases. AU110203 and AU113703 did not achieve three consecutive unprompted successful responses in phase I. As they successfully made three consecutive unprompted successful requests in the subsequent phases, we assume that they actually had the ability to achieve this in phase I. We assume that their failure in phase I was caused by the minimal number of trials (3 or 5) that the trainers conducted with them in phase I.

Table 2 lists the accuracy rate after three consecutive unprompted successful responses were achieved in each phase for each child. Six of the eight children who achieved three consecutive unprompted successful responses in phase I achieved at least 50% accuracy in phase I (Table 2). Eight of the ten children who achieved three consecutive unprompted successful responses in phase II achieved at least 50% accuracy in phase II (Table 2). Four of the eight children who achieved three consecutive unprompted successful responses in phase III achieved at least 50% accuracy in phase III (Table 2). Four of the seven children who achieved three consecutive unprompted successful responses in phase IVA achieved at least 50% accuracy in phase IVA (Table 2). Three of the four children who achieved three consecutive unprompted successful responses in phase IVB achieved at least 50% accuracy in phase IVB (Table 2). All of the three children who achieved three consecutive unprompted successful responses in phase V achieved at least 50% accuracy in phase V (Table 2).

Seven children achieved at least 50% accuracy in at least two of the five phases (Table 2 and Additional file 2: Figure S1). AU112103, AU112303, and AU113203 achieved at least 50% accuracy in only one phase (Table 2 and Additional file 2: Figure S1). AU112103 and AU112303 achieved at least 50% accuracy in phase I. AU113203 achieved at least 50% accuracy in phase II. Two children (AU112003 and AU110003) achieved at least 50% accuracy in all of the phases in which they were trained (Table 2 and Additional file 2: Figure S1). AU69603 and AU112603 achieved at least 50% accuracy in phase IVA but not in phase IVB (Table 2 and Additional file 2: Figure S1).

Discussion

To address the lack of AAC mobile Apps for minimally verbal children with ASD in Mainland China, we developed a flexible and customizable App named Yuudee that runs on mobile touchscreen devices. We evaluated the training effectiveness of making requests with Yuudee in ten minimally verbal children with ASD in Mainland China. All of the children improved in their ability to make requests with Yuudee during training. These ten children achieved three consecutive unprompted successful responses in at least three of the five training phases and at least 50% accuracy in at least one of the five training phases. The design of the training phases was strongly influenced by typical PECS phases and sought to introduce the various functions of Yuudee. The training procedures used in this study improved the requesting skills of minimally verbal children with ASD.

Both single-step and multiple-step requesting skills were targeted in this study. Phases I and II aimed to enable children to touch the pictures on the screen to request favorable items; a single-step process to make a request. Phases III and V addressed the advanced functions of Yuudee. As the distances between the child, the device, and the communication partner increased in phase IV, the child was required to move to and then take the device. Thus, phases III, IV, and V were

Table 2 Accuracy rates after three consecutive unprompted successful responses

ID	Phase I	Phase II	Phase III	Phase IVA	Phase IVB	Phase V
AU069603	38.23%	92.50%	72.41%	56.71%	N	100%
AU112103	60.61%	47.05%	27.41%	–	49.25%	–
AU112003	52.17%	97.14%	80%	100%	50%	–
AU110003	100%	64.70%	64.0%	–	74.11%	80%
AU112603	100%	56.15%	–	66.67%	N	N
AU113203	45.83%	78.14%	27.55%	28.57%	N	–
AU110203	N	91.67%	17.64%	85.71%	60%	–
AU113703	N	85%	89.25%	42.85%	N	100%
AU112303	50%	9.56%	N	36.06%	N	–
AU131703	63.49%	84%	17.12%	N	–	–

Gray shading indicates that the trained children achieved at least 50% accuracy in these phases. –: The child was not offered training in this phase; *N*: The child did not achieve three consecutive unprompted successful responses in this phase

multiple-step processes. Four children achieved at least 50% accuracy in both phases I and II. Four children achieved at least 50% accuracy in at least two of the three phases from phase III to phase V. Therefore, our multi-session training process for Yuudee improved both single-step and multiple-step requesting skills of minimally verbal children with ASD.

For the trained children who did not achieve three consecutive unprompted successful responses in phases III, IV, and V, the numbers of trials conducted with them were close to or more than the average number of trials conducted with the children who achieved three consecutive unprompted successful responses in these phases. We thus conclude that these phases were difficult for them. For children who obtained a low accuracy after the achievement of three consecutive unprompted successful responses, they usually needed prompts to initiate or correctly complete the requests in many trials. Therefore, the accuracy rates in a sense reflected the speed at which they were able to master these particular phases. The numbers of phases in which they reached at least 50% accuracy appears to reflect the training effectiveness of the training process.

Recall that we used the achievement of 50% accuracy as an evaluation criterion in this study. In phase II, discrimination was initially made between one preferred item and one non-preferred/unrelated item. For all ten of the children, at least six unprompted successful requests were made during eight consecutive trials. This suggested that pictures were not chosen by chance when there were only two pictures on the screen.

Two of the children (AU112103 and AU110003) were not offered training for phase IVA but were directly trained for phase IVB. This was an oversight of the trainers. AU112103 and AU110003 both achieved three consecutive unprompted successful responses and achieved 49.25 and 74.11% accuracy, respectively, in phase IVB. Among the eight other children (i.e., those who were initially trained for phase IVA), four children achieved at least 50% accuracy in phase IVA, and two children achieved at least 50% accuracy in phase IVB. Therefore, it seems that directly offering training for phase IVB was also effective in increasing the spontaneity of the children.

The present study had several limitations. First, there were no follow-up sessions. Although all ten of these children made progress in requesting items during the training, it would be valuable to measure the maintenance of their requesting skills through follow-up sessions in future studies. Second, the training sessions and evaluations were conducted in a classroom. It would be important in future studies to evaluate how their requesting behaviors may be generalized outside of the classroom. Third, in the present study, we did not collect data on whether and how much the parents trained their children to use Yuudee at home between the official training sessions. Training conducted by the parents at home, if it existed, may have affected the training effectiveness that we evaluated. Fourth, there was no control group in the present study, which limited the possible analyses. In future studies, we will add a control group of children who will undertake the same behavior intervention but with no training with Yuudee or training with other AACs. Finally, in addition to the above, more subjects are needed to associate training effectiveness with pre-training factors. Training effectiveness varied considerably between these ten children. It is worth noting that AU112003, who had the lowest expressive age equivalent score among these children, obtained relatively better training effectiveness. AU112003 achieved three consecutive unprompted successful responses and at least 50% accuracy in all of the phases (phases I–IV) in which he was trained. Neither standard scores nor age equivalent scores for the four domains of the Vineland Adaptive Behavior Scales-Chinese version were significantly correlated with the number of training phases for which the children were able to achieve at least 50% accuracy (p value >0.1, Pearson's correlation). This may relate to the small sample size. It is conceivable that conducting a combined analysis of additional phenotypic factors with the training data collected from more children could help to identify any strong influences related to the impressive performance of children like AU112003. The identification of pre-training characteristics that are associated with training effectiveness could enable us to predict which children may respond particularly well to Yuudee training.

The feature of turning off the speech outputs was added to Yuudee based on the advice of experienced trainers who teach children with autism who have limited functional speech. Testing whether or not turning off the speech outputs could promote the spontaneous speech of children was not one of the primary aims of this study. However, we did make some interesting observations about how three particular children behaved when the speech outputs were turned off in a few trials. AU110003 and AU110203 spoke the name of the reinforcers when they found that no speech was broadcast after they touched a picture. In two trials, AU110003 said the name of another item that he was not asking for after he touched the target picture with no speech output. AU069603 touched the picture of another reinforcer when no speech was broadcast. During training, AU110003 and AU110203 often echoed the phrases outputted by the iPads but AU069603 seldom did.

Each child was assessed using the aberrant behavior checklist (Chinese version) before and after Yuudee training [40]. These children obtained significantly improved scores on the lethargy/social withdrawal subscale after Yuudee training (p value $= 0.04$, one-sided Wilcoxon rank sum test). However, because of the lack of a control group, we were not able to ascertain whether the improvements were the result of Yuudee training as these ten children also attended ABA (applied behavior analysis) training during the 5-week period when they underwent training for making requests with Yuudee.

The parents of some children who were not among the ten trained children in the main study trained their child (with limited spoken language) to make requests with Yuudee at home under the direction of trainers involved in the present study. A 5-year-old boy with ASD who had little spoken language was trained to use Yuudee by his mother at home. The mother reported an event that made her realize that Yuudee could help her son to communicate. One day, the boy cried continually even though she had given him many of his preferred toys. She suddenly thought of Yuudee. After she gave the iPad to the boy, the boy touched the picture "I want the playdough." When she gave him the playdough the boy calmed down. As reported by the mother, her child could, after a period of sustained training, spontaneously find and use the iPad to make requests at home.

Yuudee is the first AAC mobile App in Mainland China, and in this study, we demonstrated the effectiveness of Yuudee at improving the requesting skills of minimally verbal children with ASD. Because of the widespread use of mobile touchscreen devices, Yuudee is easily available and accessible. Yuudee can be adapted to a wide variety of situations in which children have communication needs. It is conceivable that its use could be included as a natural part of daily life. Considering the free availability of Yuudee and the large number of minimally verbal individuals with ASD in Mainland China and the large global population of Chinese speakers, Yuudee could (in theory) benefit a great many children with ASD and their families. Given what has been reported in studies using other SGDs, it is possible that the sustained use of Yuudee may be helpful for improving spoken language or other functional communication skills (e.g., commenting skills) in children with ASD. Moreover, Yuudee may also be helpful for minimally verbal children with other disabilities.

Conclusions

We developed an AAC mobile App named Yuudee for minimally verbal children with ASD in Mainland China. The large built-in library of Yuudee has 39 categories of pictures with corresponding spoken phrases that represent the various communication needs of minimally verbal children. Yuudee can be easily customized according to the specific communication needs of the child and the level at which the child operates Yuudee. Yuudee is freely available and runs on iPads and Android phones. The training for making requests with Yuudee consists of five phases that were designed based on the training phases of PECS and the functionalities of Yuudee. All ten of the minimally verbal children with ASD who received Yuudee training achieved three consecutive unprompted successful responses in at least three of the five phases. Three children achieved at least 50% accuracy in only one phase; the other seven children achieved at least 50% accuracy in at least two of the five phases. Two children achieved at least 50% accuracy in all of the phases in which they were trained. Therefore, the use of Yuudee with the training procedures adapted from the PECS training procedures was effective at improving the requesting skills of minimally verbal children with ASD.

Abbreviations

AAC: Augmentative and alternative communication; ADOS: Autism Diagnostic Observation Schedule; ASD: Autism spectrum disorder; IOA: Interobserver agreement; PECS: Picture Exchange Communication System; SGDs: Speech-generating devices

Acknowledgements

We would like to thank all of the families who participated in this study. We would also like to thank the trainers from Beijing Stars and Rain Educational Institute who conducted the training for making requests with Yuudee. We are also grateful to Jiandong Gao for his advice on the design of Yuudee and to Wenfang Ma who collected the data as an independent observer.

Funding

This work was supported by the Beijing Municipal Science and Technology Commission (no. Z131100006813046). The funders had no role in the study design, data collection, data analysis, manuscript preparation, or publication decisions.

Authors' contributions

LW designed and coordinated the study and wrote and revised the manuscript. SA participated in the design of Yuudee, the design of the training, data collection and analysis, and the writing and revision of the manuscript. XF and YD participated in the design of Yuudee and the development of the iOS Version of Yuudee. Line drawings in the built-in library were drawn by ML's team. JW and XL participated in the design of the user interface of Yuudee. CG and CL developed the Android version of Yuudee. HB and XW participated in the design of the training and led their team to conduct the training. All of the authors read and approved the final manuscript.

Competing interests

The authors declare that they have no competing interests.

Author details

[1]School of Life Sciences, Beijing Normal University, No. 19, XinJieKouWai St., HaiDian District, Beijing 100875, China. [2]National Institute of Biological Sciences, No. 7, Science Park Road, ZhongGuanCun Life Science Park, ChangPing District, Beijing 102206, China. [3]AppChina, Bejing, China. [4]Beijing Stars and Rain Education Institute, No. 18, ShuangQiao East Road, Beijing 100121, China. [5]Academy of Arts and Design, Tsinghua University, No. 1, QingHuaYuan Road, HaiDai District, Beijing 100084, China. [6]Inway Design, Beijing, China. [7]G-Wearables, Inc., Beijing, China. [8]Center for Bioinformatics, State Key Laboratory of Protein and Plant Gene Research, School of Life Sciences, Peking University, No. 5, YiHeYuan Road, HaiDian District, Beijing 100871, China.

References

1. Association AP. Diagnostic and statistical manual of mental disorders. 5th ed. Arlington: American Psychiatric Publishing; 2013.
2. Norrelgen F, Fernell E, Eriksson M, Hedvall A, Persson C, Sjolin M, Gillberg C, Kjellmer L. Children with autism spectrum disorders who do not develop phrase speech in the preschool years. Autism. 2015;19(8):934–43.
3. Anderson DK, Lord C, Risi S, DiLavore PS, Shulman C, Thurm A, Welch K, Pickles A. Patterns of growth in verbal abilities among children with autism spectrum disorder. J Consult Clin Psychol. 2007;75(4):594–604.
4. Tager-Flusberg H, Kasari C. Minimally verbal school-aged children with autism spectrum disorder: the neglected end of the spectrum. Autism Res. 2013;6(6):468-78.
5. Kasari C, Brady N, Lord C, Tager-Flusberg H. Assessing the minimally verbal school-aged child with autism spectrum disorder. Autism Res. 2013:n/a-n/a.
6. Bondy AS, Frost LA. The picture exchange communication system. Focus Autism Other Dev Disabl. 1994;9(3):1–19.
7. Bondy A, Frost L. The picture exchange communication system. Behav Modif. 2001;25(5):725–44.
8. Frost LA, Bondy AS. The picture exchange communication system training manual. 2nd ed. Newark: Pyramid Educational Consultants Inc.; 2002.
9. Ganz JB, Davis JL, Lund EM, Goodwyn FD, Simpson RL. Meta-analysis of PECS with individuals with ASD: investigation of targeted versus non-targeted outcomes, participant characteristics, and implementation phase. Res Dev Disabil. 2012;33(2):406–18.
10. Flippin M, Reszka S, Watson LR. Effectiveness of the Picture Exchange Communication System (PECS) on communication and speech for children with autism spectrum disorders: a meta-analysis. Am J Speech Lang Pathol. 2010;19(2):178–95.
11. Preston D, Carter M. A review of the efficacy of the picture exchange communication system intervention. J Autism Dev Disord. 2009;39(10): 1471–86.
12. Howlin P, Gordon RK, Pasco G, Wade A, Charman T. The effectiveness of Picture Exchange Communication System (PECS) training for teachers of children with autism: a pragmatic, group randomised controlled trial. J Child Psychol Psychiatry. 2007;48(5):473–81.
13. Boesch MC, Wendt O, Subramanian A, Hsu N. Comparative efficacy of the Picture Exchange Communication System (PECS) versus a speech-generating device: effects on requesting skills. Res Autism Spectr Disord. 2013;7(3):480–93.
14. Tincani M, Crozier S, Alazetta L. The Picture Exchange Communication System: effects on manding and speech development for school-aged children with autism. Edu Train Dev Disab. 2006:177–84.
15. Kravits TR, Kamps DM, Kemmerer K, Potucek J. Brief report: increasing communication skills for an elementary-aged student with autism using the Picture Exchange Communication System. J Autism Dev Disord. 2002;32(3):225–30.

16. Charlop-Christy MH, Carpenter M, Le L, LeBlanc LA, Kellet K. Using the picture exchange communication system (PECS) with children with autism: assessment of PECS acquisition, speech, social-communicative behavior, and problem behavior. J Appl Behav Anal. 2002;35(3):213–31.
17. Yoder P, Stone WL. A randomized comparison of the effect of two prelinguistic communication interventions on the acquisition of spoken communication in preschoolers with ASD. J Speech Lang Hear Res. 2006; 49(4):698–711.
18. Choi H, O'Reilly M, Sigafoos J, Lancioni G. Teaching requesting and rejecting sequences to four children with developmental disabilities using augmentative and alternative communication. Res Dev Disabil. 2010;31(2):560–7.
19. Olive ML, de la Cruz B, Davis TN, Chan JM, Lang RB, O'Reilly MF, Dickson SM. The effects of enhanced milieu teaching and a voice output communication aid on the requesting of three children with autism. J Autism Dev Disord. 2007;37(8):1505–13.
20. Sigafoos J, Drasgow E, Halle JW, O'Reilly M, Seely-York S, Edrisinha C, Andrews A. Teaching VOCA use as a communicative repair strategy. J Autism Dev Disord. 2004;34(4):411–22.
21. van der Meer LA, Rispoli M. Communication interventions involving speech-generating devices for children with autism: a review of the literature. Dev Neurorehabil. 2010;13(4):294–306.
22. Kasari C, Kaiser A, Goods K, Nietfeld J, Mathy P, Landa R, Murphy S, Almirall D. Communication interventions for minimally verbal children with autism: a sequential multiple assignment randomized trial. J Am Acad Child Adolesc Psychiatry. 2014;53(6):635–46.
23. Almirall D, DiStefano C, Chang YC, Shire S, Kaiser A, Lu X, Nahum-Shani I, Landa R, Mathy P, Kasari C. Longitudinal effects of adaptive interventions with a speech-generating device in minimally verbal children with ASD. J Clin Child Adolesc Psychol. 2016;45(4):442–56.
24. Sennott S, Bowker A. Autism, aac, and proloquo2go. Perspect Augment altern commun. 2009;18(4):137–45.
25. Sampath H, Indurkhya B, Sivaswamy J: A communication system on smart phones and tablets for non-verbal children with autism. In: 13th International Conference, ICCHP: July 11-13, 2012; Linz, Austria. Computers Helping People with Special Needs: Springer 2012: 323-30.
26. Mirenda P. Promising innovations in AAC for individuals with autism spectrum disorders. Perspect Augment altern commun. 2009;18:112-3.
27. Achmadi D, Kagohara DM, van der Meer L, O'Reilly MF, Lancioni GE, Sutherland D, Lang R, Marschik PB, Green VA, Sigafoos J. Teaching advanced operation of an iPod-based speech-generating device to two students with autism spectrum disorders. Res Autism Spectr Disord. 2012;6(4):1258–64.
28. Sigafoos J, Lancioni GE, O'Reilly MF, Achmadi D, Stevens M, Roche L, Kagohara DM, van der Meer L, Sutherland D, Lang R, et al. Teaching two boys with autism spectrum disorders to request the continuation of toy play using an iPad®-based speech-generating device. Res Autism Spectr Disord. 2013;7(8):923–30.
29. King ML, Takeguchi K, Barry SE, Rehfeldt RA, Boyer VE, Mathews TL. Evaluation of the iPad in the acquisition of requesting skills for children with autism spectrum disorder. Res Autism Spectr Disord. 2014;8(9):1107–20.
30. van der Meer L, Kagohara D, Achmadi D, Green VA, Herrington C, Sigafoos J, O'Reilly MF, Lancioni GE, Lang R, Rispoli M. Teaching functional use of an iPod-based speech-generating device to individuals with developmental disabilities. Journal of Special Education Technology. 2011;26(3):1–11.
31. Waddington H, Sigafoos J, Lancioni GE, O'Reilly MF, van der Meer L, Carnett A, Stevens M, Roche L, Hodis F, Green VA, et al. Three children with autism spectrum disorder learn to perform a three-step communication sequence using an iPad(R)-based speech-generating device. Int J Dev Neurosci. 2014;39:59–67.
32. Lorah ER, Tincani M, Dodge J, Gilroy S, Hickey A, Hantula D. Evaluating picture exchange and the iPad™ as a speech generating device to teach communication to young children with autism. J Dev Phys Disabil. 2013; 25(6):637–49.
33. Sun X, Allison C, Matthews FE, Sharp SJ, Auyeung B, Baron-Cohen S, Brayne C. Prevalence of autism in mainland China, Hong Kong and Taiwan: a systematic review and meta-analysis. Mol Autism. 2013;4(1):7.
34. Zablotsky B, Black LI, Maenner MJ, Schieve LA, Blumberg SJ. Estimated prevalence of autism and other developmental disabilities following questionnaire changes in the 2014 National Health Interview Survey. Natl Health Stat Report. 2015;87:1–20.
35. Thurm A, Manwaring SS, Swineford L, Farmer C. Longitudinal study of symptom severity and language in minimally verbal children with autism. J Child Psychol Psychiatry. 2015;56(1):97–104.
36. Fournier KA, Hass CJ, Naik SK, Lodha N, Cauraugh JH. Motor coordination in autism spectrum disorders: a synthesis and meta-analysis. J Autism Dev Disord. 2010;40(10):1227–40.
37. Lord CRS, Lambrecht L, et al. The autism diagnostic observation schedule-generic: a standard measure of social and communication deficits associated with the spectrum of autism. J Autism Dev Disord. 2000;30(3):205–23.
38. Lord C, Rutter M, Couteur AL. Autism diagnostic interview-revised: a revised version of a diagnostic interview for caregivers of individuals with possible pervasive developmental disorders. J Autism Dev Disord. 1994;24(5):659–85.
39. Wu WT, Cheng CF, Lu HH, Chiu SC. Vineland adaptive behavior scale-- Chinese version. Taipei: Psychological Publishing; 2004.
40. Ma J, Guo Y, Jia M, Li X, Liu J. Reliability and validity of the Chinese version of the Aberrant Behavior Checklist (ABC) in children with autism. Chin Ment Health J. 2011;25(001):14–9.

16

Attitudes toward risk and ambiguity in patients with autism spectrum disorder

Junya Fujino[1,2], Shisei Tei[1,2,3,4], Ryu-ichiro Hashimoto[1,5], Takashi Itahashi[1], Haruhisa Ohta[1,6], Chieko Kanai[1], Rieko Okada[1], Manabu Kubota[1,2,7], Motoaki Nakamura[1,8], Nobumasa Kato[1] and Hidehiko Takahashi[1,2*]

Abstract

Although the ability to make optimal decisions under uncertainty is an integral part of everyday life, individuals with autism spectrum disorder (ASD) frequently report that they experience difficulties with this skill. In behavioral economics, researchers distinguish two types of uncertainty to understand decision-making in this setting: risk (known probabilities) and ambiguity (unknown probabilities). However, it remains unclear how individuals with ASD behave under risk and ambiguity, despite growing evidence of their altered decision-making under uncertainty. We therefore extended previous research by studying the attitudes of those with ASD toward risk and ambiguity in both positive and negative contexts (i.e., gain and loss). In gain contexts, no significant difference was observed between the groups in risk attitudes, but ambiguity aversion was attenuated in ASD. In loss contexts, ambiguity attitudes did not significantly differ between the groups, but the ASD participants were less risk-seeking compared with the controls. In addition, insensitivity to the context change under risk and ambiguity in ASD was both significantly associated with poor social skills. These results improve our understanding of altered decision-making under uncertainty by disentangling the attitudes toward risk and ambiguity in ASD individuals. Applying behavioral economic tools may provide insights into the mechanisms underlying behavioral disturbances in ASD.

Keywords: Autism spectrum disorder, Decision-making, Risk, Ambiguity, Uncertainty, Gain, Loss

Introduction

Decision-making under uncertainty is central to daily functions, because our lives are filled with incomplete, ambiguous, and unpredictable components. Individuals with autism spectrum disorder (ASD), which is characterized by altered social interaction and atypical interests, frequently report having trouble making optimal decisions when faced with such uncertainty [1–3]. This, in turn, can negatively impact their social functioning. Improving our understanding of this problem could provide useful information to help develop practical interventions to improve quality of life in those with ASD.

In recent years, the field of behavioral economics has been expanding rapidly. Researchers in this field distinguish between two types of uncertainty: risk and ambiguity [4, 5]. Under "risk," the precise probabilities of certain outcomes can be estimated (e.g., gambling on a roulette wheel). However, in real-life situations, the probabilities of outcomes often cannot be estimated (e.g., the likelihood of a terrorist attack is unpredictable), and this latter type of uncertainty is referred to as "ambiguity." Previous studies of healthy populations have revealed high variability in individual attitudes toward risk and ambiguity, with little correlation between these measures across individuals [5, 6]. This suggests that attitudes toward risk and ambiguity independently contribute to decision-making under uncertainty. Please see Additional file 1 (Supplementary Introduction) for details regarding risk and ambiguity attitudes.

To date, it has been indicated that individual risk and ambiguity attitudes are linked to various types of behavior, including self-insurance and risk-taking behavior [7, 8]. Using tools of behavioral economics, recent studies have begun to investigate risk and ambiguity attitudes with the aim of better understanding altered decision-making under uncertainty in specific clinical populations. For example, a previous study showed that ambiguity aversion

* Correspondence: hidehiko@kuhp.kyoto-u.ac.jp
[1]Medical Institute of Developmental Disabilities Research, Showa University, 6-11-11 Kita-karasuyama, Setagaya-ku, Tokyo, Japan
[2]Department of Psychiatry, Graduate School of Medicine, Kyoto University, 54 Shogoin-Kawaracho, Sakyo-ku, Kyoto, Japan

was increased in individuals with obsessive-compulsive disorder [9], while another study reported it was attenuated in those with schizophrenia [10]. Findings from these studies laid the groundwork needed to improve the diagnosis and treatment of these psychiatric disorders.

These research findings raise a relevant question: how do individuals with ASD behave under risk and ambiguity? However, to the best of our knowledge, no study has investigated the attitudes of patients with ASD toward uncertainty by clearly distinguishing between risk and ambiguity. Several experimental studies have investigated decision-making under uncertainty in those with ASD, using the Iowa Gambling Task (IGT), which is a well-known behavioral task involving uncertainty [11]. For example, Yechiam et al. reported that patients with ASD did not continue to increase their choices from advantageous decks at the same rate during the IGT when compared with healthy controls [12]. However, an important consideration with the IGT is that the probability distribution is unknown to the participants at the beginning of the test, and they gradually learn this from feedbacks during the task. Therefore, the IGT is a complex measure with elements of decision-making under both risk and ambiguity, where poor performance may partially reflect dysfunctional learning abilities [9, 13].

From a different perspective, De Martino et al. examined the framing effect on monetary decisions in ASD [14]. The framing effect is a well-known decision bias in which people react differently to a particular choice depending on whether it is presented in a positive context (gain) or in a negative one (loss) [15, 16]. Compared with neurotypical participants, adults with ASD demonstrated less susceptibility to the framing effect and made more consistent choices (the results have recently been replicated [2]). The authors proposed that this insensitivity to contextual frame, although enhancing economic rationality, may come at a cost of impaired social skills in ASD [14]. From this perspective, it is crucial to assess attitudes toward risk and ambiguity in both positive and negative contexts (gain and loss) and to investigate the sensitivity to the context change under risk and ambiguity to get a comprehensive picture of these attitudes among patients with ASD.

In this research, we studied risk and ambiguity attitudes in both gain and loss contexts in participants with ASD, using an economic task that clearly distinguished risk and ambiguity containing no feedback learning [6, 7, 9, 17]. Based on the studies mentioned, we hypothesized that ASD participants would exhibit distinctly altered behavioral patterns under risk and ambiguity. In addition, recent studies have shown the association of altered decision-making with the levels of autistic traits [3, 18]. Thus, we also administered the Autism-Spectrum Quotient (AQ) test [19, 20] to quantify ASD-related symptoms and exploratively performed correlation analyses between the task measures and AQ scores among ASD participants.

Methods

Participants

Twenty-seven adults with ASD and 27 healthy controls participated in this study. The sample size was determined based on previous studies on psychiatric disorders that used a similar task [9, 10]. Patients were recruited from a database of volunteers who had received a clinical diagnosis of ASD in outpatient units of the Showa University Karasuyama Hospital. The diagnostic procedure to identify patients with ASD was the same as in our previous studies [21–23]. Briefly, at least three experienced psychiatrists and a clinical psychologist assessed all the patients using the criteria of the Diagnostic and Statistical Manual of Mental Disorders, fourth edition text revision (DSM-IV-TR). The assessment consisted of participant interviews about developmental history, present illness, life history, and family history. Patients were also asked to bring suitable informants who had known them in early childhood. This process required approximately 3 h. A diagnosis of ASD was made only when there was a consensus between the psychiatrists and clinical psychologist. At the time of testing, an experienced psychiatrist evaluated psychiatric comorbidity using the Structured Clinical Interview for DSM-IV Axis I Disorders (SCID). No ASD participants satisfied the diagnostic criteria for substance use disorder, bipolar disorder, or schizophrenia. The controls were recruited through advertisements and acquaintances. They did not meet the criteria for any psychiatric disorders according to SCID performed by an experienced psychiatrist. No participants (ASD participants or controls) had any history of head trauma, serious medical or surgical illness, or substance abuse.

The intelligence quotient (IQ) scores of all ASD participants had been evaluated before the study using either the Wechsler Adult Intelligence Scale-Third Edition (WAIS-III) or the WAIS-Revised (WAIS-R). Each participant with ASD was considered to be high functioning because his or her full-scale IQ score was above 80. Although there are several minor changes in WAIS-III from WAIS-R (e.g., more items), the number of core items remained largely unchanged. Therefore, we considered that the WAIS-R and WAIS-III were essentially the same with regard to measuring the full-scale IQ score of individuals with ASD. The IQ scores of the controls were estimated using a Japanese version of the National Adult Reading Test (JART), based on the previous findings that JART successfully predicted the full-scale IQ score in the healthy population [24, 25].

Three ASD participants and one control were excluded from the analyses due to their poor performance in the numeracy test or the decision quality measures, which suggested that they did not understand the task (details are described in Additional file 1: Supplementary Methods). Thus, data from 24 ASD participants and 26 controls were analyzed (age: 20–45 years). In total, 12 ASD participants were administered the following psychotropic drugs: anxiolytics (n = 3), antidepressants (n = 6), antipsychotics (n = 3), antiepileptics (n = 2), sleep-inducing drugs (n = 6), and other psychotropic drugs (n = 3). Although gender, handedness, current smoking status, and estimated full-scale IQ levels were matched between the groups, the control group was slightly younger than the ASD group (Table 1).

This study was approved by the Committee on Medical Ethics of Kyoto University and the institutional review board of Showa University Karasuyama Hospital and was conducted in accordance with The Code of Ethics of the World Medical Association. After a complete description of the study, written informed consent was obtained from all participants.

Autism-Spectrum Quotient

All participants completed the Japanese version of the Autism-Spectrum Quotient (AQ) test, which has high reliability and validity [19, 20]. The AQ is a brief and self-administered measure that includes items covering both social and nonsocial aspects of behavior and cognition [19, 20]. Therefore, it has been widely used to quantify autistic traits in research and clinical practice. To characterize specific autistic traits of each participant, we computed the three factors: "social skills," "details/patterns," and "communication/mindreading" based on the previous studies [26]. Example items are as follows: the social skills factor ("I frequently find that I don't know how to keep a conversation going" and "I find it hard to make new friends"), the details/patterns factor ("I notice patterns in things all the time" and "I am fascinated by numbers"), and the communication/mindreading factor ("When I'm reading a story, I find it difficult to work out the characters' intentions" and "I am often the last to understand the point of a joke"). The AQ was scored using the collapsed scoring system [19, 20, 26]. Higher scores for each factor indicated higher autistic traits (e.g., poor social skills).

Table 1 Demographic and clinical characteristics of participants

	Control group (N = 26)	ASD group (N = 24)	Statistics p
Age (years)	25.7 (6.8)	29.5 (4.3)	0.01[a]
Gender (female)	2 (7.7%)	3 (12.5%)	0.57[b]
Handedness (right)	2 (7.7%)	2 (8.3%)	0.93[b]
Smoking (current smoker)	2 (7.7%)	3 (12.5%)	0.57[b]
Estimated full-scale IQ	105.5 (9.3)	108.0 (12.1)	0.57[a]
AQ total	16.2 (7.0)	34.4 (5.2)	< 0.01[a]
Social skills	2.7 (2.9)	8.8 (3.0)	< 0.01[a]
Details/patterns	3.5 (1.7)	4.7 (2.2)	0.04[a]
Communication/mindreading	1.1 (1.5)	4.3 (1.3)	< 0.01[a]

Standard deviations or percentages in parentheses
AQ Autism-Spectrum Quotient, *IQ* intelligence quotient
[a]Mann–Whitney test
[b]Two-tailed chi-square test

Economic task

We modified a task used in the previous studies [6, 7, 9, 17]. The current task consisted of two sessions (gain trials and loss trials sessions). Participants were asked to make a series of choices between pairs of different monetary options. In each trial, participants could choose between a fixed monetary amount and a lottery. The fixed monetary amount did not change from trial to trial, but either the outcome probability or the ambiguity level associated with the lottery option could vary from trial to trial.

In the gain trials, participants chose between a guaranteed gain of ¥200 (about $2) and a lottery that might pay more than ¥200 but might also pay ¥0. The lottery appeared on the screen in the form of a bowl containing 24 red- and blue-colored chips. If the bowl was chosen, one chip was drawn, and participants had the right to win the amount allocated to the color of the drawn chip. In risky lotteries, the entire bowl was visible (Fig. 1a). In ambiguous lotteries, we used a black occluder to hide the center of the bowl (Fig. 1b). For instance, as shown in Fig. 1a, if participants choose the left side, they will win ¥200. If they choose the right side, they will win ¥850 if a red chip is drawn, but they will win ¥0 if a blue chip is drawn. In risky lotteries, five winning probabilities were used in the bowl (0.125, 0.25, 0.375, 0.5, and 0.75; Fig. 1c), and in ambiguous lotteries, three ambiguity levels were used in the bowl (0.25, 0.5, and 0.75; Fig. 1d). Probability and ambiguity levels were communicated to the participants using visual displays of lottery bowls before starting the experiment. In addition, we explained that the ambiguous bowls were filled before the experiment began and remained sealed during the experiment, according to the previous studies [6, 7, 9, 17]. It should be noted that the true probability of winning across all ambiguous lotteries was 0.5 because the true probability of winning in each ambiguous lottery was selected at random and fixed throughout a session and because half of all trials paid-off on red and the other half paid-off on blue [6, 7, 9, 17]. Five winning amounts (¥200, ¥350, ¥850, ¥2200, ¥5200) were used per risk and ambiguity level. All lottery situations during the task are shown in Additional file 2 (Tables S1 and S2).

Similarly, the loss trials were performed after the gain trials. In the loss trials, participants chose between a

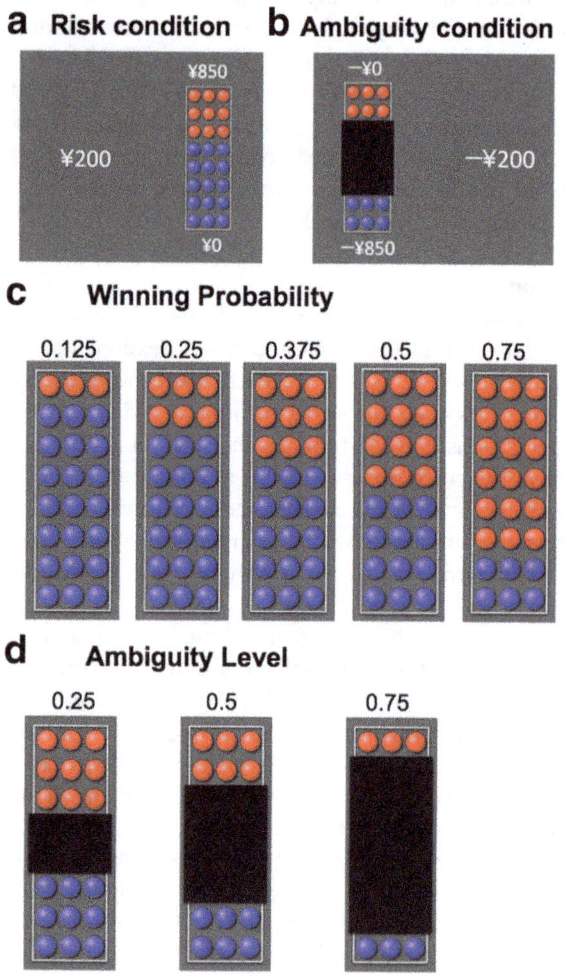

Fig. 1 Experimental design. **a** Examples of the stimuli in the risk condition. **b** Examples of the stimuli in the ambiguity condition. In the gain (loss) trials, participants chose between a guaranteed gain (loss) of ¥200 and a lottery that might pay (could yield losses of) more than ¥200 but might also pay ¥0 (could also yield no loss). For instance, as can be seen in **a**, if participants choose the left side, they will win ¥200. If they choose the right side, they will win ¥850 if a red chip is drawn, but they will win ¥0 if a blue chip is drawn. As shown in **b**, if participants choose the left side, they will lose ¥0 if a red chip is drawn, but they will lose ¥850 if a blue chip is drawn. If they choose the right side, they will lose ¥200. **c** The stimuli of the five winning probabilities are shown (red is the winning color). **d** The stimuli of the three ambiguity levels are shown

guaranteed loss of ¥200 and a lottery that could yield losses of more than ¥200, but that could also yield no loss (¥0). The probability and ambiguity levels of the lotteries were the same as those in the gain trials. Five losing amounts (−¥200, −¥250, −¥350, −¥850, and −¥2200) were used per risk and ambiguity level.

In both gain and loss trial sessions, each unique lottery was presented four times, counterbalancing the winning color and the side it appeared on-screen, resulting in a total of 160 trials, that is, 5 amounts × (5 risk + 3 ambiguity) × 4 = 160 trials (320 trials, summing the gain and loss trials). These trials were separated into four blocks. Each block included 40 trials (i.e., 5 amounts × [5 risk + 3 ambiguity]) and was performed in a pseudorandom order that was unique to each block. During each trial, participants had 6 s to indicate their choice. The interval between successive trials was 2.5 s. Participants could rest between the blocks, and it was up to them to decide when to begin each block. No feedback of the outcome was provided after each choice.

Before starting the task, we performed a numeracy test to assess the participants' numeracy skills and understanding of numbers (see Additional file 1: Supplementary Methods). All participants were quizzed about how well they understood the task (Additional file 1: Supplementary Methods) and practiced at least once on a short version of the task. Only after they successfully completed the quiz were they allowed to proceed to the experiment. We explained that their winnings were defined referring to the outcomes of three gain trials and three loss trials after they had finished (in reality, we paid a maximum pre-defined participation fee of ¥6000), based on the previous studies [5, 27]. The experiment was presented using E-Prime software (Psychology Software Tools, Inc., Pittsburgh, PA, USA).

Statistical analyses

Because some of our continuous measures were not normally distributed (Shapiro–Wilk test, $p < 0.05$), we chose Mann–Whitney tests to compare group differences and Spearman's rank correlations for the correlation analyses. Data were analyzed using SPSS 21 (IBM Corp., Armonk, NY, USA). Statistical significance was set at $p < 0.05$ (two-tailed).

We estimated the participants' attitudes toward risk and ambiguity based on the previous studies [6, 7, 9, 17]. Under risk, a risk-neutral decision maker would choose the option of the higher expected value (EV; the product of probability and amount) in the gain contexts and the option of the lower EV in the loss contexts. In our task, such a decision maker should choose risky lotteries over the guaranteed payoff 60% of the time in both gain and loss contexts (see Additional file 2: Tables S3 and S4). Participants who chose risky lotteries less or more were termed risk-averse or risk-seeking, respectively. Thus, the risk attitude will be positive for a risk-averse decision maker and negative for a risk-seeking decision maker, when using the following equation:

$$\text{risk attitude (gain, loss)} = 0.6 - \frac{\text{number of risky lotteries chosen}}{\text{total number of risky lotteries}}$$

Concerning ambiguity, an ambiguity-neutral decision maker would make the same choices regardless of the ambiguity level. Because the range of possible outcome probabilities was centered at 0.5 in all of the ambiguity trials, such a decision-maker should make the same choices in ambiguous trials and in risky trials in which the outcome probability was 0.5. To estimate ambiguity attitudes, we therefore compared each participant's choices in the ambiguous lotteries to his or her choices in the risky lotteries with a 0.5 outcome probability. Participants who chose ambiguous lotteries less or more often than they chose 0.5 risky lotteries with the same potential reward were termed ambiguity-averse or ambiguity-seeking, respectively. Thus, the ambiguity attitude will be positive for decision makers who are ambiguity-averse and negative for decision-makers who are ambiguity-seeking when using the following equation:

$$\text{ambiguity attitude (gain, loss)} = \frac{\text{number of 50\%risky lotteries chosen}}{\text{total number of 50\%risky lotteries}} - \frac{\text{number of ambiguous lotteries chosen}}{\text{total number of ambiguous lotteries}}$$

In addition, we further estimated sensitivity to the context change among participants by taking the difference in their risk and ambiguity attitudes to losses from those to gains. Greater sensitivity was denoted by a larger value.

Finally, we performed correlation analyses between these measures (risk attitudes [gain and loss], ambiguity attitudes [gain and loss], and sensitivity to the context change [risk and ambiguity]) and the three factors of the AQ (social skills, details/patterns, and communication/mindreading) among ASD participants.

Results

Overall, the participants (N = 50 [control 26, ASD 24]) performed the task well, missing an average of only 0.58 ± 1.30 (mean ± standard deviation [SD]) trials. There were no significant differences between the two groups in the decision quality measures, or in reaction time under risk and ambiguity in the gain and loss contexts (see Additional file 1: Supplementary Methods and Additional file 2: Tables S5 and S6). Because the order of sessions in the task was not counterbalanced (the loss trial session followed the gain trial session for all participants), we compared measures related to comprehension/attention and the effect of time on these measures between gain and loss trials in both groups. We found no significant difference between gain and loss trials in terms of decision quality. Details are described in Additional file 1 (Supplementary Results).

Attitudes toward risk and ambiguity under gain

Figure 2a, b depicts the attitudes toward risk and ambiguity in the gain contexts in both groups. Although no significant difference was found in attitudes toward risk (control 0.25 ± 0.17, ASD 0.28 ± 0.20; U = 280.50, Z = −0.61, p = 0.54, effect size r = − 0.09), the ASD group showed attenuated ambiguity aversion (control 0.18 ± 0.18, ASD 0.07 ± 0.14; U = 203.50, Z = − 2.11, p = 0.03, effect size r = − 0.30). Because several ASD participants took psychotropic drugs, we compared the behavioral data of ASD participants without psychotropic drugs (N = 12) with those of the controls. The analyses did not materially change the results (Additional file 2: Table S7). Please also see Additional file 1 (Supplementary Results), Additional file 3 (Figure S1), and Additional file 4 (Figure S2) for details regarding the distribution of task measures and potential outliers.

Attitudes toward risk and ambiguity under loss

Figure 3a, b depicts the attitudes toward risk and ambiguity in the loss contexts in both groups [please also see Additional file 1 (Supplementary Results), Additional file 3 (Figure S1), and Additional file 4 (Figure S2)]. No significant difference was observed in attitudes toward ambiguity (control 0.01 ± 0.11, ASD 0.02 ± 0.13; U = 285.50, Z = − 0.52, p = 0.61, effect size r = − 0.07), but ASD participants were less risk-seeking compared with the controls (control − 0.06 ± 0.12, ASD 0.01 ± 0.13; U = 200.50, Z = − 2.17, p = 0.03, effect size r = − 0.31). The analyses after excluding the data on ASD with psychotropic medication did not materially change the results (Additional file 2: Table S7).

Sensitivity to the context change

We estimated sensitivity to the context change under risk and ambiguity in both groups. Although the difference in sensitivity to the context change under risk did not reach statistical significance between the groups (control 0.32 ± 0.19, ASD 0.27 ± 0.21; U = 277.00, Z = − 0.68, p = 0.50, effect size r = − 0.10), this measure under ambiguity was significantly reduced in the ASD group compared with the control group (control 0.16 ± 0.18, ASD 0.05 ± 0.14; U = 195.50, Z = − 2.27, p = 0.02, effect size r = − 0.32). The analyses after excluding the data on ASD with psychotropic medication did not materially change the results (Additional file 2: Table S7). Details are described in Additional file 1 (Supplementary Results), Additional file 3 (Figure S1), and Additional file 4 (Figure S2).

Correlation analyses

In the correlation analyses, we found no significant relationship between attitudes toward risk or ambiguity and the AQ factors among ASD participants, except for a negative correlation between risk attitudes to gains and the communication/mindreading factor (rho = − 0.43, p = 0.03) (Additional file 2: Table S8). Sensitivity to the context change under risk and ambiguity was both significantly and negatively correlated with the social skills

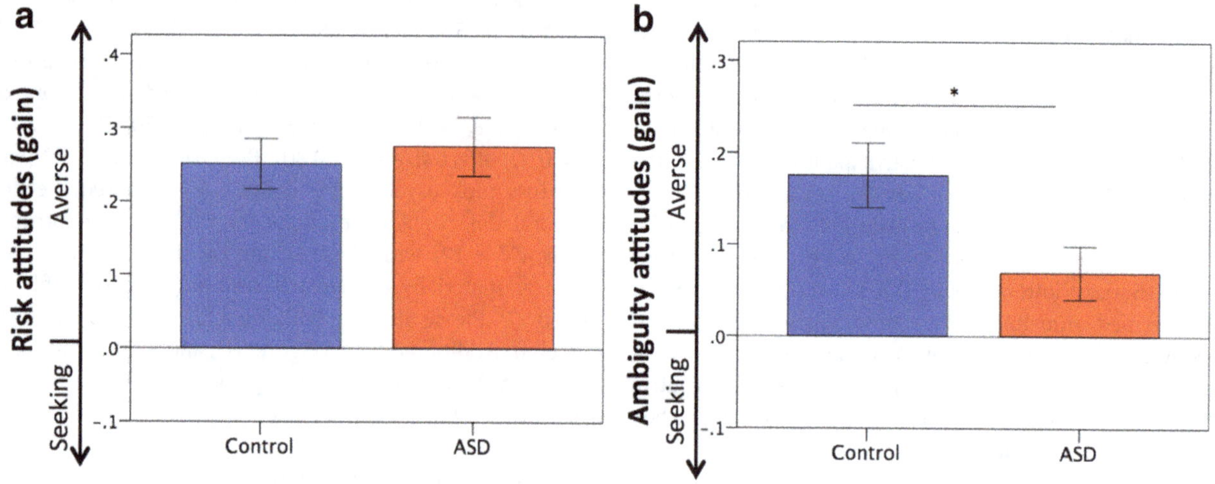

Fig. 2 Attitudes toward risk and ambiguity under gain. **a** No significant difference was observed in attitudes toward risk between the groups. **b** The ASD group showed reduced ambiguity aversion compared with the controls. Error bars indicate ± standard errors. $^*p < 0.05$

factor of AQ (*rho* = − 0.44, p = 0.03 and *rho* = − 0.50, p = 0.01, respectively; Fig. 4).

Discussion

To the best of our knowledge, this is the first study to investigate risk and ambiguity attitudes in both gain and loss contexts in participants with ASD. The results provide new insights into altered decision-making under uncertainty that occurs in patients with ASD.

As in previous studies [6, 7, 9, 17], our healthy controls were, on an average, risk averse in the gain context and risk seeking in the loss context; they were also ambiguity averse in the gain context but largely ambiguity neutral in the loss context.

In gain contexts, no significant difference was observed between the groups in risk attitudes, but ambiguity aversion was attenuated in the ASD group. This suggests that they had greater tolerance for options with consequences that had unknown probabilities under positive circumstances. In loss contexts, ambiguity attitudes did not significantly differ between the groups, but the ASD participants were less risk-seeking compared with the controls, indicating that they avoided risk-taking around potential negative outcomes when outcome probabilities were known. These dissociated behavioral patterns, which were altered under risk and ambiguity, might make it difficult to assess behavioral disturbances of this patient group in clinical settings. Previous studies using the IGT have yielded inconsistent results concerning altered decision-making under uncertainty in those with ASD; some studies reported poor performance of IGT in ASD while other studies did not [12, 28–30]. The distinct behavioral

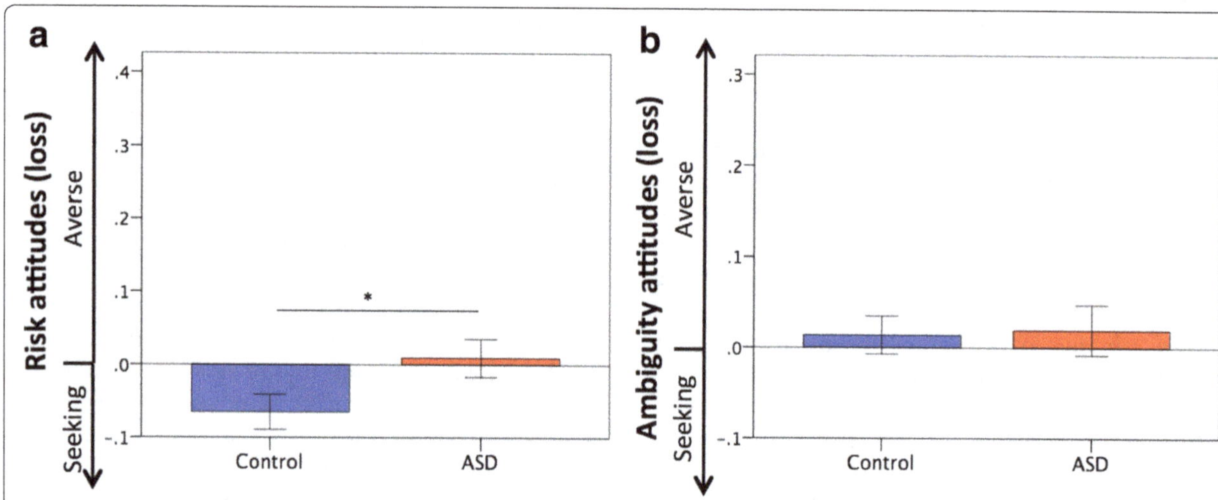

Fig. 3 Attitudes toward risk and ambiguity under loss. **a** The ASD participants were less risk-seeking to losses compared with the controls. **b** Ambiguity attitudes to losses did not differ between the groups. Error bars indicate ± standard errors. $^*p < 0.05$

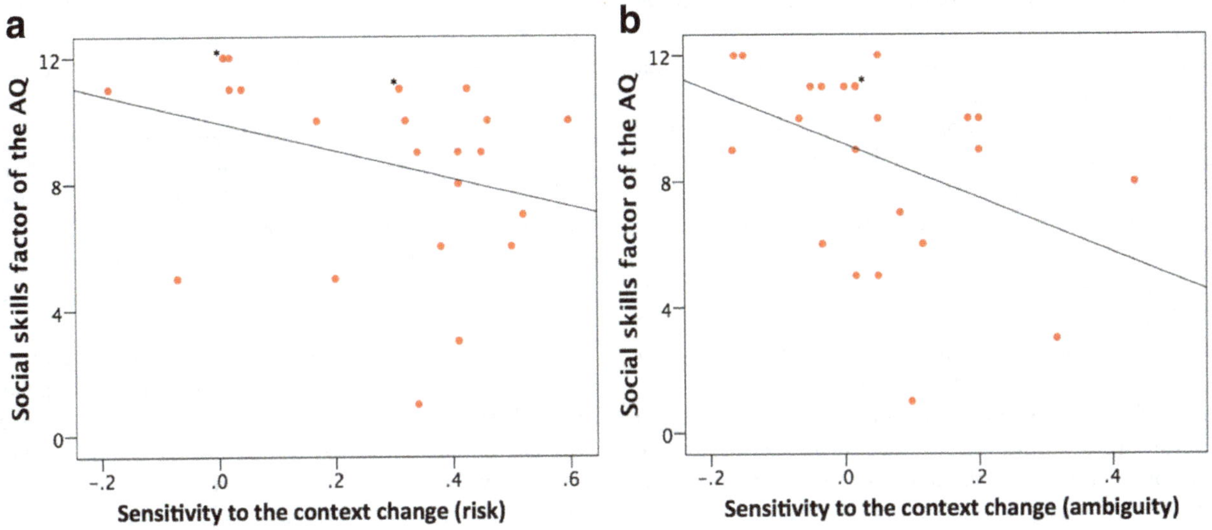

Fig. 4 Correlations between sensitivity to the context change under risk and ambiguity and social skills factor of the AQ among ASD participants. **a** Correlations between sensitivity to the context change under risk and the social skills factor of the AQ (*rho* = – 0.44, *p* = 0.03). **b** Correlations between sensitivity to the context change under ambiguity and the social skills factor of the AQ (*rho* = – 0.50, *p* = 0.01). Asterisk, overlapping data point

patterns altered by risk and ambiguity in our study, along with the mixed results of previous IGT studies, emphasize that it is critical to distinguish risk and ambiguity in order to understand altered decision-making under uncertainty in ASD clearly. We found no significant relationship between either the risk or the ambiguity attitudes and the AQ factors, except for the negative correlation between risk attitudes to gains and the communication/mindreading factor. Therefore, we could not infer the mechanisms underlying the altered attitudes toward risk and ambiguity in ASD. However, our findings should provide an impetus for future neuroimaging studies that elucidate the mechanisms of altered attitudes toward risk and ambiguity in those with ASD.

It is important to note that sensitivity to the context change under both risk and ambiguity was significantly and negatively correlated with the social skills factor of the AQ in ASD participants (although the difference in this measure under risk did not reach statistical significance between the groups, it served as important individual difference variables within the ASD group). It is well known that individuals react to a particular choice in a different manner under risk depending on whether it is presented as a gain or as a loss (referred to as the "framing effect") [15, 16]. Furthermore, a recent study demonstrated that the framing effect also existed during decision-making under ambiguity [31]. This effect is economically irrational but seems to play a key role in making optimal decisions under uncertain situations [15]. Previous studies have examined the framing effect on monetary decisions in individuals with ASD [2, 14]. These studies have shown that ASD individuals are less susceptible to the framing effect and make more consistent choices, and the authors have proposed that ASD confers enhanced logical consistency, which clinically presents as reduced behavioral flexibility. More recently, Farmer et al. compared a series of choices regarding consumer products between ASD participants and controls [18] and showed that participants' preferences between a given pair of options frequently switched when the third item in the set was changed. This tendency was reduced among ASD participants, indicating more consistent and conventionally rational choices [a comparison of people with low- vs high-levels of autistic traits assessed by AQ (drawn from the general population) also revealed a weaker version of the same effect]. The authors have proposed that the price ASD individuals pay for this resistance to contextual influence may be a reduction in the potentially adaptive updating of beliefs about optimum choices that come from using local comparisons to inform decision-making. Taken together, our results, using a different experimental paradigm, supported these previous findings [2, 14, 18] and suggested that a difficulty to adapt behavioral strategies according to the valence of the context under both risk and ambiguity might be related with poor social skills in individuals with ASD.

As for the clinical implications of this study, our findings support the notion that behavioral economics is a promising method for objectively evaluating behavioral disturbance in patients with psychiatric disorders [9, 17]. Rodgers and colleagues have elegantly demonstrated that intolerance of uncertainty plays an important role in understanding anxiety symptoms in ASD [32–36]. Although the jargon used in psychology and economics is not necessarily identical and careful interpretation is needed, a previous study reported a possible link between ambiguity intolerance and ambiguity aversion in healthy population [37]. The behavioral economics tools are relatively affordable and easy to administer, and thus, applying these tools may provide insights into the mechanisms underlying behavioral disturbances under uncertain environment in ASD.

There are several limitations to this study. First, half the individuals with ASD were administered psychotropic medication, which means that we cannot exclude the possibility of a medication effect. For example, previous studies have shown that dopaminergic and serotoninergic agents influence risk-taking behaviors [38]. In addition, Beninger et al. found an association between antipsychotic drug use status and better performance on the gambling task in patients with schizophrenia [39]. Unfortunately, the medicated participants with ASD in our study were administered different types of psychotropic drugs, hampering further analysis of the effect of medication on our behavioral results. However, we still found significant differences between the groups with regard to the three measures (i.e., risk attitudes [loss], ambiguity attitudes [gain], and sensitivity to the context change [ambiguity]) when analyzing the data, excluding those of the ASD participants administered psychotropic medication. Our findings should be replicated in future research that recruits more individuals with ASD who are not taking medication. Second, the order of sessions in our task was not counterbalanced (the loss trial session followed the gain trial session for all participants). Thus, factors related to the order of testing (e.g., fatigue) have the possibility of causing confounding. However, to minimize the influence of fatigue on the task performance, we allowed sufficient rest time between each block. The experimenter also observed participants during the task, and the post-task interview confirmed that their concentration throughout the task was good. Furthermore, we found no significant difference between gain and loss sessions in terms of decision quality for both groups. Before data collection, we took steps to ensure that task instructions were understood; in these steps, the participants were required to pass the numeracy test and comprehension quizzes. Thus, we believe that our study can provide a good foundation for future studies. Third, although the difference was small, the healthy controls were younger. A previous study investigated risk and ambiguity attitudes in both gain and loss contexts in healthy subjects aged 12–90 years and found no significant differences in these attitudes between the young adults group (21–25 years) and the midlife adults group (30–50 years) [6]. Therefore, given the age range of our sample (20–45 years), we believe that our findings will be useful for obtaining a better understanding of decision-making under uncertainty in ASD. Fourth, emotional factors, including interoception, have recently been reported to play a key role in decision-making [2, 40, 41]. For example, Shah et al. have demonstrated that framing effects are associated with interoception and alexithymia in the neurotypical population but that emotional and interoceptive signals have less impact on decision-making processes in ASD [2]. However, we did not measure factors, such as alexithymia, in the current study. Future studies should comprehensively take social and emotional factors into account and investigate the contribution of such factors in risk and ambiguity attitudes in ASD. Fifth, because of the exploratory nature of this study, no correction was applied for multiple comparisons during the group comparisons of the task measures (Mann–Whitney tests) and the correlation analyses between these measures and the AQ factors. Thus, our preliminary findings should be interpreted cautiously and need to be carefully replicated in future research. Nevertheless, the current results may serve as an indication of the fruitfulness of research in this area and motivate future research on a wider scale.

Conclusions

In conclusion, the current results extend previous findings by disentangling the attitudes toward risk and ambiguity in individuals with ASD. Applying behavioral economic tools may provide insights into the mechanisms underlying behavioral disturbances in ASD.

Additional files

Additional file 1: Supporting information concerning the task measures. Detailed explanations regarding risk and ambiguity attitudes are included in the Supplementary Introduction. Details concerning the exclusion criteria, numeracy test, quiz, and decision quality measures are described in the Supplementary Methods. The distribution of the task measures, potential outliers, and decision quality in gain and loss trials are explained in the Supplementary Results.

Additional file 2: Tables showing the details of the task measures. **Table S1.** All lottery situations in the gain trials. Table S2. All lottery situations in the loss trials. Table S3. Probability of choosing a lottery for a risk-neutral decision maker in the gain contexts. Table S4. Probability of choosing a lottery for a risk-neutral decision maker in the loss contexts. Table S5. Measures of decision quality. Table S6. Reaction time (ms) in risk and ambiguity conditions. **Table S7.** Results of additional analyses between ASD participants without psychotropic medication and controls. Table S8. Correlation coefficients between risk and ambiguity attitudes and the three factors of the Autism-Spectrum Quotient (AQ) among ASD participants.

Additional file 3: Distribution of the task measures (**Figure S1.**) **Figure S1.** depicts the distribution of each of the task measures (risk attitudes [gain and loss], ambiguity attitudes [gain and loss], and sensitivity to the context change [risk and ambiguity]). Because some of the task measures were not normally distributed (Shapiro–Wilk test, $p < 0.05$), we chose Mann–Whitney tests to compare group differences. Concerning the task measures that were normally distributed, we also compared the group difference using two-sample t-tests, which did not materially change the results.

Additional file 4 Analyses of the task measures after excluding the potential outliers (**Figure S2.**) To confirm our conclusion of this study, we also reanalyzed the group comparison of the task measures (risk attitudes [gain and loss], ambiguity attitudes [gain and loss], and sensitivity to the context change [risk and ambiguity]) after excluding the potential outliers of each task measure (> 2 SD from the group mean). These analyses did not materially change the results.

Abbreviations

AQ: Autism-Spectrum Quotient; ASD: Autism spectrum disorder; DSM-IV-TR: Diagnostic and Statistical Manual of Mental Disorders fourth edition text revision; EV: Expected value; IGT: Iowa Gambling Task; IQ: Intelligence quotient; JART: Japanese version of the National Adult Reading Test; SCID: Structured Clinical Interview for DSM-IV Axis I Disorders; SD: Standard deviation; WAIS-III: Wechsler Adult Intelligence Scale-Third Edition; WAIS-R: Wechsler Adult Intelligence Scale-Revised

Acknowledgements

The authors wish to extend their gratitude to the research team of the Medical Institute of Developmental Disabilities Research at Showa University for their assistance in data acquisition.

Funding

This work was supported by grants-in-aid for scientific research A (24243061) and on Innovative Areas (23120009, 16H06572), from the Ministry of Education, Culture, Sports, Science and Technology of Japan (MEXT); Grants-in-Aid for Start-up (16H07194) and Young Scientists B (17K16398) from the Japan Society for the Promotion of Science (JSPS); and Takeda Science Foundation. A part of this study is the result of Development of BMI Technologies for Clinical Application carried out under the Strategic Research Program for Brain Sciences by MEXT, "Research and development of technology for enhancing functional recovery of elderly and disabled people based on non-invasive brain imaging and robotic assistive devices", the Commissioned Research of National Institute of Information and Communications Technology, JAPAN, and the Joint Usage/Research Program of Medical Institute of Developmental Disabilities Research, Showa University.

Authors' contributions

JF, ST, RH, HO, CK, MK, MN, NK, and HT designed the research; JF, ST, TI, and RO participated in the data acquisition; JF, HO, CK, MN, and NK were in charge of the clinical assessment. JF and ST analyzed data; HO, CK, RO, MN, and NK helped with the interpretation of data. JF, ST, RH, TI, MK, and HT wrote the paper. All authors have made intellectual contribution to the work and approved the final version of the manuscript for submission.

Competing interests

The authors declare that they have no competing interests.

Author details

[1]Medical Institute of Developmental Disabilities Research, Showa University, 6-11-11 Kita-karasuyama, Setagaya-ku, Tokyo, Japan. [2]Department of Psychiatry, Graduate School of Medicine, Kyoto University, 54 Shogoin-Kawaracho, Sakyo-ku, Kyoto, Japan. [3]Institute of Applied Brain Sciences, Waseda University, 2-579-15 Mikajima, Tokorozawa, Saitama, Japan. [4]School of Human and Social Sciences, Tokyo International University, 2509 Matoba, Kawagoe, Saitama, Japan. [5]Department of Language Sciences, Graduate School of Humanities, Tokyo Metropolitan University, 1-1 Minami-Osawa, Hachioji-shi, Tokyo, Japan. [6]Department of Psychiatry, School of Medicine, Showa University, 6-11-11 Kita-karasuyama, Setagaya-ku, Tokyo, Japan. [7]Department of Functional Brain Imaging Research, National Institute of Radiological Sciences, National Institutes for Quantum and Radiological Science and Technology, 4-9-1 Anagawa, Inage-ku, Chiba, Japan. [8]Kanagawa Psychiatric Center, 2-5-1 Serigaya, Yokohama, Kanagawa, Japan.

References

1. Luke L, Clare IC, Ring H, Redley M, Watson P. Decision-making difficulties experienced by adults with autism spectrum conditions. Autism. 2012;16:612–21.
2. Shah P, Catmur C, Bird G. Emotional decision-making in autism spectrum disorder: the roles of interoception and alexithymia. Mol Autism. 2016;7:43.
3. Robic S, Sonie S, Fonlupt P, Henaff M-A, Touil N, Coricelli G, et al. Decision-making in a changing world: a study in autism spectrum disorders. J Autism Dev Disord. 2015;45:1603–13.
4. Camerer C, Weber M. Recent developments in modeling preferences: uncertainty and ambiguity. J Risk Uncertainty. 1992;5:325–70.
5. Levy I, Snell J, Nelson AJ, Rustichini A, Glimcher PW. Neural representation of subjective value under risk and ambiguity. J Neurophysiol. 2010;103:1036–47.
6. Tymula A, Belmaker LAR, Ruderman L, Glimcher PW, Levy I. Like cognitive function, decision making across the life span shows profound age-related changes. Proc Natl Acad Sci U S A. 2013;110:17143–8.
7. Tymula A, Belmaker LAR, Roy AK, Ruderman L, Manson K, Glimcher PW, et al. Adolescents' risk-taking behavior is driven by tolerance to ambiguity. Proc Natl Acad Sci U S A. 2012;109:17135–40.
8. Alary D, Gollier C, Treich N. The effect of ambiguity aversion on insurance and self-protection. Econ J. 2013;123:1188–202.
9. Pushkarskaya H, Tolin D, Ruderman L, Kirshenbaum A, Kelly JM, Pittenger C, et al. Decision-making under uncertainty in obsessive–compulsive disorder. J Psychiatr Res. 2015;69:166–73.
10. Fujino J, Hirose K, Tei S, Kawada R, Tsurumi K, Matsukawa N, et al. Ambiguity aversion in schizophrenia: an fMRI study of decision-making under risk and ambiguity. Schizophr Res. 2016;178:94–101.
11. Bechara A, Damasio AR, Damasio H, Anderson SW. Insensitivity to future consequences following damage to human prefrontal cortex. Cognition. 1994;50:7–15.
12. Yechiam E, Arshavsky O, Shamay-Tsoory SG, Yaniv S, Aharon J. Adapted to explore: reinforcement learning in autistic spectrum conditions. Brain Cogn. 2010;72:317–24.
13. Buckert M, Schwieren C, Kudielka BM, Fiebach CJ. Acute stress affects risk taking but not ambiguity aversion. Front Neurosci. 2014;8:82.
14. De Martino B, Harrison NA, Knafo S, Bird G, Dolan RJ. Explaining enhanced logical consistency during decision making in autism. J Neurosci. 2008;28:10746–50.
15. De Martino B, Kumaran D, Seymour B, Dolan RJ. Frames, biases, and rational decision-making in the human brain. Science. 2006;313:684–7.
16. Tversky A, Kahneman D. The framing of decisions and the psychology of choice. Science. 1981;211:453–8.
17. Ruderman L, Ehrlich DB, Roy A, Pietrzak RH, Harpaz-Rotem I, Levy I. Posttraumatic stress symptoms and aversion to ambiguous losses in combat veterans. Depress Anxiety. 2016;33:606–13.
18. Farmer G, Baron-Cohen S, Skylark W. People with autism spectrum conditions make more consistent decisions. Psychol Sci. 2017;28:1067–76.
19. Baron-Cohen S, Wheelwright S, Skinner R, Martin J, Clubley E. The autism-spectrum quotient (AQ): evidence from asperger syndrome/high-functioning autism, malesand females, scientists and mathematicians. J Autism Dev Disord. 2001;31:5–17.
20. Wakabayashi A, Baron-Cohen S, Wheelwright S, Tojo Y. The Autism-Spectrum Quotient (AQ) in Japan: a cross-cultural comparison. J Autism Dev Disord. 2006;36:263–70.
21. Itahashi T, Yamada T, Watanabe H, Nakamura M, Ohta H, Kanai C, et al. Alterations of local spontaneous brain activity and connectivity in adults with high-functioning autism spectrum disorder. Mol Autism. 2015;6:1.
22. Itahashi T, Yamada T, Nakamura M, Watanabe H, Yamagata B, Jimbo D, et al. Linked alterations in gray and white matter morphology in adults with high-functioning autism spectrum disorder: a multimodal brain imaging study. Neuroimage Clin. 2015;7:155–69.
23. Yamada T, Itahashi T, Nakamura M, Watanabe H, Kuroda M, Ohta H, et al. Altered functional organization within the insular cortex in adult males with high-functioning autism spectrum disorder: evidence from connectivity-based parcellation. Mol Autism. 2016;7:41.

24. Matsuoka K, Kim Y. Japanese Adult Reading Test (JART). Tokyo: Shinkou-Igaku publishers; 2006.
25. Matsuoka K, Uno M, Kasai K, Koyama K, Kim Y. Estimation of premorbid IQ in individuals with Alzheimer's disease using Japanese ideographic script (Kanji) compound words: Japanese version of national adult reading test. Psychiatry Clin Neurosci. 2006;60:332–9.
26. Hurst R, Mitchell J, Kimbrel N, Kwapil T, Nelson-Gray R. Examination of the reliability and factor structure of the Autism Spectrum Quotient (AQ) in a non-clinical sample. Pers Individ Dif. 2007;43:1938–49.
27. Tanaka Y, Fujino J, Ideno T, Okubo S, Takemura K, Miyata J, et al. Are ambiguity aversion and ambiguity intolerance identical? A neuroeconomics investigation. Front Psychol. 2014;5:1550.
28. South M, Chamberlain PD, Wigham S, Newton T, Le Couteur A, McConachie H, et al. Enhanced decision making and risk avoidance in high-functioning autism spectrum disorder. Neuropsychology. 2014;28:222–8.
29. Johnson SA, Yechiam E, Murphy RR, Queller S, Stout JC. Motivational processes and autonomic responsivity in Asperger's disorder: evidence from the Iowa Gambling Task. J Int Neuropsychol Soc. 2006;12:668–76.
30. Mussey JL, Travers BG, Klinger LG, Klinger MR. Decision-making skills in ASD: performance on the Iowa Gambling Task. Autism Res. 2015;8:105–14.
31. Osmont A, Cassotti M, Agogué M, Houdé O, Moutier S. Does ambiguity aversion influence the framing effect during decision making? Psychon Bull Rev. 2015;22:572–7.
32. Boulter C, Freeston M, South M, Rodgers J. Intolerance of uncertainty as a framework for understanding anxiety in children and adolescents with autism spectrum disorders. J Autism Dev Disord. 2014;44:1391–402.
33. Chamberlain PD, Rodgers J, Crowley MJ, White SE, Freeston MH, South M. A potentiated startle study of uncertainty and contextual anxiety in adolescents diagnosed with autism spectrum disorder. Mol Autism. 2013;4:31.
34. Rodgers J, Glod M, Connolly B, McConachie H. The relationship between anxiety and repetitive behaviours in autism spectrum disorder. J Autism Dev Disord. 2012;42:2404–9.
35. Wigham S, Rodgers J, South M, McConachie H, Freeston M. The interplay between sensory processing abnormalities, intolerance of uncertainty, anxiety and restricted and repetitive behaviours in autism spectrum disorder. J Autism Dev Disord. 2015;45:943–52.
36. Keefer A, Kreiser NL, Singh V, Blakeley-Smith A, Duncan A, Johnson C, Klinger L, Meyer A, Reaven J, Vasa RA. Intolerance of uncertainty predicts anxiety outcomes following CBT in youth with ASD. J Autism Dev Disord. 2016; in press
37. Sherman R. The psychological difference between ambiguity and risk. Q J Econ. 1974;88:166–9.
38. Rogers RD. The roles of dopamine and serotonin in decision making: evidence from pharmacological experiments in humans. Neuropsychopharmacology. 2011;36:114–32.
39. Beninger RJ, Wasserman J, Zanibbi K, Charbonneau D, Mangels J, Beninger BV. Typical and atypical antipsychotic medications differentially affect two nondeclarative memory tasks in schizophrenic patients: a double dissociation. Schizophr Res. 2003;61:281–92.
40. Shah P, Catmur C, Bird G. From heart to mind: linking interoception, emotion, and theory of mind. Cortex 2017;93:220–3.
41. Ondobaka S, Kilner J, Friston K. The role of interoceptive inference in theory of mind. Brain Cogn. 2017;112:64–8.

17

Prenatal levonorgestrel exposure induces autism-like behavior in offspring through ERβ suppression in the amygdala

Yuanlin Zou[1,2†], Qiaomei Lu[1,2†], Dan Zheng[3†], Zhigang Chu[4], Zhaoyu Liu[1,2], Haijia Chen[5], Qiongfang Ruan[4], Xiaohu Ge[5], Ziyun Zhang[1,2], Xiaoyan Wang[5], Wenting Lou[4], Yongjian Huang[2], Yifei Wang[5], Xiaodong Huang[4], Zhengxiang Liu[1,2], Weiguo Xie[4*], Yikai Zhou[3*] and Paul Yao[1,2,4*]

Abstract

Background: Autism spectrum disorder (ASD) is characterized by impairments in social communication and restricted or repetitive behaviors or interests. ASD is now diagnosed in more than one out of 100 children and is biased towards males by a ratio of at least 4:1. Many possible explanations and potential causative factors have been reported, such as genetics, sex, and environmental factors, although the detailed mechanisms of ASD remain unclear.

Methods: The dams were exposed through oral contraceptives to either vehicle control (VEH) alone, levonorgestrel (LNG) alone, ethinyl estradiol (EE) alone, or a combination of LNG/EE for 21 days during their pregnancy. The subsequent 10-week-old offspring were used for autism-like behavior testing, and the limbic tissues were isolated for analysis. In another experimental group, 8-week-old male offspring were treated by infusion of ERβ overexpression/knockdown lentivirus in the amygdala, and the offspring were analyzed after 2 weeks.

Results: We show that prenatal exposure of either LNG alone or a LNG/EE combination, but not EE alone, results in suppression of ERβ (estrogen receptor β) and its target genes in the amygdala with autism-like behavior in male offspring, while there is a much smaller effect on female offspring. However, we find that there is no effect on the hippocampus and hypothalamus. Further investigation shows that ERβ suppression is due to LNG-mediated altered methylation on the ERβ promoter and results in tissue damage with oxidative stress and the dysfunction of mitochondria and fatty acid metabolism, which subsequently triggers autism-like behavior. Overexpression of ERβ in the amygdala completely restores LNG-induced ERβ suppression and autism-like behaviors in offspring, while ERβ knockdown mimics this effect, indicating that ERβ expression in the amygdala plays an important role in autism-like behavior development.

Conclusions: We conclude that prenatal levonorgestrel exposure induces autism-like behavior in offspring through ERβ suppression in the amygdala. To our knowledge, this is the first time the potential effect of oral contraceptives on the contribution of autism-like behavior in offspring has been discovered.

Keywords: Amygdala, Autism-like behavior, Estrogen receptor β, Oral contraceptives, Oxidative stress

* Correspondence: wgxie@hotmail.com; zhouyk@mails.tjmu.edu.cn; vasilis112@yahoo.com
†Equal contributors
[4]Institute of Burns, Tongren Hospital of Wuhan University, Wuhan 430060, People's Republic of China
[3]Institute of Environmental Medicine, Tongji Medical College, Huazhong University of Science and Technology, Wuhan 430030, People's Republic of China
[1]Internal Medicine of Tongji Hospital, Tongji Medical College, Huazhong University of Science and Technology, Wuhan 430030, People's Republic of China
Full list of author information is available at the end of the article

Background

Autism spectrum disorder (ASD) is characterized by impairments in social communication and restricted or repetitive behaviors or interests [1]. ASD is now diagnosed in more than one out of 100 children [2]. The identified prevalence of ASD has increased in a short period of time with an epidemic proportion in the world. The detailed mechanism of ASD remains unclear [3], and many possible explanations and potential causative factors have been reported. A three-hit theory, which includes the combination of genetic/epigenetic, environmental, and sex factors for the mechanism of ASD, has been widely accepted [4]. Interestingly, ASD is biased towards males by a ratio of at least 4:1, suggesting that fetal or perinatal exposure to elevated male hormones may increase susceptibility towards autism [5–7]. On the other hand, there is a hypothesis that estrogen, especially ethinyl estradiol (EE) from COC (combined oral contraceptives), may play a role in ASD development [8], although current literatures have not reached a conclusion [9].

ERβ (estrogen receptor β) is the principal estrogen receptor expressed in brain areas [3, 10, 11]. An earlier study has found a significant association of the ERβ gene with scores on the Autism Spectrum Quotient and the Empathy Quotient in ASD subjects, and in the ERβ gene, the C allele in rs1271572 and rs1152582 were associated with higher AQ in the typical population and were also found to be more frequent in cases than in controls [12]. Moreover, ERβ mediates some of the effects on anxiety, locomotor activity, fear responses, and learning behavior in mice [13]. It has been recently reported that the ERβ expression in the middle frontal gyrus of ASD subjects is decreased, indicating that ERβ expression in the brain may play a role in the development of ASD [14].

We have previously reported that ERβ is responsible for the basal expression of superoxide dismutase (SOD2) [15] and estrogen-related receptor α (ERRα) [16], where ERRα expression regulates mitochondrial function and fatty acid metabolism and SOD2 regulates oxidative stress [17, 18]. Therefore, ERβ suppression may bring potential damage and disorders to the brain tissues through SOD2 suppression-mediated oxidative stress and DNA break as well as ERRα suppression-mediated dysfunction of mitochondria and fatty acid metabolism.

Oral contraceptive hormones, including EE and levonorgestrel (LNG), have been the mainstay contraceptive hormones for the last four decades and have potential effects on behavior and the central nervous system [19]. We hypothesize that prenatal exposure of oral contraceptive hormones may contribute to ASD development in offspring. Previous studies demonstrate that 10 μg/rat/day EE and 20 μg/rat/day LNG are the lowest individual doses found to inhibit ovulation in intact rodents [20–23]. In order to find the best dose for the treatment of our dams, we tried two combination doses, with the low dose of 10 μg EE/20 μg LNG and high dose of 30 μg EE/60 μg LNG per rat each day, as recommended by a recent study [19]. Our preliminary data showed that high doses brought many problems to the dams, including abnormal pregnancy, such as bleeding, or, in some case, the pregnancy was prevented or interrupted even though a vaginal plug was found after mating. Therefore, we chose the dosage of 10 μg EE/20 μg to be the final treatment for the dams.

In this study, we show that prenatal exposure of either LNG alone or combined LNG/EE treatment induces significant ERβ suppression in the amygdala and autism-like behavior in offspring, while EE2 treatment alone shows no effect. Further investigation shows that ERβ suppression is due to LNG-mediated altered methylation on the ERβ promoter. Overexpression of ERβ in the amygdala completely restores LNG-mediated autism-like behavior in offspring, while ERβ knockdown mimics this effect. This suggests that prenatal LNG exposure may play a dominant role in oral contraceptive-mediated autism-like behavior through ERβ suppression in the amygdala.

Methods

Materials

The antibodies for ERRα (ab37438), H2AX (ab20669) and γH2AX (ab2893), H3K9me2 (ab1220), and H3K9me3 (ab8898) and H3K27me3 (ab6002) were obtained from Abcam. Antibodies for β-actin (sc-47,778), ERβ (sc-137,381), and SOD2 (sc-30,080) were obtained from Santa Cruz Biotechnology. LNG and EE were obtained from Sigma. 3-Nitrotyrosine (3-NT) was measured using the 3-Nitrotyrosine ELISA Kit (ab116691 from Abcam) per manufacturers' instructions. The mitochondrial fraction was isolated using a Pierce Mitochondria Isolation Kit (Pierce Biotechnology) per manufacturers' instructions. Nuclear extracts were prepared using the NE-PER Nuclear and Cytoplasmic Extraction Reagents Kit (Pierce Biotechnology). Protein concentration was measured using the Coomassie Protein Assay Kit (Pierce Biotechnology).

Generation of lentivirus

Rat ERβ expression lentivirus. The rat complementary DNA (cDNA) for ERβ was obtained from Open Biosystems. The cDNA for rat ERβ was subcloned into the pLVX-Puro vector (from Clontech) with the restriction sites of Xho1 and Xba1 using the below primers: ERβ forward primer: 5′-gtac-**ctcgag**-atg aca ttc tac agtcctgct-3′ (Xho1) and ERβ reverse primer: 5′-gtac-**tctaga**-tcactg agactg tag gttctg-3′ (Xba1). The ERβ or empty control (CTL) was expressed through Lenti-X™ Lentiviral

Expression Systems (from Clontech) per manufacturers' instructions.

Rat ERβ shRNA lentivirus. According to our preliminary data from in vitro cell culture experiments, the following sequence was confirmed as the most effective in knockdown rat ERβ: 5′-GGT CAT GTG AAG GAT GTA AGG-3′. The shRNA template for ERβ or scrambled was designed (sense strand + loop + antisense strand), and the related double strand DNA (dsDNA) was synthesized and annealed. They were then inserted into the pLVX-shRNA1 vector (from Clontech) using BamH1/EcoR1 restriction sites. The Scrambled (CTL) or shERβ lentivirus was then expressed through Lenti-X™ shRNA Expression Systems (from Clontech) per manufacturers' instructions.

In vivo rat experiments

Sprague–Dawley rats (Wuhan, China) were maintained under standard 12-h light/dark cycles and given ad libitum access to food and water. The animal protocol conformed to the US NIH guidelines (Guide for the Care and Use of Laboratory Animals, No. 85–23, revised 1996) and was reviewed and approved by the Institutional Animal Care and Use Committee from Tongji Medical College and Wuhan University.

Rat protocol 1

Adult (3 months old) female Sprague–Dawley rats were monitored for estrous cycles with daily vaginal smears. Only rats with at least two regular 4- to 5-day estrous cycles were included in the studies. The females were caged with proven males, and pregnancy was verified by observation of a sperm plug, which was designated as day 0 of pregnancy. Dams were randomly assigned to the following drug conditions: LNG (20 μg levonorgestrel), EE (10 μg ethinyl estradiol), or LNG/EE (20 μg LNG and 10 μg EE combination), and VEH rats received the same volume of vehicle. Drugs were suspended in 5% ethanol in organic sesame oil, and 0.1 ml were given daily through subcutaneous injection at the nape starting from day 1 until pup delivery for ~21 days. The same individuals handled the rats for injections, and experimenters were naive to drug conditions. The male and female offspring were separated from the dams on day 21 and fed until 9–10 weeks old for further experiments. Parts of 9- to 10-week-old offspring were then used for behavior tests, including autism-like and anxiety-like behavior testing. After that, the offspring were sacrificed, and the different brain tissues, including the amygdala, hypothalamus, and hippocampus, were isolated, flash frozen in dry ice, and then stored in a −80 °C freezer for the analysis of gene expression, SOD2 activity, superoxide anion release, DNA damage, mitochondrial function, and fatty acid metabolism. In addition, other parts of the offspring were used for the isolation of primary amygdala neurons.

Rat protocol 2

The male offspring (8 weeks old) from the VEH and LNG groups in *rat protocol 1* were anesthetized with a mixture of ketamine (90 mg/kg) and xylazine (2.7 mg/kg) and implanted with a guide cannula targeting the amygdala (26 gauge; Plastics One). The following coordinates were chosen for the amygdala: −2.0 mm posterior to the bregma, ±4.2 mm from the midline, and −7.2 mm from the skull surface on which it was based. Cannula was attached to the skull with dental acrylic and jeweler's screws and closed with an obturator [24]. An osmotic minipump (Alzet model 2002; flow rate 0.5 μl/h; Cupertino, CA) connected to a 26-gauge internal cannula that extended 1 mm below the guide was implanted and used to deliver ERβ overexpression (↑ERβ), ERβ knockdown (shERβ), or empty (EMP) lentivirus. Vehicle consisting of artificial cerebrospinal fluid (aCSF; 140 mM NaCl, 3 mM KCl, 1.2 mM Na_2HPO_4, 1 mM $MgCl_2$, 0.27 mM NaH_2PO_4, 1.2 mM $CaCl_2$, and 7.2 mM dextrose, pH 7.4) was used for the infusion of the lentivirus. Infusion (flow rate 0.5 μl/h) begun immediately after placement of the minipump. 0.5 μl of total 2×10^3 cfu of lentivirus was infused for 1 h. Rats received the infusion of lentivirus to either knockdown or overexpress ERβ. The experimental rats were separated into four groups (10 per group): group 1, VEH offspring with empty control lentivirus infusion (VEH/EMP); group 2, LNG offspring with empty control lentivirus infusion (LNG/EMP); group 3, LNG offspring with ERβ expression lentivirus infusion (LNG/↑ERβ); and group 4, VEH offspring with ERβ knockdown lentivirus infusion (VEH/shERβ); cannula placement was verified histologically postmortem by the injection of 0.5 μl of India ink (volume matched drug delivery in the experiments). Rats whose dye injections were not located in the amygdala were excluded from the data analysis. Two weeks after the lentivirus infusion, the offspring were used for behavior tests followed by biomedical analysis, as indicated in rat protocol 1.

Animal behavior test

The animal behavior test of offspring was carried out at 10 weeks of age. Female offspring were tested in the diestrus phase, which was confirmed by vaginal smears. Autism-like behavior was evaluated using the marbles burying test (MBT), social interaction (SI) test, elevated plus maze (EPM), and open-field test [25, 26].

Marbles burying test

In brief, each rat is placed in a clean cage ($35 \times 23 \times 19$ cm^3) filled with wood chip bedding to a depth of 5 cm containing

20 colored glass marbles (1 cm diameter) placed in a 5 × 4 arrangement. The number of marbles buried (>50% covered by bedding material) in 30 min was hand-scored by the experimenter [25, 27].

Social interaction test

In short, the subjects (test and stranger) were separately habituated to the arena for 5 min before the test. During each test, the rats were placed into the apparatus over a period of 20 min and the time spent following, mounting, grooming, and sniffing any body parts of the other rat was taken as an indicator of social engagement, and was hand-scored by the experimenter. The animal used as the "stranger" was used only once and was a Sprague–Dawley rat of the same gender, weight, and age, with no previous contact with the test rats [25, 27].

Elevated plus maze

All behavioral tests were performed when the rats were 10 weeks old. To investigate the presence of anxiety-like behavior in male and female offspring, the EPM test, a well-established rodent model used to characterize anxiety-like behavior, was performed. The Elevated Plus Maze Package with IR Beam Detection for Rat (Cat #: MED-ELVM-1R) was obtained from Med Associates Inc. The maze is comprised of two open and two closed arms. Dual sensors at the entrance to each goal runway allow software to differentiate between runway exploration and entrance, resulting in more accurate position detection. The rats were placed in the junction area, and their movements were measured for 5 min using infrared beams installed on each arm and automatically registered by the MED-PC software (Cat #: SOF-735, Med Associates) for further analysis [24].

Open-field test

Immediately following the EPM, the rats were tested in an open-field arena using the Open Field Starter Package for Rat (Cat #: MED-OFA-RSU, Med Associates Inc.). The open-field arena consists of fixed position walls mounted to the system base. Animal movement is tracked using three of 16 beam IR arrays. IR beams are located on both the *X* and *Y* axes for positional tracking and the *Z* axis for rearing detection. The animals were placed in the center of an open field, and exploration was assessed for 30 min. The dimensions of the arena were 40 cm × 40 cm, of which the peripheral 10 cm were considered the peripheral zone and the central 20 cm were considered the central zone [24].

In vitro primary culture of amygdala neurons

Ten-week-old offspring were used for the preparation of primary amygdala neurons. Amygdala tissues were dissected from rat offspring that were humanely sacrificed through cervical dislocation. The tissues were treated with 0.05% trypsin EDTA for 15 min at 37 °C. Trypsin EDTA was replaced with soybean trypsin inhibitor (Sigma) for 5 min at 37 °C to stop the reaction. This was then replaced with supplemented Neurobasal A (Invitrogen) followed by mechanical dissociation. The cells were then resuspended in culture media, including Neurobasal A, B27, 1×GlutaMAX and 100 U/ml Pen/Strep (from Invitrogen), and then, the cells were incubated at 37 °C, 5% CO_2 [28]. The isolated amygdala neurons were used for the analysis of DNA methylation, epigenetic changes by chromatin immunosuppression (ChIP) assay on the ERβ promoter, and in vitro fatty acid lipid uptake.

RT reaction and real-time quantitative PCR

Total RNA from the amygdala was extracted using the RNeasy Micro Kit (Qiagen), and the RNA was reverse-transcribed using an Omniscript RT kit (Qiagen). All the primers were designed using Primer 3 Plus software with the Tm at 60 °C, the primer size of 21 bp, and the product length in the range of 140–160 bp (see Additional file 1: Table S1). The primers were validated with the amplification efficiency in the range of 1.9–2.1, and the amplified products were confirmed with agarose gel. The real-time quantitative PCR was run on iCycleriQ (Bio-Rad) with the Quantitect SYBR green PCR kit (Qiagen). The PCR was performed by denaturation at 95 °C for 8 min, followed by 45 cycles of denaturation at 95 °C, annealing at 60 °C, and extension at 72 °C for 10 s, respectively. One microliter of each cDNA was used to measure target genes. The β-actin was used as the housekeeping gene for transcript normalization, and the mean values were used to calculate relative transcript levels with the $^{\Delta\Delta}$CT method per instructions from Qiagen. In brief, the amplified transcripts were quantified by the comparative threshold cycle method using β-actin as a normalizer. Fold changes in gene messenger RNA (mRNA) expression were calculated as $2^{-\Delta\Delta CT}$ with CT = threshold cycle, ΔCT = CT (target gene)-CT (β-actin), and the ΔΔCT = ΔCT (experimental)-ΔCT (reference).

Western blotting

The amygdala tissues were lysed in an ice-cold lysis buffer (0.137 M NaCl, 2 mM EDTA, 10% glycerol, 1% NP-40, 20 mM Tris base, pH 8.0) with protease inhibitor cocktail (Sigma). The proteins were separated in 10% SDS-PAGE and further transferred to the PVDF membrane. The membrane was incubated with appropriate antibodies and washed and incubated with HRP-labeled secondary antibodies, and then, the blots were visualized using the ECL+plus Western Blotting Detection System (Amersham). The blots were quantitated by IMAGE-QUANT, and the results were normalized by β-actin.

SOD2 activity assay

The SOD2 was obtained from the mitochondrial fraction that was isolated using a Pierce Mitochondria Isolation Kit (Pierce) per manufacturers' instructions. The SOD activity was measured as described previously [29]. In brief, a stable O_2^- source was generated through the conversion action of XOD (xanthine oxidase) from xanthine and was mixed with chemiluminescent (CL) reagents to achieve a stable light emission. The SOD2 sample injection can scavenge O_2^-, and the subsequent decrease of chemiluminescent response is proportional to SOD2 activity. This system can have a detection limit of 0.001 U ml^{-1} with the linear range of 0.03 ~ 2.00 U ml^{-1}. The results were normalized by protein concentration and were expressed as units per milligram proteins (U/mg).

In vivo superoxide anion (O_2^-) release

Superoxide anion release from the amygdala tissue was determined by a luminol-EDTA-Fe enhanced chemiluminescence (CL) system supplemented with DMSO-TBAC (dimethyl sulfoxide-tetrabutyl ammonium chloride) solution for extraction of released O_2^- from tissues, as described previously. The superoxide levels were calculated from the standard curve generated by the xanthine/xanthine oxidase reaction [30].

Measurement of DNA breaks

The 8-OHdG formation was measured using an OxiSelect™ Oxidative DNA Damage ELISA Kit (Cat No. STA320, from Cell Biolabs Inc.) per manufacturers' instructions. The formation of γH2AX was measured from nuclear extracts by western blotting using H2AX as the input control.

Evaluation of mitochondrial function

Mitochondrial DNA copies. The genomic DNA was extracted from the amygdala tissue using a QIAamp DNA Mini Kit (Qiagen), and the mitochondrial DNA was extracted using the REPLI-g Mitochondrial DNA Kit (Qiagen). The purified DNA was used for the analysis of genomic β-actin (marker of the nuclear gene) and ATP6 (ATP synthase F0 subunit 6, marker of the mitochondrial gene), respectively, using the qPCR method mentioned above. The primers for genomic β-actin: forward 5′-acc aca gct gag agg gaa atc-3′ and reverse 5′-att gcc gat agt gat gac ctg-3′. The primers for ATP6 are forward 5′- tag ggc ttc ttc ccc ata cat-3′ and reverse 5′-tta gtg aga tgg ggg ttc ctt-3′. The mitochondrial DNA copies were obtained from relative ATP6 copies that were normalized by β-actin copies using the $^{\Delta\Delta}$CT method.

Intracellular ATP level. The intracellular ATP level was determined using the luciferin-/luciferase-induced bioluminescence system. An ATP standard curve was generated at concentrations of 10^{-12} to 10^{-3} M. Intracellular ATP levels were calculated and expressed as nanomole per milligram protein [30].

DNA methylation analysis

We developed a real-time PCR-based method for methylation-specific PCR (MSP) analysis on the rat ERβ promoter according to the previously described method with some modifications [31–33]. The rat genomic DNA from the amygdala was extracted and purified and then treated by bisulfite modification using the EpiJET Bisulfite Conversion Kit (#K1461, Fisher). The modified DNA was then amplified using methylated and unmethylated primers for MSP that were designed using the Methprimer software (http://www.urogene.org/cgi-bin/methprimer/methprimer.cgi) with the below details: methylated primer forward 5′-TTT TTT TTA GGT TTT TAA AAG ACG T-3′, reverse 5′-ATA CCA ATA ACA ACA CCA ACC G-3′, unmethylated primer forward 5′-TTT TTT TTA GGT TTT TAA AAG ATG T-3′, and reverse 5′-AAT ACC AAT AAC AAC ACC AAC CAC T-3′, the product size 194 bp (methylated) and 195 bp (unmethylated), CpG island size 134 bp, and Tm 68–70 °C. The final methylation readout was normalized by unmethylated input PCR, the PCR products were confirmed by electrophorese using 2% agarose gel, and the DNA bands were imaged.

Chromatin immunoprecipitation

Cells were washed and crosslinked using 1% formaldehyde for 20 min and terminated by 0.1 M glycine. Cell lysates were sonicated and centrifuged. Five hundred micrograms of protein were pre-cleared by BSA/salmon sperm DNA with preimmune IgG and a slurry of protein A agarose beads. Immunoprecipitations were performed with the indicated antibodies, BSA/salmon sperm DNA, and a 50% slurry of protein A agarose beads. Input and immunoprecipitates were washed and eluted, then incubated with 0.2 mg/ml proteinase K for 2 h at 42 °C, followed by 6 h at 65 °C to reverse the formaldehyde crosslinking. DNA fragments were recovered by phenol/chloroform extraction and ethanol precipitation. A 140 bp fragment in the range of −200~0 from the transcription start site on the rat ERβ promoter was amplified by real-time PCR (qPCR) using the below primers: forward 5′-ggg tgt ccc tag tgg atg act-3′ and reverse 5′-aaa aga gtg tgg gag ggt agc-3′.

Evaluation of fatty acid metabolism

In vitro *lipid transport assay.* Primary amygdala neurons were seeded in a 12-well plate and grew until they were 80% confluent. After treatment, 0.5 mCi $well^{-1}$ of ^{14}C oleic acid (OA) from PerkinElmer was added. After 4 h of incubation, the cells were washed and harvested, and the total radioactivity was quantitated by scintillation counting [34].

Rate of fatty acid oxidation from tissues. The fatty acid oxidation (FAO) rate was measured by evaluation of palmitate oxidation using published methods with minor modifications [35, 36]. In brief, the amygdala tissue was homogenized, and 30 μl of tissue homogenate were then incubated in 370 μl of DMEM containing 0.5% BSA/ 0.2 mM palmitate/0.5 μCi/ml 1-^{14}C-palmitate at 37 °C for 2 h. The incubation was stopped by the injection of 0.2 ml of 40% perchloric acid into the tube to acidify the medium and liberate the CO_2. The CO_2 was trapped by a filter paper saturated with 20 μL of 1 M NaOH located on the top of the cap. After overnight isotopic equilibration at room temperature, the filter was removed, and the trapped $^{14}CO_2$ and ^{14}C acid-soluble products generated by the oxidation of [^{14}C] palmitate were counted to calculate the total palmitate oxidation. The protein concentrations were measured, and the results were expressed as nanomole per milligram proteins per hour (nmol/mg/h).

Statistical analysis

The data was given as mean ± SEM, and all the experiments were performed at least in quadruplicate unless indicated otherwise. In order to evaluate the effects of different hormonal treatments on the examined parameters in both males and females, the two-way analysis of variance (ANOVA) followed by the Bonferroni post hoc test was used; to evaluate the effects of hormonal treatments on the examined parameters in either males or females only, the one-way ANOVA followed by the Tukey –Kramer test was used to determine statistical significance of different groups by SPSS 22 software, and a P value of <0.05 was considered significant.

Results

Prenatal levonorgestrel exposure suppresses ERβ expression and its target genes in the amygdala in male offspring (10 weeks old) and has less of an effect on female offspring

We first evaluated the effect of prenatal exposure of COC on the expression of ERβ and its target genes in the limbic system in the offspring. Three-month-old pregnant dams were exposed to LNG (20 μg levonorgestrel), EE (10 μg ethinyl estradiol), LNG/EE (20 μg LNG and 10 μg EE combination), or VEH (the same volume of vehicle) through subcutaneous daily injections of 0.1 ml for 21 days until pup delivery. The limbic system, including the hypothalamus, hippocampus, and amygdala, were isolated for the analysis of gene expression. In Additional file 1: Table S2, we measured the gene expression of AR (androgen receptor), ERα (estrogen receptor α), and GPER1 (G protein-coupled estrogen receptor-1) from the hypothalamus, hippocampus, and amygdala, the brain areas known to be involved in the regulation of mood behavior. The results showed that there was no difference in expression in either male or female offspring. We also measured the gene expression of ERβ and its target genes, including SOD2 and ERRα in the hypothalamus and hippocampus from both male and female offspring (see Additional file 1: Figure S1), and found that there was no difference in those genes. We then measured the mRNA expression of ERβ (see Fig. 1a) and its target genes SOD2 (see Fig. 1b) and ERRα (see Fig. 1c) in the amygdala. We found that treatment of either LNG alone or LNG/EE combination significantly suppressed the expression of ERβ, SOD2, and ERRα in male offspring, and EE alone had no effect. On the other hand, in female offspring, LNG alone could still significantly suppress these genes but had a much smaller effect compared to that in male offspring, and EE alone and LNG/EE combination had no effect. We then measured the protein levels in the amygdala from both male and female offspring. The results showed that protein levels of ERβ and its target genes SOD2 and ERRα were suppressed significantly in male offspring by treatment of LNG alone and LNG/EE combination, and EE alone had no effect (see Fig. 1d, e). On the other hand, there was much less of an effect in female offspring. LNG alone slightly decreased protein expression, while LNG/EE combination and EE alone showed no effect on protein expression (see Fig. 1f, g). We finally measured the SOD2 activity (see Fig. 1h), and similar patterns, like SOD2 protein expression, were observed. SOD2 activity decreased significantly in LNG and LNG/EE treatment in male offspring, while in female offspring, only LNG alone slightly decreased activity, and LNG/EE and EE treatment showed no effect (see detailed statistical information in Additional file 1: Data S1). Our results suggest that LNG may play a dominant role in prenatal exposure of COC-induced ERβ suppression in the amygdala in offspring, while EE seems to have no effect, and that females are less responsive to prenatal LNG exposure, compared to male offspring.

Prenatal levonorgestrel exposure induces ERβ suppression in the amygdala through increased methylation on the ERβ promoter, while EE has no effect

We measured DNA methylation on the ERβ promoter using methylation-specific PCR (MSP) analysis. In Fig. 2a, b, both LNG and LNG/EE treatments significantly increased DNA methylation on the ERβ promoter in amygdala neurons from both male and female offspring (10 weeks old), while EE treatment had no effect. On the other hand, there was much less of an effect on DNA methylation with the LNG/EE treatment in females compared in males. We then measured the epigenetic changes on the ERβ promoter using ChIP techniques. The results showed significantly

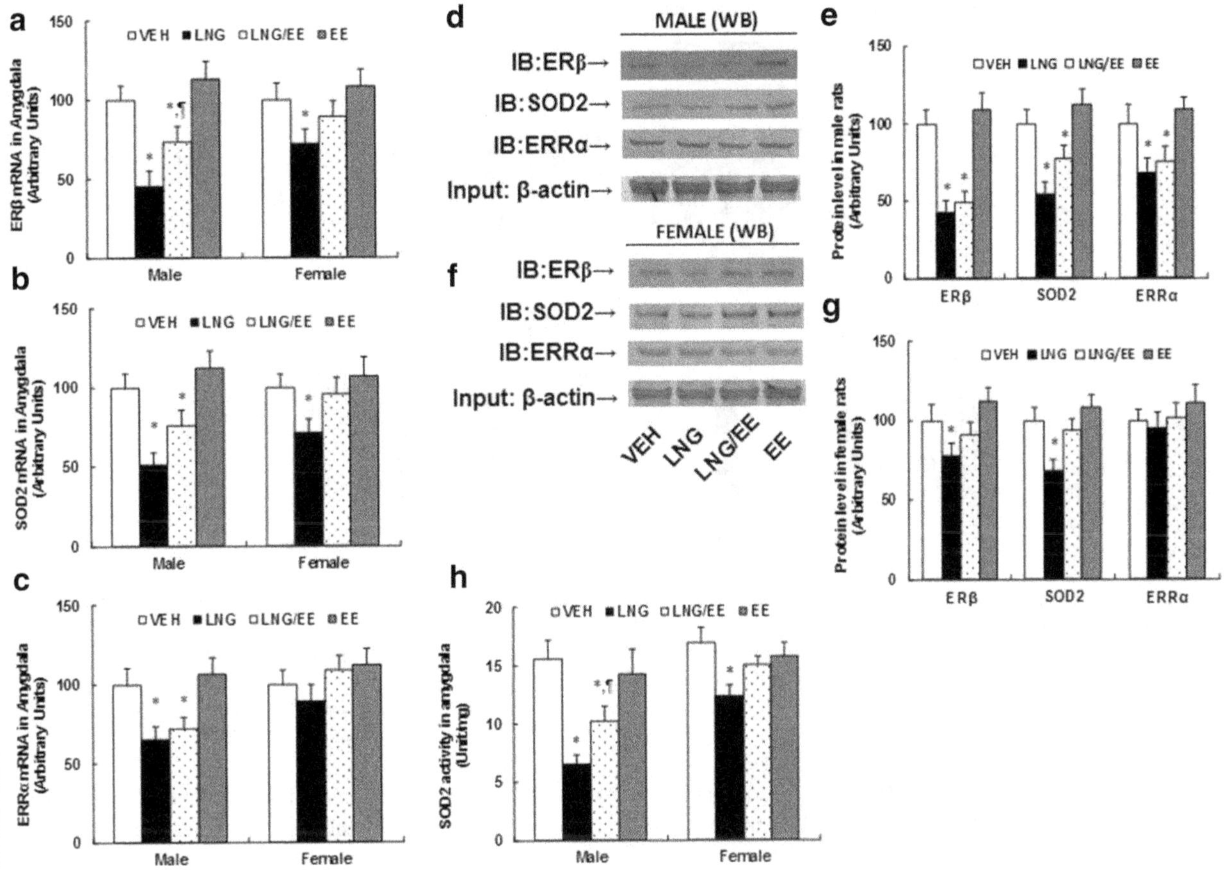

Fig. 1 Prenatal levonorgestrel exposure suppresses ERβ expression and its target genes in the amygdala in male offspring (10 weeks old) and has less of an effect in females. Three-month-old pregnant dams were exposed to LNG (20 μg levonorgestrel), EE (10 μg ethinyl estradiol), LNG/EE (20 μg LNG and 10 μg EE combination), or VEH (vehicle, 5% ethanol in organic sesame oil) by subcutaneous daily injection of 0.1 ml for 21 days until pup delivery. Both male and female offspring were sacrificed at 10 weeks of age to isolate the amygdala for further analysis. mRNA levels in the amygdala for genes of **a** ERβ, **b** SOD2, and **c** ERRα, $n = 5$. **d** The representative pictures of protein levels of male offspring by western blotting. **e** Protein expression quantitation for **d**, $n = 5$. **f** The representative pictures for protein levels of female offspring by western blotting. **g** Protein expression quantitation for **f**, $n = 5$. **h** SOD2 activities for both male and female offspring in the amygdala, $n = 6$. *$P < 0.05$ vs. VEH group; $P < 0.05$ vs. LNG group. Results are expressed as mean ± SEM

increased H3K9 di-methylation (H3K9me2) and H3K27 tri-methylation (H3K27me3) on the ERβ promoter from both male (see Fig. 2c) and female offspring (see Fig. 2d) with LNG alone and LNG/EE combination treatment, while EE had no effect (see detailed statistical information in Additional file 1: Data S2). Our results indicate that prenatal levonorgestrel exposure-induced ERβ suppression in amygdala neurons is due to increased DNA methylation on the ERβ promoter.

Prenatal levonorgestrel exposure induces ROS generation and DNA damage, along with dysfunction of mitochondria and fatty acid metabolism in the amygdala in male offspring (10 weeks old), while there is less of an effect in female offspring

We evaluated the molecular consequences of prenatal levonorgestrel exposure-induced ERβ suppression in the amygdala in both male and female offspring. We showed that prenatal levonorgestrel exposure (both LNG and LNG/EE treatment) significantly increased superoxide anion (O_2^-) release from amygdala tissues (see Fig. 3a), 3-nitrotyrosine formation (see Fig. 3b), 8-OHdG formation (see Fig. 3c), and DNA damage with γH2AX formation (see Fig. 3d, e); it also suppressed mitochondrial function, including decreased mitochondrial DNA copies (see Fig. 3f) and intracellular ATP level (see Fig. 3g). Furthermore, it suppresses fatty acid metabolism, including decreased in vivo fatty acid oxidation (see Fig. 3h) and in vitro fatty acid uptake (see Fig. 3i). Interestingly, there was much less damage in the amygdala in female offspring than in male offspring, which is consistent with the ERβ expression in the amygdala (see detailed statistical information in Additional file 1: Data S3). These results indicate that prenatal levonorgestrel exposure-induced ERβ suppression in both male and female offspring (10 months old) may contribute to LNG-mediated molecular damage in the amygdala.

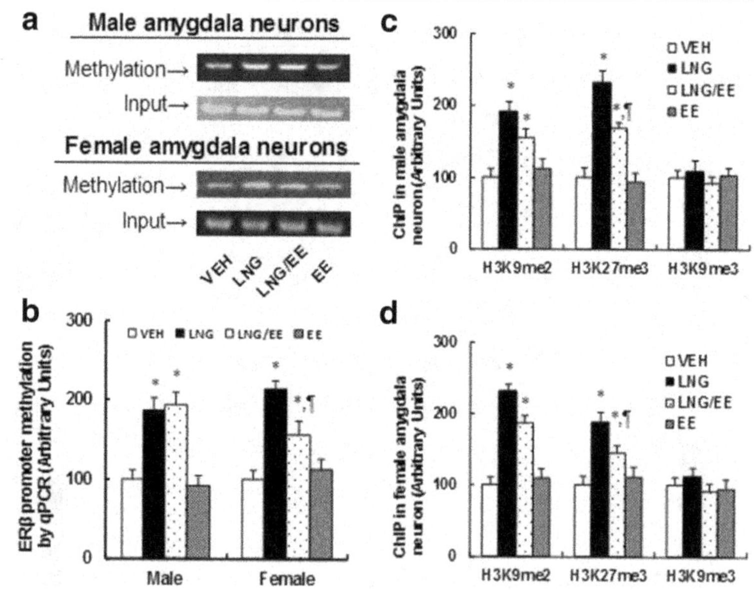

Fig. 2 Prenatal levonorgestrel exposure induces ERβ suppression in amygdala neurons through increased methylation on the ERβ promoter, while EE has no effect. **a** The amygdala neurons were isolated from 10-week-old male/female offspring for in vitro cell culture analysis. The representative bands for ERβ methylation in amygdala neurons from both male (*upper panel*) and female (*lower panel*) offspring. **b** DNA methylation on ERβ by real-time PCR-based methylation-specific PCR (MSP) analysis in amygdala neurons, $n = 5$. **c** ChIP analysis on the ERβ promoter in male amygdala neurons, $n = 5$. **d** ChIP analysis on ERβ promoter in female amygdala neurons, $n = 5$. $^*P < 0.05$ vs. VEH group; $P < 0.05$ vs. LNG group. Results are expressed as mean ± SEM

Prenatal levonorgestrel exposure induces autism-like behavior in male offspring (10 weeks old), while there is less of an effect in female offspring

We measured the effect of prenatal levonorgestrel exposure on autism-like behavior in offspring. The male offspring that received the LNG and LNG/EE treatment had significant less buried marbles (see Fig. 4a) and interaction time (see Fig. 4b) and spent significantly less time in the open arm (see Fig. 4c) and more time in the closed arm (see Fig. 4d) in the EPM (elevated plus maze) test compared to the vehicle-treated animals (VEH). Also, the male offspring spent less time in the central area (see Fig. 4e) and more time in the peripheral area (see Fig. 4f) but without changes in total horizontal locomotor activity (see Fig. 4g) in the open-field test. On the other hand, the female offspring were less responsive, as LNG treatment only slightly induced autism-like behavior, while LNG/EE and EE treatment showed little effect. Our results indicate that male offspring are more sensitive to prenatal levonorgestrel exposure-induced autism-like behavior. The detailed statistical information is shown below:

In Fig. 4a, two-way ANOVA revealed significant effect of sex [F (1, 56) = 4.594, P = 0.031] and a significant effect on treatment [F (3, 56) = 5.918, P < 0.01], and there was a significant interaction [F (3, 56) = 4.110, P = 0.042]. Subsequent post hoc analysis revealed that LNG and LNG/EE decreased buried marbles in male offspring (−50%, −40% vs. VEH group, respectively, p < 0.01), and the female offspring had significant less response in VEH and EE treatments compared to male offspring (p < 0.01).

In Fig. 4b, two-way ANOVA revealed significant effect of sex [F (1, 56) = 3.849, P = 0.041] and a significant effect on treatment [F (3, 56) = 5.101, P = 0.019], and there was a significant interaction [F (3, 56) = 3.917, P = 0.027]. Subsequent post hoc analysis revealed that LNG and LNG/EE decreased interaction time in male offspring (−26%, −33% vs. VEH group, respectively, p < 0.05); LNG decreased interaction time in female offspring (−35% vs. VEH group, p < 0.01), and the female offspring had significant less response in LNG/EE treatment compared to the male offspring (p < 0.01).

In Fig. 4c, two-way ANOVA revealed no significant effect of sex [F (1, 56) = 2.194, P = 0.061] and a significant effect on treatment [F (3, 56) = 3.691, P = 0.037], no significant interaction [F (3, 56) = 2.114, P = 0.167]. Subsequent post hoc analysis revealed that LNG and LNG/EE decreased time in open arm in male offspring (−22%, −16% vs. VEH group, respectively, p < 0.05), and LNG decreased time in open arm in female offspring (−15% vs. VEH group, p < 0.05).

In Fig. 4d, two-way ANOVA revealed significant effect of sex [F (1, 56) = 4.195, P = 0.023] and a significant effect on treatment [F (3, 56) = 6.348, P < 0.01], and there was a significant interaction [F (3, 56) = 3.987, P = 0.023]. Subsequent post hoc analysis revealed that LNG and LNG/EE increased time in closed arm in male

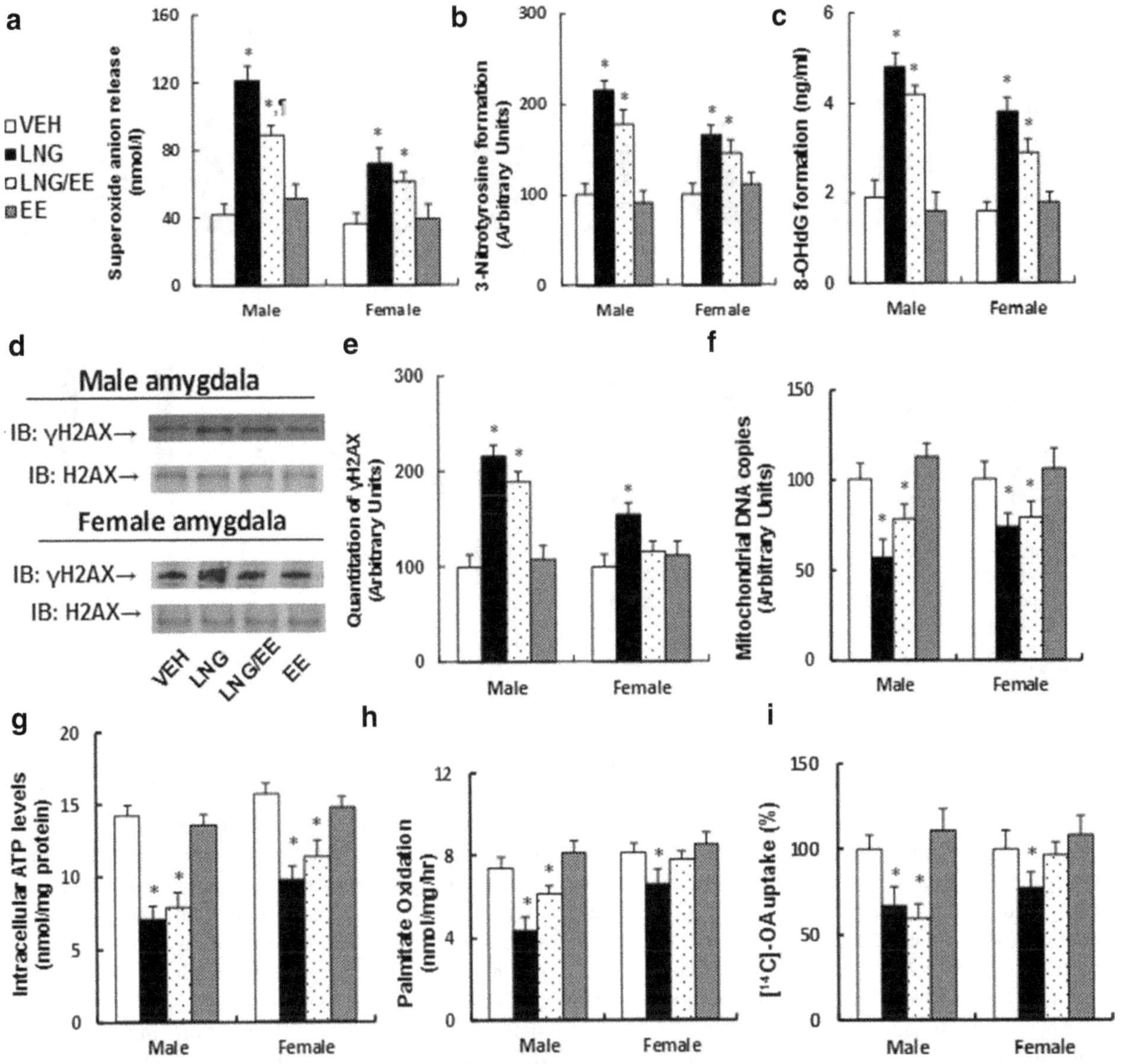

Fig. 3 Prenatal levonorgestrel exposure induces ROS generation and DNA damage and dysfunction of mitochondria and fatty acid metabolism from the amygdala in male offspring (10 weeks old), while there is less of an effect in females. **a**–**h** The amygdala tissues were isolated from 10-week-old male/female offspring for further analysis. **a** In vivo superoxide anion release, $n = 6$. **b** Quantitation of 3-nitrotyrosine (3-NT) formation, $n = 5$. **c** 8-OHdG formation, $n = 5$. **d** Representative γH2AX western blotting band for both male (*upper panel*) and female (*down panel*) offspring. **e** Quantitation of γH2AX formation for **d**, $n = 5$. **f** Mitochondrial DNA copies, $n = 4$. **g** Intracellular ATP levels, $n = 5$. **h** The in vivo palmitate oxidation rate, $n = 5$. **i** The amygdala neurons were isolated from 10-week-old male/female offspring for in vitro ^{14}C–OA fatty acid uptake, $n = 5$. *$P < 0.05$ vs. VEH group; $P < 0.05$ vs. LNG group. Results are expressed as mean ± SEM

offspring (+186%, +164% vs. VEH group, respectively, $p < 0.05$); and LNG increased time in closed arm in female offspring (+146% vs. VEH group, $p < 0.05$), and the female offspring had significant less response in LNG/EE treatment compared to male offspring ($p < 0.05$).

In Fig. 4e, two-way ANOVA revealed significant effect of sex [F (1, 64) = 3.447, P = 0.042] and a significant effect on treatment [F (3, 64) = 3.915, P = 0.036], and there was no significant interaction [F (3, 64) = 2.138, P = 0.194]. Subsequent post hoc analysis revealed that LNG and LNG/EE decreased central time in male offspring (−17%, −27% vs. VEH group, respectively, $p < 0.05$); LNG decreased central time in female offspring (−21% vs. VEH group, $p < 0.05$), and the female offspring had significant less response in LNG/EE treatment compared to male offspring ($p < 0.05$).

In Fig. 4f, two-way ANOVA revealed significant effect of sex [F (1, 64) = 3.461, P = 0.043] and a significant effect on treatment [F (3, 64) = 3.612, P = 0.037], and there was a significant interaction [F (3, 64) = 4.016,

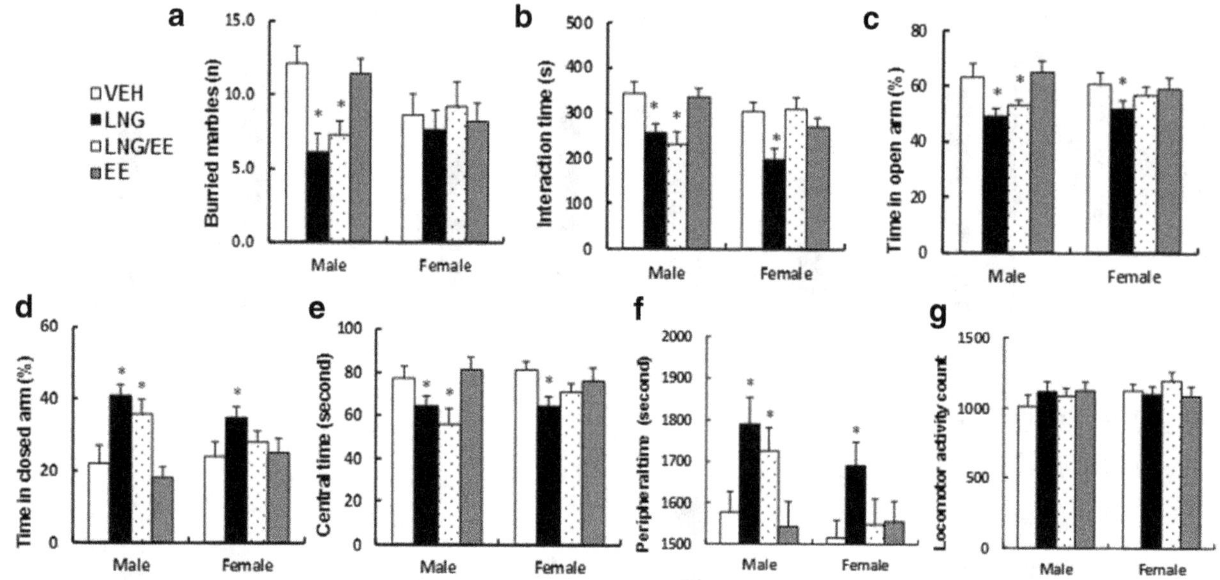

Fig. 4 Prenatal levonorgestrel exposure induces autism-like behavior in male offspring (10 weeks old), while there is less of an effect in females. Three-month-old pregnant dams were exposed to LNG (20 μg levonorgestrel), EE (10 μg ethinyl estradiol), LNG/EE (20 μg LNG and 10 μg EE combination), or VEH (vehicle, 5% ethanol in organic sesame oil) through 0.1 ml of subcutaneous daily injection for 21 days until pup delivery. Both male and female offspring were used for autism-like behavior tests at 10 weeks old. **a** Buried marbles tests, $n = 8$. **b** Interaction time, $n = 8$. Time spent in **c** open and **d** closed arms in EPM test, $n = 8$. Time spent in **e** central and **f** peripheral area and **g** locomotor activity in the open-field test, $n = 9$. $^*P < 0.05$ vs. VEH group. Results are expressed as mean ± SEM

$P = 0.031$]. Subsequent post hoc analysis revealed that LNG and LNG/EE increased peripheral time in male offspring (+13%, +9% vs. VEH group, respectively, $p < 0.05$); LNG increased peripheral time in female offspring (+11% vs. VEH group, $p < 0.05$), and the female offspring had significant less response in LNG/EE treatment compared to male offspring ($p < 0.05$).

In Fig. 4g, two-way ANOVA revealed no significant effect of sex [F (1, 64) = 1.021, $P = 0.561$] and no significant effect on treatment [F (3, 64) = 1.014, $P = 0.947$] and no interaction [F (3, 64) = 0.948, $P = 1.041$].

Overexpression of ERβ in the amygdala restores prenatal levonorgestrel exposure-induced ROS generation and DNA damage, along with dysfunction of mitochondria and fatty acid metabolism in 10-week-old offspring, while ERβ knockdown mimics the effect

The 8-week-old male offspring from dams that were treated by either VEH or LNG received either EMP, ERβ overexpression (↑ERβ), or knockdown (shERβ) lentivirus infusion to the amygdala, and the offspring were sacrificed at 10 weeks of age for analysis of gene expression and the subsequent molecular consequences. Our results showed that the gene expression of ERβ and its target genes SOD2 and ERRα, including mRNA (see Fig. 5a) and protein levels (see Fig. 5b, c), decreased significantly in LNG/EMP treatment compared to that in the VEH/EMP group, and the expression increased in the LNG/↑ERβ group but decreased in the VEH/shERβ group. We also measured SOD2 activity (see Fig. 5d), and the results showed that LNG/EMP and VEH/shERβ treatment decreased SOD2 activity, while LNG/↑ERβ group increased SOD2 activity. Our results indicate that the manipulation of ERβ gene expression in the amygdala through lentivirus infusion was successful and efficient. We then measured the molecular consequences from the male offspring treated by ERβ lentivirus. Our results showed that LNG/EMP treatment significantly increased ROS formation, including superoxide anion release (see Fig. 5e), 3-nitrotyrosine formation (see Fig. 5f), and DNA damage, including 8-OHdG formation (see Fig. 5g) and γH2AX formation (see Fig. 5h, i). Overexpression of ERβ (LNG/↑ERβ group) completely normalized this effect compared to the VEH/EMP control group, while ERβ knockdown (VEH/shERβ group) mimicked the LNG effect. We then measured the function of mitochondria and fatty acid metabolism. Our results showed that LNG treatment (LNG/EMP group) significantly decreased mitochondrial DNA copies (see Fig. 5j), intracellular ATP levels (see Fig. 5k), in vivo palmitate oxidation rate (see Fig. 5l), and in vitro ^{14}C–OA fatty acid uptake (see Fig. 5m) compared to the VEH/EMP control group. Again, ERβ expression (LNG/↑ERβ group) completely normalized the effect, and ERβ knockdown (VEH/shERβ group) mimicked the effect (see detailed statistical information in Additional file 1: Data S4). Our results

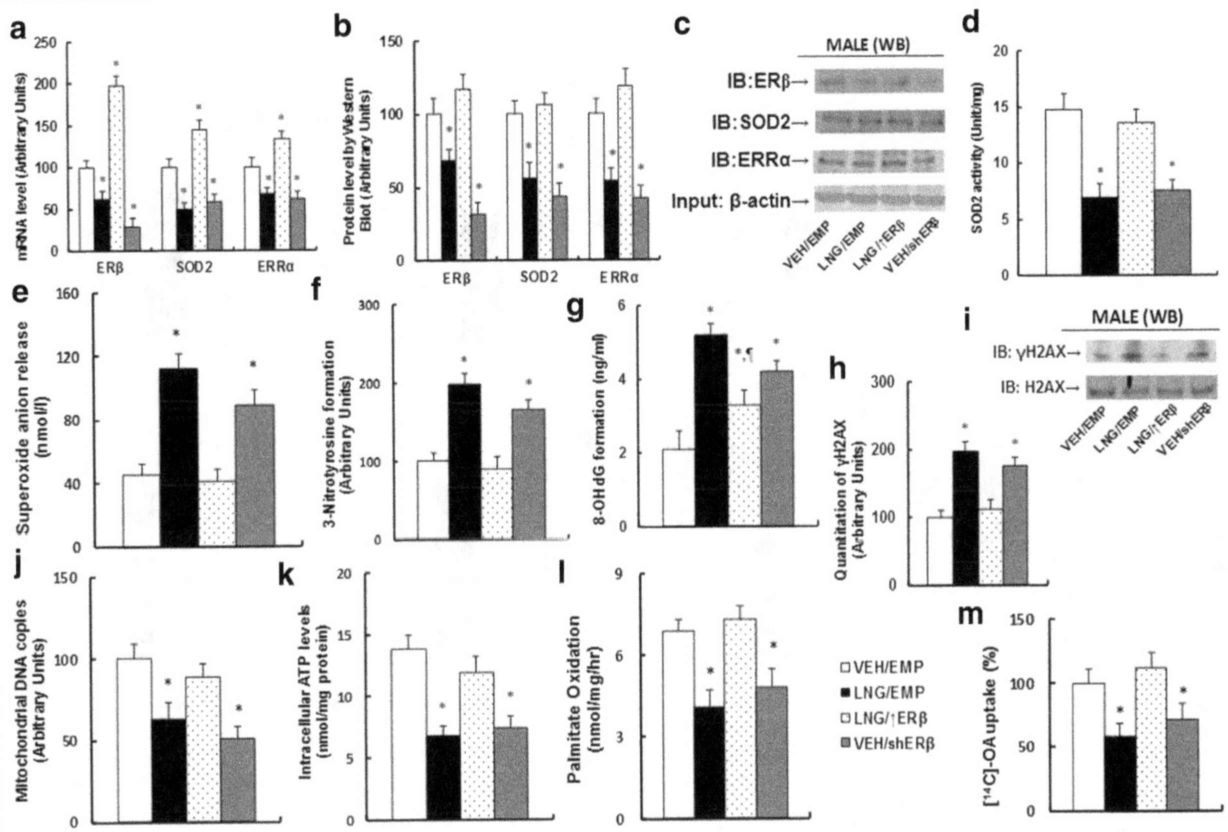

Fig. 5 Overexpression of ERβ in the amygdala restores prenatal levonorgestrel exposure-induced ROS generation and DNA damage, along with dysfunction of mitochondria and fatty acid metabolism in 10-week-old offspring, while ERβ knockdown mimics the effect. The 8-week-old male offspring from the VEH group received either empty control (VEH/EMP) or ERβ knockdown (VEH/shERβ) lentivirus infusion, and the male offspring from the LNG group received either empty control (LNG/EMP) or ERβ expression (LNG/↑ERβ) lentivirus infusion, and the offspring were sacrificed at 10 weeks of age. **a**–**l** The amygdala tissues were isolated from 10-week-old treated male offspring for further analysis. **a** The mRNA levels for gene expression, $n = 4$. **b** The quantitation of protein levels, $n = 5$. **c** Representative bands for western blots. **d** SOD2 activity, $n = 5$. **e** In vivo superoxide anion release, $n = 6$. **f** Quantitation of 3-nitrotyrosine (3-NT) formation, $n = 5$. **g** 8-OHdG formation, $n = 5$. **h** Quantitation of γH2AX formation, $n = 5$. **i** Representative γH2AX western blotting band. **j** Mitochondrial DNA copies, $n = 4$. **k** Intracellular ATP levels, $n = 5$. **l** The in vivo palmitate oxidation rate, $n = 5$. **m** The amygdala neurons were isolated from 10-week-old treated male offspring for in vitro ^{14}C–OA fatty acid uptake, $n = 5$. *$P < 0.05$ vs. VEH group; $P < 0.05$ vs. LNG group. Results are expressed as mean ± SEM

indicate that ERβ expression in the amygdala plays a major role in prenatal levonorgestrel exposure-mediated molecular dysfunction in offspring.

Overexpression of ERβ in the amygdala restores prenatal levonorgestrel exposure-induced autism-like behavior in 10-week-old offspring, while ERβ knockdown mimics the effect

We measured the effect of ERβ expression on prenatal levonorgestrel exposure-induced autism-like behavior in offspring. The male offspring from the LNG/EMP treatment had significant less buried marbles (see Fig. 6a) and interaction time (see Fig. 6b) and spent significantly less time in the open arm (see Fig. 6c) and more time in the closed arm (see Fig. 6d) in the EPM test compared to that in the VEH/EMP control group. The offspring also spent less time in the central area (see Fig. 6e) and more time in the peripheral area (see Fig. 6f), but without changes in total horizontal locomotor activity (see Fig. 6g) in the open-field test. Overexpression of ERβ (LNG/↑ERβ group) completely normalized the effect, while ERβ knockdown (VEH/shERβ) mimicked it. Our results indicate that prenatal levonorgestrel exposure-induced autism-like behavior in offspring is due to ERβ suppression in the amygdala. The detailed statistical information is shown below:

In Fig. 6a, for buried marbles, one-way ANOVA revealed a significant effect [F (3, 31) = 8.162, $P < 0.01$]. Subsequent Tukey analysis revealed that LNG decreased buried marbles (−59% vs. VEH group, $p < 0.01$); ↑ERβ increased (+181% vs. EMP group, $p < 0.01$), while shERβ decreased (−38% vs. EMP group, $p < 0.01$) buried marbles.

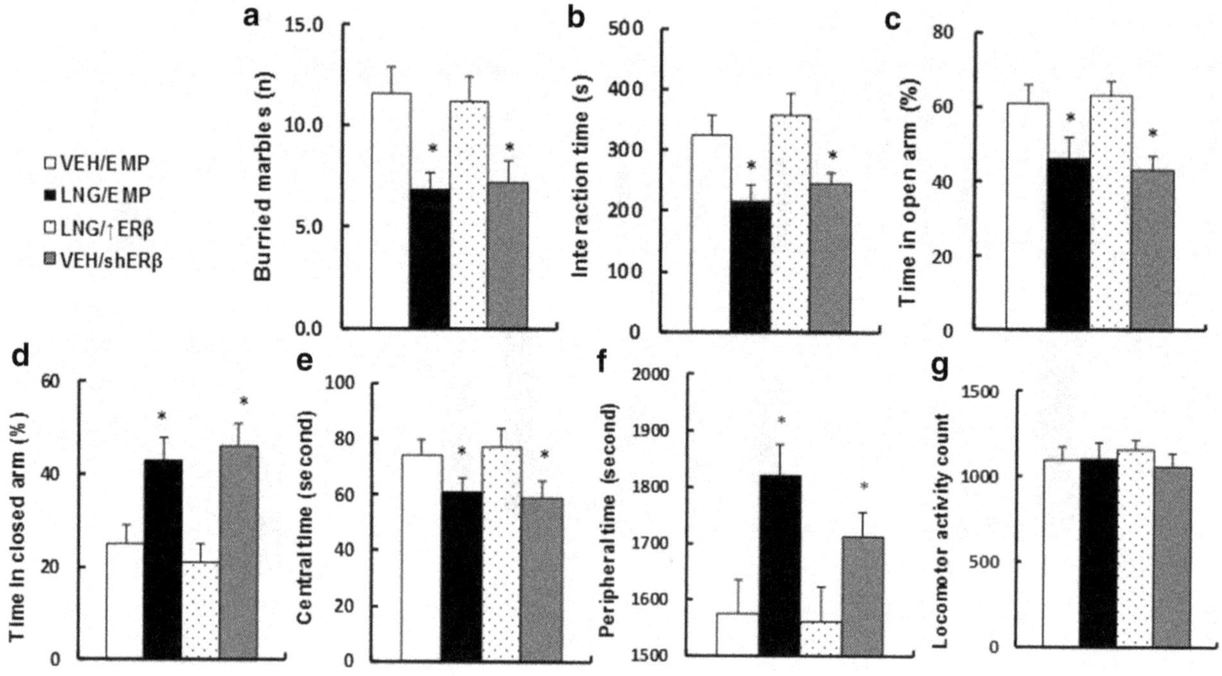

Fig. 6 Overexpression of ERβ in the amygdala restores prenatal levonorgestrel exposure-induced autism-like behavior in 10-week-old offspring, while ERβ knockdown mimics the effect. The 8-week-old male offspring from the VEH group received either empty control (VEH/EMP) or ERβ knockdown (VEH/shERβ) lentivirus infusion, and the male offspring from the LNG group received either empty control (LNG/EMP) or ERβ expression (LNG/↑ERβ) lentivirus infusion. At 10 weeks of age, the offspring were used for autism-like behavior testing. **a** Buried marbles tests, $n = 8$. **b** Interaction time, $n = 8$. **c, d** Time spent in **c** open and **d** closed arms in the EPM test, $n = 9$. **e–g** Time spent in **e** central and **f** peripheral area and **g** locomotor activity in the open-field test, $n = 9$. $^*P < 0.05$ vs. VEH group. Results are expressed as mean ± SEM

In Fig. 6b, for interaction time, one-way ANOVA revealed a significant effect [F (3, 31) = 7.694, $P < 0.01$]. Subsequent Tukey analysis revealed that LNG decreased interaction time (−34% vs. VEH group, $p < 0.01$); ↑ERβ increased (+174% vs. EMP group, $p < 0.01$), while shERβ decreased (−25% vs. EMP group, $p = 0.024$) interaction time.

In Fig. 6c, for time in open arm, one-way ANOVA revealed a significant effect [F (3, 35) = 4.367, $P = 0.032$]. Subsequent Tukey analysis revealed that LNG decreased time in open arm (−25% vs. VEH group, $p = 0.021$); ↑ERβ increased (+137% vs. EMP group, $p < 0.01$), while shERβ decreased (−30% vs. EMP group, $p = 0.024$) time in open arm.

In Fig. 6d, for time in closed arm, one-way ANOVA revealed a significant effect [F (3, 35) = 8.127, $P < 0.01$]. Subsequent Tukey analysis revealed that LNG increased time in closed arm (+172% vs. VEH group, $p < 0.01$); ↑ERβ decreased (−52% vs. EMP group, $p < 0.01$), while shERβ increased (+187% vs. EMP group, $p < 0.01$) time in closed arm.

In Fig. 6e, for central time, one-way ANOVA revealed a significant effect [F (3, 35) = 4.361, $P = 0.037$]. Subsequent Tukey analysis revealed that LNG decreased central time (−18% vs. VEH group, $p = 0.036$); ↑ERβ increased (+126% vs. EMP group, $p = 0.039$), while shERβ decreased (−21% vs. EMP group, $p = 0.037$) central time.

In Fig. 6f, for peripheral time, one-way ANOVA revealed a significant effect [F (3, 35) = 3.794, $P = 0.044$]. Subsequent Tukey analysis revealed that LNG increased peripheral time (+115% vs. VEH group, $p = 0.034$); ↑ERβ decreased (−14% vs. EMP group, $p = 0.041$), while shERβ increased (+109% vs. EMP group, $p = 0.043$) peripheral time.

In Fig. 6g, for locomotor activity, one-way ANOVA revealed no significant effect [F (3, 35) = 0.594, $P = 0.791$].

Discussion

In this study, we show that the compound LNG used in COC modifies the fetal condition during the prenatal period through altered methylation with ERβ suppression in the amygdala. ERβ suppression results in decreased expression of SOD2 and ERRα, and subsequently triggers damage in amygdala tissue through oxidative stress and the dysfunction of mitochondria and fatty acid metabolism, and eventually contributes to autism-like behavior in offspring.

The amygdala is responsible for storing memories of events for future recognition. It assists in the development of memories, fear emotion, and plays a major role in pleasure and sexual arousal, and many reports have shown that the amygdala is involved in ASD symptoms [37–39]. The functional significance of the changes only localized to the amygdala is social fear and/or anxiety learning [24, 40]. Our results show that prenatal LNG exposure induces ERβ suppression in the amygdala with autism-like behavior in offspring [12], and overexpression of ERβ completely restores this effect. This indicates that ERβ suppression in the amygdala may be a causative factor for autism-like behavior development. Furthermore, suppression of ERβ and its target genes, including SOD2 and ERRα, results in oxidative stress [41] and dysfunction of mitochondria and fatty acid metabolism [42–44], which may directly or indirectly contribute to tissue damage and the subsequent autism-like behavior development.

Association of oral contraceptives and autism

The increase in the prevalence of oral contraceptive use in the past 60 years coincides with the recent dramatic rise in autism and ASD prevalence [8], indicating a link between oral contraceptive and ASD. The incidence of mild to moderate depressive syndrome among women taking oral contraceptives is ~10 to 40% [45], and several studies demonstrated that oral contraceptives have a negative effect on anxiety, mood, and emotional well-being in women [46–49]. It has been reported that long-term administration of combined LNG and EE, two of the most widely used steroids in oral contraceptive pills, is associated with a reduction in social behavior [50]. It is reasonable that the neurochemical changes induced by LNG/EE treatment may contribute to some of the emotional disorders observed in hormonal contraceptive users. The combined oral contraceptive, especially LNG, is used by women to prevent pregnancy after birth control failure. This medication is a progestin hormone that works primarily by preventing the release of an egg (ovulation) during the menstrual cycle. The suppression of ovulation produced by oral contraceptives is an indisputable abnormality [8], while to date, there is no comprehensive research on the potential neurodevelopmental effects of oral contraceptive use on oocyte and progeny. Our study shows that prenatal LNG exposure induces ERβ suppression in the amygdala in offspring with autism-like behavior, which includes significantly less buried marbles and interaction time in the social behavior test and spending much less time in the open arm and more time in the closed arm in the EPM test, as well as spending less time in the central area and more time in the peripheral area in the open-field test. This indicates that prenatal exposure to oral contraceptives may be a potential risk factor for ASD or related neurodevelopment abnormalities in offspring. On the other hand, we must emphasize that because of the high doses of the hormones administered, as well as the long duration of time, the applicability of these findings to the human condition is limited.

ERβ suppression may contribute to male predominance in autism

ASD is much more common in males than in females, with a ratio of 4:1. It has been reported that high levels of testosterone during early fetal development may be a risk factor for ASD. This is supported by many studies reporting an association between fetal testosterone levels and autistic features [24, 51, 52], while the related mechanism is still unknown. ERβ is largely expressed in brain tissues [53], and it has been recently reported that there are alterations in ERβ expression in the brain of ASD subjects [14]. ERβ-deficient mice also show increased anxiety [13], indicating that ERβ may play an important role in ASD development [54]. Our results show that prenatal exposure of EE has no effect on autism-like behavior, which is consistent with previous observations that estrogen is a neuroprotective hormone [55]. On the other hand, prenatal exposure to oral contraceptive LNG induces ERβ suppression with autism-like behavior in offspring. Furthermore, we show that male offspring are more susceptible to LNG-induced ERβ suppression with higher autism-like behavior ratio. This may be due to the following reasons: (a) higher endogenous estrogen levels in female offspring partly normalize the testosterone effect of LNG; (b) the female offspring have a higher basal expression of ERβ compared to male offspring, which is more resistant to LNG-induced ERβ suppression; and (c) higher estrogen levels in female offspring could activate ERβ and upregulate its target genes SOD2 and ERRα and subsequently ameliorate tissue damage [15, 16] with less responsiveness to autism-like behavior development. In this study, the LNG/EE treatment induces effects like those of LNG in many of the biochemical and behavioral parameters examined, while sometimes in female offspring, the LNG/EE shows an effect to that of EE instead of LNG alone. This may be due to that the potential effect of LNG is partly normalized or antagonized by estrogen.

Potential oral contraceptive exposure from the environment

Increasing evidence shows that the environment also plays an important role in the etiology of ASD [4]. It has been reported that the concordance rate for ASD in dizygotic twins is around 30% [56], which is much higher than the 8–17% concordance rate for non-twin siblings [57], indicating that environmental factors significantly contribute to ASD. Recently, specific environmental factors, including prenatal and perinatal exposure factors, have been reported to contribute to increased ASD risk [24, 58]. In our study, prenatal LNG exposure in dams during pregnancy induces autism-like behavior in offspring, indicating that oral contraceptive exposure may be an important environmental factor in ASD development. Currently in China, other than the intentional uptake of oral contraceptive pills for birth control, another important increasing source of prenatal LNG exposure comes from seafood contaminated with COC. COC has been widely used in China in the seafood industry to prevent the pregnancy of female organisms, such as fish and shrimp, so that they can grow more quickly and become fatter without pregnancy. This may be an important reason for why there is continuously increasing incidence of ASD in China. Pregnant women must be especially careful to avoid eating oral contraceptive-contaminated seafood.

Conclusions

Altogether, we show that prenatal exposure to oral contraceptive LNG alters DNA methylation on the ERβ promoter with ERβ suppression in the amygdala. This subsequently results in tissue damage with oxidative stress and dysfunction of mitochondria and fatty acid metabolism and triggers autism-like behavior in offspring. Meanwhile, EE seems to have no effect, and male offspring are more susceptible than female offspring. Overexpression of ERβ restores LNG-mediated effects, while ERβ knockdown mimics the effect. This is the first time the potential effect of prenatal exposure to oral contraceptives on the contribution of autism-like behavior in offspring is discovered.

Abbreviations

AR: Androgen receptor; ASD: Autism spectrum disorder; ChIP: Chromatin immunoprecipitation; COC: Combined oral contraceptives; EE: Ethinyl estradiol; EMP: Empty control; EPM: Elevated plus maze; ERR: Estrogen-related receptor α; ERα: Estrogen receptor α; ERβ: Estrogen receptor β; GPER1: G protein-coupled estrogen receptor-1; LNG: Levonorgestrel; MBT: Marbles burying test; SI: Social interaction; SOD2: Mitochondrial superoxide dismutase; VEH: Vehicle control

Acknowledgements

Not applicable.

Funding

This study was financially supported by the National Natural Science Foundation of China, Project #: 81,501,667& 81,273,024; the Wuhan Science and Technology Innovation, Project #: 2,015,070,404,010,214; the Hubei Science & Technology Development, Project #: 2016CFB589& 2016CFB473; the 2013 International Science and Technology Cooperation Project of Ministry of Education (China) #: 2013 DFA31400; and the Science and Technology Planning Project of Guangdong Province (China) #: 2016B090918040.

Authors' contributions

PY, YZ, and WX designed, interpreted the experiments, and wrote the paper. ZC, QR, WL, and XH performed the rat surgery and social behavior testing. ZYL, ZZ, YH, and ZXL performed the steroid measurement, virus preparation, and western blots analysis. HC, XG, XY, and YW performed the amygdala isolation and analysis. YZ, QL, and DZ performed the remaining experiments. All authors read, edited, and approved the final manuscript.

Competing interests

The authors declare that they have no competing interests.

Author details

[1]Internal Medicine of Tongji Hospital, Tongji Medical College, Huazhong University of Science and Technology, Wuhan 430030, People's Republic of China. [2]Tongji Wenchang Hospital, Huazhong University of Science and Technology, Wenchang 571321, People's Republic of China. [3]Institute of Environmental Medicine, Tongji Medical College, Huazhong University of Science and Technology, Wuhan 430030, People's Republic of China. [4]Institute of Burns, Tongren Hospital of Wuhan University, Wuhan 430060, People's Republic of China. [5]SALIAI Stem Cell Institute of Guangdong, Guangzhou SALIAI Stem Cell Science and Technology Co. LTD, Guangzhou 510055, People's Republic of China.

References

1. Wang T, Guo H, Xiong B, Stessman HA, Wu H, Coe BP, Turner TN, Liu Y, Zhao W, Hoekzema K, et al. De novo genic mutations among a Chinese autism spectrum disorder cohort. Nat Commun. 2016;7:13316.
2. Abrahams BS, Geschwind DH. Advances in autism genetics: on the threshold of a new neurobiology. Nat Rev Genet. 2008;9(5):341–55.
3. Bodo C, Rissman EF. New roles for estrogen receptor beta in behavior and neuroendocrinology. Front Neuroendocrinol. 2006;27(2):217–32.
4. Schaafsma SM, Pfaff DW. Etiologies underlying sex differences in autism spectrum disorders. Front Neuroendocrinol. 2014;35(3):255–71.
5. Baron-Cohen S, Knickmeyer RC, Belmonte MK. Sex differences in the brain: implications for explaining autism. Science. 2005;310(5749):819–23.
6. Auyeung B, Taylor K, Hackett G, Baron-Cohen S. Foetal testosterone and autistic traits in 18 to 24-month-old children. Mol Autism. 2010;1(1):11.
7. Sarachana T, Xu M, Wu RC, Hu VW. Sex hormones in autism: androgens and estrogens differentially and reciprocally regulate RORA, a novel candidate gene for autism. PLoS One. 2011;6(2):e17116.
8. Strifert K. The link between oral contraceptive use and prevalence in autism spectrum disorder. Med Hypotheses. 2014;83(6):718–25.
9. Jamnadass ES, Keelan JA, Hollier LP, Hickey M, Maybery MT, Whitehouse AJ. The perinatal androgen to estrogen ratio and autistic-like traits in the general population: a longitudinal pregnancy cohort study. J Neurodev Disord. 2015;7(1):17.

10. Phan A, Suschkov S, Molinaro L, Reynolds K, Lymer JM, Bailey CD, Kow LM, MacLusky NJ, Pfaff DW, Choleris E. Rapid increases in immature synapses parallel estrogen-induced hippocampal learning enhancements. Proc Natl Acad Sci U S A. 2015;112(52):16018–23.
11. Ervin KS, Lymer JM, Matta R, Clipperton-Allen AE, Kavaliers M, Choleris E. Estrogen involvement in social behavior in rodents: rapid and long-term actions. Horm Behav. 2015;74:53–76.
12. Chakrabarti B, Dudbridge F, Kent L, Wheelwright S, Hill-Cawthorne G, Allison C, Banerjee-Basu S, Baron-Cohen S. Genes related to sex steroids, neural growth, and social-emotional behavior are associated with autistic traits, empathy, and Asperger syndrome. Autism Res. 2009;2(3):157–77.
13. Krezel W, Dupont S, Krust A, Chambon P, and Chapman PF. Increased anxiety and synaptic plasticity in estrogen receptor beta-deficient mice. Proc Natl Acad Sci U S A 2001;98(21):12278-82.
14. Crider A, Thakkar R, Ahmed AO, Pillai A. Dysregulation of estrogen receptor beta (ERbeta), aromatase (CYP19A1), and ER co-activators in the middle frontal gyrus of autism spectrum disorder subjects. Mol Autism. 2014;5(1):46.
15. Liu Z, Gou Y, Zhang H, Zuo H, Zhang H, Liu Z, Yao D. Estradiol improves cardiovascular function through up-regulation of SOD2 on vascular wall. Redox Biol. 2014;3(0):88–99.
16. Li H, Liu Z, Gou Y, Yu H, Siminelakis S, Wang S, Kong D, Zhou Y, Liu Z, Ding Y, et al. Estradiol mediates vasculoprotection via ERRα-dependent regulation of lipid and ROS metabolism in the endothelium. J Mol Cell Cardiol. 2015; 87:92–101.
17. Kong D, Zhan Y, Liu Z, Ding T, Li M, Yu H, Zhang L, Li H, Luo A, Zhang D, et al. SIRT1-mediated ERβ suppression in the endothelium contributes to vascular aging. Aging Cell. 2016;15:1092-1102.
18. Zhan Y, Liu Z, Li M, Ding T, Zhang L, Lu Q, Liu X, Zhang Z, Vlessidis A, Aw TY, et al. ERβ expression in the endothelium ameliorates ischemia/reperfusion-mediated oxidative burst and vascular injury. Free Radic Biol Med. 2016;96:223–33.
19. Simone J, Bogue EA, Bhatti DL, Day LE, Farr NA, Grossman AM, Holmes PV. Ethinyl estradiol and levonorgestrel alter cognition and anxiety in rats concurrent with a decrease in tyrosine hydroxylase expression in the locus coeruleus and brain-derived neurotrophic factor expression in the hippocampus. Psychoneuroendocrinology. 2015;(62):265–78.
20. Andrews P, Freyberger A, Hartmann E, Eiben R, Loof I, Schmidt U, Temerowski M, Folkerts A, Stahl B, Kayser M. Sensitive detection of the endocrine effects of the estrogen analogue ethinylestradiol using a modified enhanced subacute rat study protocol (OECD test guideline no. 407). Arch Toxicol. 2002;76(4):194–202.
21. Coelingh Bennink HJ, Skouby S, Bouchard P, Holinka CF. Ovulation inhibition by estetrol in an in vivo model. Contraception. 2008;77(3):186–90.
22. Kumar N, Koide SS, Tsong Y, Sundaram K. Nestorone: a progestin with a unique pharmacological profile. Steroids. 2000;65(10–11):629–36.
23. Genazzani AR, Gambacciani M, Simoncini T, Schneider HP, International Menopause S. "Controversial issues in climacteric medicine" series 3rd Pisa workshop "HRT in climacteric and aging brain". Pisa, Italy, 15-18 march 2003. Maturitas. 2003;46(1):7–26.
24. Hu M, Richard JE, Maliqueo M, Kokosar M, Fornes R, Benrick A, Jansson T, Ohlsson C, Wu X, Skibicka KP, et al. Maternal testosterone exposure increases anxiety-like behavior and impacts the limbic system in the offspring. Proc Natl Acad Sci U S A. 2015;112(46):14348–53.
25. Bahi A. Hippocampal BDNF overexpression or microR124a silencing reduces anxiety- and autism-like behaviors in rats. Behav Brain Res. 2017;326:281–90.
26. White SW, Oswald D, Ollendick T, Scahill L. Anxiety in children and adolescents with autism spectrum disorders. Clin Psychol Rev. 2009;29(3):216–29.
27. Bahi A. Sustained lentiviral-mediated overexpression of microRNA124a in the dentate gyrus exacerbates anxiety- and autism-like behaviors associated with neonatal isolation in rats. Behav Brain Res. 2016;311:298–308.
28. Hay CW, Shanley L, Davidson S, Cowie P, Lear M, McGuffin P, Riedel G, McEwan IJ, MacKenzie A. Functional effects of polymorphisms on glucocorticoid receptor modulation of human anxiogenic substance-P gene promoter activity in primary amygdala neurones. Psychoneuroendocrinology. 2014;47:43–55.
29. Yao D, Vlessidis AG, Gou Y, Zhou X, Zhou Y, Evmiridis NP. Chemiluminescence detection of superoxide anion release and superoxide dismutase activity: modulation effect of *Pulsatilla chinensis*. Anal Bioanal Chem. 2004;379(1):171–7.
30. Yao D, Shi W, Gou Y, Zhou X, Yee Aw T, Zhou Y, Liu Z. Fatty acid-mediated intracellular iron translocation: a synergistic mechanism of oxidative injury. Free Radic Biol Med. 2005;39(10):1385–98.
31. Ogino S, Kawasaki T, Brahmandam M, Cantor M, Kirkner GJ, Spiegelman D, Makrigiorgos GM, Weisenberger DJ, Laird PW, Loda M, et al. Precision and performance characteristics of bisulfite conversion and real-time PCR (MethyLight) for quantitative DNA methylation analysis. J Mol Diagn. 2006; 8(2):209–17.
32. Eads CA, Danenberg KD, Kawakami K, Saltz LB, Blake C, Shibata D, Danenberg PV, Laird PW. MethyLight: a high-throughput assay to measure DNA methylation. Nucleic Acids Res. 2000;28(8):E32.
33. Nosho K, Irahara N, Shima K, Kure S, Kirkner GJ, Schernhammer ES, Hazra A, Hunter DJ, Quackenbush J, Spiegelman D, et al. Comprehensive biostatistical analysis of CpG island methylator phenotype in colorectal cancer using a large population-based sample. PLoS One. 2008;3(11):e3698.
34. Hagberg CE, Falkevall A, Wang X, Larsson E, Huusko J, Nilsson I, van Meeteren LA, Samen E, Lu L, Vanwildemeersch M, et al. Vascular endothelial growth factor B controls endothelial fatty acid uptake. Nature. 2010; 464(7290):917–21.
35. Taib B, Bouyakdan K, Hryhorczuk C, Rodaros D, Fulton S, Alquier T. Glucose regulates hypothalamic long-chain fatty acid metabolism via AMP-activated kinase (AMPK) in neurons and astrocytes. J Biol Chem. 2013;288(52):37216–29.
36. Huynh FK, Green MF, Koves TR, Hirschey MD. Measurement of fatty acid oxidation rates in animal tissues and cell lines. Methods Enzymol. 2014;542: 391–405.
37. Huang WC, Chen Y, Page DT. Hyperconnectivity of prefrontal cortex to amygdala projections in a mouse model of macrocephaly/autism syndrome. Nat Commun. 2016;7:13421.
38. Kleinhans NM, Reiter MA, Neuhaus E, Pauley G, Martin N, Dager S, Estes A. Subregional differences in intrinsic amygdala hyperconnectivity and hypoconnectivity in autism spectrum disorder. Autism Res. 2016;9(7):760–72.
39. Schumann CM, Hamstra J, Goodlin-Jones BL, Lotspeich LJ, Kwon H, Buonocore MH, Lammers CR, Reiss AL, Amaral DG. The amygdala is enlarged in children but not adolescents with autism; the hippocampus is enlarged at all ages. J Neurosci. 2004;24(28):6392–401.
40. Twining RC, Vantrease JE, Love S, Padival M, Rosenkranz JA. An intra-amygdala circuit specifically regulates social fear learning. Nat Neurosci. 2017;20(3):459–69.
41. Rossignol DA, Frye RE. Evidence linking oxidative stress, mitochondrial dysfunction, and inflammation in the brain of individuals with autism. Front Physiol. 2014;5:150.
42. Clark-Taylor T, Clark-Taylor BE. Is autism a disorder of fatty acid metabolism? Possible dysfunction of mitochondrial beta-oxidation by long chain acyl-CoA dehydrogenase. Med Hypotheses. 2004;62(6):970–5.
43. Macfabe D. Autism: metabolism, mitochondria, and the microbiome. Glob Adv Health Med. 2013;2(6):52–66.
44. Villafuerte S. Suggestive evidence on the genetic link between mitochondria dysfunction and autism. Acta Psychiatr Scand. 2011;123(2):95.
45. Epperson CN, Wisner KL, Yamamoto B. Gonadal steroids in the treatment of mood disorders. Psychosom Med. 1999;61(5):676–97.
46. Welling LL. Psychobehavioral effects of hormonal contraceptive use. Evol Psychol. 2013;11(3):718–42.
47. Bottcher B, Radenbach K, Wildt L, Hinney B. Hormonal contraception and depression: a survey of the present state of knowledge. Arch Gynecol Obstet. 2012;286(1):231–6.
48. Segebladh B, Borgstrom A, Odlind V, Bixo M, Sundstrom-Poromaa I. Prevalence of psychiatric disorders and premenstrual dysphoric symptoms in patients with experience of adverse mood during treatment with combined oral contraceptives. Contraception. 2009;79(1):50–5.
49. Hall KS, White KO, Rickert VI, Reame N, Westhoff C. Influence of depressed mood and psychological stress symptoms on perceived oral contraceptive side effects and discontinuation in young minority women. Contraception. 2012;86(5):518–25.
50. Santoru F, Berretti R, Locci A, Porcu P, Concas A. Decreased allopregnanolone induced by hormonal contraceptives is associated with a reduction in social behavior and sexual motivation in female rats. Psychopharmacology. 2014;231(17):3351–64.
51. Auyeung B, Knickmeyer R, Ashwin E, Taylor K, Hackett G, Baron-Cohen S. Effects of fetal testosterone on visuospatial ability. Arch Sex Behav. 2012; 41(3):571–81.

52. Pfaff DW, Rapin I, Goldman S. Male predominance in autism: neuroendocrine influences on arousal and social anxiety. Autism Res. 2011; 4(3):163–76.
53. Mitra SW, Hoskin E, Yudkovitz J, Pear L, Wilkinson HA, Hayashi S, Pfaff DW, Ogawa S, Rohrer SP, Schaeffer JM, et al. Immunolocalization of estrogen receptor beta in the mouse brain: comparison with estrogen receptor alpha. Endocrinology. 2003;144(5):2055–67.
54. Wang L, Andersson S, Warner M, Gustafsson JA. Estrogen receptor (ER)beta knockout mice reveal a role for ERbeta in migration of cortical neurons in the developing brain. Proc Natl Acad Sci U S A. 2003;100(2):703–8.
55. Behl C. Oestrogen as a neuroprotective hormone. Nat Rev Neurosci. 2002; 3(6):433–42.
56. Hallmayer J, Cleveland S, Torres A, Phillips J, Cohen B, Torigoe T, Miller J, Fedele A, Collins J, Smith K, et al. Genetic heritability and shared environmental factors among twin pairs with autism. Arch Gen Psychiatry. 2011;68(11):1095–102.
57. Constantino JN, Zhang Y, Frazier T, Abbacchi AM, Law P. Sibling recurrence and the genetic epidemiology of autism. Am J Psychiatry. 2010;167(11): 1349–56.
58. Gardener H, Spiegelman D, Buka SL. Perinatal and neonatal risk factors for autism: a comprehensive meta-analysis. Pediatrics. 2011;128(2):344–55.

18

Bengali translation and characterisation of four cognitive and trait measures for autism spectrum conditions in India

Alokananda Rudra[1,2], Jai Ranjan Ram[3], Tom Loucas[1], Matthew K. Belmonte[4,5] and Bhismadev Chakrabarti[1*]

Abstract

Background: Autism is characterised by atypical social-communicative behaviour and restricted range of interests and repetitive behaviours. These features exist in a continuum in the general population. Behavioural measures validated across cultures and languages are required to quantify the dimensional traits of autism in these social and non-social domains. Bengali is the seventh most spoken language in the world. However, there is a serious dearth of data on standard measures of autism-related social and visual cognition in Bengali.

Methods: Bengali translations of two measures related to social-communicative functioning (the Children's Reading the Mind in the Eyes Test (RMET) and a facial emotion recognition test with stimuli taken from the Karolinska Directed Emotional Faces database), one measure of visual perceptual disembedding (the Embedded Figures Test), and a questionnaire measure (the Children's Empathy Quotient) were tested in 25 children with autism spectrum conditions (ASC) and 26 control children (mean age = 10.7 years) in Kolkata, India. Group differences were analysed by *t* test and multiple regression (after accounting for potential effects of gender, IQ, and age).

Results: Behavioural and trait measures were associated with group differences in the expected directions: ASC children scored lower on the Children's Empathy Quotient and the RMET, as well as on facial emotion recognition, but were faster and more accurate on the Embedded Figures Test. Distributional properties of these measures within groups are similar to those reported in Western countries.

Conclusions: These results provide an empirical demonstration of cross-cultural generalisability and applicability of these standard behavioural and trait measures related to autism, in a major world language.

Keywords: Autism, Theory of mind, Central coherence, Perceptual construal, Assessment, Behaviour, Translation, Validity, India, Bengali

Background

The atypicalities in social interaction, restricted range of interests or repetitive behaviour, and sensory perceptual dysmodulation that define and characterise autism [1] are expressed in varied degrees in different individuals, making the broad phenotype of autism a spectrum of conditions. DSM-5 accordingly proposes the replacement of the single disorder in favour of the autism spectrum concept, indicating differing grades of severity of one single diagnosis [1].

Autism spectrum conditions (ASC) can be identified as early as 18 months of age [2], and numerous psychological screening and diagnostic tests have been developed to identify ASC. Most of the screening tests include self-report or parent-report questionnaires, while diagnostic measures tend to involve observation within a semi-structured clinical interview setting. The standard screening and diagnostic tools have been developed in English, which often poses a drawback for countries where English is not the primary language. Autism research in South Asia suffers from a lack of availability of well-characterised tasks and questionnaires in local languages, and culture-specific norms. There are some tools that capture neurodevelopmental conditions in India but

* Correspondence: b.chakrabarti@reading.ac.uk
[1]School of Psychology and Clinical Language Sciences, University of Reading, Reading, UK

none are specific to autism. Data on the validity of standardised questionnaires relevant to autism are vital in order to establish a common toolkit for global research and to build research capacity in low-resource settings. In a recent paper, we have taken a first step in this direction by characterising and validating translated versions of standard screening and diagnostic tools for autism (specifically, the Social Communication Disorder Checklist (SCDC), Social Communication Questionnaire (SCQ), Autism Spectrum Quotient (AQ), and the Autism Diagnostic Observation Schedule (ADOS)) [3].

Behavioural/performance measures constitute the next step in this sequence to characterise the autistic phenotype. These involve direct participation of the individual under study and so complement questionnaire- or interview-based measures. The data from these tasks tend to be continuously distributed, which make them good candidates for the proposed dimensional approach of studying psychopathology using the Research Domain Criteria (RDoC) framework [4], across categorical diagnostic boundaries.

The specific measures of interest in this study relate to core domains in which atypicalities have been observed in ASC, namely social-emotional function and perceptual/low-level sensory function.

The Reading the Mind in the Eyes Test (RMET) is one of the best validated measures of emotion recognition from limited facial cues (eye region only) and is associated with deficits in autism [5]. While it has been translated into several languages worldwide, no data are available on this task in South Asia. The original task was developed for adult participants [6], but a modified version adapted for children has shown similar group differences between autism and neurotypicals [5]. Several of the emotions depicted in the RMET are complex and can be associated with cultural differences in recognition. Thus, it is vital to test the cultural generalisability of the data obtained from this task. The second task related to social-emotional function is a basic emotion recognition task using stimuli from the Karolinska Directed Emotional Faces (KDEF) database [7]. A version of this task has been used in adults and shown to be associated with clear differences between individuals with and without ASC [8]. While cultural differences in this task are not expected due to near-universality of basic emotion expressions, all stimuli in this task are faces of white Caucasian actors. Emotion recognition is influenced by the ethnicity of the stimuli [9, 10] (but can be robust to some differences [11], especially given cultural exposure [12]), and hence, it is of particular interest to test children with and without ASC from a non-white ethnic background with limited exposure to other ethnicities on this task. The third measure related to social-emotional functioning is the child version of the Empathy Quotient (EQ-C), which has been associated with robust group differences between children with and without ASC [9]. EQ-C has been translated to five languages in Europe and America, but the lack of availability of this instrument in any South Asian language limits its comparability and generalisability.

To measure an aspect of sensory perceptual functioning, we administered the Embedded Figures Test (EFT) [10], a measure of perceptual disembedding or, equivalently, field independence or level of construal. Individuals with ASC perform faster and more accurately than matched controls in this task [11–14]. Cultural differences in visual perceptual tasks have been noted in both autism spectrum [15] and typical [16, 17–21] populations and are reflected in cognitive neurophysiology [22, 23]. The aim of the current study was thus to translate into Bengali this battery of four measures related to key autism symptom domains and to characterise them in a sample of children from Kolkata, India, with and without ASC. Bengali is spoken by more than 193 million people as a first or second language around the world, with the majority of speakers in India and Bangladesh (www.ethnologue.com). Characterising these tools in India can indicate the degree to which the behavioural profile of children with or without autism is similar or variable across languages and cultures and will create a vital resource for future research in autism in low-resource settings of South Asia.

Methods

Translation

Translators who were bilingual (fluent in English and Bengali) with expertise in autism were identified and approached and explained the nature of the study. Translation was followed by blind back-translation into English by individuals fluent in English and Bengali. This back-translated English version was then matched with the original English version by two bilingual expert raters (AR and BC). This procedure was iterated until rater consensus was reached regarding the usability of the back-translated Bengali version.

Participants

Twenty-five ASC children aged 9 to 11 years were recruited from multiple clinics in Kolkata. All of them had a certified diagnosis of an autism spectrum disorder (Asperger syndrome or high-functioning autism) using DSM-IV TR criteria from a recognised clinician and confirmed by a clinician-administered ADOS. Furthermore, all ASC children scored above 76 on the Autism Spectrum Quotient: Children's Version (AQ-C). A score of 76 or above on AQ-C is indicative of ASD [24] and thus provided a further confirmation of the diagnostic status. All ASC children attended schools or special education centres that cater to students from middle or low-middle socio-economic status (SES). Control children were recruited from two mainstream schools: a co-educational school with children of low-middle SES and a girls' school with children of middle SES (see Table 1 for demographics). The choice of these schools was governed by the prior familiarity of the experimenter. The inclusion criterion for cases was a confirmed diagnosis of ASC, while that for the controls was the absence of any mental health condition, as reported by the parents. Both groups were matched for gender. However, the limited availability of high-functioning autism cases in this age group who were willing to take part in research did not allow us to match the two groups for age or intelligence quotient (IQ).

Tools

The EQ-C, a short parent-report questionnaire comprising 27 items [9], is intended to measure how easily one can pick up on other people's feelings and how strongly one is affected by them. Children scoring less than 30 show difficulties in identifying and/or responding appropriately to others' emotions. For the EQ-C, a 'slightly agree' or 'slightly disagree' response endorsing an empathic trait or behaviour scores one point, 'definitely agree' or 'definitely disagree' endorsing an empathic trait or behaviour scores two points, and all responses not endorsing empathic behaviour score zero. The maximum possible score is 54. The EQ-C has shown high test–retest reliability, with an intra-class correlation coefficient of 0.86, ($p < 0.001$) [9].

The AQ-C was administered solely to confirm the clinical diagnosis of the ASC participants. The AQ-C is a parent-report questionnaire comprising 50 questions quantifying autistic traits in 4- to 11-year-olds. Children with ASC score high on the AQ-C as compared to typically developing children [24]. The translated and validated version of the AQ-C in Bengali was used for this study [3]. The EQ-C and AQ-C were filled in by the parents of the children selected for the study.

Three behavioural measures were applied:

1. The RMET-Child [5] comprises 28 images of the eye region of the face, each representing a mental state. Each picture is flanked by four words as candidate labels for the depicted emotion. The participant has to indicate the correct answer by pointing. During the process of iterative translation/back-translation, a few of the option words were translated into short phrases (rather than single words) to allow for easy understanding in everyday language. A direct dictionary-based translation from English in such cases would often result in complex words that are not typically used. In order to make the test materials as closely matched to those used worldwide, no stimulus was discarded from the RMET. The RMET stimuli contain just the eye region and not the entire face and are presented in black and white—which can potentially reduce the impact of the ethnicity-related differences that influence emotion perception.
2. The KDEF database, developed in 1998 by Daniel Lundqvist and colleagues in Stockholm (http://www.emotionlab.se/resources/kdef), consists of photographs of facial expressions of basic emotions. In the task based on these stimuli, participants choose amongst seven basic emotion words written below each picture (happy, sad, angry, surprised, disgusted, afraid, and neutral). An online version of this task demonstrates differences in performance between individuals with and without ASC [8]. Both the RMET-Child and the KDEF were printed on A4-sized laminated paper. Twenty-eight faces from the KDEF database (4 faces for each of 7 emotions) were selected. The KDEF stimuli were presented in black and white for reasons described above.
   Before beginning the KDEF and RMET-C tests, the children were provided with a glossary containing all the words/phrases in Bengali. They were asked to familiarise themselves with the words and were given explanations where necessary. The pictures for the RMET-Child and the KDEF were shown to the children one by one. Participants were told to identify the emotion and to say or point to the correct answer with either their index finger or a pen as they preferred. No time limit was imposed.
3. The standard child Embedded Figures Test (EFT) [10] consists of pictures of complex shapes, each of which contains a target simple shape. Twenty-five EFT images were printed and laminated on photographic paper. A fixed set of simple patterns was shown and explained prior to the test. The experimenter first showed the complex design for 15 s, asking the participants to describe it, then revealed the simple shape for 10 s. Then the complex design was presented again and a stopwatch started immediately. The participant was told to look for the simple shape in the complex figure and to trace its lines with their finger or a pencil. Each child was given 1 min to identify and to trace the simple pattern and the response time was noted (as soon as the tracing

Table 1 Participant demographics

Participant	Gender	Number	Mean age (s.d.)	Mean verbal IQ (s.d.)
ASC	Male	20	11.56 (1.84)	87.8 (2.1)
	Female	5	11.60 (2.21)	88.4 (1.9)
Control	Male	21	9.89 (0.96)	102.0 (4.6)
	Female	5	10.01 (1.3)	95.8 (1.6)

was completed). The designs were presented in a fixed order, beginning with a practice item followed by the 25 test items. Subjects were encouraged with positive comments if they failed to identify in the first minute. A wrong answer or a 'pass' by the participant was taken as an indicator to move on to the next image. The instructions were given in simple Bengali sentences. Responses were recorded by the experimenter and coded for accuracy (if the correct shape was traced). Reaction time was noted using a stopwatch.

All subjects were tested either in their homes or in a quiet room in the clinic or special school. All data were collected in 2013–2014.

Since compliance with a lengthy testing regimen would have been difficult for many subjects with autism (the total administration time for Malin's Intelligence Scale for Children (MISIC) is 2.5 h on average), only the verbal subtests of MISIC, the Indian adaptation of the Wechsler Intelligence Scale for Children [25], were administered prior to the experiment.

All the tests were administered in person in less than 2 h. Parents of both cases and controls were administered the paper versions of the EQ-C and AQ-C.

Analysis

Mean scores of the cases and controls were calculated for each tool, separately for each gender. Simple effects of group were assayed by t test. In light of significant deviations from normal distribution, Spearman's correlation coefficients were calculated between all measurements. Multiple regression for each of the dependent measures tested effects of group, gender, age, and verbal IQ.

Results

Twenty-five ASC children and 26 controls participated. Of the ASC participants, 25.5% attended special schools, 23.5% inclusive schools, and the rest attended special education centres. All control children attended mainstream schools. Mean age for the ASC group was 11.57 (S.D. = 1.8), for the control group 9.92 (S.D. = 1.1). The range of IQ scores for the controls and cases was between 80 and 120. The mean verbal IQ for cases was 87.9 (S.D. = 2.04) and for controls was 100.8 (S.D. = 4.8). Cases and controls were gender matched (Table 1).

Table 2 shows the mean scores obtained by cases and controls on AQ, EQ, KDEF, and the Child Eyes test and the accuracy-adjusted response time on the Child-EFT (CEFT), separately for each gender. All ASC participants and none of the controls scored above the cut-off of 76 on AQ-C. ASC and control groups differed highly significantly ($p < 0.001$) on all measures (data presented in Table 3). Figure 1 shows the distribution of scores received on all the measures.

Correlations between measurements

Spearman's rank order correlation was computed as the data were not normally distributed. Across the whole sample, the scores on the EQ-C were negatively correlated with that on the AQ-C (Spearman's rho = −0.776, $p < 0.001$). The EQ-C scores significantly positively correlated with the total accuracy score for the KDEF (Spearman's rho = 0.780) and the RMET-Child (Spearman's rho = 0.829), both $p < 0.001$.

Within the control group, EQ-C scores correlated negatively with AQ-C (Spearman's rho = −0.397, p = 0.045) and positively with total accuracy for the KDEF (Spearman's rho = 0.411, p = 0.037). RMET correlated with EQ-C scores (Spearman's rho = 0.224, p = 0.272).

Within the ASC group, EQ-C was not significantly correlated with the AQ-C (Spearman's rho = 0.271, p = 0.190), the KDEF (Spearman's rho = −0.273, p = 0.186), or the RMET-Child (Spearman's rho = 0.354, p = 0.083).

Table 2 Mean scores obtained by cases and controls on AQ, EQ, KDEF, RMET-Child, and the accuracy-adjusted response time on CEFT according to gender

Behavioural measures	ASC				Control			
	Male		Female		Male		Female	
	Mean	S.D.	Mean	S.D.	Mean	S.D.	Mean	S.D.
Accuracy (Child Eyes test)	0.09	0.03	0.12	0.03	0.58	0.15	0.68	0.1
Accuracy (KDEF)	0.38	0.07	0.41	0.09	0.82	0.12	0.81	0.05
Accuracy (CEFT)	0.78	0.04	0.78	0.04	0.76	0.02	0.75	0.01
Accuracy-adjusted response time (CEFT)	688.23	79.21	683.17	34	973.09	50.4	985.6	53.2
Child-AQ score	85.30	7.6	87.8	5.02	39.67	7.9	39	6.9
Child-EQ score	11.35	2.3	13.40	2.3	46.62	1.9	46.6	0.9

Accuracy is calculated as the total number of correct responses divided by the total number of items. Accuracy-adjusted response time is calculated as the reaction time for a correct response, divided by accuracy

Table 3 Group mean scores on each measure and *t* test statistics for the comparison between cases and controls

Cognitive measures	Mean (S.D.)		*t* test	Effect size Cohen's d
	ASC	Control		
RMET-C (accuracy)	0.09 (0.04)	0.6 (0.15)	16.5***	4.6
KDEF (accuracy)	0.39 (0.07)	0.82 (0.11)	16.3***	4.7
CEFT (RT for correct responses)	687.26 (71.9)	975.49 (50.11)	16.7***	4.7
Child-AQ	85.8 (7.14)	39.54 (7.5)	22.4***	6.3
Child-EQ	11.76 (2.4)	46.62 (1.7)	60.01***	16.8

***Denotes significance at $p < 0.001$

Multiple regression analysis with gender, age, and IQ as predictors

As the groups differed in IQ and age, a multiple regression analysis was carried out (Table 4). This analysis showed a significant effect of group for each of the measures after accounting for potential effects of age and IQ (RMET-C accuracy scores: $\beta = 0.956$ $p < 0.001$; CEFT accuracy-adjusted reaction time scores: $\beta = 0.958$, $p < 0.001$; KDEF accuracy scores: $\beta = 0.870$, $p < 0.001$; EQ-C: $\beta = 0.955$, $p < 0.001$). There was no significant interaction between group*verbal IQ, group*age, or age*verbal IQ. To avoid common confounds associated with ANCOVA [26, 27], these analyses were re-run without including IQ and age in the model. No significant changes in the test statistics were observed.

Discussion

We tested Bengali translations of four trait and behavioural measures related to autism in a sample of children in Kolkata, India. The measures pertaining to socio-emotional functioning include two behavioural tests: complex facial emotion recognition using the 'Reading the Mind in the Eyes Test'-Child Version (RMET-C) and a basic facial emotion recognition task using stimuli from the Karolinska Directed Emotional Faces (KDEF) database. The trait measure related to social cognition was the Children's Empathy Quotient (EQ-C) [9]. The behavioural test related to sensory perceptual functioning was the Child-EFT. All of these tools showed group differences between ASC and controls in the expected direction, similar to those in the original reports. These

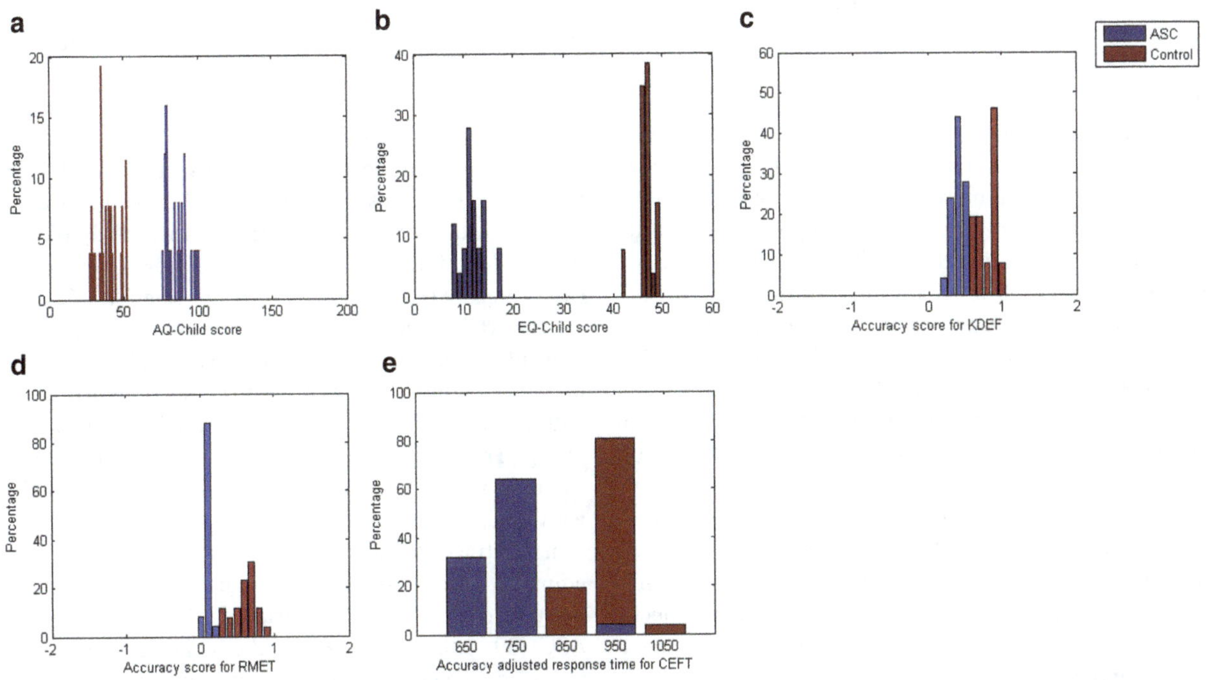

Fig. 1 The top panels (**a**–**c**) show the distribution of raw scores for AQ, EQ, and KDEF for cases and controls. The bottom panels (**d**, **e**) show the distribution of raw scores for RMET-C and CEFT for cases and controls

Table 4 Multiple regression analysis to test the effect of effect of group, gender, age, and verbal IQ on all measures

Predictors	RMET-C total accuracy score		KDEF total accuracy score		CEFT total response time for correct responses		Child-AQ		Child-EQ	
	β	p	β	p	β	p	β	p	β	p
Group	0.956	<0.001	0.870	<0.001	0.958	<0.001	0.904	<0.001	0.955	<0.001
Gender	0.091	0.128	0.025	0.683	0.003	0.964	0.007	0.877	0.027	0.112
Age	0.009	0.894	0.044	0.512	0.088	0.178	0.017	0.328	0.037	0.053
Verbal IQ	0.035	0.772	0.082	0.508	0.091	0.447	0.049	0.600	0.689	0.494

results thus provide evidence for generalisability for these tools and suggest their usability for research in people speaking Bengali (>193 million).

Children with ASC responded significantly less accurately in RMET-C scores compared to the control children. Notably, the maximum number of correct answers obtained by ASC participants was 4 out of 29. This is not significantly higher than chance [5]. In contrast, the controls in our study had an accuracy of 60%, similar to that reported in the original study in the same age range [5]. Similar to the Persian version [28], and in conformity with a sign test of published studies of the original English and translated RMET versions in which no study's male mean RMET score exceeded its female mean RMET score [29], females scored higher than males on the RMET. The low verbal IQ in the ASC group in our sample may account for the low accuracy in the RMET-C: the ASC group may have found it difficult to identify complex verbal phrases defining emotions. In contrast to the RMET-C, the emotion words in the basic emotion recognition task are simpler, and hence, the ASC group performed comparatively better on this task than on the RMET-C.

It is known that people from East Asia, who are more often studied than South Asian populations, are more prone than are North Americans to explain behaviour using social contexts rather than individuals' internal states [30, 31]. Furthermore, RMET scores of people born in East Asia are lower than those of people born in North America [32], reinforcing the result that attention to context impairs the detail-orientated analysis necessary to recognise social and other visual information from still pictures [33]. At least a portion of the difference in RMET scores between languages and cultures may stem not from artefacts of languages and translations but actually from real differences in the ways in which visual attention is allocated within social (and non-social) scenes. In this regard, differences in psychological distance and associated level of construal [34] might describe not only cognitive and perceptual differences associated with short-term social psychological manipulations but also long-term effects of culture and biological and cultural effects associated with sex and gender [35].

Similar to the RMET-C, the KDEF task accuracy differed significantly between the ASC and control groups (Table 2). This result is similar to those previously reported by Sucksmith et al. [8] in an adult sample. Most ASC children were able to recognise the 'happy' emotion more accurately than negative emotions, as has been previously observed in adults [36]. Similar to this study, deficits in emotion recognition have also been seen between ASC and controls on negative basic emotions in a study by Ashwin et al. on male adults [37]. However, it is possible that this observed lack of differences for recognition of non-negative emotions is driven by the inclusion of just one positive emotion (happy) in the set of emotions tested. The similarity of our results with those obtained in Caucasian samples suggests that the emotion recognition performance, and group differences thereof as seen in ASC, are relatively unaffected by the ethnicity of the actors.

On the EQ-C, ASC children scored considerably lower than the control sample (ASC mean score = 11.76, control mean score = 46.62) (see Table 2). These scores are comparable to those reported in the original British sample (ASC 13.97, S.D. 6.82; controls 37.7, S.D. 9.81) [13]. The observed pattern of sex differences in the scores for both cases and controls also replicated those reported in the original report.

EQ-C scores showed the expected pattern of correlations in the whole sample, i.e. low EQ-C scorers were less accurate in identifying emotions on the KDEF and the RMET-C. A positive correlation between EQ-C and RMET-C has been previously noted in a study of 6- to 9-year-old children [38]. Total EQ-C scores were significantly negatively correlated with the total AQ-C scores for the whole sample. EQ-C scores in controls were significantly negatively correlated to AQ-C, also replicating previous results in adults [6]. Interestingly, however, this pattern of correlations was not observed within the ASC group. This lack of covariation could reflect the limited variation within this group of higher-functioning children with ASC.

In contrast to measures of emotion recognition and empathy, tasks of sensory perceptual function have often been associated with an advantage in individuals with ASC [39, 40]. On the EFT, ASC children are typically faster in detecting simple patterns in complex figures [13]. As predicted, the total response time for ASC children on the CEFT was lower than that for controls, replicating previous results [41, 42]. However, there was no significant difference in the total mean accuracy score between cases and controls, again replicating previous results [12].

Limited resources precluded confirmation of clinical diagnoses by a psychiatrist or with an additional research ADOS administration. However, all the ASC participants had certified diagnostic reports based on DSM-IV (TR)/ ICD-10 from recognised clinicians and had a suprathreshold score on the AQ-C. A second limitation is that time constraints precluded measurement of full-scale IQ, which was instead estimated by adding 6% to the verbal test quotients as suggested in the MISIC manual [25]. Third, the verbal component of two of the tasks (KDEF and RMET-C) meant that we could only test high-functioning verbal ASD children. Future studies should develop tasks that can be used in children with a wide range of verbal abilities, including nonverbal children with ASC. Finally, since the participant pool was drawn from mainstream and special schools that serve a largely middle SES urban population, it is difficult to extrapolate these results to the extreme low end of SES or to rural populations. Future studies should attempt to address these limitations by more complete phenotyping in larger, more representative samples.

Conclusions

We translated and tested three behavioural measures and one trait measure related to various aspects of autistic cognition in Bengali-speaking children in Kolkata, India. We find strong evidence of cultural generalisability for these tools, as well as for group differences between ASC and controls. These results provide the first evidence for the usability of these tools in a major regional language of South Asia and constitute a vital step to standardise measurement of autism-related symptomatology globally.

Abbreviations

AQ-C: Autism Spectrum Quotient: Children's Version; ASC: Autism spectrum conditions; EFT: Embedded Figures Test; EQ-C: Children's Empathy Quotient; IQ: Intelligence quotient; KDEF: Karolinska Directed Emotional Faces (database); SES: Socio-economic status

Acknowledgements

The authors thank Patricia Riddell, Merry Barua, Nidhi Singhal, and Shaneel Mukerji for their valuable input. AR was supported by the Felix foundation. BC was supported by the Medical Research Council UK. MKB was supported by a Fulbright-Nehru Senior Research Fellowship from the United States–India Educational Foundation, funded by the governments of India and the USA.

Authors' contributions

AR and BC designed the study. AR collected and analysed the data. JRR and TL provided clinical guidance. AR, MKB, and BC wrote the paper. All authors revised the manuscript for critical intellectual content and approved the final version of the manuscript.

Competing interests

The authors declare that they have no competing interests.

Author details

[1]School of Psychology and Clinical Language Sciences, University of Reading, Reading, UK. [2]Ben Gurion University of the Negev, Beer-Sheva, Israel. [3]Mental Health Foundation, Kolkata, India. [4]The Com DEALL Trust, Bangalore, India. [5]Nottingham Trent University, Nottingham, UK.

References

1. American Psychiatric Association. Diagnostic and Statistical Manual of Mental Disorders (5th ed.). Arlington: American Psychiatric Publishing; 2013.
2. Baird G, Charman T, Baron-Cohen S, Cox A, Swettenham J, Wheelwright S, et al. A screening instrument for autism at 18 months of age: a 6-year follow-up study. J Am Acad Child Adolesc Psychiatry. 2000;39:694–702.
3. Rudra A, Banerjee S, Singhal N, Barua M, Mukerji S, Chakrabarti B. Translation and usability of autism screening and diagnostic tools for autism spectrum conditions in India: translation of autism screening tools in India. Autism Res. 2014;7:598–607.
4. Insel T, Cuthbert B, Garvey M, Heinssen R, Pine DS, Quinn K, et al. Research Domain Criteria (RDoC): toward a new classification framework for research on mental disorders. Am J Psychiatry. 2010;167:748–51.
5. Baron-Cohen S, Wheelwright S, Spong A, Scahill V, Lawson J. Are intuitive physics and intuitive psychology independent? A test with children with Asperger syndrome. J Dev Learn Disord. 2001;5:47–78.
6. Baron-Cohen S, Wheelwright S. The empathy quotient: an investigation of adults with Asperger syndrome or high functioning autism, and normal sex differences. J Autism Dev Disord. 2004;34:163–75.
7. Lundqvist D, Flykt A, Öhman A. The Karolinska Directed Emotional Faces - KDEF, CD ROM from Department of Clinical Neuroscience, Psychology section, Karolinska Institutet, ISBN 91-630-7164-9. http://www.emotionlab.se/resources/kdef.
8. Sucksmith E, Allison C, Baron-Cohen S, Chakrabarti B, Hoekstra RA. Empathy and emotion recognition in people with autism, first-degree relatives, and controls. Neuropsychologia. 2013;51:98–105.
9. Lee K-U, Khang HS, Kim K-T, Kim Y-J, Kweon Y-S, Shin Y-W, et al. Distinct processing of facial emotion of own-race versus other-race. Neuroreport. 2008;19:1021–5.
10. Hu CS, Wang Q, Han T, Weare E, Fu G. Differential emotion attribution to neutral faces of own and other races. Cogn Emot. 2017;32(2):360–368.
11. Hejmadi A, Davidson RJ, Rozin P. Exploring Hindu Indian emotion expressions: evidence for accurate recognition by Americans and Indians. Psychol Sci. 2000;11:183–7.
12. Elfenbein HA, Ambady N. When familiarity breeds accuracy: cultural exposure and facial emotion recognition. J Pers Soc Psychol. 2003;85:276.
13. Auyeung B, Wheelwright S, Allison C, Atkinson M, Samarawickrema N, Baron-Cohen S. The children's Empathy Quotient and Systemizing Quotient: sex differences in typical development and in autism spectrum conditions. J Autism Dev Disord. 2009;39:1509–21.
14. Shah A, Frith U. An islet of ability in autistic children: a research note. J Child Psychol Psychiatry. 1983;24:613–20.
15. Koh HC, Milne E. Evidence for a cultural influence on field-independence in autism spectrum disorder. J Autism Dev Disord. 2012;42:181–90.
16. Witkin HA, Oltman PK, Raskin E, Karp SA. Embedded figures test, children's embedded figures test, group embedded figures test: manual. Palo Alto: Consulting Psychologists Press; 1971.
17. Richardson BS, Chan HL, Lee A, Teo ST. The Müller-Lyer illusion: a cross-cultural study in Singapore. Ergonomics. 1972;15:293–8.
18. Segall MH, Campbell DT, Herskovits MJ. Cultural differences in the perception of geometric illusions. Science. 1963;139:769–71.
19. Nisbett RE, Miyamoto Y. The influence of culture: holistic versus analytic perception. Trends Cogn Sci. 2005;9:467–73.
20. Cantrell L, Kuwabara M, Smith LB. Set size and culture influence children's attention to number. J Exp Child Psychol. 2015;131:19–37.
21. Kuwabara M, Smith LB. Cultural differences in visual object recognition in 3-year-old children. J Exp Child Psychol. 2016;147:22–38.
22. Goh JO, Park DC. Culture sculpts the perceptual brain. Prog Brain Res. 2009; 178:95–111.
23. Gutchess AH, Welsh RC, Boduroğlu A, Park DC. Cultural differences in neural function associated with object processing. Cogn Affect Behav Neurosci. 2006;6:102–9.

24. Auyeung B, Baron-Cohen S, Wheelwright S, Allison C. The Autism Spectrum Quotient: Children's Version (AQ-Child). J Autism Dev Disord. 2008;38:1230–40.
25. Malin AJ. Malin Intelligence Scale for Indian Children. Indian J Mental Retard. 1971;4:15–25.
26. Miller GA, Chapman JP. Misunderstanding analysis of covariance. J Abnorm Psychol. 2001;110:40.
27. Mayers A. Introduction to statistics and SPSS in psychology. London: Pearson Education limited; 2013.
28. Khorashad BS, Baron-Cohen S, Roshan GM, Kazemian M, Khazai L, Aghili Z, Afkhamizadeh M. The "Reading the Mind in the Eyes" test: investigation of psychometric properties and test–retest reliability of the persian version. J Autism Dev Disord. 2015;45(9):2651–2666.
29. Vellante M, Baron-Cohen S, Melis M, Marrone M, Petretto DR, Masala C, et al. The "Reading the Mind in the Eyes" test: systematic review of psychometric properties and a validation study in Italy. Cognit Neuropsychiatry. 2013;18: 326–54.
30. Morris MW, Peng K. Culture and cause: American and Chinese attributions for social and physical events. J Pers Soc Psychol. 1994;67:949.
31. Nisbett RE, Peng K, Choi I, Norenzayan A. Culture and systems of thought: holistic versus analytic cognition. Psychol Rev. 2001;108:291–310.
32. Prevost M, Carrier M-E, Chowne G, Zelkowitz P, Joseph L, Gold I. The Reading the Mind in the Eyes test: validation of a French version and exploration of cultural variations in a multi-ethnic city. Cognit Neuropsychiatry. 2014;19:189–204.
33. Mesquita B, Tanida S, Anxin Leu J. Placing the face in context: cultural differences in the perception of facial emotion. J Pers Soc Psychol. 2008;94: 365–81.
34. Trope Y, Liberman N. Construal-level theory of psychological distance. Psychol Rev. 2010;117:440.
35. Belmonte MK. The autism spectrum as a source of cognitive and cultural diversity. Ranchi Instit Neuro Psychiatry Allied Sci J. 2011;3:S46–54.
36. Calvo MG, Lundqvist D. Facial expressions of emotion (KDEF): identification under different display-duration conditions. Behav Res Methods. 2008;40: 109–15.
37. Ashwin C, Chapman E, Colle L, Baron-Cohen S. Impaired recognition of negative basic emotions in autism: a test of the amygdala theory. Soc Neurosci. 2006;1:349–63.
38. Chapman E, Baron-Cohen S, Auyeung B, Knickmeyer R, Taylor K, Hackett G. Fetal testosterone and empathy: evidence from the empathy quotient (EQ) and the "reading the mind in the eyes" test. Soc Neurosci. 2006;1:135–48.
39. Happé F, Frith U. The weak coherence account: detail-focused cognitive style in autism spectrum disorders. J Autism Dev Disord. 2006;36:5–25.
40. Wang L, Mottron L, Peng D, Berthiaume C, Dawson M. Local bias and local-to-global interference without global deficit: a robust finding in autism under various conditions of attention, exposure time, and visual angle. Cogn Neuropsychol. 2007;24:550–74.
41. Jarrold C, Gilchrist ID, Bender A. Embedded figures detection in autism and typical development: preliminary evidence of a double dissociation in relationships with visual search. Dev Sci. 2005;8:344–51.
42. Jolliffe T, Baron-Cohen S. Are people with autism and Asperger syndrome faster than normal on the Embedded Figures Test? J Child Psychol Psychiatry. 1997;38:527–34.

19

Blood–brain barrier and intestinal epithelial barrier alterations in autism spectrum disorders

Maria Fiorentino[1,4*], Anna Sapone[1,2], Stefania Senger[1,4], Stephanie S. Camhi[1,3], Sarah M. Kadzielski[4], Timothy M. Buie[4], Deanna L. Kelly[5], Nicola Cascella[6] and Alessio Fasano[1,3,4]

Abstract

Background: Autism spectrum disorders (ASD) are complex conditions whose pathogenesis may be attributed to gene–environment interactions. There are no definitive mechanisms explaining how environmental triggers can lead to ASD although the involvement of inflammation and immunity has been suggested. Inappropriate antigen trafficking through an impaired intestinal barrier, followed by passage of these antigens or immune-activated complexes through a permissive blood–brain barrier (BBB), can be part of the chain of events leading to these disorders. Our goal was to investigate whether an altered BBB and gut permeability is part of the pathophysiology of ASD.

Methods: *Postmortem* cerebral cortex and cerebellum tissues from ASD, schizophrenia (SCZ), and healthy subjects (HC) and duodenal biopsies from ASD and HC were analyzed for gene and protein expression profiles. Tight junctions and other key molecules associated with the neurovascular unit integrity and function and neuroinflammation were investigated.

Results: Claudin (*CLDN*)-5 and -12 were increased in the ASD cortex and cerebellum. *CLDN-3*, *tricellulin*, and *MMP-9* were higher in the ASD cortex. *IL-8*, *tPA*, and *IBA-1* were downregulated in SCZ cortex; *IL-1b* was increased in the SCZ cerebellum. Differences between SCZ and ASD were observed for most of the genes analyzed in both brain areas. CLDN-5 protein was increased in ASD cortex and cerebellum, while CLDN-12 appeared reduced in both ASD and SCZ cortexes. In the intestine, 75% of the ASD samples analyzed had reduced expression of barrier-forming TJ components (*CLDN-1*, *OCLN*, *TRIC*), whereas 66% had increased pore-forming CLDNs (*CLDN-2*, *-10*, *-15*) compared to controls.

Conclusions: In the ASD brain, there is an altered expression of genes associated with BBB integrity coupled with increased neuroinflammation and possibly impaired gut barrier integrity. While these findings seem to be specific for ASD, the possibility of more distinct SCZ subgroups should be explored with additional studies.

Keywords: Blood–brain barrier, Autism spectrum disorders, Gut–brain axis, Gut permeability, Schizophrenia, Neuroinflammation, Postmortem brain, Duodenal biopsies

* Correspondence: mrfiorentino@mgh.harvard.edu
[1]Mucosal Immunology and Biology Research Center, Massachusetts General Hospital for Children, Boston, MA, USA
[4]Department of Pediatrics, Harvard Medical School, Boston, MA, USA
Full list of author information is available at the end of the article

Background

Autism spectrum disorders (ASD) are neurodevelopmental diseases with complex symptoms and whose neurobiological basis remains poorly understood. Research suggests that a combination of genetic, autoimmune, environmental, and perhaps in utero risk factors leading to neuroinflammation can contribute to the pathogenesis of ASD [1–6] as well as other neurobehavioral and/or neuropsychiatric disorders including schizophrenia (SCZ) [7–13]. Over-expression of acute phase proteins in the serum, brain, and cerebrospinal fluid of ASD as well as SCZ individuals suggests that inflammation is involved in the pathophysiology of these diseases [4, 6, 14–21]. Autoimmune diseases have been associated with increased risk of ASD and SCZ [10, 22–28] suggesting altered or inappropriate immune responses.

Furthermore, many ASD patients experience gastrointestinal (GI) symptoms and/or dysfunctions [29–38]. Clinical observations describe increased intestinal permeability in ASD [39–42], and permeability to food antigens derived from the partial digestion of wheat (gliadorphins) and cow's milk (casomorphins) has been reported in both ASD and SCZ [41, 43–46].

Despite research efforts, there are no defined explanations of how environmental triggers can lead to these neurobehavioral conditions. One hypothesis, based on the interconnectivity of the gut–brain axis, suggests that inappropriate antigen trafficking through an impaired intestinal barrier, followed by passage of antigens or activated immune complexes through a permissive blood–brain barrier (BBB), can be part of the chain of events leading to neuroinflammation and thereby subsequent disease.

Table 1 List of primers used for RT-qPCR

Gene	Accession number	5′ OLIGO	3′ OLIGO	Gene function in the brain/gut context
CLDN-1	NM_021101	GTGATAGCAATCTTTGTGGC	ACTAAAATAGCCAGACCTGC	Barrier-forming claudin
CLDN-5	NM_001130861	GAACTTCCTGAAGTGGTGTC	CCAGACCTCTCAATCTTCAC	Barrier-forming claudin; endothelial cell-specific
CLDN-12	NM_001185072	GAGAAGCAGGCTCAGATTAT	AGATTCAGAACTTCCCTGTG	Function at BBB unknown
OCLN	U53823	CACACCACACCTACACTC	TCCAAGATAAACCAATCTGCT	Barrier-forming component of the TJs
VE-Cad	X79981	AGTTCTTCCGAGTCACAAAA	TCAGGTTATACCAGGGGTAG	Main integral membrane protein of endothelial AJs; controls endothelial cell survival, stabilization of blood vessel assembly, and vascular permeability
MMP-9	NM_004994	TGTACCGCTATGGTTACACTCG	GGCAGGGACAGTTGCTTCT	Metalloprotease involved in local proteolysis of the extracellular matrix and in leukocyte migration
MMP-2	NM_004530	TACAGGATCATTGGCTACACACC	GGTCACATCGCTCCAGACT	Metalloprotease involved in local proteolysis of the extracellular matrix and in leukocyte migration
tPA	NM_001319189	CCGGCTACGGCAAGCA	AGCGGCTGGATGGGTACA	Serine protease involved in the synthesis of MMPs and BBB damage
18S	X03205	AGAAACGGCTACCACATCCA	CCCTCCAATGGATCCTCGTT	Ribosomal RNA (control gene for qPCR)
CLDN-2	NM_001171092	QIAGEN		Pore-forming claudin; regulates paracellular ion and water flow
CLDN-3	NM_001306	QIAGEN		Barrier-forming component of the TJs
CLDN-10	NM_001160100	QIAGEN		Pore-forming claudin; regulates paracellular ion flow
CLDN-15	NM_001185080 NM_014343 NM_138429	QIAGEN		Pore-forming claudin; regulates paracellular ion flow
TRIC	NM_001038603	QIAGEN		Barrier-forming component of the TJs
IL-1b	NM_000576	QIAGEN		Pro-inflammatory cytokine involved in increased BBB permeability
IL-6	NM_000600	QIAGEN		Pro-inflammatory cytokine
IL-8	NM_000584	QIAGEN		Pro-inflammatory cytokine
IL-10	NM_000572	QIAGEN		Anti-inflammatory cytokine
TSPO	NM_000714	QIAGEN		Mitochondrial protein expressed on reactive glial cells; biomarker for inflammation in the brain
tTG6	NM_001254734	QIAGEN		Marker of gluten-related neuroinflammation
MSFD2A	NM_001136493	QIAGEN		Key regulator of BBB function; required for the establishment of a functional BBB
IBA-1	NM_001623	QIAGEN		Marker of microglia activation

Table 2 Demographic and clinical characteristics of subjects analyzed in this study

						Cortex and CBL	
MBC #	Age	Race	Sex	Diagnosis	PMI	Cause of death	Additional clinical information
585	42	AA	M	SCZ	16	Pulmonary embolism	Tox (at death): doxepin
612	45	W	M	SCZ	24	Suicide, doxepin intoxication	N/A
628	59	W	M	SCZ	13	Pulmonary thromboembolia	Tox (at death): ETOH, diphenhydramine
664	53	W	M	SCZ	11	ASCVD	Tox (at death): olanzapine
705	47	W	M	SCZ	16	Deep vein thrombosis	N/A
737	55	W	M	SCZ	12	ASCVD	N/A
741	40	W	M	SCZ	14	Motor vehicle accident	Tox (at death): cocaine
751	28	W	M	SCZ	34	Suicide, GSW to chest	Tox (at death): olanzapine
783	53	W	M	SCZ	19	Manner undetermined	N/A
831	53	W	M	SCZ	14	ASCVD	N/A
4334	11	H	M	ASD	27	Acute hemorrhagic tracheobronchitis	History of epilepsy. Brain edema, acute, mild. Otherwise normal brain
4999	20	W	M	ASD	14	Cardiac arrythmia	PDD, autism, and severe mental retardation. Naltrexone
5027	37	AA	M	ASD	26	Obstruction of bowel due to adhesion	Risperdal and Luvox
5115	46	W	M	ASD	29	Complications of pseudomyxoma peritonei	Adult brain with moderate atherosclerosis
5144	7	W	M	ASD	3	Cancer, complication of	Rhabdomyosarcoma
5176	22	AA	M	ASD	18	Subdural hemorrhage	Risperdal
5308	4	W	M	ASD	21	Skull fractures	Struck by a car. Multifocal subarachnoid hemorrhage
5403	16	W	M	ASD	35	Cardiac arrhythmia	Developmental delays. GI evaluations
1464	42	W	M	Control	19	Pulmonary embolism	Chest and abdominal pain, pale, and diaphoretic
1829	25	W	M	Control	21	Electrocution	N/A
1831	44	W	M	Control	17	CO_2 inhalation complicating ASCVD	History of hypertension. Complained of headaches
1936	46	W	M	Control	13	ASCVD	History of HBP. Had been experiencing chest pain
5024	56	W	M	Control	10	ASCVD; diabetes mellitus	Smoker, no drinking of ETOH. History of prescription drug abuse. On insulin, metformin, oxycodone, Levaquin, and Lyrica
5185	21	W	M	Control	26	Car accident	Drink ETOH prior to death
5189	40	W	M	Control	14	Cardiac arrhythmia complicated by drowning	Severe stomach pains, chest palpitations, and nausea
5276	22	W	M	Control	18	Heroin intoxication	Asthma and drug abuse; smoker
5237	52	W	M	Control	13	HASCVD	ETOH and cocaine abuse. Clean for 30 days and not feeling well
5349	24	W	M	Control	16	Combined drug intoxication	Drug use
5553	54	W	M	Control	17	Hypertensive atherosclerosis heart disease	History of HTN and daily ETOH intake
5615	50	W	M	Control	19	N/A	N/A
4337	8	AA	M	Control	16	Blunt force neck injury. Car accident	Asthma. Brain petechiae, fresh
4670	4	W	M	Control	17	Commotio cordis (struck by a ball in the sternum)	N/A
5334	12	H	M	Control	15	Hanging/suicide	N/A

					Duodenum (biopsies)	
Study #	Age	Race	Sex	Diagnosis	GI symptoms	Additional clinical information
GBA #2	8	W	M	ASD	Non-apparent	Food allergies, GFCF diet, probiotics
GBA #3	11	W	M	ASD	GERD, vomiting, bloating	Asperger's. No milk diet
GBA #6	19	W	M	ASD	Regurgitation after each meal, constipation	History of aggressive behaviors

Table 2 Demographic and clinical characteristics of subjects analyzed in this study *(Continued)*

GBA #7	21	W	F	ASD	GERD, erosive esophagitis, IBS, severe constipation, occasional diarrhea	GFCF diet
GBA #10	9	W	M	ASD	EoE, GERD, constipation, vomiting	Asthma, somewhat loose stools. Dairy-free diet
GBA #12	6	AA	M	ASD	Non-apparent	Eats only pureed food
GBA #13	5	AA	M	ASD	Severe constipation, GERD, abdominal pain, runny stools	Asthma, food allergies
GBA #14	3	W	M	ASD	Chronic constipation	History of obesity, restricted diet (yogurt, milk, juice)
GBA #15	11	W	F	ASD	GERD, constipation	Macrocephaly, sleep disorder
GBA #16	6	W	M	ASD	Gastroesophageal reflux, constipation	Food and seasonal allergies, asthma
GBA #18	16	W	F	ASD	Constipation, abdominal pain, heartburn, regurgitation	Acute mono, weight loss
GBA #20	6	AA	F	ASD	GERD with esophagitis, constipation	ADHD, asthma. Vegetarian
GBA #5	10	HL	M	HC	Abdominal pain, nausea, vomiting, sometimes diarrhea	Lactose-free diet
GBA #8	16	W	F	HC	Constipation, abdominal pain, burping, bloating	GFCG diet, some FODMAP diet
GBA #9	16	W	F	HC	Dysphagia, abdominal pain, regurgitation	
GBA #11	15	W	F	HC	Abdominal pain, GERD	Seasonal allergies, lactose intolerance, dairy-free and nut-free diet, ADHD, obesity
GBA #17	21	W	F	HC	Nausea, vomiting, upset stomach, GERD. Abdominal pain	Previous duodenitis and gastritis, hepatic adenoma
GBA #19	6.5	N/A	M	HC	GERD, constipation	Hydronephrosis, nephrocalcinosis, clubfoot, seasonal allergies, asthma
GBA #21	15	W	M	HC	Dysphagia, esophagitis	Asthma
GBA #23	15	W	M	HC	Abdominal pain, IBS-like constipation	N/A
GBA #24	4	W	M	HC	Reflux	History of constipation. Dairy-free diet

W white, *AA* African-American, *HL* Hispanic-Latino, *M* male, *F* female, *HC* healthy control, *ASD* autism spectrum disorder, *GBA* gut–brain axis study; *GERD* gastroesophageal reflux disease, *GFCF* gluten-free casein-free, *PMI* postmortem interval, *ADD/ADHD* attention-deficit/hyperactivity disorder, *ASCVD* atherosclerotic cardiovascular disease, *HASCVD* hypertensive arteriosclerotic cardiovascular disease, *PDD/PDD-NOS* pervasive developmental disorder/not otherwise specified, *OCD* obsessive-compulsive disorder

The BBB plays a critical role in the central nervous system (CNS) defense through limiting the access of circulating solutes, macromolecules, and cells that could negatively impact neuronal activity. Dysfunctions of the BBB have been associated with numerous neurological disorders, such as stroke, epilepsy, multiple sclerosis, and Parkinson's and Alzheimer's disease [47–56].

The overall goal of this study was to assess whether a dysfunctional BBB or gut barrier could contribute pathophysiologically to ASD. To address this, we conducted an in-depth molecular analysis of the components associated with the BBB and gut barrier integrity in postmortem brain tissue and small intestinal biopsies obtained from ASD subjects. In addition, we assessed changes in the BBB integrity of patients with SCZ as SCZ is a psychiatric illness in which the involvement of inflammation, immunity and altered BBB integrity have been postulated [22, 23, 57, 58].

Methods

Postmortem tissues

Human frozen postmortem brain tissue blocks (1 to 2 cm^3) from the frontal cortex (Brodmann's area 45) and cerebellum (CBL) of 15 HC and eight ASD subjects were obtained from the NICHD Brain and Tissue Bank for Developmental Disorders at the University of Maryland, Baltimore, MD, USA, which is a Brain and Tissue Repository of the NIH NeuroBioBank. Additionally, the Maryland Brain Collection of the Maryland Psychiatric Research Center at the University of Maryland School of Medicine, Baltimore, USA, provided ten SCZ samples from each of the two aforementioned brain areas of interest.

Duodenal biopsies

Biopsy specimens were taken from the second portion of the duodenum from ASD ($n = 12$) and control ($n = 9$) patients with GI symptoms undergoing esophagogastroduodenoscopy (EGD) for clinically indicated reasons. All study subjects provided written informed consent for the collection of additional biopsies, for the purpose of this study, during the procedure. This study was approved by the Partners Human Research Committee (PHRC) at Massachusetts General Hospital and performed in accordance with the ethical standards and regulatory requirements set forth by the Declaration of Helsinki.

Gene expression profile analysis

Total RNA was isolated from samples (~100 mg) using Trizol (Life Technologies, Carlsbad, CA) and/or Direct-zol RNA miniprep spin columns (Zymo Research, Irvine, CA) following the manufacturers' instructions. RNA concentrations and A260/A280 and A260/A230 ratios were measured with the NanoDrop spectrophotometer (Thermo Scientific) before 2 μg total RNA were reverse transcribed using random hexamer primers and Maxima universal first strand cDNA synthesis kit #1661 (Thermo Fisher Scientific, Waltham, MA). Real-time quantitative PCR (qPCR) was used to measure gene expression levels and was performed in an iCycler96X detection system (Bio-Rad, Hercules, CA) according to the manufacturer's protocol. In brain tissues, we analyzed the expression level of genes associated with the formation, integrity, and function of the BBB and neuroinflammation, as follows: Claudin(*CLDN)*-1, *CLDN-3*, *CLDN-5*, and *CLDN-12*; occludin (*OCLN*); tricellulin (*TRIC*); vascular endothelial cadherin (*VE-Cad*); interleukin (*IL*)-1b, *IL-6*, *IL-8*, and *IL-10*; the microglia activation marker ionized calcium-binding adaptor molecule (*IBA*)-1; the translocator protein 18 kDa (*TSPO*); matrix metalloprotease (*MMP*)-2 and *MMP-9*; tissue transglutaminase (*tTG*)-6; tissue plasminogen activator (*tPA*); and the major facilitator super family domain containing 2A (*MFSD2A*). Duodenal biopsies were evaluated for the expression of *CLDN-1*, *CLDN-2*, *CLDN-10*, *CLDN-15*, *TRIC*, and *OCLN*. *18S* housekeeping gene was chosen as internal control. *CLDN-2*, *CLDN-3*, *CLDN-10*, *CLDN-15*, *TRIC*, *IL-1b*, *IL-6*, *IL-8*, *IL-10*, *tTG-6*, *IBA-1*, *TSPO*, and *MSFD2A* primers were purchased from Qiagen (RT^2 qPCR or Quantitect Primer Assay). The other primer sets used were purchased by IDT (Integrated DNA Technologies, Coralville, IA), and their sequences together with gene function in the context of the BBB and/or gut are listed in Table 1. The sequence specificity of synthesized primers (IDT) were determined by the online Blast program from the National Center for Biotechnology Information website (http://www.ncbi.nlm.nih.gov/blast/Blast.cgi) and compared with the GenBank database. Differences in gene expression profiles were evaluated applying the $2^{(-ddCT)}$ method [59].

Protein detection

Western blot analysis was performed as routinely described. Brain tissues (~100 mg) were homogenized on ice in lysis buffer [RIPA Buffer (Sigma, S. Louis, MO)] containing protease inhibitor cocktail (Complete Mini,

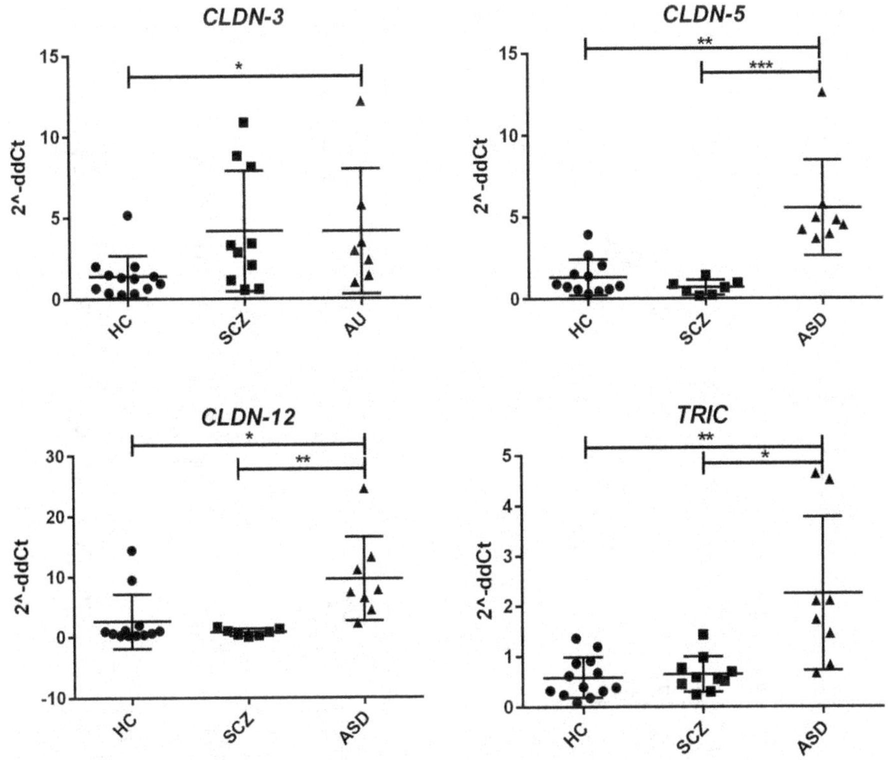

Fig. 1 Altered gene expression level of TJ components in the cortex of ASD subjects. Each *dot* represents data from a single subject. Gene expression level is reported as 2^{-ddCT} with normalization of mRNA expression to the endogenous control *18S*. Mean ± SEM are reported for each group. One-way ANOVA test has been used to evaluate statistical significance. *$p < 0.05$; **$p < 0.01$; ***$p < 0.001$

Roche). Homogenates were centrifuged at 14 K rpm for 30 min at 4 °C in a benchtop centrifuge. The supernatant, representing total protein lysate, was collected, and protein concentration was determined by Lowry protein assay (DC, BioRad, Hercules, CA) using bovine serum albumin (BSA) as a protein standard. Protein lysates were mixed with loading buffer and reducing agent (both from Life Technologies, Carlsbad, CA) and heated at 99 °C for 5 min. The lysates were then loaded on 4–20% Tris-Glycine gels (Life Technologies, Carlsbad, CA) and after gel electrophoresis transferred onto PVDF membranes. The membranes were blocked with 5% BSA in Tris buffered saline with 0.1% Tween 20 (TBST), and incubated with primary antibody overnight at 4 °C. Actin was used as loading control while ACTA2, also known as alpha-smooth muscle actin (in this paper reported as SMA), was used for quantitative analysis normalization for tight junction (TJ) proteins. The membranes were washed three times with TBST and incubated with secondary antibody (diluted 1:5000 in 5% BSA-TBST) for 1 h at room temperature. Western blot signal was visualized using a LI-COR Odyssey infrared scan (LI-COR Biosciences, Lincoln, NE). Results were quantified with the ImageJ 1.47 software (NIH). The protein levels were

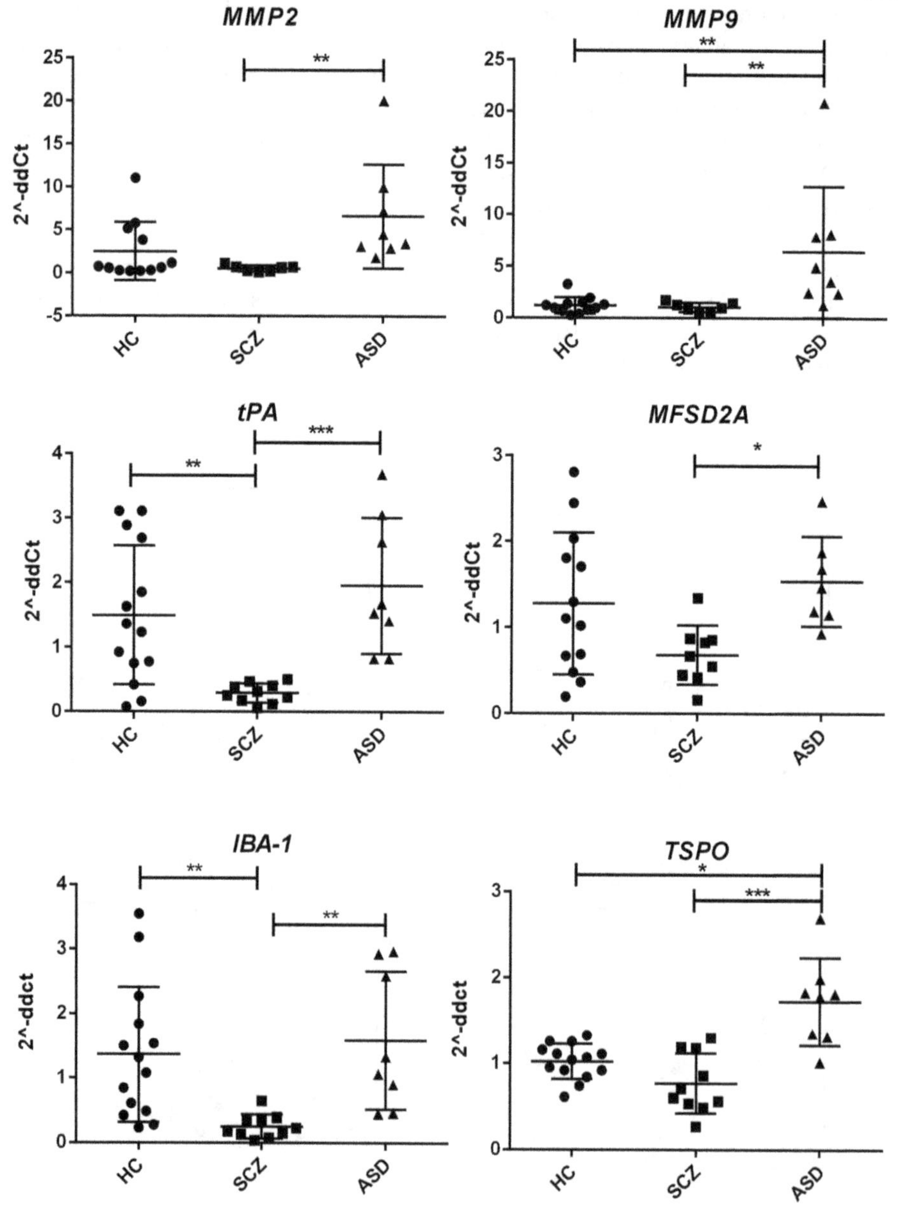

Fig. 2 Gene expression profile of BBB function associated components in the cortex of HC, ASD, and SCZ subjects. Each *dot* represents data from a single subject. Gene expression level is reported as 2^{-ddCT} with normalization of mRNA expression to the endogenous control *18S*. Mean ± SEM are reported for each group. One-way ANOVA test has been used to evaluate statistical significance. *$p < 0.05$; **$p < 0.01$; ***$p < 0.001$

normalized as ratio to actin or SMA, as internal controls. Data represent the average of a minimum of two independent experiments.

Antibodies

Mouse anti-claudin-5 (cat # 35–2500; 1:500) antibody was purchased from Life Technologies, (Carlsbad, CA). Mouse anti-actin protein antibody (cat # 82353; 1:2000) was purchased from Thermo Fisher Scientific (Waltham, MA). Rabbit anti-claudin-12 (cat # NBP1-87450; 1:500) was purchased from Novus Biologicals (Littleton, CO). Rabbit anti-alpha-smooth muscle actin (SMA) antibody (#Ab5694; 1:1000) was purchased from Abcam (Cambridge, MA). LI-COR IRDye800 anti-rabbit (LI-COR Biosciences, Lincoln, NE; cat # 92632211) and Alexa Fluor 680 goat anti-mouse (Thermo Fisher Scientific, Waltham, MA; cat # A21057) were used as secondary antibodies in WB analysis.

Statistics

Data were analyzed by using the GraphPad (San Diego, CA) software. Comparisons among groups were made by the one-way ANOVA (Kruskal–Wallis *H* test; Dunn's test for multiple comparisons). Differences between two groups were calculated by the unpaired *t* test (Mann–Whitney). All data with $p < 0.05$ were considered significant.

Results

Subjects

A total of 33 brain sections from the three subject groups were studied. No drug abuse or gunshot wounds were reported for ASD subjects. Two of the ASD individuals were on therapy with one antipsychotic and/or antidepressant. Those ASD cases whose cause of death was drowning were not considered for the brain study to eliminate the damaging effects on brain and vasculature caused by hypoxia/anoxia [60, 61]. Of the ten SCZ individuals, no medical records were available. The only existing information was collected at autopsy: the post-mortem toxicological analysis showed that three had used antipsychotics and/or antidepressants, one had used cocaine and one had ingested alcohol prior to death. Similar to ASD patients, no gunshot wounds at the head region were reported for SCZ subjects. The control cases had no known neurological disorder or known neuropathology. Three HC out of 15 had a history of drugs and/or alcohol abuse. Biopsies from the second portion of the duodenum were collected from the ASD ($n = 12$) and control ($n = 8$) patients with gastrointestinal symptoms. The available clinical characteristics of the analyzed subjects, together with demographic data are summarized in Table 2.

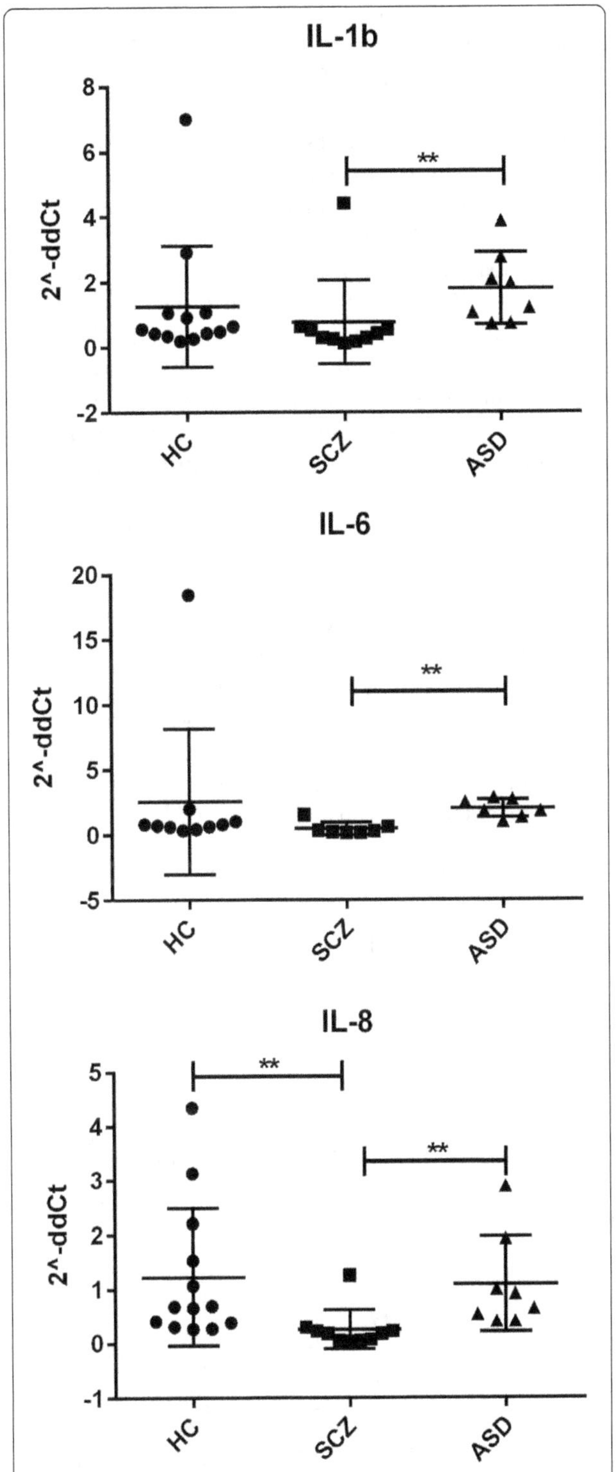

Fig. 3 Gene expression profile of some pro-inflammatory cytokines in the cortex of HC, ASD, and SCZ subjects. Each *dot* represents data from a single subject. Gene expression level is reported as 2^{-ddCT} with normalization of mRNA expression to the endogenous control *18S*. Mean ± SEM are reported for each group. One-way ANOVA test has been used to evaluate statistical significance. $^{**}p < 0.01$

Genes associated with BBB integrity and function are differentially regulated in the brain of ASD subjects

To assess the integrity of the BBB, we measured the gene expression levels of the major components of the brain microvascular endothelial tight junctions (TJs) by qRT-PCR, in the cortex and CBL of HC ($n = 15$), ASD ($n = 8$), and SCZ ($n = 10$) subjects. In the cortex, *CLDN-3, -5,* and *-12* and *TRIC* were upregulated in ASD subjects compared to controls (Fig. 1). Neither *CLDN-1, OCLN,* nor *VE-Cad* were differentially expressed in the cortex in any of the groups analyzed (not shown). Gene expression profiles of *tPA, IBA-1, TSPO, MFSD2A,* pro-inflammatory cytokines, and members of the matrix metalloprotease (MMP) family, described to be linked to BBB function disruption and/or neuroinflammation, were also analyzed. Results showed that in the cortex of ASD subjects, *MMP-9* and *TSPO* were significantly upregulated compared to those of the HC, whereas *tPA* and *IBA-1* appeared downregulated in SCZ compared in HC (Fig. 2). None of the pro-inflammatory cytokines analyzed were differentially regulated in ASD compared in HC. While *IL-8* appeared significantly reduced in SCZ vs. HC, all cytokines evaluated were expressed at a lower level in SCZ compared to ASD (Fig. 3). *IL-10* and *tTG6* expressions were below detection levels. In the CBL, similar to our findings in the cortex, *CLDN-5, −12* and *TSPO* were found to be elevated in ASD subjects when compared to HC (Fig. 4). Among the other genes analyzed, *IL-1b* appeared significantly higher in SCZ vs. HC (Fig. 4). As a general observation, unlike ASD, SCZ subjects clustered well together for most of the genes analyzed in both brain areas. The gene expression fold changes relative to HC (=1) and the corresponding *p* values are summarized in Table 3.

BBB tight junction proteins are altered in ASD and SCZ subjects

To understand whether our gene expression results correlated with levels of protein produced, we performed western blotting analysis of tissue lysates using commercially available antibodies against some TJ components in both the cortex and CBL of HC, ASD, and SCZ subjects. Consistent with the gene expression profile, we observed a significant higher level of CLDN-5 in the cortex of ASD subjects, compared in HC (Fig. 5). Interestingly and in this case in opposition to gene expression results, CLDN-12 was reduced in the cortex of ASD and also showed a reduced trend in SCZ subjects (Fig. 5).

In the CBL (Fig. 6), the production of CLDN-5 in ASD appeared slightly higher than in HC ($p = 0.1$), whereas its level in SCZ was reduced compared to

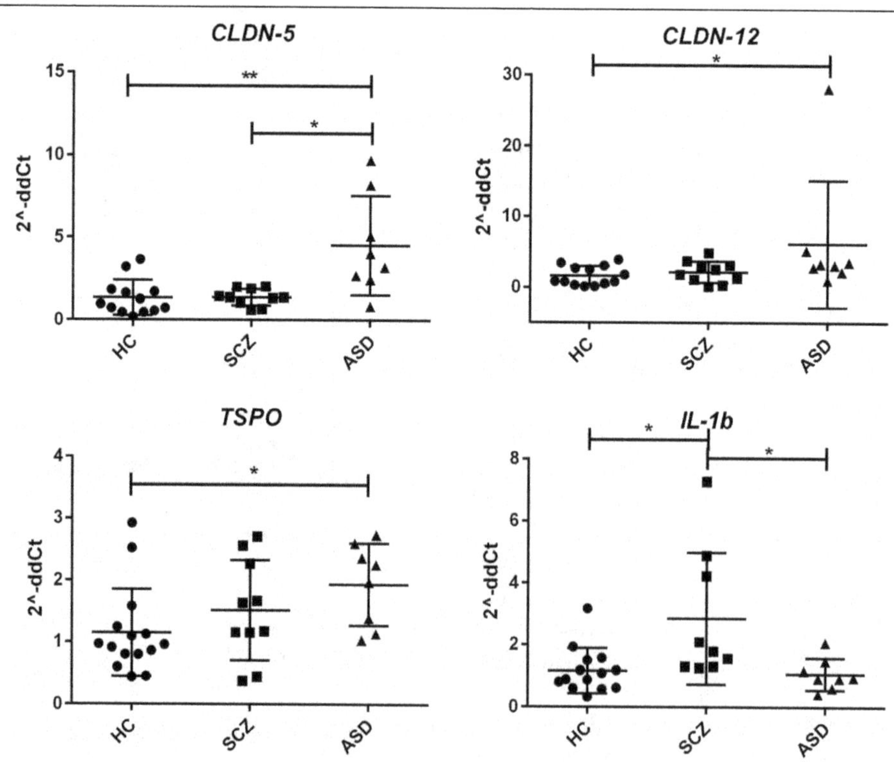

Fig. 4 Increased claudins and inflammatory markers gene expression levels in the cerebellum of HC, ASD, and SCZ subjects. Each *dot* represents data from a single subject. Gene expression level is reported as 2^{-ddCT} with normalization of mRNA expression to the endogenous control *18S*. Mean ± SEM are reported for each group. One-way ANOVA test has been used to evaluate statistical significance. $^*p < 0.05$; $^{**}p < 0.01$

Table 3 Summary of gene expression profiling by RT-qPCR

Gene	Fold change		*p* values		
			Cortex		
	SCZ	ASD	HC vs. SCZ	HC vs. ASD	ASD vs. SCZ
CLDN-1	0.7	2.3	ns	ns	ns
CLDN-3	2.7	3.0	<0.05	<0.05	ns
CLDN-5	0.5	5.1	ns	<0.0001	<0.0001
CLDN-12	0.5	7.7	ns	<0.01	<0.001
IBA-1	0.2	1.2	<0.01	ns	<0.01
IL-1b	0.4	1.5	ns	ns	<0.01
IL-6	0.3	1.9	ns	ns	<0.01
IL-8	0.2	1.1	<0.01	ns	<0.01
IL-10	0.5	3.9	ns	ns	ns
MMP-9	0.9	4.5	ns	<0.001	<0.001
MMP-2	0.4	4.9	ns	<0.05	<0.001
MSFD2A	0.6	1.5	ns	ns	ns
OCLN	1.2	1.4	ns	ns	ns
tPA	0.2	1.7	<0.001	ns	<0.01
TRIC	1.3	1.8	ns	<0.001	<0.01
TSPO	0.7	1.7	ns	<0.05	<0.001
VE-Cad	0.8	1.3	ns	ns	ns
			Cerebellum		
CLDN-1	1.3	1.8	ns	ns	ns
CLDN-3	0.6	1.2	ns	ns	ns
CLDN-5	1.3	3.6	ns	0.01	<0.05
CLDN-12	1.5	3.7	ns	<0.05	ns
IBA-1	1.0	1.2	ns	ns	ns
IL-1b	2.3	1.0	0.01	ns	<0.05
IL-6	1.1	0.3	ns	ns	ns
IL-8	1.8	0.9	ns	ns	ns
IL-10	1.3	0.9	ns	ns	ns
MMP-9	1.0	1.9	ns	ns	ns
MMP-2	0.7	2.8	ns	ns	ns
OCLN	1.2	1.5	ns	ns	ns
tPA	1.2	1.5	ns	ns	ns
TRIC	0.6	0.9	ns	ns	ns
TSPO	1.3	1.8	ns	<0.05	ns
VE-Cad	1.4	1.3	ns	ns	ns
			Duodenum (biopsies)		
CLDN-1	N/A	1.7	N/A	ns	N/A
CLDN-2	N/A	2.3	N/A	ns	N/A
CLDN-10	N/A	4.0	N/A	ns	N/A
CLDN-15	N/A	1.6	N/A	ns	N/A
OCLN	N/A	1.2	N/A	ns	N/A
TRIC	N/A	1.6	N/A	ns	N/A

Gene expression levels are presented as fold change vs. HC (=1) using the formula $2(-\Delta\Delta Ct)$. Statistical difference among groups is calculated by the one-way ANOVA (Kruskal–Wallis *H* test). Differences between two groups are calculated by the Mann–Whitney unpaired *t* test. All data with $p < 0.05$ were considered significant
ns non-significant, *N/A* not applicable

that in HC ($p = 0.07$), although data did not reach statistical significance. No differences were observed for CLDN-12 among the groups.

Increased pore-forming CLDNs and decreased barrier-forming TJ components expression in the intestine of ASD patients

To corroborate our hypothesis of a possible involvement of a dysfunctional intestinal barrier in the pathogenesis of ASD, we analyzed small intestinal biopsies of ASD and HC subjects for TJ defects (Fig. 7). Our results showed that 75% (9 out of 12) of the samples analyzed had a decreased expression of at least one barrier-forming TJ component (*CLDN-1, OCLN, TRIC*), whereas about 66% (eight out of 12) showed increased levels of pore-forming CLDNs, described to increase intestinal permeability (*CLDN-2, CLDN-10, CLDN-15*) ([62–65]).

Discussion

To the best of our knowledge, this is the first study addressing the molecular signature of BBB dysfunctions in ASD and SCZ in human samples. In spite of the obvious small sample number, due to the nature of the samples and the consequent procurement difficulty, we observed statistically significant differences among the study groups. However, it is also worthwhile to acknowledge that the small sample number may have affected some otherwise possibly significant results, which could have emerged if a larger number of tissues had been available.

Our molecular analysis of the BBB integrity and function shows an altered BBB in the ASD subjects evaluated. Indeed, the increased gene expression of MMP-9 we detected in ASD subjects supports our hypothesis of an impaired BBB, most likely associated with neuroinflammation. Several pieces of evidence indicate that MMP-9 secretion induces BBB disruption and this is an important step in the development of inflammatory diseases of the nervous system [66–74]. Although we did not observe elevated gene expression levels of pro-inflammatory cytokines in the ASD subjects analyzed in this study, we found a significantly high expression of *TSPO* in the ASD brain. *TSPO* increased expression level in activated microglia and reactive astrocytes [75–81] is

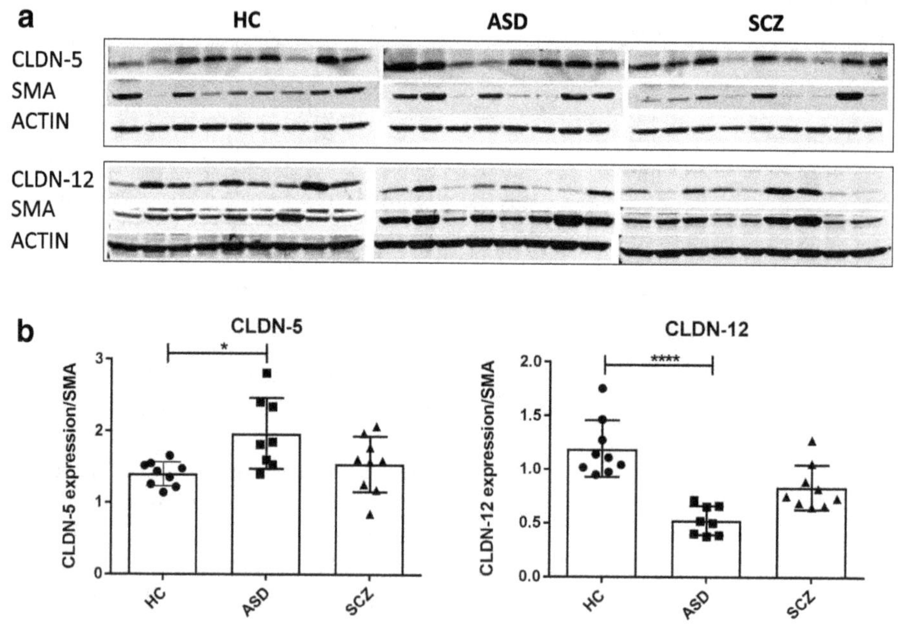

Fig. 5 Increased CLDN-5 and decreased CLDN-12 expression in the cortex of ASD subjects. **a** Brain tissues were lysed and immunoblotted with anti-claudin-5, anti-claudin-12, SMA or actin antibody. **b** Densitometry analysis of the results from the western blots is shown, where the data are normalized against SMA expression and are expressed as the mean ± standard error. Quantitative results represent the average of three independent experiments.$^{*}p < 0.05$; $^{****}p < 0.0001$

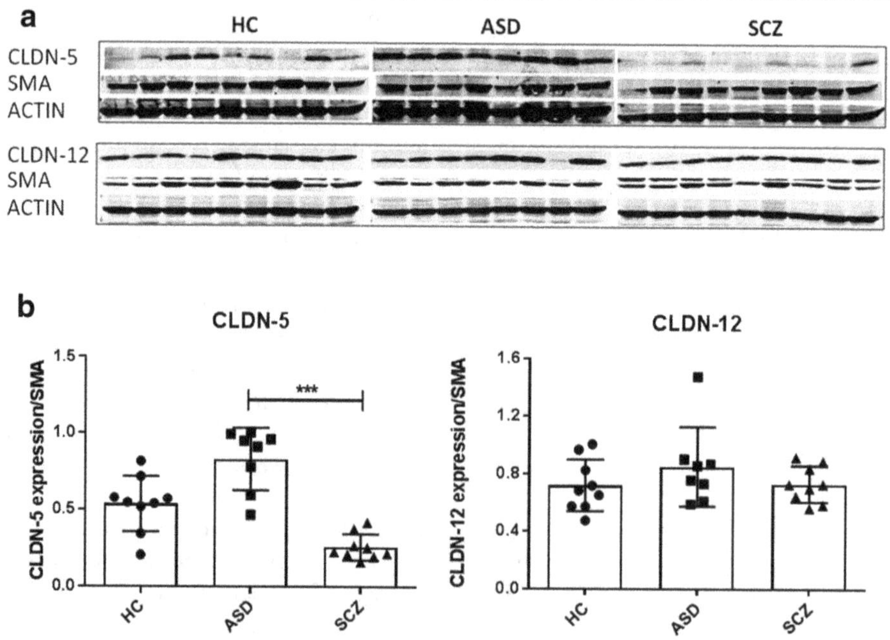

Fig. 6 Increased CLDN-5 expression in the cerebellum of ASD subjects. **a** Western blots of brain lysates immunoblotted with anti-claudin-5, anti-claudin-12, SMA or actin antibody. **b** Densitometry analysis of the results from the western blots is shown, where the data are normalized against SMA expression and are expressed as the mean ± standard error. Quantitative results represent the average of three independent experiments. $^{***}p < 0.001$

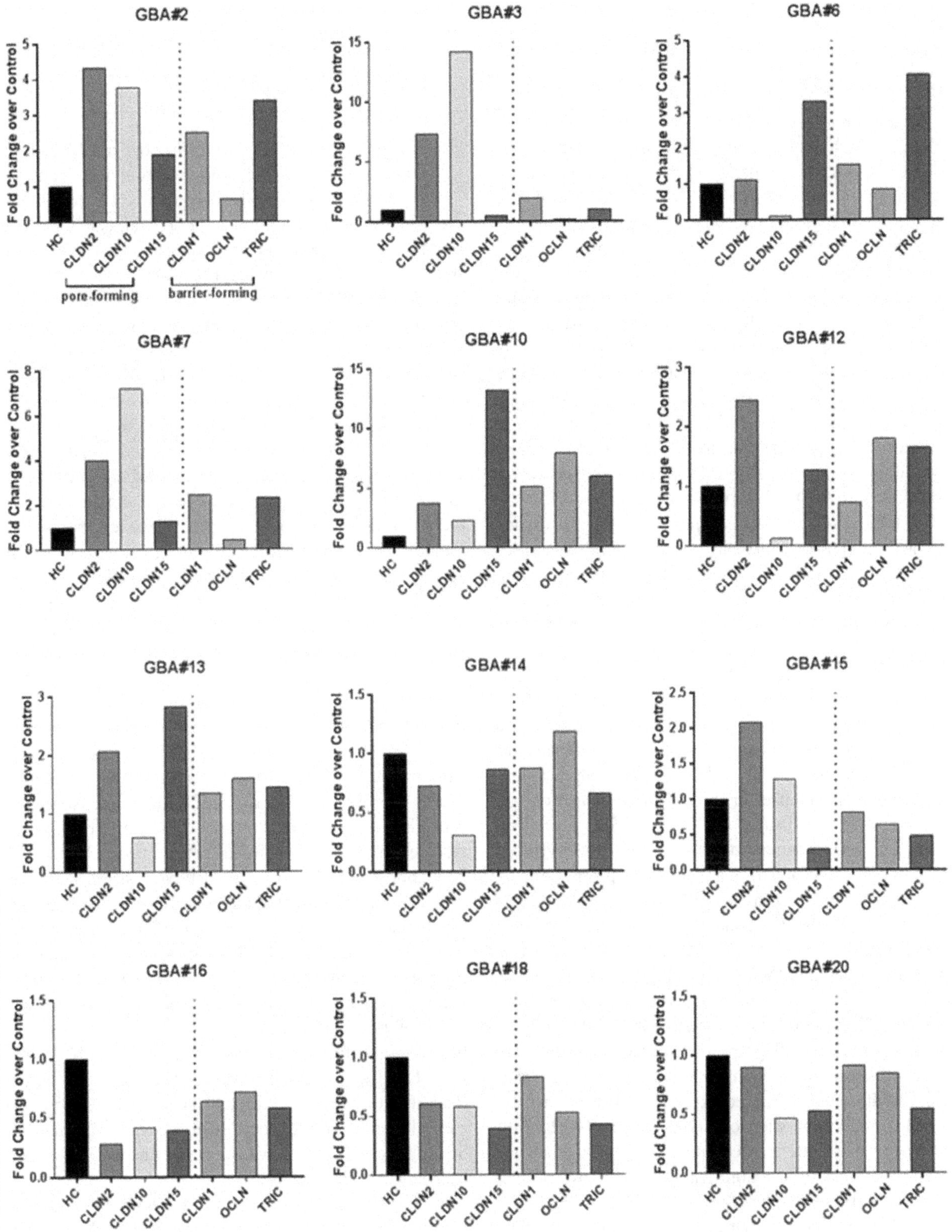

Fig. 7 (See legend on next page.)

(See figure on previous page.)

Fig. 7 Increased pore-forming claudins and decreased barrier-forming TJ components expression in the small intestine of HC and ASD subjects. Gene expression levels of TJ components in duodenal biopsies from HC ($n = 9$) and ASD patients ($n = 12$). *CLDN-2*, *-10* and/or *-15* levels are higher in eight out of 12 ASD samples, compared in controls. *CLDN-1*, *OCLN*, and/or *TRIC* levels are decreased in nine out of 12 ASD samples over controls. Each graph represents single patient results. Data are expressed as fold change over the averaged controls

associated with brain injury and neuroinflammation, making TSPO a reliable marker of brain inflammation.

Of the four claudins (i.e., *CLDN-1*, *-3*, *-5* and *-12*) that to date are thought to be incorporated in the BBB [82–85], we found that two were significantly more expressed in the ASD brain as compared in HC. *CLDN-5*, the major and more abundant cell adhesion molecule of TJs in brain endothelial cells, is expressed 5.1 and 3.6 times higher in the cortex and CBL of ASD subjects, respectively, than in those of HC (Table 3). Similarly, *CLDN-12* is expressed about 7.7 and 3.6 times more in the ASD cortex and CBL, respectively, than in the control group. *CLDN-3*, on the other hand, appears elevated by about 2.7 and 3.0 times in the cortex of both SCZ and ASD subjects, respectively, compared in that of HC. *TRIC*, another component of the TJs associated with increased epithelial tightness and decreased permeability to macromolecules [86], appears significantly elevated in the ASD cortex, suggesting either a more competent BBB or a compensatory mechanism for disrupted endothelial barrier integrity.

At the protein level, CLDN-5 is elevated in the ASD cortex, consistent with its mRNA expression, whereas, on the other hand, CLDN-12 is significantly reduced. An increased gene expression of sealing TJ components (*CLDN-5*, *-12*, and *-3* and *TRIC*) should imply a tighter BBB and a better control in the diffusion of macromolecules. However, our data on *MMP9* and *TSPO* expression compatible with ongoing neuroinflammation suggest a compensatory mechanism to repair a compromised BBB. Another plausible explanation for the CLDN-5 data is that, once produced, the protein is not capable of being incorporated into the TJ complex because of impaired trafficking to the endothelial cell–cell interface or because the protein has some mutations that prevent it from establishing homophilic and/or heterophilic protein–protein interactions, leading to a sustained compensatory gene expression and protein accumulation. On the other hand, the discrepancy between gene upregulation and decreased protein expression observed for CLDN-12 might suggest the existence of a compensatory mechanism for post-translational destruction/degradation of the protein itself. While the sealing function of CLDN-5 in BBB TJs is well established [83, 87], that of CLDN-3 and -12 are less understood. CLDN-1 and -3 sequences are highly homologous to CLDN-5, suggesting similar properties. Indeed, several studies strongly suggest that CLDN-3 contributes to BBB tightness [85, 88–90]. Conversely, CLDN-12 sequence is quite dissimilar from those of CLDN-1 and -3, and this might indicate a different function. Piontek et al. [91] showed that CLDN-12 cannot form homophilic trans-interactions or homopolymeric strands in vitro, suggesting that "heterophilic cis- and/or trans-interactions with another TJ-protein are necessary for the incorporation of CLDN-12 in strands." It may be hypothesized that the increased CLDN-5 we observed in ASD subjects might be compensatory to a decreased CLDN-12 in a heterophilic cis- and/or trans-interaction between the two claudins.

Our cohort of SCZ individuals did not show major changes in the genes analyzed compared to HC, except for an increased *IL-1b* in the CBL and significantly reduced levels of tPA and *IBA-1* in the cortex. Whereas we do not know the physiological relevance of downregulated IBA-1, our results are in agreement with data from other studies indicating activation of pro-inflammatory networks and reduced tPA activity in SCZ [92–102], this latter feature leading to a dysfunctional coagulation system and increased risk of thrombotic events in SCZ patients [101]. Other genes analyzed in SCZ appeared to follow a trend similar to ASD subjects (i.e., increased *CLDN-3* and reduced CLDN-12 protein level in the cortex). Furthermore, although non-statistically significant ($p = 0.07$), we did observe a trend toward reduced CLDN-5 protein level in the SCZ CBL as well, suggesting a possibly leaking BBB. Previous clinical and postmortem research in SCZ has suggested that an impaired BBB could be a contributing factor to the pathogenesis of the disease in only a subgroup of SCZ patients [103–105]. It is important to mention that the SCZ and ASD subjects studied were not selected on the basis of specific immune biomarkers and, therefore, may represent a mixed group of patients, which thereby limits the statistical significance of some of our findings. A sample stratification approach based on specific immunological features might be a better way of analyzing pathways of interest, and this may be particularly true for SCZ, a disorder characterized by marked clinical and neurobiological heterogeneity. Alternatively, SCZ physiopathology may lie in subtle changes that chronically affect brain function.

As for the intestine, due to the high heterogeneity intrinsic of ASD, our goal was to elucidate the TJ component profile from a functional perspective. Toward this aim, we have analyzed the expression level of TJ elements dividing them into two major functional groups: pore-forming (*CLDN-1*, *OCLN*, *TRIC*) and barrier-forming components (*CLDN-2, -10, -15*). These results, showing increased expression levels of pore-forming (66% of the ASD samples) and decreased levels of barrier-forming (75% of the ASD samples) TJ components in the duodenal samples, suggest an impaired gut barrier and serve as a proof of concept to support the hypothesis of a gut–brain axis dysfunction in a subgroup of ASD patients. According to this hypothesis, non-self antigens crossing a damaged intestinal barrier elicit a local and/or systemic inflammatory reaction that,

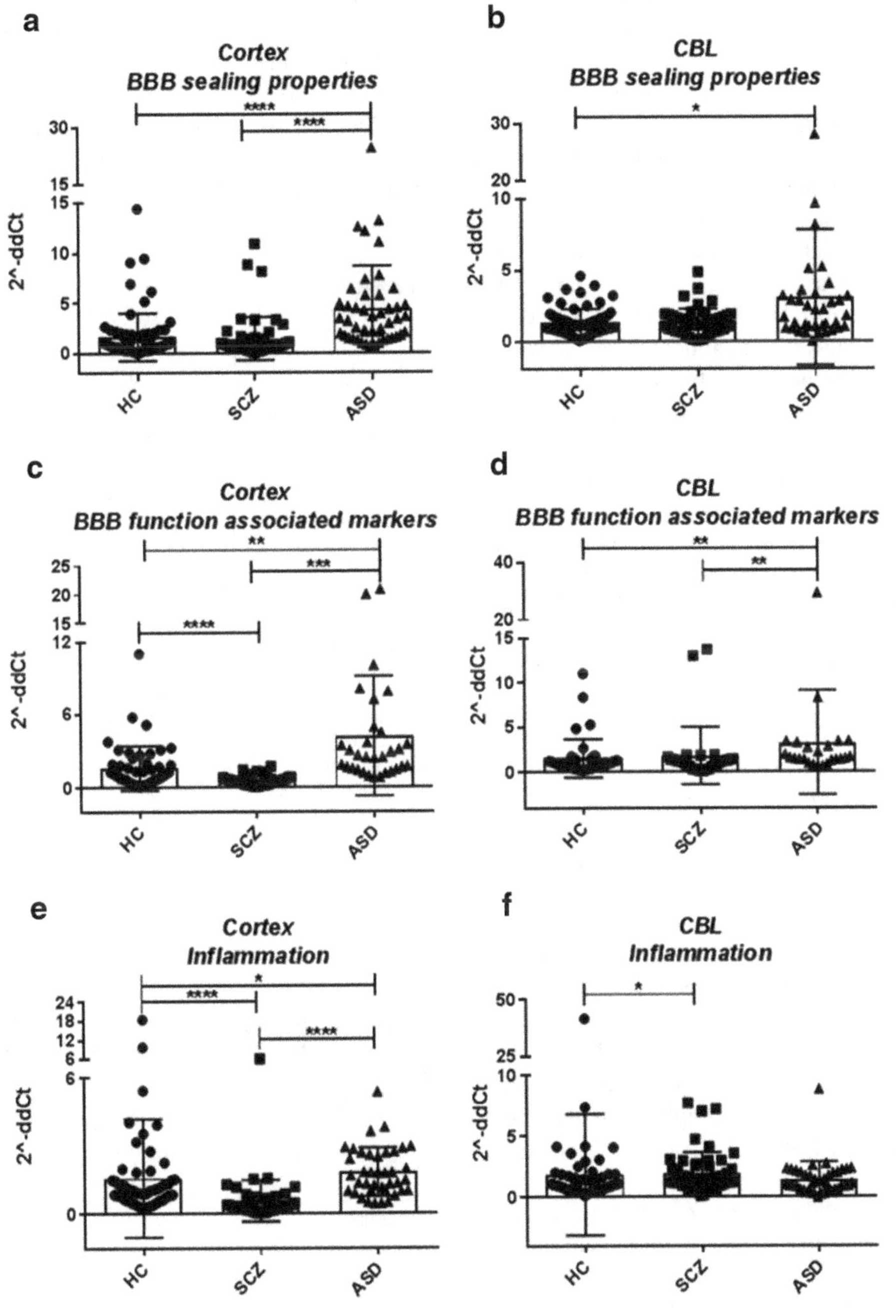

Fig. 8 Gene expression in the cortex and cerebellum (CBL) of HC, ASD, and SCZ subjects clustered by functional category. Results are represented as scatter plots where each *dot* represents data obtained from one subject sample. **a** Cortex *BBB sealing properties* group includes *CLDN-3*, *-5*, and *-12*, *TRIC*, and *OCLN*. **b** CBL "BBB sealing properties" group includes *CLDN-3*, *-5*, and *-12*, *TRIC*, and *OCLN*. **c** Cortex *BBB function associated markers* group includes *tPA*, *MMP2/9*, and *MSFD2A*. **d** CBL *BBB function associated markers* group includes *tPA* and *MMP-2/9*. **e** Cortex *Inflammation* group includes *IL-1b*, *IL-6*, and *IL-8*; *TSPO*; and *IBA-1*. **f** CBL *Inflammation* group includes *IL-1b*, *IL-6*, and *IL-8*; *TSPO*; *IBA-1*. Gene expression level is reported as 2^{-ddCT} with normalization of mRNA expression to the endogenous control *18S*. Mean ± SEM are reported for each group. One-way ANOVA test has been used to evaluate statistical significance. $^{*}p < 0.05$; $^{**}p < 0.01$; $^{***}p < 0.001$; $^{****}p < 0.0001$

associated with a breach of the BBB, may lead to ASD in genetically predisposed subjects.

This study addressed for the first time, at the molecular level, some relevant and still open questions regarding the gut–brain axis in neurobehavioral disorders and furthermore demonstrated that both the BBB and gut barrier may be affected in ASD. However, these findings present with a few limitations. The first lies in the postmortem nature of the samples with potential confounding factors deriving from tissue preservation and the personal history of each subject, including exposure to medications, health conditions, cause of death, and postmortem interval (PMI). Our statistical analysis of the PMI showed no differences among groups suggesting that PMI might not have affected our results. Similarly, data from medical records or postmortem toxicology analysis showed that about the same number of subjects in ASD and SCZ groups were on antipsychotics/antidepressants, so it is unlikely that the differences we observed among groups could be explained by the effects of the drugs. For clarity, a few studies addressing the impact of antipsychotics on the BBB function do suggest a disturbance effect on its sealing property [106, 107], whereas other studies on the blood–cerebrospinal (BCS) fluid barrier show divergent results [103, 108]. Furthermore, there are numerous studies reporting the suppressing effect of antipsychotics on the blood cytokine profile in SCZ and ASD [98, 109–118], as well as on microglia activation [119, 120], that could explain our data on *IBA-1* and the cytokine gene expression profiles. However, our *IBA*-1 results are well in agreement with the published studies on postmortem brain tissues showing no significant changes in its expression in ASD [121].

The second limitation of this study is represented by its descriptive nature that does not allow us to draw conclusions on the causality of a breach of the intestinal/BBB integrity supporting neuroinflammation and ASD and SCZ symptoms. However, our data is in line with animal studies suggesting causality between loss of barrier function and neurobehavioral changes compatible with ASD [122–124]. Finally, as already mentioned, a third limitation is represented by the small number of samples analyzed due to limited availability which might impact on the statistical significance of some of our results. However, given the complexity of the studies performed and the difficulty associated with the procurement of these samples, our study represents a solid foundation to justify a more robust sample collection and analysis to further investigate the gut–brain axis in ASD.

Conclusions

In conclusion, our results seem to point to a dysfunctional gut–brain axis associated with neuroinflammation in ASD. When clustered together by functional groups (barrier properties, pro-inflammatory markers, and enzymatic activity), our data support the notion that in ASD, there is a differential regulation of the pathways associated with our hypothesis of a gut–brain axis dysfunction involving the intestinal barrier, BBB integrity/function, and neuroinflammation (Fig. 8). Certainly, more in-depth molecular studies, possibly in animal or in vitro cell culture models, are necessary to understand the specific mechanisms behind the BBB disturbance we have herein reported. These studies will allow for patient stratification and personalized interventions (precision medicine) to target specific pathways involved in the pathogenesis of ASD.

Abbreviations

AJ: Adherens junction; ASD: Autism spectrum disorders; BBB: Blood–brain barrier; BCS: Blood–cerebrospinal; CBL: Cerebellum; CLDN: Claudin; CNS: Central nervous system; GBA: Gut–brain axis study; GI: Gastrointestinal; HC: Healthy controls; IBA-1: Ionized calcium-binding adaptor molecule 1; IL: Interleukin; INF: Interferon; MSFD2A: Major facilitator super family domain containing 2A; MMP: Matrix metalloprotease; NICHD: National Institute of Child Health and Human Development; OCLN: Occludin; PMI: Postmortem interval; SCZ: Schizophrenia; TJ: Tight junction; TNF: Tumor necrosis factor; tPA: Tissue plasminogen activator; tTG6: Tissue transglutaminase 6; TRIC: Tricellulin; TSPO: Translocator protein; VE-Cad: Vascular endothelial cadherin; ZO-1: Zonula occludens-1

Acknowledgements

The authors would like to thank the NICHD Brain and Tissue Bank for Developmental Disorders at the University of Maryland, Baltimore, MD, which is a Brain and Tissue Repository of the NIH NeuroBioBank, and the Maryland Brain Collection Steering Committee for their help in the brain acquisition and characterization. We would like to thank the tissue donors and their families for contributing to the advancement of brain research through the donation of tissue belonging to their self or their loved one.

Funding

The authors did not receive any funding for the study.

Authors' contributions

MF, AS, AF, and NC conceived the study. MF and AS conceived and designed the experiments. MF, AS, and SS performed the experiments. MF and AS analyzed the data. MF drafted the manuscript. AF, NC, AS, SS, and DLK helped with the interpretation of the data. AF, NC, DLK, SSC, and SS assisted in writing and/or editing the manuscript. SSC, SMK, and TMB actively contributed to the procurement of the duodenal biopsies and to the critical reading of the manuscript. All authors read and approved the final manuscript.

Competing interests

The authors declare that they have no competing interests.

Ethics approval and consent to participate

The human postmortem tissue collection, medical records, and family contact have been approved by the University of Maryland and Department of Health and Mental Hygiene Institutional Review Boards (IRBs). In addition, the specific collection was approved by the Maryland Psychiatric Research Center (MPRC), Maryland Brain Collection Steering Commitee, and the NIH NeuroBioBank Tissue Access Commitee. The specimens were collected under specific protocols, and the family consent was collected for the tissue to be used for scientific purposes including publication. Study procedures for the collection of the duodenal biopsies were reviewed and approved by the Partners Human Research Committee (PHRC) at Massachusetts General Hospital and performed in accordance with the Declaration of Helsinki. The PHRC operates in full compliance with all applicable federal, state, and local laws and regulations to protect the rights and welfare of the human subjects. Written informed consent was obtained from all the subjects at the time of enrollment.

Author details

[1]Mucosal Immunology and Biology Research Center, Massachusetts General Hospital for Children, Boston, MA, USA. [2]Department of Medicine, Celiac Center, Division of Gastroenterology, Beth Israel Deaconess Medical Center and Harvard Medical School, Boston, MA, USA. [3]Center for Celiac Research and Division of Pediatric Gastroenterology and Nutrition, Massachusetts General Hospital for Children, Boston, MA, USA. [4]Department of Pediatrics, Harvard Medical School, Boston, MA, USA. [5]Maryland Psychiatric Research Center, University of Maryland School of Medicine, Baltimore, MD, USA. [6]Neuropsychiatry Program, Sheppard Pratt Health System, Baltimore, MD, USA.

References

1. Nelson KB, Grether JK, Croen LA, Dambrosia JM, Dickens BF, Jelliffe LL, Hansen RL, Phillips TM. Neuropeptides and neurotrophins in neonatal blood of children with autism or mental retardation. Ann Neurol. 2001;49(5):597–606.
2. Vargas DL, Nascimbene C, Krishnan C, Zimmerman AW, Pardo CA. Neuroglial activation and neuroinflammation in the brain of patients with autism. Ann Neurol. 2005;57(1):67–81.
3. Zimmerman AW, Connors SL, Matteson KJ, Lee LC, Singer HS, Castaneda JA, Pearce DA. Maternal antibrain antibodies in autism. Brain Behav Immun. 2007;21(3):351–7.
4. Zimmerman AW, Jyonouchi H, Comi AM, Connors SL, Milstien S, Varsou A, Heyes MP. Cerebrospinal fluid and serum markers of inflammation in autism. Pediatr Neurol. 2005;33(3):195–201.
5. Chez MG, Dowling T, Patel PB, Khanna P, Kominsky M. Elevation of tumor necrosis factor-alpha in cerebrospinal fluid of autistic children. Pediatr Neurol. 2007;36(6):361–5.
6. Pardo CA, Vargas DL, Zimmerman AW. Immunity, neuroglia and neuroinflammation in autism. Int Rev Psychiatry. 2005;17(6):485–95.
7. Kinney DK, Hintz K, Shearer EM, Barch DH, Riffin C, Whitley K, Butler R. A unifying hypothesis of schizophrenia: abnormal immune system development may help explain roles of prenatal hazards, post-pubertal onset, stress, genes, climate, infections, and brain dysfunction. Med Hypotheses. 2010;74(3):555–63.
8. Carter CJ. Schizophrenia: a pathogenetic autoimmune disease caused by viruses and pathogens and dependent on genes. J Pathog. 2011;2011:128318.
9. Barch DM, Carter CS. Amphetamine improves cognitive function in medicated individuals with schizophrenia and in healthy volunteers. Schizophr Res. 2005;77(1):43–58.
10. Eaton WW, Byrne M, Ewald H, Mors O, Chen CY, Agerbo E, Mortensen PB. Association of schizophrenia and autoimmune diseases: linkage of Danish national registers. Am J Psychiatry. 2006;163(3):521–8.
11. Avramopoulos D, Pearce BD, McGrath J, Wolyniec P, Wang R, Eckart N, Hatzimanolis A, Goes FS, Nestadt G, Mulle J, et al. Infection and inflammation in schizophrenia and bipolar disorder: a genome wide study for interactions with genetic variation. PLoS One. 2015;10(3):e0116696.
12. Gantert M, Kreczmanski P, Kuypers E, Jellema R, Strackx E, Bastian N, Gavilanes AW, Zimmermann LJ, Garnier Y, Schmitz C, et al. Effects of in utero endotoxemia on the ovine fetal brain: a model for schizophrenia? Front Biosci (Elite Ed). 2012;4:2845–53.
13. Hope S, Dieset I, Agartz I, Steen NE, Ueland T, Melle I, Aukrust P, Andreassen OA. Affective symptoms are associated with markers of inflammation and immune activation in bipolar disorders but not in schizophrenia. J Psychiatr Res. 2011;45(12):1608–16.
14. Yang Y, Wan C, Li H, Zhu H, La Y, Xi Z, Chen Y, Jiang L, Feng G, He L. Altered levels of acute phase proteins in the plasma of patients with schizophrenia. Anal Chem. 2006;78(11):3571–6.
15. Wan C, La Y, Zhu H, Yang Y, Jiang L, Chen Y, Feng G, Li H, Sang H, Hao X, et al. Abnormal changes of plasma acute phase proteins in schizophrenia and the relation between schizophrenia and haptoglobin (Hp) gene. Amino Acids. 2007;32(1):101–8.
16. Ashwood P, Wakefield AJ. Immune activation of peripheral blood and mucosal CD3+ lymphocyte cytokine profiles in children with autism and gastrointestinal symptoms. J Neuroimmunol. 2006;173(1–2):126–34.
17. Cascella NG, Santora D, Gregory P, Kelly DL, Fasano A, Eaton WW. Increased prevalence of transglutaminase 6 antibodies in sera from schizophrenia patients. Schizophr Bull. 2013;39(4):867–71.
18. Cohly HH, Panja A. Immunological findings in autism. Int Rev Neurobiol. 2005;71:317–41.
19. Singh VK. Phenotypic expression of autoimmune autistic disorder (AAD): a major subset of autism. Ann Clin Psychiatry. 2009;21(3):148–61.
20. Kliushnik TP, Androsova LV, Simashkova NV, Zozulia SA, Otman IN, Koval'-Zaitsev AA. [Innate and adaptive immunity in children with psychotic forms of autism-spectrum disorders]. Zh Nevrol Psikhiatr Im S S Korsakova. 2011;111(8 Pt 1):41–5.
21. Estes ML, McAllister AK. Immune mediators in the brain and peripheral tissues in autism spectrum disorder. Nat Rev Neurosci. 2015;16(8):469–86.
22. Chen SJ, Chao YL, Chen CY, Chang CM, Wu EC, Wu CS, Yeh HH, Chen CH, Tsai HJ. Prevalence of autoimmune diseases in in-patients with schizophrenia: nationwide population-based study. Br J Psychiatry. 2012;200(5):374–80.
23. Kalaydjian AE, Eaton W, Cascella N, Fasano A. The gluten connection: the association between schizophrenia and celiac disease. Acta Psychiatr Scand. 2006;113(2):82–90.
24. Wu S, Ding Y, Wu F, Li R, Xie G, Hou J, Mao P. Family history of autoimmune diseases is associated with an increased risk of autism in children: a systematic review and meta-analysis. Neurosci Biobehav Rev. 2015;55:322–32.
25. Billeci L, Tonacci A, Tartarisco G, Ruta L, Pioggia G, Gangemi S. Association between atopic dermatitis and autism spectrum disorders: a systematic review. Am J Clin Dermatol. 2015;16:371–88.
26. Kohane IS, McMurry A, Weber G, MacFadden D, Rappaport L, Kunkel L, Bickel J, Wattanasin N, Spence S, Murphy S, et al. The co-morbidity burden of children and young adults with autism spectrum disorders. PLoS One. 2012;7(4):e33224.
27. Zerbo O, Leong A, Barcellos L, Bernal P, Fireman B, Croen LA. Immune mediated conditions in autism spectrum disorders. Brain Behav Immun. 2015;46:232–6.
28. Magalhaes ES, Pinto-Mariz F, Bastos-Pinto S, Pontes AT, Prado AE, deAzevedo LC. Immune allergic response in Asperger syndrome. J Neuroimmunol. 2009; 216(1–2):108–12.
29. Gorrindo P, Williams KC, Lee EB, Walker LS, McGrew SG, Levitt P. Gastrointestinal dysfunction in autism: parental report, clinical evaluation, and associated factors. Autism Res. 2012;5(2):101–8.
30. Valicenti-McDermott MD, McVicar K, Cohen HJ, Wershil BK, Shinnar S. Gastrointestinal symptoms in children with an autism spectrum disorder and language regression. Pediatr Neurol. 2008;39(6):392–8.
31. Buie T, Campbell DB, Fuchs 3rd GJ, Furuta GT, Levy J, Vandewater J, Whitaker AH, Atkins D, Bauman ML, Beaudet AL, et al. Evaluation, diagnosis, and treatment of gastrointestinal disorders in individuals with ASDs: a consensus report. Pediatrics. 2010;125 Suppl 1:S1–18.
32. Lightdale JR, Hayer C, Duer A, Lind-White C, Jenkins S, Siegel B, Elliott GR, Heyman MB. Effects of intravenous secretin on language and behavior of children with autism and gastrointestinal symptoms: a single-blinded, open-label pilot study. Pediatrics. 2001;108(5), E90.
33. Horvath K, Papadimitriou JC, Rabsztyn A, Drachenberg C, Tildon JT. Gastrointestinal abnormalities in children with autistic disorder. J Pediatr. 1999;135(5):559–63.
34. Horvath K, Perman JA. Autism and gastrointestinal symptoms. Curr Gastroenterol Rep. 2002;4(3):251–8.
35. Horvath K, Perman JA. Autistic disorder and gastrointestinal disease. Curr Opin Pediatr. 2002;14(5):583–7.
36. Kang V, Wagner GC, Ming X. Gastrointestinal dysfunction in children with autism spectrum disorders. Autism Res. 2014;7(4):501–6.
37. Torrente F, Anthony A, Heuschkel RB, Thomson MA, Ashwood P, Murch SH. Focal-enhanced gastritis in regressive autism with features distinct from Crohn's and Helicobacter pylori gastritis. Am J Gastroenterol. 2004;99(4):598–605.

38. Torrente F, Ashwood P, Day R, Machado N, Furlano RI, Anthony A, Davies SE, Wakefield AJ, Thomson MA, Walker-Smith JA, et al. Small intestinal enteropathy with epithelial IgG and complement deposition in children with regressive autism. Mol Psychiatry. 2002;7(4):375–82. 334.
39. D'Eufemia P, Celli M, Finocchiaro R, Pacifico L, Viozzi L, Zaccagnini M, Cardi E, Giardini O. Abnormal intestinal permeability in children with autism. Acta Paediatr. 1996;85(9):1076–9.
40. de Magistris L, Familiari V, Pascotto A, Sapone A, Frolli A, Iardino P, Carteni M, De Rosa M, Francavilla R, Riegler G, et al. Alterations of the intestinal barrier in patients with autism spectrum disorders and in their first-degree relatives. J Pediatr Gastroenterol Nutr. 2010;51(4):418–24.
41. de Magistris L, Picardi A, Siniscalco D, Riccio MP, Sapone A, Cariello R, Abbadessa S, Medici N, Lammers KM, Schiraldi C, et al. Antibodies against food antigens in patients with autistic spectrum disorders. Biomed Res Int. 2013;2013:729349.
42. Dalton N, Chandler S, Turner C, Charman T, Pickles A, Loucas T, Simonoff E, Sullivan P, Baird G. Gut permeability in autism spectrum disorders. Autism Res. 2014;7(3):305–13.
43. Niebuhr DW, Li Y, Cowan DN, Weber NS, Fisher JA, Ford GM, Yolken R. Association between bovine casein antibody and new onset schizophrenia among US military personnel. Schizophr Res. 2011;128(1–3):51–5.
44. Jackson J, Eaton W, Cascella N, Fasano A, Warfel D, Feldman S, Richardson C, Vyas G, Linthicum J, Santora D, et al. A gluten-free diet in people with schizophrenia and anti-tissue transglutaminase or anti-gliadin antibodies. Schizophr Res. 2012;140(1–3):262–3.
45. Severance EG, Dickerson FB, Halling M, Krivogorsky B, Haile L, Yang S, Stallings CR, Origoni AE, Bossis I, Xiao J, et al. Subunit and whole molecule specificity of the anti-bovine casein immune response in recent onset psychosis and schizophrenia. Schizophr Res. 2010;118(1–3):240–7.
46. Jackson J, Eaton W, Cascella N, Fasano A, Santora D, Sullivan K, Feldman S, Raley H, McMahon RP, Carpenter Jr WT, et al. Gluten sensitivity and relationship to psychiatric symptoms in people with schizophrenia. Schizophr Res. 2014;159(2–3):539–42.
47. Moor AC, de Vries HE, de Boer AG, Breimer DD. The blood–brain barrier and multiple sclerosis. Biochem Pharmacol. 1994;47(10):1717–24.
48. Hemmer B, Cepok S, Zhou D, Sommer N. Multiple sclerosis—a coordinated immune attack across the blood brain barrier. Curr Neurovasc Res. 2004;1(2):141–50.
49. Yang Y, Rosenberg GA. Blood–brain barrier breakdown in acute and chronic cerebrovascular disease. Stroke. 2011;42(11):3323–8.
50. Weissberg I, Reichert A, Heinemann U, Friedman A. Blood–brain barrier dysfunction in epileptogenesis of the temporal lobe. Epilepsy Res Treat. 2011;2011:143908.
51. de Vries HE, Kuiper J, de Boer AG, Van Berkel TJ, Breimer DD. The blood–brain barrier in neuroinflammatory diseases. Pharmacol Rev. 1997;49(2):143–55.
52. Heinemann U, Kaufer D, Friedman A. Blood–brain barrier dysfunction, TGFbeta signaling, and astrocyte dysfunction in epilepsy. Glia. 2012; 60(8):1251–7.
53. Seiffert E, Dreier JP, Ivens S, Bechmann I, Tomkins O, Heinemann U, Friedman A. Lasting blood–brain barrier disruption induces epileptic focus in the rat somatosensory cortex. J Neurosci. 2004;24(36):7829–36.
54. Gray MT, Woulfe JM. Striatal blood–brain barrier permeability in Parkinson's disease. J Cereb Blood Flow Metab. 2015;35(5):747–50.
55. Bell RD, Zlokovic BV. Neurovascular mechanisms and blood–brain barrier disorder in Alzheimer's disease. Acta Neuropathol. 2009;118(1):103–13.
56. Lee H, Pienaar IS. Disruption of the blood–brain barrier in Parkinson's disease: curse or route to a cure? Front Biosci (Landmark Ed). 2014;19:272–80.
57. Eaton W, Mortensen PB, Agerbo E, Byrne M, Mors O, Ewald H. Coeliac disease and schizophrenia: population based case control study with linkage of Danish national registers. BMJ. 2004;328(7437):438–9.
58. Hanson DR, Gottesman II. Theories of schizophrenia: a genetic-inflammatory-vascular synthesi. BMC Med Genet. 2005;6:7.
59. Schmittgen TD, Livak KJ. Analyzing real-time PCR data by the comparative C(T) method. Nat Protoc. 2008;3(6):1101–8.
60. Al Ahmad A, Gassmann M, Ogunshola OO. Involvement of oxidative stress in hypoxia-induced blood–brain barrier breakdown. Microvasc Res. 2012;84(2):222–5.
61. Engelhardt S, Al-Ahmad AJ, Gassmann M, Ogunshola OO. Hypoxia selectively disrupts brain microvascular endothelial tight junction complexes through a hypoxia-inducible factor-1 (HIF-1) dependent mechanism. J Cell Physiol. 2014;229(8):1096–105.
62. Amasheh S, Meiri N, Gitter AH, Schoneberg T, Mankertz J, Schulzke JD, Fromm M. Claudin-2 expression induces cation-selective channels in tight junctions of epithelial cells. J Cell Sci. 2002;115(Pt 24):4969–76.
63. Gunzel D, Stuiver M, Kausalya PJ, Haisch L, Krug SM, Rosenthal R, Meij IC, Hunziker W, Fromm M, Muller D. Claudin-10 exists in six alternatively spliced isoforms that exhibit distinct localization and function. J Cell Sci. 2009;122(Pt 10):1507–17.
64. Inai T, Kamimura T, Hirose E, Iida H, Shibata Y. The protoplasmic or exoplasmic face association of tight junction particles cannot predict paracellular permeability or heterotypic claudin compatibility. Eur J Cell Biol. 2010;89(7):547–56.
65. Tamura A, Hayashi H, Imasato M, Yamazaki Y, Hagiwara A, Wada M, Noda T, Watanabe M, Suzuki Y, Tsukita S. Loss of claudin-15, but not claudin-2, causes Na + deficiency and glucose malabsorption in mouse small intestine. Gastroenterology. 2011;140(3):913–23.
66. Leppert D, Ford J, Stabler G, Grygar C, Lienert C, Huber S, Miller KM, Hauser SL, Kappos L. Matrix metalloproteinase-9 (gelatinase B) is selectively elevated in CSF during relapses and stable phases of multiple sclerosis. Brain. 1998;121(Pt 12):2327–34.
67. Kandagaddala LD, Kang MJ, Chung BC, Patterson TA, Kwon OS. Expression and activation of matrix metalloproteinase-9 and NADPH oxidase in tissues and plasma of experimental autoimmune encephalomyelitis in mice. Exp Toxicol Pathol. 2012;64(1–2):109–14.
68. Minagar A, Alexander JS. Blood–brain barrier disruption in multiple sclerosis. Mult Scler. 2003;9(6):540–9.
69. Nygardas PT, Hinkkanen AE. Up-regulation of MMP-8 and MMP-9 activity in the BALB/c mouse spinal cord correlates with the severity of experimental autoimmune encephalomyelitis. Clin Exp Immunol. 2002;128(2):245–54.
70. Yong VW, Zabad RK, Agrawal S, Goncalves Dasilva A, Metz LM. Elevation of matrix metalloproteinases (MMPs) in multiple sclerosis and impact of immunomodulators. J Neurol Sci. 2007;259(1–2):79–84.
71. Chiu PS, Lai SC. Matrix metalloproteinase-9 leads to blood–brain barrier leakage in mice with eosinophilic meningoencephalitis caused by Angiostrongylus cantonensis. Acta Trop. 2014;140:141–50.
72. Dal-Pizzol F, Rojas HA, dos Santos EM, Vuolo F, Constantino L, Feier G, Pasquali M, Comim CM, Petronilho F, Gelain DP, et al. Matrix metalloproteinase-2 and metalloproteinase-9 activities are associated with blood–brain barrier dysfunction in an animal model of severe sepsis. Mol Neurobiol. 2013;48(1):62–70.
73. Lee MA, Palace J, Stabler G, Ford J, Gearing A, Miller K. Serum gelatinase B, TIMP-1 and TIMP-2 levels in multiple sclerosis. A longitudinal clinical and MRI study. Brain. 1999;122(Pt 2):191–7.
74. Waubant E. Biomarkers indicative of blood–brain barrier disruption in multiple sclerosis. Dis Markers. 2006;22(4):235–44.
75. Lavisse S, Guillermier M, Herard AS, Petit F, Delahaye M, Van Camp N, Ben Haim L, Lebon V, Remy P, Dolle F, et al. Reactive astrocytes overexpress TSPO and are detected by TSPO positron emission tomography imaging. J Neurosci. 2012;32(32):10809–18.
76. Wang M, Wang X, Zhao L, Ma W, Rodriguez IR, Fariss RN, Wong WT. Macroglia-microglia interactions via TSPO signaling regulates microglial activation in the mouse retina. J Neurosci. 2014;34(10):3793–806.
77. Rupprecht R, Papadopoulos V, Rammes G, Baghai TC, Fan J, Akula N, Groyer G, Adams D, Schumacher M. Translocator protein (18 kDa) (TSPO) as a therapeutic target for neurological and psychiatric disorders. Nat Rev Drug Discov. 2010;9(12):971–88.
78. Karlstetter M, Nothdurfter C, Aslanidis A, Moeller K, Horn F, Scholz R, Neumann H, Weber BH, Rupprecht R, Langmann T. Translocator protein (18 kDa) (TSPO) is expressed in reactive retinal microglia and modulates microglial inflammation and phagocytosis. J Neuroinflammation. 2014;11:3.
79. Chen MK, Guilarte TR. Translocator protein 18 kDa (TSPO): molecular sensor of brain injury and repair. Pharmacol Ther. 2008;118(1):1–17.
80. Cosenza-Nashat M, Zhao ML, Suh HS, Morgan J, Natividad R, Morgello S, Lee SC. Expression of the translocator protein of 18 kDa by microglia, macrophages and astrocytes based on immunohistochemical localization in abnormal human brain. Neuropathol Appl Neurobiol. 2009;35(3):306–28.
81. Vowinckel E, Reutens D, Becher B, Verge G, Evans A, Owens T, Antel JP. PK11195 binding to the peripheral benzodiazepine receptor as a marker of microglia activation in multiple sclerosis and experimental autoimmune encephalomyelitis. J Neurosci Res. 1997;50(2):345–53.
82. Morita K, Sasaki H, Furuse M, Tsukita S. Endothelial claudin: claudin-5/TMVCF constitutes tight junction strands in endothelial cells. J Cell Biol. 1999;147(1):185–94.

83. Nitta T, Hata M, Gotoh S, Seo Y, Sasaki H, Hashimoto N, Furuse M, Tsukita S. Size-selective loosening of the blood–brain barrier in claudin-5-deficient mice. J Cell Biol. 2003;161(3):653–60.
84. Liebner S, Fischmann A, Rascher G, Duffner F, Grote EH, Kalbacher H, Wolburg H. Claudin-1 and claudin-5 expression and tight junction morphology are altered in blood vessels of human glioblastoma multiforme. Acta Neuropathol. 2000;100(3):323–31.
85. Wolburg H, Wolburg-Buchholz K, Kraus J, Rascher-Eggstein G, Liebner S, Hamm S, Duffner F, Grote EH, Risau W, Engelhardt B. Localization of claudin-3 in tight junctions of the blood–brain barrier is selectively lost during experimental autoimmune encephalomyelitis and human glioblastoma multiforme. Acta Neuropathol. 2003;105(6):586–92.
86. Krug SM, Amasheh S, Richter JF, Milatz S, Gunzel D, Westphal JK, Huber O, Schulzke JD, Fromm M. Tricellulin forms a barrier to macromolecules in tricellular tight junctions without affecting ion permeability. Mol Biol Cell. 2009;20(16):3713–24.
87. Ohtsuki S, Yamaguchi H, Katsukura Y, Asashima T, Terasaki T. mRNA expression levels of tight junction protein genes in mouse brain capillary endothelial cells highly purified by magnetic cell sorting. J Neurochem. 2008;104(1):147–54.
88. Liebner S, Corada M, Bangsow T, Babbage J, Taddei A, Czupalla CJ, Reis M, Felici A, Wolburg H, Fruttiger M, et al. Wnt/beta-catenin signaling controls development of the blood–brain barrier. J Cell Biol. 2008;183(3):409–17.
89. Schrade A, Sade H, Couraud PO, Romero IA, Weksler BB, Niewoehner J. Expression and localization of claudins-3 and -12 in transformed human brain endothelium. Fluids Barriers CNS. 2012;9:6.
90. Milatz S, Krug SM, Rosenthal R, Gunzel D, Muller D, Schulzke JD, Amasheh S, Fromm M. Claudin-3 acts as a sealing component of the tight junction for ions of either charge and uncharged solutes. Biochim Biophys Acta. 2010; 1798(11):2048–57.
91. Piontek J, Fritzsche S, Cording J, Richter S, Hartwig J, Walter M, Yu D, Turner JR, Gehring C, Rahn HP, et al. Elucidating the principles of the molecular organization of heteropolymeric tight junction strands. Cell Mol Life Sci. 2011;68(23):3903–18.
92. Theodoropoulou S, Spanakos G, Baxevanis CN, Economou M, Gritzapis AD, Papamichail MP, Stefanis CN. Cytokine serum levels, autologous mixed lymphocyte reaction and surface marker analysis in never medicated and chronically medicated schizophrenic patients. Schizophr Res. 2001;47(1):13–25.
93. Song XQ, Lv LX, Li WQ, Hao YH, Zhao JP. The interaction of nuclear factor-kappa B and cytokines is associated with schizophrenia. Biol Psychiatry. 2009;65(6):481–8.
94. Erbagci AB, Herken H, Koyluoglu O, Yilmaz N, Tarakcioglu M. Serum IL-1beta, sIL-2R, IL-6, IL-8 and TNF-alpha in schizophrenic patients, relation with symptomatology and responsiveness to risperidone treatment. Mediators Inflamm. 2001;10(3):109–15.
95. Coelho FM, Reis HJ, Nicolato R, Romano-Silva MA, Teixeira MM, Bauer ME, Teixeira AL. Increased serum levels of inflammatory markers in chronic institutionalized patients with schizophrenia. Neuroimmunomodulation. 2008;15(2):140–4.
96. Zakharyan R, Boyajyan A. Inflammatory cytokine network in schizophrenia. World J Biol Psychiatry. 2014;15(3):174–87.
97. Potvin S, Stip E, Sepehry AA, Gendron A, Bah R, Kouassi E. Inflammatory cytokine alterations in schizophrenia: a systematic quantitative review. Biol Psychiatry. 2008;63(8):801–8.
98. Miller BJ, Buckley P, Seabolt W, Mellor A, Kirkpatrick B. Meta-analysis of cytokine alterations in schizophrenia: clinical status and antipsychotic effects. Biol Psychiatry. 2011;70(7):663–71.
99. Goldsmith DR, Rapaport MH, Miller BJ. A meta-analysis of blood cytokine network alterations in psychiatric patients: comparisons between schizophrenia, bipolar disorder and depression. Mol Psychiatry. 2016;21(12):1696–709.
100. Al-Asmari AK, Khan MW. Inflammation and schizophrenia: alterations in cytokine levels and perturbation in antioxidative defense systems. Hum Exp Toxicol. 2014;33(2):115–22.
101. Hoirisch-Clapauch S, Nardi AE. Low activity of plasminogen activator: a common feature of non-iatrogenic comorbidities of schizophrenia. CNS Neurol Disord Drug Targets. 2015;14(3):325–30.
102. Hoirisch-Clapauch S, Nardi AE. Markers of low activity of tissue plasminogen activator/plasmin are prevalent in schizophrenia patients. Schizophr Res. 2014;159(1):118–23.
103. Kirch DG, Alexander RC, Suddath RL, Papadopoulos NM, Kaufmann CA, Daniel DG, Wyatt RJ. Blood-CSF barrier permeability and central nervous system immunoglobulin G in schizophrenia. J Neural Transm Gen Sect. 1992;89(3):219–32.
104. Uranova NA, Zimina IS, Vikhreva OV, Krukov NO, Rachmanova VI, Orlovskaya DD. Ultrastructural damage of capillaries in the neocortex in schizophrenia. World J Biol Psychiatry. 2010;11(3):567–78.
105. Bechter K, Benveniste H. Quinckes' pioneering 19th centuries CSF studies may inform 21th centuries research. Neurol Psychiatry Brain Res. 2015;21(2):79–81.
106. Muller N, Riedel M, Hadjamu M, Schwarz MJ, Ackenheil M, Gruber R. Increase in expression of adhesion molecule receptors on T helper cells during antipsychotic treatment and relationship to blood–brain barrier permeability in schizophrenia. Am J Psychiatry. 1999;156(4):634–6.
107. Elmorsy E, Smith PA. Bioenergetic disruption of human micro-vascular endothelial cells by antipsychotics. Biochem Biophys Res Commun. 2015;460(3):857–62.
108. Zetterberg H, Jakobsson J, Redsater M, Andreasson U, Palsson E, Ekman CJ, Sellgren C, Johansson AG, Blennow K, Landen M. Blood-cerebrospinal fluid barrier dysfunction in patients with bipolar disorder in relation to antipsychotic treatment. Psychiatry Res. 2014;217(3):143–6.
109. Al-Amin MM, Nasir Uddin MM, Mahmud Reza H. Effects of antipsychotics on the inflammatory response system of patients with schizophrenia in peripheral blood mononuclear cell cultures. Clin Psychopharmacol Neurosci. 2013;11(3):144–51.
110. Borovcanin M, Jovanovic I, Radosavljevic G, Djukic Dejanovic S, Stefanovic V, Arsenijevic N, Lukic ML. Antipsychotics can modulate the cytokine profile in schizophrenia: attenuation of the type-2 inflammatory response. Schizophr Res. 2013;147(1):103–9.
111. Tourjman V, Kouassi E, Koue ME, Rocchetti M, Fortin-Fournier S, Fusar-Poli P, Potvin S. Antipsychotics' effects on blood levels of cytokines in schizophrenia: a meta-analysis. Schizophr Res. 2013;151(1–3):43–7.
112. Song C, Lin A, Kenis G, Bosmans E, Maes M. Immunosuppressive effects of clozapine and haloperidol: enhanced production of the interleukin-1 receptor antagonist. Schizophr Res. 2000;42(2):157–64.
113. Ajami A, Abedian F, Hamzeh Hosseini S, Akbarian E, Alizadeh-Navaei R, Taghipour M. Serum TNF-alpha, IL-10 and IL-2 in schizophrenic patients before and after treatment with risperidone and clozapine. Iran J Immunol. 2014;11(3):200–9.
114. Cazzullo CL, Sacchetti E, Galluzzo A, Panariello A, Adorni A, Pegoraro M, Bosis S, Colombo F, Trabattoni D, Zagliani A, et al. Cytokine profiles in schizophrenic patients treated with risperidone: a 3-month follow-up study. Prog Neuropsychopharmacol Biol Psychiatry. 2002;26(1):33–9.
115. Noto C, Ota VK, Gouvea ES, Rizzo LB, Spindola LM, Honda PH, Cordeiro Q, Belangero SI, Bressan RA, Gadelha A et al. Effects of risperidone on cytokine profile in drug-naive first-episode psychosis. Int J Neuropsychopharmacol. 2015;18(4).
116. MacDowell KS, Garcia-Bueno B, Madrigal JL, Parellada M, Arango C, Mico JA, Leza JC. Risperidone normalizes increased inflammatory parameters and restores anti-inflammatory pathways in a model of neuroinflammation. Int J Neuropsychopharmacol. 2013;16(1):121–35.
117. Tobiasova Z, van der Lingen KH, Scahill L, Leckman JF, Zhang Y, Chae W, McCracken JT, McDougle CJ, Vitiello B, Tierney E, et al. Risperidone-related improvement of irritability in children with autism is not associated with changes in serum of epidermal growth factor and interleukin-13. J Child Adolesc Psychopharmacol. 2011;21(6):555–64.
118. Choi JE, Widjaja F, Careaga M, Bent S, Ashwood P, Hendren RL. Change in plasma cytokine levels during risperidone treatment in children with autism. J Child Adolesc Psychopharmacol. 2014;24(10):586–9.
119. Kato T, Monji A, Hashioka S, Kanba S. Risperidone significantly inhibits interferon-gamma-induced microglial activation in vitro. Schizophr Res. 2007;92(1–3):108–15.
120. Zhu F, Zheng Y, Ding YQ, Liu Y, Zhang X, Wu R, Guo X, Zhao J. Minocycline and risperidone prevent microglia activation and rescue behavioral deficits induced by neonatal intrahippocampal injection of lipopolysaccharide in rats. PLoS One. 2014;9(4):e93966.
121. Edmonson C, Ziats MN, Rennert OM. Altered glial marker expression in autistic post-mortem prefrontal cortex and cerebellum. Mol Autism. 2014;5(1):3.
122. de Theije CG, Koelink PJ, Korte-Bouws GA, Lopes da Silva S, Korte SM, Olivier B, Garssen J, Kraneveld AD. Intestinal inflammation in a murine model of autism spectrum disorders. Brain Behav Immun. 2014;37:240–7.
123. Hsiao EY, McBride SW, Hsien S, Sharon G, Hyde ER, McCue T, Codelli JA, Chow J, Reisman SE, Petrosino JF, et al. Microbiota modulate behavioral and physiological abnormalities associated with neurodevelopmental disorders. Cell. 2013;155(7):1451–63.
124. Braniste V, Al-Asmakh M, Kowal C, Anuar F, Abbaspour A, Toth M, Korecka A, Bakocevic N, Ng LG, Kundu P, et al. The gut microbiota influences blood–brain barrier permeability in mice. Sci Transl Med. 2014;6(263):263ra158.

Permissions

All chapters in this book were first published in MA, by BioMed Central; hereby published with permission under the Creative Commons Attribution License or equivalent. Every chapter published in this book has been scrutinized by our experts. Their significance has been extensively debated. The topics covered herein carry significant findings which will fuel the growth of the discipline. They may even be implemented as practical applications or may be referred to as a beginning point for another development.

The contributors of this book come from diverse backgrounds, making this book a truly international effort. This book will bring forth new frontiers with its revolutionizing research information and detailed analysis of the nascent developments around the world.

We would like to thank all the contributing authors for lending their expertise to make the book truly unique. They have played a crucial role in the development of this book. Without their invaluable contributions this book wouldn't have been possible. They have made vital efforts to compile up to date information on the varied aspects of this subject to make this book a valuable addition to the collection of many professionals and students.

This book was conceptualized with the vision of imparting up-to-date information and advanced data in this field. To ensure the same, a matchless editorial board was set up. Every individual on the board went through rigorous rounds of assessment to prove their worth. After which they invested a large part of their time researching and compiling the most relevant data for our readers.

The editorial board has been involved in producing this book since its inception. They have spent rigorous hours researching and exploring the diverse topics which have resulted in the successful publishing of this book. They have passed on their knowledge of decades through this book. To expedite this challenging task, the publisher supported the team at every step. A small team of assistant editors was also appointed to further simplify the editing procedure and attain best results for the readers.

Apart from the editorial board, the designing team has also invested a significant amount of their time in understanding the subject and creating the most relevant covers. They scrutinized every image to scout for the most suitable representation of the subject and create an appropriate cover for the book.

The publishing team has been an ardent support to the editorial, designing and production team. Their endless efforts to recruit the best for this project, has resulted in the accomplishment of this book. They are a veteran in the field of academics and their pool of knowledge is as vast as their experience in printing. Their expertise and guidance has proved useful at every step. Their uncompromising quality standards have made this book an exceptional effort. Their encouragement from time to time has been an inspiration for everyone.

The publisher and the editorial board hope that this book will prove to be a valuable piece of knowledge for researchers, students, practitioners and scholars across the globe.

List of Contributors

Dorothea L. Floris
Autism Research Centre, Department of Psychiatry, University of Cambridge, Cambridge, UK
Department of Child and Adolescent Psychiatry, the Child Study Center, New York University Langone Medical Center, New York, NY, USA

Anita D. Barber, Mary Beth Nebel, Mary Martinelli, Deana Crocetti and Stewart H. Mostofsky
Center for Neurodevelopmental and Imaging Research, Kennedy Krieger Institute, Baltimore, MD, USA
Department of Neurology, Johns Hopkins School of Medicine, Baltimore, MD, USA
Department of Psychiatry and Behavioral Sciences, Johns Hopkins School of Medicine, Baltimore, MD, USA

Meng-Chuan Lai
Child, Youth and Family Services, Centre for Addiction and Mental Health and Department of Psychiatry, University of Toronto, Toronto, Canada
Department of Psychiatry, College of Medicine, National Taiwan University Hospital, Taipei City, Taiwan

John Suckling
Cambridgeshire and Peterborough NHS Foundation Trust, Cambridge, UK
National Institute of Health Research, Cambridge Biomedical Research Centre, Cambridge, UK
Behavioural and Clinical Neuroscience Institute, University of Cambridge, Cambridge, UK
Brain Mapping Unit, Department of Psychiatry, University of Cambridge, Cambridge, UK

James J. Pekar
F.M. Kirby Research Center for Functional Brain Imaging, Kennedy Krieger Institute, Baltimore, USA
Department of Radiology, Johns Hopkins School of Medicine, Baltimore, USA
Center for Neurodevelopmental and Imaging Research, Kennedy Krieger Institute, Baltimore, MD, USA

Simon Baron-Cohen
Cambridgeshire and Peterborough NHS Foundation Trust, Cambridge, UK
National Institute of Health Research, Cambridge Biomedical Research Centre, Cambridge, UK
Behavioural and Clinical Neuroscience Institute, University of Cambridge, Cambridge, UK
Brain Mapping Unit, Department of Psychiatry, University of Cambridge, Cambridge, UK
Autism Research Centre, Department of Psychiatry, University of Cambridge, Cambridge, UK

William J. Skylark
Department of Psychology, University of Cambridge, Cambridge CB2 3EB, UK

Simon Baron-Cohen
Department of Psychology, University of Cambridge, Cambridge CB2 3EB, UK
Autism Research Centre, Department of Psychiatry, University of Cambridge, Cambridge CB2 8AH, UK

Ting Ting Lee
Department of Psychiatry, The University of Melbourne, Parkville, Australia
Centre for Neural Engineering, The University of Melbourne, Parkville, Australia

Daniela Zantomio
Department of Clinical Haematology, Austin Hospital, Heidelberg, Australia

Gursharan Chana
Department of Medicine, The University of Melbourne, Parkville, Australia Department of Psychiatry, The University of Melbourne, Parkville, Australia
Centre for Neural Engineering, The University of Melbourne, Parkville, Australia
Florey Institute of Neuroscience and Mental Health, The University of Melbourne, Parkville, Australia

Christos Pantelis
Melbourne Neuropsychiatry Centre, The University of Melbourne & Melbourne Health, Parkville, Australia
Florey Institute of Neuroscience and Mental Health, The University of Melbourne, Parkville, Australia
Department of Psychiatry, The University of Melbourne, Parkville, Australia
Centre for Neural Engineering, The University of Melbourne, Parkville, Australia

Efstratios Skafidas
Florey Institute of Neuroscience and Mental Health, The University of Melbourne, Parkville, Australia
Department of Psychiatry, The University of Melbourne, Parkville, Australia
Centre for Neural Engineering, The University of Melbourne, Parkville, Australia

Ian Everall
The Institute of Psychiatry, Psychology and Neuroscience, King's College London, London, UK
Florey Institute of Neuroscience and Mental Health, The University of Melbourne, Parkville, Australia
Department of Psychiatry, The University of Melbourne, Parkville, Australia
Centre for Neural Engineering, The University of Melbourne, Parkville, Australia

Mirella Dottori
Illawarra Health and Medical Research Institute, University of Wollongong, Wollongong, Australia
Department of Biomedical Engineering, The University of Melbourne, Parkville, Australia
Centre for Neural Engineering, The University of Melbourne, Parkville, Australia

Attia Anwar and Sabah Pasha
Warwick Medical School, University of Warwick, Clinical Sciences Research Laboratories, University Hospital, Coventry, UK

Provvidenza Maria Abruzzo, Alessandra Bolotta and Marina Marini
Department of Experimental, Diagnostic and Specialty Medicine, School of Medicine, University of Bologna, Via Belmeloro 8, 40126 Bologna, Italy
Don Carlo Gnocchi Foundation ONLUS, IRCCS "S. Maria Nascente", Via Alfonso Capecelatro 66, 20148 Milan, Italy

Alessandro Ghezzo
Department of Experimental, Diagnostic and Specialty Medicine, School of Medicine, University of Bologna, Via Belmeloro 8, 40126 Bologna, Italy

Kashif Rajpoot
Department of Computer Science, University of Birmingham, Birmingham, UK

Paola Visconti
Child Neurology and Psychiatry Unit, IRCCS Institute of Neurological Sciences, Via Altura, 3, 40139 Bologna, Italy

Annio Posar
Child Neurology and Psychiatry Unit, IRCCS Institute of Neurological Sciences, Via Altura, 3, 40139 Bologna, Italy
Department of Biomedical and Neuromotor Sciences, University of Bologna, Via Altura 3, 40139 Bologna, Italy

Paul J. Thornalley
Zeeman Institute for Systems Biology & Infectious Disease Epidemiology Research, Senate House, University of Warwick, Coventry CV4 7AL, UK
Warwick Medical School, University of Warwick, Clinical Sciences Research Laboratories, University Hospital, Coventry, UK

Naila Rabbani
Research Technology Platform–Proteomics, University of Warwick, Coventry, UK
Attia Anwar, Sabah Pasha, Paul J. Thornalley and Naila Rabbani Warwick Medical School, University of Warwick, Clinical Sciences Research Laboratories, University Hospital, Coventry, UK
Zeeman Institute for Systems Biology & Infectious Disease Epidemiology Research, Senate House, University of Warwick, Coventry CV4 7AL, UK
Warwick Medical School, University of Warwick, Clinical Sciences Research Laboratories, University Hospital, Coventry, UK

Heidi Elisabeth Nag
Frambu Resource Centre for Rare Disorders, Siggerud, Norway
University of Stavanger, Stavanger, Norway

Ann Nordgren and Britt-Marie Anderlid
Karolinska Centre for Rare Diseases, Karolinska University Hospital, Solna, Sweden

Terje Nærland
NevSom, Department of Rare Disorders and Disabilities, Oslo University Hospital, Oslo, Norway
KG Jebsen Centre for Psychosis Research, NORMENT, University of Oslo, Oslo, Norway

Gregor Kohls
Department of Child and Adolescent Psychiatry, Psychosomatics and Psychotherapy, RWTH Aachen University, Aachen, Germany

Ligia Antezana
Department of Psychology, Virginia Polytechnic Institute and State University, Blacksburg, VA, USA

Maya G. Mosner
Department of Psychology, University of North Carolina at Chapel Hill, Chapel Hill, NC, USA

Robert T. Schultz
Center for Autism Research, The Children's Hospital of Philadelphia, 3535 Market Street, Ste 860, Philadelphia, PA 19104, USA
Pediatrics Department, Perelman School of Medicine, University of Pennsylvania, Philadelphia, PA, USA
Psychiatry Department, Perelman School of Medicine, University of Pennsylvania, Philadelphia, PA, USA

Benjamin E. Yerys
Center for Autism Research, The Children's Hospital of Philadelphia, 3535 Market Street, Ste 860, Philadelphia, PA 19104, USA
Psychiatry Department, Perelman School of Medicine, University of Pennsylvania, Philadelphia, PA, USA

Fu-Sun Lo and Reha S. Erzurumlu
Department of Anatomy and Neurobiology, University of Maryland School of Medicine, 22 Penn Street HSFII-S259, Baltimore, MD 21201, USA

Kit San Yeung, Christopher Chun Yu Mak, Gordon Ka Chun Leung, Mandy Ho Yin Tsang, Dingge Ying, Steven Lim Cho Pei and Wanling Yang
Department of Paediatrics and Adolescent Medicine, The University of Hong Kong, Pok Fu Lam, Hong Kong, China

Winnie Wan Yee Tso and So Lun Lee
Department of Paediatrics and Adolescent Medicine, The Duchess of Kent Children's Hospital, Pok Fu Lam, Hong Kong, China

Brian Hon-Yin Chung
Department of Paediatrics and Adolescent Medicine, The University of Hong Kong, Pok Fu Lam, Hong Kong, China
Department of Paediatrics and Adolescent Medicine, The Duchess of Kent Children's Hospital, Pok Fu Lam, Hong Kong, China
Department of Radiology, Queen Mary Hospital, Room103, New Clinical Building, 102 Pokfulam Road, Pok Fu Lam, Hong Kong, China

Janice Jing Kun Ip
Department of Radiology, Queen Mary Hospital, Room103, New Clinical Building, 102 Pokfulam Road, Pok Fu Lam, Hong Kong, China

Matthias Jung, Benjamin M. Häberle, Tristan Tschaikowsky, Elli-Anna Balta, Vivien-Charlott Stadler and D. Chichung Lie
Institute of Biochemistry, Emil Fischer Center, Friedrich-Alexander-Universität Erlangen-Nürnberg, 91054 Erlangen, Germany

Christiane Zweier
Institute of Human Genetics, Friedrich-Alexander-Universität Erlangen-Nürnberg, Erlangen, Germany

Marie-Theres Wittmann
Institute of Biochemistry, Emil Fischer Center, Friedrich-Alexander-Universität Erlangen-Nürnberg, 91054 Erlangen, Germany
Institute of Human Genetics, Friedrich-Alexander-Universität Erlangen-Nürnberg, Erlangen, Germany

Arnd Dörfler
Department of Neuroradiology, University Clinic Erlangen, Friedrich-Alexander-Universität Erlangen-Nürnberg, 91054 Erlangen, Germany

Christian Johannes Gloeckner
German Center for Neurodegenerative Diseases, 72076 Tübingen, Germany
Institute for Ophthalmic Research, Center for Ophthalmology, University of Tübingen, 72076 Tübingen, Germany

Debra S. Karhson, Robin A. Libove, Jennifer M. Phillips, Antonio Y. Hardan and Karen J. Parker
Department of Psychiatry and Behavioral Sciences, Stanford University, 401 Quarry Rd., Stanford, CA 94305, USA

Karolina M. Krasinska and Allis S. Chien
Vincent Coates Foundation Mass Spectrometry Laboratory, Stanford University, 333 Campus Dr., Stanford, CA 94305, USA

Jamie Ahloy Dallaire
Department of Comparative Medicine, Stanford University, 287 Campus Dr., Stanford, CA 94305, USA

Joseph P. Garner
Department of Comparative Medicine, Stanford University, 287 Campus Dr., Stanford, CA 94305, USA
Department of Psychiatry and Behavioral Sciences, Stanford University, 401 Quarry Rd., Stanford, CA 94305, USA

Shan V. Andrews and Brooke Sheppard
Department of Epidemiology, Johns Hopkins Bloomberg School of Public Health, 615 N. Wolfe Street, Baltimore, MD 21205, USA
Wendy Klag Center for Autism and Developmental Disabilities, Johns Hopkins Bloomberg School of Public Health, 615 N. Wolfe Street, W6509, Baltimore, MD 21205, USA

Gayle C. Windham
California Department of Public Health, Environmental Health Investigations Branch, 850 Marina Bay Parkway, Richmond, CA 94804, USA

Laura A. Schieve
National Center on Birth Defects and Developmental Disabilities, Centers for Disease Control and Prevention, MS E-86, 1600 Clifton Road, Atlanta, GA 30333, USA

Stephen T. Warren
Department of Pediatrics, Emory University School of Medicine, 615 Michael Street, Atlanta, GA 30322, USA
Department of Human Genetics, Emory University School of Medicine, 615 Michael Street, Atlanta, GA 30322, USA
Department of Biochemistry, Emory University School of Medicine, 615 Michael Street, Atlanta, GA 30322, USA

Andrew P. Feinberg
Center for Epigenetics, Johns Hopkins School of Medicine, 855 N. Wolfe Street, Baltimore, MD 21205, USA
Department of Medicine, Johns Hopkins School of Medicine, 855 N. Wolfe Street, Baltimore, MD 21205, USA

Lucia Capano, Jessica Brian, Deepali Mankad, Sharon Smile and Evdokia Anagnostou
Holland Bloorview Kids Rehabilitation Hospital, University of Toronto, 150 Kilgour Road, Toronto, ON M4G 1R8, Canada

Annie Dupuis
Sick Kids, University of Toronto, 555 University Avenue, Toronto, ON M5G 1X8, Canada

Toni Lui, Dina Odrobina, Lisa Genore and Rianne Hastie Adams
Holland Bloorview Kids Rehabilitation Hospital, 150 Kilgour Road, Toronto, ON M4G 1R8, Canada

Jane A. Foster
St. Joseph's Health Care, McMaster University, 50 Charlton Avenue East, Hamilton, ON L8N 4A6, Canada

Hui-ping Li, Chun-yang Li, Chun-chun Hu and Xiu Xu
Department of Child Health Care, Children's Hospital of Fudan University, Shanghai 201102, China

Qiong Xu
Department of Child Health Care, Children's Hospital of Fudan University, Shanghai 201102, China
Department of Pediatrics, Duke University School of Medicine, Durham 27710, NC, USA

Yuan-yuan Liu and Guo-he Tan
Guangxi Key Laboratory of Regenerative Medicine & Guangxi Collaborative Innovation Center for Biomedicine, School of Preclinical Medicine, Guangxi Medical University, Nanning 530021, Guangxi, China

Xiaoming Wang
Department of Pediatrics, Duke University School of Medicine, Durham 27710, NC, USA

Samuel W. Hulbert
Department of Neurobiology, Duke University School of Medicine, Durham 27710, NC, USA

Zhi-qi Xiong
Institute of Neuroscience & State Key Laboratory of Neuroscience, CAS Center for Excellence in Brain Science and Intelligence Technology, Shanghai Institutes for iological Sciences, Chinese Academy of Sciences, Shanghai 200031, China
University of Chinese Academy of Sciences, Beijing 100049, China

Yong-hui Jiang
Department of Pediatrics, Duke University School of Medicine, Durham 27710, NC, USA
Department of Neurobiology, Duke University School of Medicine, Durham 27710, NC, USA
Program in Genetics and Genomics, Duke University School of Medicine, Durham 27710, NC, USA
Cellular Molecular Biology, Duke University School of Medicine, Durham 27710, NC, USA

Fang Liu
College of Food Science and Engineering, Ocean University of China, Qingdao, China

Kayla Horton-Sparks and Vanessa Hull
Institute for Pediatric Regenerative Medicine and Shriners Hospitals for Children Northern California, 2504 Stockton Blvd, Sacramento, CA 95817, USA

Robert W. Li
United States Department of Agriculture, Agriculture Research Service (USDA-ARS), Animal Genomics and Improvement Laboratory, Beltsville, MD, USA

Verónica Martínez-Cerdeño
Department of Pathology and Laboratory Medicine, UC Davis School of Medicine, Sacramento, CA, USA
MIND Institute, Sacramento, CA, USA
Institute for Pediatric Regenerative Medicine and Shriners Hospitals for Children Northern California, 2504 Stockton Blvd, Sacramento, CA 95817, USA

Sainan An
School of Life Sciences, Beijing Normal University, No. 19, XinJieKouWai St., HaiDian District, Beijing 100875, China
National Institute of Biological Sciences, No. 7, Science Park Road, ZhongGuanCun Life Science Park, ChangPing District, Beijing 102206, China

Xiaoping Feng and Yue Dai
AppChina, Bejing, China

Hongli Bo Xiuqing Wang
Beijing Stars and Rain Education Institute, No. 18, ShuangQiao East Road, Beijing 100121, China

Mu Li
Academy of Arts and Design, Tsinghua University, No. 1, QingHuaYuan Road, HaiDai District, Beijing 100084, China

John Zhuohao Woo and Xingmei Liang
Inway Design, Beijing, China

Cheng Guo and Charles Xingchao Liu
G-Wearables, Inc., Beijing, China

Liping Wei
Center for Bioinformatics, State Key Laboratory of Protein and Plant Gene Research, School of Life Sciences, Peking University, No. 5, YiHeYuan Road, HaiDian District, Beijing 100871, China

Takashi Itahashi, Chieko Kanai, Rieko Okada and Nobumasa Kato
Medical Institute of Developmental Disabilities Research, Showa University, 6-11-11 Kita-karasuyama, Setagaya-ku, Tokyo, Japan

Junya Fujino and Hidehiko Takahashi
Medical Institute of Developmental Disabilities Research, Showa University, 6-11-11 Kita-karasuyama, Setagaya-ku, Tokyo, Japan
Department of Psychiatry, Graduate School of Medicine, Kyoto University, 54 Shogoin-Kawaracho, Sakyo-ku, Kyoto, Japan

Shisei Tei
Medical Institute of Developmental Disabilities Research, Showa University, 6-11-11 Kita-karasuyama, Setagaya-ku, Tokyo, Japan
Department of Psychiatry, Graduate School of Medicine, Kyoto University, 54 Shogoin-Kawaracho, Sakyo-ku, Kyoto, Japan
Institute of Applied Brain Sciences, Waseda University, 2-579-15 Mikajima, Tokorozawa, Saitama, Japan
School of Human and Social Sciences, Tokyo International University, 2509 Matoba, Kawagoe, Saitama, Japan

Ryu-ichiro Hashimoto
Department of Language Sciences, Minami-Osawa, Hachioji-shi, Tokyo, Japan
Medical Institute of Developmental Disabilities Research, Showa University, 6-11-11 Kita-karasuyama, Setagaya-ku, Tokyo, Japan

Haruhisa Ohta
Department of Psychiatry, School of Medicine, Showa University, 6-11-11 Kita-karasuyama, Setagaya-ku, Tokyo, Japan
Medical Institute of Developmental Disabilities Research, Showa University,6-11-11 Kita-karasuyama, Setagaya-ku, Tokyo, Japan

Manabu Kubota
Department of Functional Brain Imaging Research, National Institute of Radiological Sciences, National Institutes for Quantum and Radiological Science and Technology, 4-9-1 Anagawa, Inage-ku, Chiba, Japan
Medical Institute of Developmental Disabilities Research, Showa University, 6-11-11 Kita-karasuyama, Setagaya-ku, Tokyo, Japan
Department of Psychiatry, Graduate School of Medicine, Kyoto University, 54 Shogoin-Kawaracho, Sakyo-ku, Kyoto, Japan

Motoaki Nakamura
Kanagawa Psychiatric Center, 2-5-1 Serigaya, Yokohama, Kanagawa, Japan
Medical Institute of Developmental Disabilities Research, Showa University, 6-11-11 Kita-karasuyama, Setagaya-ku, Tokyo, Japan

Yuanlin Zou, Qiaomei Lu, Zhaoyu Liu, Ziyun Zhang and Zhengxiang Liu
Internal Medicine of Tongji Hospital, Tongji Medical College, Huazhong
University of Science and Technology, Wuhan 430030, People's Republic of China
Tongji Wenchang Hospital, Huazhong University of Science and Technology, Wenchang 571321, People's Republic of China

Yongjian Huang
Tongji Wenchang Hospital, Huazhong University of Science and Technology, Wenchang 571321, People's Republic of China

Dan Zheng and Yikai Zhou
Institute of Environmental Medicine, Tongji Medical College, Huazhong University of Science and Technology, Wuhan 430030, People's Republic of China

Qiongfang Ruan, Wenting Lou, Xiaodong Huang, Zhigang Chu and Weiguo Xie
Institute of Burns, Tongren Hospital of Wuhan University, Wuhan 430060, People's Republic of China

Paul Yao
Internal Medicine of Tongji Hospital, Tongji Medical College, Huazhong
University of Science and Technology, Wuhan 430030, People's Republic of China
Tongji Wenchang Hospital, Huazhong University of Science and Technology, Wenchang 571321, People's Republic of China
Institute of Burns, Tongren Hospital of Wuhan University, Wuhan 430060, People's Republic of China

Haijia Chen, Xiaoyan Wang, Yifei Wang and Xiaohu Ge
SALIAI Stem Cell Institute of Guangdong, Guangzhou SALIAI Stem Cell Science and Technology Co. LTD, Guangzhou 510055, People's Republic of China

Tom Loucas and Bhismadev Chakrabarti
School of Psychology and Clinical Language Sciences, University of Reading, UK

Alokananda Rudra
Ben Gurion University of the Negev, Beer-Sheva, Israel
School of Psychology and Clinical Language Sciences, University of Reading, Reading, UK

Jai Ranjan Ram
Mental Health Foundation, Kolkata, India

Matthew K. Belmonte
The Com DEALL Trust, Bangalore, India
Nottingham Trent University, Nottingham, UK

Maria Fiorentino and Stefania Senger
Mucosal Immunology and Biology Research Center, Massachusetts General Hospital for Children, Boston, MA, USA
Department of Pediatrics, Harvard Medical School, Boston, MA, USA

Anna Sapone
Department of Medicine, Celiac Center, Division of Gastroenterology, Beth Israel Deaconess Medical Center and Harvard Medical School, Boston, MA, USA
Mucosal Immunology and Biology Research Center, Massachusetts General Hospital for Children, Boston, MA, USA

Alessio Fasano
Center for Celiac Research and Division of Pediatric Gastroenterology and Nutrition, Massachusetts General Hospital for Children, Boston, MA, USA
Mucosal Immunology and Biology Research Center, Massachusetts General Hospital for Children, Boston, MA, USA
Department of Pediatrics, Harvard Medical School, Boston, MA, USA

Stephanie S. Camhi
Center for Celiac Research and Division of Pediatric Gastroenterology and Nutrition, Massachusetts General Hospital for Children, Boston, MA, USA
Mucosal Immunology and Biology Research Center, Massachusetts General Hospital for Children, Boston, MA, USA

Sarah M. Kadzielski and Timothy M. Buie
Department of Pediatrics, Harvard Medical School, Boston, MA, USA

Deanna L. Kelly
Maryland Psychiatric Research Center, University of Maryland School of Medicine, Baltimore, MD, USA

Nicola Cascella
Neuropsychiatry Program, Sheppard Pratt Health System, Baltimore, MD, USA

Index